Psychiatric Nursing Care Plans

Fourth edition

Katherine M. Fortinash, MSN, RNCS, CNS
Certified Clinical Specialist
Adult Psychiatric–Mental Health Nursing
Clinical Nurse Specialist and Educator
Sharp HealthCare, Mesa Vista Hospital
San Diego, California

Consultant and Lecturer
San Diego, California

Patricia A. Holoday Worret, MSN, RNCS, CNS
Certified Clinical Specialist
Adult Psychiatric–Mental Health Nursing
Professor, Psychiatric Mental Health Nursing
Palomar College
San Marcos, California

Consultant
San Diego, California

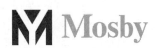

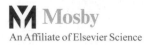
Mosby

An Affiliate of Elsevier Science

11830 Westline Industrial Drive
St. Louis, Missouri 63146

NOTICE

Psychiatric nursing is an ever-changing field. Standard safety precautions must be followed, but as new research and clinical experience broaden our knowledge, changes in treatment and drug therapy may become necessary or appropriate. Readers are advised to check the most current product information provided by the manufacturer of each drug to be administered to verify the recommended dose, the method and duration of administration, and contraindications. It is the responsibility of the licensed prescriber, relying on experience and knowledge of the patient, to determine dosages and the best treatment for each individual patient. Neither the publisher nor the editor assumes any liability for any injury and/or damage to persons or property arising from this publication.

Previous editions copyrighted 1999, 1995, 1991

Vice President, Publishing Director: Sally Shrefer
Acquisitions Editors: Terri Wood, Tom Wilhelm
Senior Developmental Editor: Robin Levin Richman
Publishing Services Manager: Peggy Fagen

Printed in the United States of America
Last digit is the print number: 9 8 7 6 5 4 3 2 1

Preface

Psychiatric Nursing Care Plans, fourth edition, represents our continued efforts to present the reader with the most current information that a psychiatric care plan text can offer. This text consists of researched information in areas of both psychiatric–mental health nursing and the psychiatric medical profession, with a strong scientific basis in both content and structure. Our goal, to unite the current discoveries in biology and technology with the interactive art of nursing, is reflected throughout this book. Many remarkable discoveries of new scientific research and interventions, which began in the "decade of the brain" (1990s) and continue to unfold in the twenty-first century, are explored in this text.

We continue to believe in the importance of a common nursing language that is distinctive to the profession and makes it easier for nurses everywhere to communicate and relate to each other and to other health care professionals. Our continued support and use of NANDA-approved nursing diagnoses reflect this belief.

As in past editions, we clarify meanings for the reader through the use of descriptive language and real-life examples, while remaining true to the professional vocabulary. The use of clear language and realistic client and family responses to the stress of mental illness helps demystify concepts that may otherwise be confusing to those who are new to psychiatric nursing and may be anxious about doing and saying the "right things" to clients and families.

Anxiety may often get in the way of learning. Anxiety may diminish the learner's appreciation for psychiatric nursing and discourage even the most gifted student from pursuing a career in psychiatric nursing. The vocabulary of a discipline distinguishes it as a profession and is a major factor in defining the profession's purpose. This is especially true for psychiatric nursing and psychiatry in general. The use of a common, unified language throughout this text helps the learner become more comfortable with psychiatric nursing, which may reduce anxiety and expedite learning.

The focus of this text is to respond to the client's psychiatric and psychosocial needs and problems with empathy and compassion and to help the client achieve and maintain psychosocial integrity at the highest possible level. The text's realistic dialogue makes it a unique clinical tool to motivate students and instructors and assist them to interact with clients and families effectively.

INTENDED USE OF THE TEXT

The primary intention of this text is to help nurses deliver professional quality care in any setting to clients with mental illness. Theory and practice are integrated to assist the learner in meeting the constant challenges of the fluctuating health care delivery systems. To maintain the text's integrity, we use the American Nurses' Association *Scope and Standards of Psychiatric and Mental Health Nursing Practice* (revised 2000), the North American Nursing Diagnosis Association (NANDA) Taxonomy II (2001–2002), and the American Psychiatric Association (APA) *Diagnostic and Statistical Manual of Psychiatric Disorders, 4th edition, text revision (DSM-IV-TR,* 2000). Nurses and physicians are inevitably at the center of client care, working with other disciplines to provide a comprehensive and cohesive therapeutic environment for clients and families. The co-mingling of *DSM-IV-TR* diagnoses and Nanda diagnoses make this text stand out as a clear, concise tool to be used by nurses everywhere.

NEW TO THIS EDITION

- Two-column, reader-friendly format for *Nursing Interventions and Rationales* results in improved clarity and comprehension.
- Completely updated and revised information on psychiatric disorders is presented in a thorough yet concise way.
- *Client and Family Teaching* boxes address the problem of shortened hospital stays and focus on discharge instructions for clients and caregivers. Boxes are in two parts: *Nurse Needs to Know* and *Teach Client and Family.*

- *Pharmacotherapy boxes* include the most recent psychotropic drug information and appropriate client care.
- A *Suicide Assessment Tool* reflects current research and practice standards (Chapter 3).
- An *Acute Confusion Care Plan* includes pain management and medications (Chapter 8).
- The free CD with the book includes a completely *interactive care plan constructor* and special *Appendixes* covering suicide assessment, the latest guidelines for seclusion and restraint, patients' rights, developmental theories, and the AA's Twelve Steps.

ORGANIZATION OF THE TEXT

Chapter 1 describes the six dynamic steps of the nursing process that guide the practice of nursing: assessment, nursing diagnosis, outcome identification, planning, implementation, and evaluation. Chapter 1 also includes the following:
- Communication skills
- Therapeutic nurse-client relationship
- Interpersonal techniques
- Client history and assessment tool
- Comprehensive case study and accompanying care plan
- Mental status examination
- Nursing Interventions Classification (NIC) and Nursing Outcome Classification (NOC)
- Clinical pathways (also known as critical pathways or care maps) currently used in the hospital, home care, and community settings

Chapters 2 through 11 cover psychiatric disorders as described in the *DSM-IV-TR,* using the most current information. The consistent format helps the learner readily and quickly locate information, with focused care plans at the end of each chapter.

ORGANIZATION OF EACH CHAPTER

Chapter organization and structure are consistent throughout, making it easier and less frustrating for students and practitioners to locate specific information, as well as helping them to prepare for clinical practice in a timely, more effective manner.

Information is presented at the beginning of each chapter and then developed into practical care plans. Each chapter begins with a concise yet comprehensive description of the mental disorders from the *DSM-IV-TR.* Clear language eliminates guesswork when identifying specific symptoms that define each disorder. All disorders are developed around the following structure:
- Introduction
- Etiology (for defined diagnoses)
- Epidemiology (statistics, research, current findings)
- Assessment and Diagnostic Criteria
- Treatment Settings

- Interventions (multiple treatment modalities, medications)
- Prognosis and Discharge Criteria

Community-based treatment is included where appropriate. Client and Family Teaching boxes provide guidelines both for nurses and for clients and families.

SELECTED NURSING DIAGNOSES

The selected nursing diagnoses reflect a wide range of client problems, most of which are frequently seen in psychiatric settings, as noted in Chapters 2, 3, and 4 on anxiety, depression, and schizophrenia, respectively. Other care plans reflect conditions less often found in psychiatric settings but equally important and challenging, such as dissociative disorders, sexual disorders, and posttraumatic stress disorder (PTSD). Gerontologic issues, including pain management and treatment, are extensively discussed in a new care plan, Acute Confusion (Chapter 8). The family and community are addressed along with the individual because the problems of one person affect the family and society as a whole. Cultural and spiritual considerations are integrated throughout because they affect each client's diagnosis and treatment in uniquely individual ways.

SELECTED CARE PLANS

The selected care plans, which appear at the end of each disorder chapter, reflect the most current psychiatric–mental health nursing theory and practice, based on sound diagnostic criteria, and encompass the following client needs and problems:
- Biologic
- Psychologic
- Spiritual
- Cultural
- Developmental
- Age specificity
- Sexual
- Family/significant others
- Community involvement
- School/work activities
- Social/relational
- Pain/comfort

Interventions used include the following modalities:
- Hospital/milieu therapy
- Psychosocial therapy
- Therapeutic nurse-client relationship
- Group therapy
- Family therapy
- Cognitive-behavioral therapy
- Medication
- Teaching/learning techniques
- Discharge information

Each care plan relates to the chapter's assessment and diagnostic criteria based on the *DSM-IV-TR* medical diagnosis. This is followed by appropriate NANDA nursing diagnoses based on NANDA's Taxonomy II conceptual framework and classification system. Accompanying focus statements briefly describe the client's behaviors. The care plan is then developed according to the remaining nursing process steps: combined *Outcome Identification* and *Evaluation, Planning* and *Implementation,* and *Nursing Intervention* and *Rationale.* The interventions and rationales in the Planning and Implementation section are presented in a two-column format to provide greater clarity and readability.

ACKNOWLEDGMENTS

The writing of any text requires an intricate mingling of ideas, concepts, and artistry. The completion of this text reflects the combined effort of many talents. We wish to thank the following for their special contributions:

- **Pauline C. Chan,** RPh, MBA, Pharmacy Manager, Sharp HealthCare, Mesa Vista Hospital, San Diego (Medication sections)
- **Phillip R. Deming,** MA, MDiv, Chaplain, Pastoral Care and Education, Grossmont Hospital Behavioral Health Partial Hospital Program, La Mesa, California (Spirituality)
- **Patricia C. Seaborg,** LCSW, MSW, doctoral student, School of Social Work, University of Southern California, Los Angeles (Client/Family Teaching)
- The people at Elsevier, Mosby, and Top Graphics.

Thanks to All!

Kathi Fortinash

Pat Worret

Contents

Detailed Contents

The Nursing Process

The nursing process continues to be the framework that guides nurses and other disciplines in clinical practice. In theory, the nursing process is a step by step problem-solving method in which client problems and needs are assessed, diagnosed, treated, and resolved in an orderly fashion. In practice, the nursing process is a more cyclic approach because of the client's changing responses to health and illness. Since the client's condition is dynamic rather than static, the nurse uses the steps of the nursing process interchangeably and continuously, according to the client's responses on the health-illness continuum. Assessment is ongoing, for example, it takes place initially; identifies the client's obvious needs and problems; and continues throughout the planning, intervention, and evaluation phases of the nursing process (Fig. 1-1). The assessment database enlarges as the client manifests other needs and problems. A client can be an individual, a family, a group, or a community.

Psychiatric–mental health nursing practice presents a unique and exciting challenge for use of the nursing process. The client's responses to mental and emotional illness are demonstrated through cognitive, affective, and behavioral domains, all of which are dynamic and subject to change. The nurse also evaluates those areas that are more constant, such as the client's culture, ethnicity, spirituality, sexuality, and developmental level. Although the psychiatric nurse focuses primarily on the client's psychosocial needs, the client's physical status and reports of pain or discomfort are also evaluated. The nursing process is also used to help psychiatric–mental health nurses make sound clinical judgments. The critical role of the nursing process as a theoretic framework is supported by the American Nurses'

Box 1-1 **Steps of the Nursing Process**

- Assessment
- Nursing diagnosis
- Outcome identification
- Planning
- Implementation
- Evaluation

Association's *Scope and Standards of Psychiatric and Mental Health Nursing Practice* (revised 2000).

The steps of the nursing process are contained in Box 1-1.

Fig. 1-2 details the nursing process in actual and risk problems.

ASSESSMENT

Assessment, the first step of the nursing process, provides the nurse with relevant data from which nursing diagnoses, the crux of treatment planning, are developed. Throughout the assessment phase the psychiatric nurse collects data through learned interactive and interviewing skills and observations of the client's behaviors and the client's reports of thoughts, feelings, and perceptions. The nurse's assessment skills are based on a broad biopsychosocial background and knowledge of normal and dysfunctional behaviors. In the discipline of psychiatric–mental health nursing, assessment takes place in many settings within the milieu.

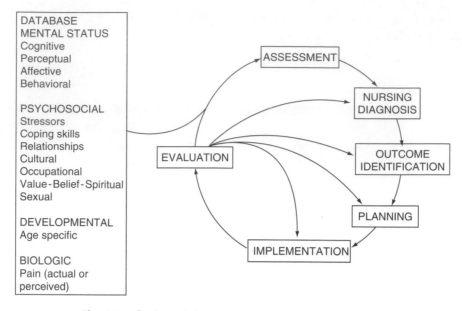

Fig. 1-1   Cyclic and dynamic nature of the nursing process.

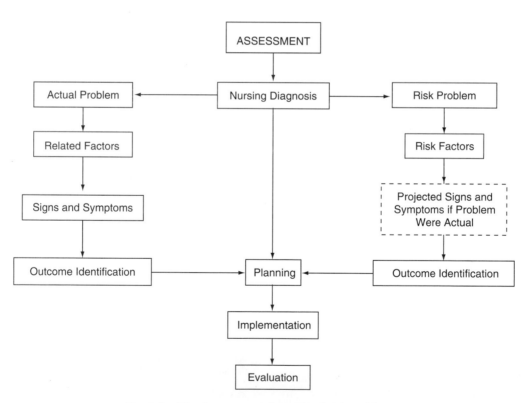

Fig. 1-2   Nursing process of actual and risk problems.

Therefore the nurse has several opportunities to observe the client and modify assessment data according to the client's continued adjustment to the milieu, as well as observe the client's progress throughout hospitalization.

Ideally, the client provides information during the assessment phase, although data may also be obtained through client records, other staff, and physicians. If the client is unable to offer a complete or accurate health history, a reliable person may be interviewed on the client's behalf, with the understanding that such information will be evaluated in terms of that person's relationship with the client.

Areas of psychiatric nursing assessment are as follows:
- Physical (including pain and comfort levels)
- Psychiatric/psychosocial
- Developmental
- Family dynamics
- Ethnicity
- Cultural
- Spiritual
- Sexual

The method of assessment includes the client's subjective reporting of symptoms and problems and the nurse's objective findings (Fig. 1-3).

Assessment of Mental Status

The psychiatric–mental health component of total client assessment is called the *mental status examination*. It is the basis for medical and nursing diagnoses and management of client care. The mental status examination is an organized collection of data that reflects an individual's level of functioning on many levels at the time of the interview, such as appearance, behavior, and attitude (Box 1-2).

The other major focus of the mental status examination is the psychosocial criteria and stressors that help define the client's strengths and capabilities for interaction with the environment. These include the ability to initiate and sustain meaningful relationships and to achieve satisfaction consistent with one's sociocultural life-style (see Box 1-2). Knowledge of the psychodynamics and psychopathology of human behavior is necessary in assessing the client's adjustment or maladjustment to internal and external life stressors.

The Interview

The client *assessment interview,* or *intake interview,* is essential in gathering critical information about the client's overall health status. It is a more meaningful, flexible method of collecting data than questionnaires or computers. The interview allows the nurse to use all the senses to explore the client's behavior, as well as specific topics and concerns. The assessment interview can take place in many settings other than the mental health facility, including the admissions/intake office, emergency department, medical-surgical unit, skilled nursing facility, crisis house, community center, alcohol/drug rehabilitation program, therapist's office, school, home, and prison.

In the mental status assessment the primary instrument of evaluation is the nurse interviewer. The success of the interview depends on the development of trust, rapport, and respect between the nurse and the client. The nurse uses essential time-proven interpersonal techniques (see later section) and communication skills, such as appropriate use of silence, reflective questioning, and offering general leads, to interact with the client and family in a therapeutic manner throughout the interview. The therapeutic qualities of the nurse are essential ingredients of the nursing process as the nurse assesses, diagnoses, and plans treatment for the client and family.

Essential Qualities for a Therapeutic Relationship

- **Genuineness.** Sincerity; verbal and behavioral congruence; authenticity. The nurse supports words with appropriate actions as long as it benefits the client. The nurse is able to meet the client's needs, but not necessarily fulfill the client's demands. For example, "I will meet with you tomorrow as we planned, but I won't bring you cigarettes." Genuineness does not mean "baring one's soul" or sharing personal problems; the client does not need further burdens.
- **Respect.** Unconditional positive regard; nonpossessive warmth; consistency and active listening. The nurse keeps appointments, shows up on time, and listens respectfully to the client's concerns while respecting the client's space and privacy.
- **Empathy.** The nurse views the world through the client's eyes but remains objective. The nurse does not identify, agree, or overly sympathize with the client but is able to focus on the client's feelings and not view the client as a stereotypic, textbook figure.
- **Concreteness/specificity.** The nurse speaks in realistic, literal terms versus vague, theoretic concepts. Clients with psychiatric disorders may have problems interpreting concepts.
- **Self-disclosure.** Appropriate disclosure of a view of one's attitudes, feelings, and beliefs. Role-modeling some shared experiences helps the client to reveal self, become more open, and feel more secure. The nurse may share feelings only when it is clear that the client will benefit from them. For example, "I have also been angry at times. Tell me how you usually manage your anger."
- **Confrontation.** The nurse approaches the client in a direct manner, usually because of perceived discrepancies in the client's behavior. Confrontation is used to help the client develop an awareness of incongruent behavior. For example, a client may say he will attend therapeutic group sessions, then not show up for group without a good reason. The nurse confronts the client by pointing out this inconsistent behavior. Confrontation needs to be done in an accepting, nonthreatening manner and only after rapport has been established.
- **Immediacy of the relationship.** The nurse focuses on the nurse-client interaction as a typical way in which the client may relate to others. The nurse needs to be careful not to share too many spontaneous feelings all at once, because divulging too many negative or personal experiences may be detrimental to the relationship, especially at the beginning.
- **Self-exploration.** The nurse helps the client vent and explore feelings during appropriate times throughout the interaction. Self-exploration may serve as a catharsis.
- **Role playing.** The nurse helps the client act out a particular event, situation, or problem to help the client gain understanding. Role playing may also be cathartic.

PSYCHIATRIC NURSING HISTORY AND ASSESSMENT

GENERAL ADMISSION INFORMATION

Client name _____   Age/Gender _____   Marital Status _____

Medical record number _____   Room number _____

Insurance company _____   Admission date _____

Address _____   Telephone _____

Significant other _____   Telephone _____

Company/school _____   Telephone _____

Fax _____   E-mail address _____

CONDITIONS OF ADMISSION (include Advance Directives)

Voluntary _____   Involuntary _____

Accompanied to facility by (family, friend, police, other) _____

Route of admission (ambulatory, wheelchair, gurney) _____

Admitted from (home, other facility, street, place of destination) _____

PAIN

Yes _____ No _____ Onset _____ Location _____

Quality (Examples: Sharp, dull, deep, aching, stabbing, radiating)

_____

Intensity _____ Origin _____

(Scale of 1-10) 1-3: mild; 4-6: moderate; 7-10: severe

What relieves pain? _____ What worsens pain? _____

Current pain meds, if any:

Prescription (Rx) _____ Over-the-counter _____

OTHER

Vital signs: P _____ B/P _____ Resp _____ Temp _____

Level of consciousness _____ Orientation (person, place, time, situation) _____

Allergies (including latex) _____ Diet _____ Height/weight _____

Place/city of residence _____ Dominant language _____

Special needs _____ Strengths/coping skills _____

Discharge to: (home, facility, other) _____ Estimated length of stay _____

Chief complaint (client's own words) _____

PREDISPOSING FACTORS

Genetic/biologic influences

Family of origin/culture (use genogram if applicable)

Present family/significant persons

Family dynamics (describe significant interpersonal relationships among family members) _____

_____

_____

MEDICAL/PSYCHIATRIC HISTORY

Client _____

_____

_____

Family members _____

_____

_____

Recent stressors (physical, emotional, psychosocial, psychiatric disorder) _____

_____

_____

Other physical, psychosocial, cultural, sexual, financial, and environmental factors relevant to current problem (physical disability, fall risk, cultural change, loss of income or bankruptcy, trauma from living in high-crime neighborhood, homelessness, abuse, domestic violence) _____

_____

_____

_____

_____

Health beliefs and practices (personal responsibility for health, wellness, special practices) _____

_____

_____

_____

Fig. 1-3   A psychiatric nursing history and assessment form.

PSYCHIATRIC NURSING HISTORY AND ASSESSMENT

MEDICAL/PSYCHIATRIC HISTORY

Religious/spiritual/values, beliefs, practices _____
_____
_____
_____

Educational/occupational background/interests _____
_____
_____
_____

Significant losses/changes/grief responses _____
_____
_____
_____

Support system (peers/friends/others) _____
_____
_____
_____

Previous patterns of coping with grief/stress
(Adaptive) _____
_____
_____

(Maladaptive) _____
_____
_____
_____

Growth and development resources (Erikson)
  Stages of development _____
  Tasks/skills mastered _____
  Tasks/skills not met _____

Contributions/areas of productivity _____
_____
_____
_____

Precipitating event (describe situation or events that influenced this hospitalization/illness/exacerbation) _____
_____
_____
_____

Client's perception of stressor/stressor event _____
_____
_____
_____

LEVEL OF ANXIETY (check one)
_____ Mild _____ Moderate _____ Severe _____ Panic

MEDICATION/DRUG HISTORY (including alcohol)
Use of prescribed drugs

Name	Dose	Reason prescribed	Results/effects

Use of over-the-counter drugs

Name	Dose	Reason taken	Results/effects

Use of street/illicit drugs/alcohol

Name	Amount used	Frequency	When last used	Effects produced

Fig. 1-3, cont'd   For legend see opposite page.

Box **1-2**   **Components of Psychiatric Nursing Assessment: Mental Status Examination and Psychosocial Criteria**

MENTAL STATUS EXAMINATION

Appearance
Dress, grooming, hygiene, cosmetics, apparent age, posture, facial expression

Behavior/activity
Hypoactivity or hyperactivity; rigid, relaxed, restless, or agitated motor movements; gait and coordination; facial grimacing; gestures; mannerisms; passive; combative; bizarre

Attitude
Interactions with interviewer: cooperative, resistive, friendly, hostile, ingratiating

Speech
Quantity: poverty of speech, poverty of content, voluminous
Quality: articulate, congruent, monotonous, talkative, repetitious, spontaneous, circumlocutory, tangential, confabulating, pressured, stereotypical
Rate: slowed, rapid

Mood and affect
Mood (intensity, depth, duration): sad, fearful, depressed, angry, anxious, ambivalent, happy, ecstatic, grandiose
Affect (intensity, depth, duration): appropriate, apathetic, constricted, blunted, flat, labile, euphoric, bizarre

Perceptions
Hallucinations, illusions, depersonalization, derealization, distortions

Thoughts
Form and content: logical vs. illogical, loose associations, flight of ideas, autistic, blocking, broadcasting, neologisms, "word salad," obsessions, ruminations, delusions, abstract vs. concrete

Sensorium/cognition
Levels of consciousness, orientation, attention span, recent and remote memory, concentration; ability to comprehend and process information; intelligence

Judgment
Ability to assess and evaluate situations, make rational decisions, understand consequences of behavior, and take responsibility for actions

Insight
Ability to perceive and understand the cause and nature of own and others' situations

PSYCHOSOCIAL CRITERIA

Stressors
Internal: psychiatric or medical illness; perceived loss, such as loss of self-concept/self-esteem
External: actual loss, such as death of a loved one, divorce, lack of support systems, job or financial loss, retirement, or dysfunctional family system

Coping skills
Adaptation to internal and external stressors; use of functional, adaptive coping mechanisms and techniques; management of activities of daily living

Relationships
Attainment and maintenance of satisfying interpersonal relationships consistent with developmental stage; includes sexual relationship as appropriate for age and status

Reliability
Interviewer's impression that individual reported information accurately and completely

Cultural
Ability to adapt and conform to prescribed norms, rules, ethics, and mores of an identified group

Spiritual (value-belief)
Presence of a self-satisfying value-belief system that the individual regards as right, desirable, worthwhile, and comforting

Occupational
Engagement in useful, rewarding activity, congruent with developmental stage and societal standards (work, school, recreation)

Principles of a Therapeutic Nurse-Client Relationship

1. Continually evaluate the client's risk for suicide using principles of suicide assessment (see Box 3-7).
2. Engage in active listening, using a warm, accepting, empathetic approach.
3. Develop an awareness of own feelings, fears, and biases regarding clients with mental disorders (autodiagnosis).
4. Discuss own fears and concerns with qualified peers.
5. Speak to the client in a moderate tone of voice, using a calm "matter-of-fact" approach and nonjudgmental attitude. Refrain from extremes of expression or responses that indicate surprise or disbelief.
6. Continue to develop trust and rapport with the client through shared time and support during the day. Use brief one-to-one contacts rather than lengthy, drawn-out conversations.
7. Remain quietly with the depressed or withdrawn client who is unable to engage in conversation at first.
8. Allow sufficient time for the client to respond, while assessing client's ability to tolerate silence and presence of nurse. Do not prolong the contact if the client is obviously uncomfortable or resistant, unless the client is troubled or suicidal and cannot be left alone.
9. Individualize the client's needs throughout contact to acknowledge client's value and worth.

The Nurse-Client Relationship

The nurse-client relationship is **therapeutic,** not social, in nature. It is always **client centered** and **goal directed.** It is **objective** rather than subjective. The intent of a professional relationship is for client behavior to change. It is a *limited* relationship, with the goal of helping the client find more satisfying behavior patterns and coping strategies and increase self-worth. It is *not* for mutual satisfaction.

In the **preorientation phase,** the nurse gathers data about the client and the client's situation and condition (chart, staff, physician). The nurse also utilizes the process of **autodiagnosis** (self-diagnosis) to determine his or her own perceptions, possible biases, and attitudes about the client. A commitment to nonjudgmentalism and the avoidance of stereotyping are imperative.

Autodiagnosis

Questions that nurses ask themselves during the self-diagnosis process (autodiagnosis) include the following:
- Do I label clients with the stereotype as a group?
- Is my need to be liked so great that I become angry or hurt when a client is rude, hostile, or uncooperative?
- Am I afraid of the responsibility I must assume in this relationship? (This fear may decrease the nurse's independent functions.)
- Do I cover feelings of inferiority with an air of superiority?
- Do I require sympathy and protection so much myself that I drown my clients with it as well?
- Do I fear closeness or identifying myself with the client to the extent of being cold and indifferent?
- Do I need to feel important and keep clients dependent on me?

Orientation phase

The purpose of the orientation phase is to become acquainted with the client, gain rapport, demonstrate genuine caring and understanding, and establish trust. The orientation phase usually lasts 2 to 10 sessions but with some clients can take many months (Box 1-3). With the current shorter lengths of stay, the phases of the relationship may not be as clear and distinct, and the nurse needs to use all her therapeutic resources to establish trust and rapport in a timely manner. Guidelines and steps in the orientation phase are as follows:

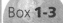 Box **1-3**   **Client Responses to Orientation Phase**

1. The client may willingly engage in therapeutic relationship.
2. May test the nurse and the limits of the nurse-client relationship.
   a. May be late for meetings.
   b. May end meetings early.
   c. May play the nurse against the staff.
3. May not remember the nurse's name or appointment time.
   a. The nurse puts information on a card and gives this to the client.
   b. Reinforces contract in early meetings and restates limits if necessary.
4. The client may attempt to shock the nurse.
   a. May use profane words.
   b. May share an experience that the client believes will shock or frighten the nurse.
   c. May use bizarre behavior.
5. May focus on the nurse in an attempt to see if the nurse is competent. The nurse refocuses on the client.

1. Build trust and security (first level of any interpersonal experience).
   a. Establish contract.
   b. Be dependable; follow contract, and keep appointments.
   c. Allow client to be responsible for contract.
   d. Convey honesty.
   e. Show caring and interest.
   f. When client is unable to control behavior, set limits and provide appropriate alternative outlets (see Box 1-3).
2. Discuss the contract: dates, times, and place of meetings; duration of each meeting; purpose of meetings; roles of both client and nurse; use of information obtained; and arrangements for notifying client/nurse if unable to keep appointment.
3. Facilitate the client's ability to verbalize his or her problem.
4. Be aware of themes.
   a. *Content:* what the client is saying.
   b. *Process:* how the client interacts.
   c. *Mood:* for example, hopeless or anxious.
   d. *Interaction:* for example, did the client ignore you? Was the client submissive? Did the client dominate conversation?
5. Observe and assess the client's strengths, limitations, and problem areas. Build on client's strengths and positive aspects of personality. Include the client in identification of client's attributes.
6. Identify client problems, nursing diagnosis, outcome criteria, and nursing interventions. Formulate nursing care plan.

Working phase

The working phase ideally begins when the client assumes responsibility to uphold the limits of the relationship. Adjustments may have to be made, depending on the client's length of stay. The purpose of the working phase is to bring about positive changes in the client's behavior, with focus on the "here and now" (Box 1-4). To achieve this, set priorities when determining the client's needs, as follows:

1. Preserve the client's life and safety. Is client suicidal, not eating, smoking in bed while medicated, or acting out behavior harmful to others?
2. Modify behavior that is unacceptable to others (e.g., acting out or hostile verbalization, bizarre behavior, withdrawal, poor hygiene, inadequate social skills).
3. Identify with the client those behaviors that the client is willing to change; set realistic goals. Make goals testable and attainable for successful experiences. This will increase the client's sense of self-worth and will help the client to accept the need for growth.

Termination phase

The purpose of the termination phase is to dissolve the relationship and assure the client that he or she can be independent in some or all of his or her functioning.

Ideally, the termination phase begins during the orientation phase. The more dependent and involved relationships may require longer time for termination. Termination normally occurs when the client has improved sufficiently for the relationship to end, but it may occur if a client is transferred or you as a nurse leave the facility (Box 1-5).

Methods of decreasing involvement
1. Space your contacts further apart (not usually necessary in student clinical experience).
2. Reduce the usual length of time you spend with client (may not be necessary lengths of stay).
3. Change the emotional tone of the interactions.
   a. Do not respond to or follow up on clues that lead to new areas to investigate (but alert staff if this occurs).
   b. Focus on future-oriented material.
4. Some clients may want to work up to the last meeting; use your judgment.

What to discuss with client about termination
1. Help the client discuss his or her feelings about termination.
2. Have the client talk about gains he or she has made (include negative aspects of sessions as well).
3. Share with the client the growth you see in the client.
4. Express benefits you have gained from the experience.
5. Express your feelings about leaving the client (be sure to keep your emotions in check).
6. *Never* give the client your address or telephone number.

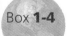 Box **1-4** **Client Responses to Working Phase***

1. The client may use less testing, less focusing on the nurse, and fewer attempts to shock the nurse.
2. May remember and anticipate appointment with the nurse.
3. May use more description and clarification to facilitate understanding; wants the nurse to know how the client feels.
4. May be more responsive in interactions.
5. May improve appearance.
6. May bring up topic that the client wants to discuss.
7. May confide more confidential material.

*The working phase is painful for the client and is reached when change occurs as the client and the nurse evaluate and discuss the client's problems.

> **Box 1-5   Client Responses to Termination**
>
> 1. The client may deny separation.
> 2. May deny significance of relationship/separation.
> 3. May express anger or hostility (overtly or covertly). Anger, openly expressed to the nurse, may be a natural and healthy response to an event. The client feels secure enough to show anger. Nurse responds in accepting, neutral manner.
> 4. May display marked change in attitude toward the nurse/therapist; may make critical remarks about the nurse or be hostile because of pending break of emotional ties. If the nurse does not understand the reason for the client's reaction, the client may react with anger or defensiveness and block the termination process.
> 5. May display a type of grief reaction. It takes time to accept the loss, which is why it is important to start the termination process early.
> 6. May feel rejected and experience increased negative self-concept.
> 7. May terminate relationship prematurely.
> 8. May regress to exhibition of previous symptoms.
> 9. May request premature discharge.
> 10. May make a suicide attempt.
> 11. May be accepting but still express regret or feel momentary resentment. This is a healthy response. Make a clean break, or you may hinder the client's realization that relationships often must, *and do*, terminate.

Impasses That Obstruct a Therapeutic Relationship

- **Resistance.** The client is reluctant to divulge information about self because he or she doubts ability to be helped. Unconditional acceptance and persistence by the nurse are critical.
- **Transference.** The client views the nurse as a significant person in the client's life and transfers feelings, emotions, and attitudes felt for that person onto the nurse. The nurse may need assistance to deal with transference issues. Clarification of the nurse-client relationship is imperative during this time.
- **Countertransference.** The nurse views the client as a significant person in the nurse's life and transfers feelings for that person onto the client. Assistance by qualified health care personnel is imperative to help the relationship regain its objective, therapeutic core.

Interpersonal Techniques

Box 1-6 lists therapeutic techniques essential to the nurse-client relationship and the successful implementation of the nursing process. Nontherapeutic interpersonal techniques are unhelpful in nursing assessment (Box 1-7).

NURSING DIAGNOSIS

Nursing diagnoses are developed through a process in which nurses interpret data collected during the assessment phase of the nursing process. Nursing diagnoses are statements that describe an individual's health state or response to illness. The diagnosis statement may be an actual or potential alteration in a person's life. The statement may reflect biologic, psychologic, sociocultural, developmental, spiritual, or sexual processes (Table 1-1).

The National Task Force for the Classification of Nursing Diagnoses was organized in 1973 by a group of nurses and is called the *North American Nursing Diagnosis Association* (NANDA). At NANDA's ninth conference in March 1990, nursing diagnosis was defined as "a clinical judgment about individual, family, or community responses to actual or potential health problems/life processes. Nursing diagnoses provide the basis for selection of nursing interventions to achieve outcomes for which the nurse is accountable."

NANDA continually collects, defines, describes, and refines nursing diagnoses (see inside back cover) submitted by interested practicing nurses and categorizes them within an organizational conceptual framework known as *Taxonomy II* (Table 1-2). The authors of this text remain true to NANDA's continuing efforts to refine and standardize nursing diagnoses. In this way, nurses everywhere can relate to a distinctive, professional language that improves communication among nurses and enhances their discipline.

Nursing Diagnoses and Medical Diagnoses

Nursing diagnoses and medical diagnoses may complement each other and still remain separate. Nursing diagnoses are based on the client's maladaptive responses, whether or not a medical diagnosis exists. In the medical model of psychiatry, "health problems" are the mental disorders as defined in the *Diagnostic and Statistical Manual of Mental Disorders*, fourth edition revised *(DSM-IV-TR)*, from which many nursing diagnoses emerge (Table 1-3).

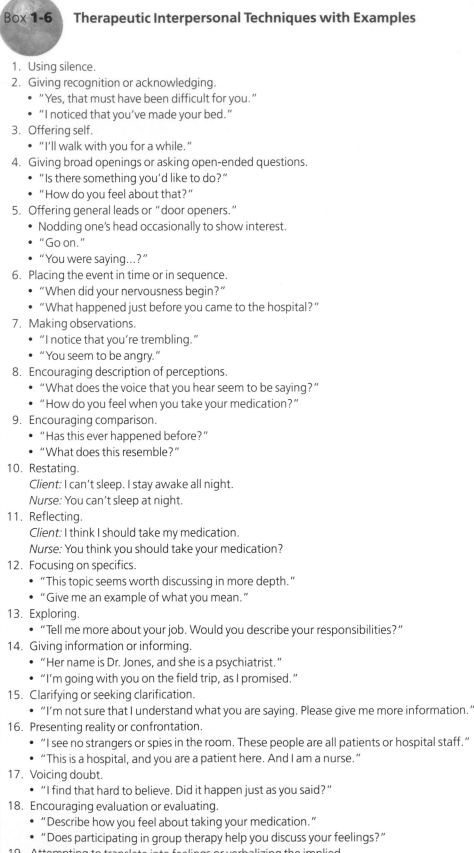

Box **1-6**   **Therapeutic Interpersonal Techniques with Examples**

1. Using silence.
2. Giving recognition or acknowledging.
   - "Yes, that must have been difficult for you."
   - "I noticed that you've made your bed."
3. Offering self.
   - "I'll walk with you for a while."
4. Giving broad openings or asking open-ended questions.
   - "Is there something you'd like to do?"
   - "How do you feel about that?"
5. Offering general leads or "door openers."
   - Nodding one's head occasionally to show interest.
   - "Go on."
   - "You were saying...?"
6. Placing the event in time or in sequence.
   - "When did your nervousness begin?"
   - "What happened just before you came to the hospital?"
7. Making observations.
   - "I notice that you're trembling."
   - "You seem to be angry."
8. Encouraging description of perceptions.
   - "What does the voice that you hear seem to be saying?"
   - "How do you feel when you take your medication?"
9. Encouraging comparison.
   - "Has this ever happened before?"
   - "What does this resemble?"
10. Restating.
    Client: I can't sleep. I stay awake all night.
    Nurse: You can't sleep at night.
11. Reflecting.
    Client: I think I should take my medication.
    Nurse: You think you should take your medication?
12. Focusing on specifics.
    - "This topic seems worth discussing in more depth."
    - "Give me an example of what you mean."
13. Exploring.
    - "Tell me more about your job. Would you describe your responsibilities?"
14. Giving information or informing.
    - "Her name is Dr. Jones, and she is a psychiatrist."
    - "I'm going with you on the field trip, as I promised."
15. Clarifying or seeking clarification.
    - "I'm not sure that I understand what you are saying. Please give me more information."
16. Presenting reality or confrontation.
    - "I see no strangers or spies in the room. These people are all patients or hospital staff."
    - "This is a hospital, and you are a patient here. And I am a nurse."
17. Voicing doubt.
    - "I find that hard to believe. Did it happen just as you said?"
18. Encouraging evaluation or evaluating.
    - "Describe how you feel about taking your medication."
    - "Does participating in group therapy help you discuss your feelings?"
19. Attempting to translate into feelings or verbalizing the implied.
    Client: I'm empty and numb.
    Nurse: Are you saying that you're not feeling anything right now, or you're not sure of your feelings?

Box 1-6 **Therapeutic Interpersonal Techniques with Examples—cont'd**

20. Suggesting collaboration.
    • "Perhaps you and your social worker can work together to plan your living arrangements after your discharge."
21. Summarizing.
    • "During the past hour we talked about your plans for the future. They include the following."
22. Encouraging formulation of a plan of action.
    • "If this situation occurs again, what options do you have?"
23. Asking direct questions.
    • "How do you feel about your hospitalization?"
    • "How do you see your progress?"

Box 1-7 **Nontherapeutic Interpersonal Techniques with Examples**

1. Reassuring (falsely).
   • "I wouldn't worry about that now."
   • "Everything will be all right."
   • "You're coming along fine."
2. Giving unwarranted approval.
   • "It sounds good to me."
   • "I'm glad that you did that."
3. Rejecting.
   • "Let's not discuss that right now."
   • "I don't want to hear about that."
4. Disapproving unnecessarily.
   • "That's bad."
   • "I'd rather you wouldn't."
5. Agreeing against better judgment.
   • "That's right."
   • "I agree with you."
6. Disagreeing unnecessarily.
   • "That's wrong."
   • "I definitely disagree with that."
   • "I don't believe that."
7. Advising without giving alternatives.
   • "I think you should do this."
   • "Why don't you do that."
8. Probing for nontherapeutic reasons.
   • "Now tell me about your sex life."
   • "Tell me your life history."
9. Challenging.
   • "But how can you possibly be president of the United States?"
   • "If you're dead, how come you're talking?"
10. Testing unnecessarily.
    • "What day is this?"
    • "Do you know what kind of a hospital this is?"
    • "Do you still have the idea that you're president?"
11. Defending.
    • "This hospital has a fine reputation."
    • "No one here would ever lie to you."
    • "Dr. B. is a very able psychiatrist. I'm sure that he has your welfare in mind when he did that."

Continued

Box **1-7** **Nontherapeutic Interpersonal Techniques with Examples—cont'd**

12. Requesting an explanation.
    - "Why do you think that?"
    - "Why do you feel this way?"
    - "Why did you do that?"
13. Indicating the existence of an external source.
    - "What makes you say that?"
    - "Who told you that you were Jesus?"
    - "What made you do that?"
14. Belittling expressed feelings.
    Client: I have nothing to live for . . . . I wish I was dead.
    Nurse: Everybody gets down in the dumps. *(or)* I've felt that way sometimes.
15. Making stereotyped comments.
    - "Nice weather we're having."
    - "I'm fine, and how are you?"
    - "It's for your own good."
    - "Keep your chin up."
    - "Just listen to your doctor and join the activities. You'll be home in no time."
16. Giving literal responses.
    Client: I'm the Wizard of Oz.
    Nurse: You don't look like him. He's much older than you.
    Client: Those people on television are talking to me.
    Nurse: Try not to watch television. *(or)* On which channel?
17. Ignoring the client's feelings or thoughts.
    Client: I'm nothing.
    Nurse: Of course you're something. Everybody is somebody.
18. Interpreting.
    - "What you really mean is that you're somebody special."
    - "Unconsciously you're saying this."
19. Introducing an unrelated topic (ignoring client's message).
    Client: I'd like to die.
    Nurse: Did you have visitors this weekend?

Table 1-1 **Nursing Diagnosis Statements in Relation to Life Processes**

Nursing Diagnosis	Life Process
Imbalanced nutrition	Biologic
Chronic low self-esteem	Psychologic
Impaired social interaction	Sociocultural
Delayed growth and development	Developmental
Spiritual distress	Spiritual
Ineffective sexuality patterns	Sexual

Components of the Nursing Diagnosis Statement

The three distinct components of an actual nursing diagnosis statement are (1) the problem, (2) etiology, and (3) signs and symptoms. The format for documentation of these components is known as the *PES format*.

Table 1-2 **NANDA Taxonomy II**

Human Response Patterns	Definitions
1 Exchanging	Mutual giving and receiving
2 Communicating	Sending messages
3 Relating	Establishing bonds
4 Valuing	Assigning of relative worth
5 Choosing	Selection of alternatives
6 Moving	Activity
7 Perceiving	Reception of information
8 Knowing	Meaning associated with information
9 Feeling	Subjective awareness of information

Table 1-3	Comparison of DSM-IV-TR and NANDA Diagnoses
DSM-IV-TR Diagnosis	NANDA Diagnosis
Generalized Anxiety Disorder	Anxiety Ineffective coping
Bipolar I Disorder	Risk for violence Defensive coping
Schizophrenia	Disturbed thought processes Disturbed sensory perception
Major Depressive Disorder	Hopelessness Powerlessness
Obsessive-Compulsive Disorder	Impaired social interaction
Posttraumatic Stress Disorder	Rape-trauma syndrome

Table 1-4	Examples of NANDA Diagnoses and Qualifying Statements
NANDA Diagnosis	Qualifying Statement
Imbalanced nutrition	Less than body requirements
Self-care deficit	Bathing, dressing/grooming, feeding, total
Noncompliance	Medication, milieu activities
Deficient knowledge	Medications, treatments

P = Problem

The *problem* is a concise statement of the client's actual or potential response to health problems or life processes, also known as the *diagnostic label* of the response. Problem statements come from the list of approved NANDA nursing diagnoses, such as *ineffective coping*.

Many diagnoses are accompanied by *definitions* that more clearly describe or explain the health problem. This feature is especially useful to students, who may need more specific clarification of the problem than the label conveys. For example, the definition that accompanies the diagnosis *social isolation* stipulates that it is a condition of aloneness experienced by the individual, who perceives it as being imposed by others and as a negative or threatening state. The definition distinguishes social isolation from the situation in which the individual prefers to be alone and becomes isolated by choice.

For additional clarity, some nursing diagnoses require *qualifying statements* based on the nature of the health problems as demonstrated in the particular client response or situation (Table 1-4).

E = Etiology

The etiology is the second part of the PES format and is the source from which the nursing diagnosis emerges. Etiologies, also known as *related factors* or *contributing factors,* are considered to be the cause of the problem to the

Table 1-5	Example of NANDA Diagnosis and Etiologies
NANDA Diagnosis	Etiology (Related Factors)
Anxiety	Threat to biologic, psychologic, or social integrity Ineffective use of coping mechanisms Depletion of coping strategies

extent that cause can be determined. Nursing diagnoses are often accompanied by several etiologic factors that interact to produce the health problem. These factors may be psychologic, biologic, relational, environmental, situational, developmental, or sociocultural, but all are associated with the problem in some way (Table 1-5).

Many etiologic factors are broad categories or examples that require more specific information based on the nature of the problem and the individual client. For example, the first etiology listed in Table 1-5 is "threat to biologic, psychologic, or social integrity." Considering the source of anxiety in a particular client, the nurse needs to be more precise in specifying which aspects of biologic, psychologic, or social integrity are threatened: recent illness or injury *(biologic);* loss of job or status, either actual or a perceived feeling of abandonment or isolation *(psychologic);* or divorce, separation, or dysfunctional relationship *(social).*

Etiologies: the focus of treatment

Etiologies may be treated by nurses independently or in collaboration with other health care professionals, as determined by the client's needs. The nurse, however, is primarily responsible for constructing the client's treatment plan and selecting etiologies that are both specific to the client's identified problem and managed and treated primarily by nurses. The treatment plan for any given nursing diagnosis must include interventions aimed at managing or resolving etiologic factors, as well as the health problem.

Nursing diagnoses as etiologies

Nursing diagnoses can also be appropriately used as etiologies for other nursing diagnoses. Examples include the following:

1. Anxiety—related to powerlessness
2. Impaired social interactions—related to chronic low self-esteem
3. Ineffective coping—related to anxiety

Medical diagnoses as etiologies

It is considered inadvisable to list medical diagnoses as etiologies for nursing diagnoses because the client's health problem (nursing diagnosis, etiologic factors) is primarily treated by *nursing* interventions and therapies.

However, many symptoms and behaviors resulting from mental disorders and medical conditions are of great concern to nurses and readily respond to treatment by nurses, such as the following:

1. Disturbed thought processes as a result of the schizophrenic process

2. Imbalanced nutrition: less than body requirements as a result of anorexia nervosa

The nurse should isolate the aspects that contribute to the symptoms or pathology and can be modified or treated by nursing interventions, citing these as etiologic factors, as in the following:

1. Disturbed thought processes related to:
   • Increased internal and external stressors
   • Impaired ability to process internal and external stimuli
2. Imbalanced nutrition: less than body requirements related to:
   • Inadequate intake and hypermetabolic need
   • Loss of appetite secondary to constipation

S = Signs and symptoms

The signs and symptoms, also known as *defining characteristics,* are the observable, measurable manifestations of a client's response to the identified health problem. Defining characteristics are listed for every nursing diagnosis. As with the problem statement and etiologies, they often require more specific descriptions to better represent the needs of the client being diagnosed.

For example, the diagnosis *ineffective coping* has the critical defining characteristic *ineffective problem solving.* As the nurse constructs this diagnostic statement for the benefit of clinical use, specific examples that describe the client's impaired problem solving should be cited. Often the nurse can clarify the "defining characteristic" statements by quoting the client, as in the following examples of ineffective problem solving:

• "I can't decide if I should stay with my family or move to a board and care home."
• "I can't decide what to do first—get a job or begin day treatment."

It is helpful when *major* characteristics are present in the nurse's assessment criteria to give some validity to the health problem that is being diagnosed. For example, major characteristics of the diagnosis *chronic low self-esteem* are those that are persistent, long-standing, and include the following:

1. Self-negating comments
2. Expression of shame or guilt
3. Evaluates self as unable to deal with events
4. Rationalizes away or rejects positive feedback

Other, *noncritical* ("minor") characteristics may be added as defining characteristics. Major defining characteristics have been tested for reliability as predictors of the diagnosis based on research and extensive clinical experience.

Risk Nursing Diagnosis
Risk factors

Risk factors are used in assessing potential health problems to describe existing health states that may contribute to the potential problem becoming an actual problem. Thus, in a risk nursing diagnosis, there are *no defining characteristics* because the actual problem has not been manifested. Also, there is *no etiologic factor* in a potential (risk) problem because cause cannot exist without effect.

Therefore a **risk** nursing diagnosis carries a *two-part statement,* whereas an **actual** nursing diagnosis consists of a *three-part statement,* as in the following:

Risk problem
Part 1: *Nursing diagnosis*
• Risk for other-directed violence
Part 2: *Risk factors* (predictors of risk problems)
• History of violence
• Panic state
• Hyperactivity, secondary to manic state
• Low impulse control

Actual problem
Part 1: *Nursing diagnosis*
• Posttrauma response
Part 2: *Etiology* (related factors)
Overwhelming anxiety secondary to:
• Rape or other assault
• Catastrophic illness
• Disasters/war
Part 3: *Defining characteristics* (signs/symptoms)
• Reexperience of traumatic events (flashbacks)
• Repetitive dreams or nightmares
• Intrusive thoughts about traumatic event

Risk factors as predictors of risk problems

The prediction of a risk health problem in a particular client requires an estimation of probability of occurrence. Risk problems can be ascribed to most individuals whose health is compromised. For example, a client taking a tricyclic antidepressant medication may be at risk for several potential problems or conditions as a result of the actions of these drugs on many body systems, such as risk for injury (hypotension, dizziness, blurred vision), risk for constipation, risk for urinary retention, and risk for impaired oral mucous membranes (dry mouth). It is nonproductive for the nurse to construct a treatment plan that lists all these diagnoses with outcome criteria and interventions without considering the probabilities.

The nurse should first assess the client's overall health state and identify factors that place the individual at a higher risk for the health problem than the general population. For example, the client taking tricyclic antidepressants who is poorly hydrated, refuses to drink juice or water, and has a low-fiber diet is at a higher risk for constipation than the general population. Therefore the *risk* diagnosis of constipation must be stated on the client's individualized treatment plan as follows:

Part 1: *Nursing diagnosis*
• Risk for constipation
Part 2: *Risk factors*
• Effects of tricyclic antidepressants
• Poor hydration and diet
• Noncompliance with high-fiber diet

This risk diagnosis was specifically selected to remind the nurse that although the focus of this text is psychiatric nursing, *all* body systems are considered during management of client care.

OUTCOME IDENTIFICATION

In the outcome identification phase of the nursing process, the nurse identifies *outcomes,* which are specific indicators derived from the nursing diagnosis. The nurse identifies expected client outcomes and individualizes them to the client and the situation. In the *evaluation* phase, nurses examine outcomes to determine whether the actual problem was resolved or reduced, or if the risk problem ever occurred.

Outcomes are measurable and mutually developed among the nurse, client, and other caregivers. When possible, outcomes are realistic and achievable in relation to the client's current and potential capabilities and available resources and support system (Box 1-8).

Outcomes provide direction for continued effective management of care and may include a time estimate for attainment based on the nurse's knowledge and experience as to when specific outcomes are typically achieved. An *outcome statement* is a projected influence that nursing interventions will have on the client in relation to the identified problem. Outcomes are *not* client goals or nursing goals and should *not* describe nursing interventions.

With risk problems such as self-directed violence, actual signs and symptoms are absent. Therefore risk problem statements are accompanied by risk factors that may be precursors to the signs and symptoms, should the problem become actual. Outcome criteria are then developed from what would be the signs and symptoms if the risk problem were to become actual (see Fig. 1-2).

PLANNING

In the planning phase of the nursing process, the nurse develops a plan of care that prescribes **interventions** with accompanying **rationale** to achieve expected client outcomes. Nurses individualize care plans to accommodate the client's condition, needs, and situation, based on actual problems or risk factors. The process of planning includes the following:

1. Collaboration by the nurse with the client, family, significant others, and treatment team
2. Identification of signs, symptoms, risk factors, and priorities of care
3. Decisions regarding use of psychotherapeutic principles and practices
4. Coordination and delegation of responsibilities according to the treatment team's expertise as it relates to client needs

Plans reflect current nursing practices and generally include input from other disciplines involved in the treatment. Nursing care plans, regardless of the format, should provide for continuity and efficiency of client care management and progress.

Clinical Pathways

A clinical pathway, also known as a **critical pathway, care path,** or **care map,** is a standardized format used to monitor client care and progress through the case management interdisciplinary health care delivery system. Although nursing is a primary proponent of the critical pathway method, other disciplines responsible for client care in the psychiatric setting are strongly involved in the planning and developing of each critical pathway. Disciplines involved in the critical pathway include the following:

- Nursing
- Psychiatry
- Social services
- Occupational therapy
- Therapeutic recreation
- Dietary services

In developing the clinical pathway, the interdisciplinary team may use the following health professionals as consultants:

- Family practice physicians
- Psychologists
- Chaplain

A clinical pathway refers primarily to a written clinical process that identifies projected caregiver behaviors and interventions and expected client outcomes. It is based on the client's mental disorder as defined in the *DSM-IV-TR,* which is in line with the *International Classification of Diseases,* tenth edition. The pathway is mapped out along a continuum that depicts chronologic milestones or timelines, which are generally the number of days of the client's estimated length of stay for each specific diagnosis.

The pathway is a projection of the client's entire hospital stay, detailing multidisciplinary interventions (processes) and client outcomes each day of hospitalization, from admission through discharge. A pathway may be extended to include the client's transfer to home care or another type of treatment facility. The pathway would then continue for as long as necessary. Clinical pathways may also be developed for clients in a home care setting by the interdisciplinary home care team.

> Box **1-8**   **Examples of Outcome Identification: Risk for Self-Directed Violence**
>
> - The client demonstrates absence of suicidal thoughts and gestures.
> - Interprets environmental stimuli accurately.
> - Interacts socially with other clients and staff.
> - Demonstrates absence of violent behaviors.

Key client outcomes

Clinical pathways may identify key outcomes to be achieved by the client that are considered critical to the client's recovery or prognosis. These outcomes generally require several interventions specifically intended to assist the client to achieve the identified key outcome. For example, in a client experiencing *mania,* a phase of bipolar disorder, key client outcomes would be identified as follows:

- Demonstrates reduction in movement, racing thoughts, grandiosity, euphoria, and irritability
- Sleeps 4 to 6 hours a night
- Lithium level within therapeutic range

The therapeutic range of lithium is generally about 1.0 mEq/L, the usual level at which a client safely functions in a nonmanic and nontoxic state. Lithium is the primary treatment for clients in the manic phase of bipolar disorder. Because a major focus in pathway implementation is linking key interventions (processes) with key outcomes, critical interventions are needed for the client to achieve these outcomes. These interventions should be progressively documented along the pathway and include the following for clients with mania:

1. Initiate lithium level to determine baseline admission level.
2. Administer lithium and other relevant medications according to protocol.
3. Teach the client and family about effects of lithium and importance of compliance.
4. Help the client and family to recognize manic symptoms and to link them with precipitating events.
5. Check lithium levels for therapeutic range.
6. Assess and reassess for lithium toxicity.
7. Continue to check lithium levels until desired level and stable mood are achieved.

Noncritical outcomes are related to the client's secondary levels of treatment, such as attending special occupational or recreational groups or performing grooming skills. Although such tasks are important in the client's overall treatment regimen and reflect a general functional level, they may not be key or critical outcomes for the client's overall diagnosis and prognosis.

Variances

Variances, also known as **outliers,** occur when a client's response to interventions differs from the expected response. A variance may be considered an *unexpected* or *aberrant* client response that "falls off" the pathway, requiring separate documentation and further investigation by the interdisciplinary team.

Causes of pathway variances may be related to the client and family, caregivers, hospital, community, and payer, including insurance companies, health maintenance organizations, and managed care organizations. A variance may be positive or negative and affect the client's length of stay and outcomes. An example of a *positive variance* is a client who responds more rapidly to medication or other forms of treatment than expected and leaves the hospital before the estimated length of stay. An example of a *negative variance* is a client who fails to achieve the desired nonmanic state or therapeutic lithium level according to the timeline designated on the clinical pathway continuum (generally by date of discharge) and whose length of stay is therefore prolonged.

The clinical pathways of case management help to ensure the following:

- Accountability for care by all disciplines
- Coordination of care
- Prevention of complications
- Timely lengths of stay
- Cost effectiveness
- Continued quality improvement

Fig. 1-4 is a clinical pathway describing a client who is experiencing mania. The client's length of stay is 8 days, the average stay for the designated related group of this category of mental disorders. In reviewing the pathway format, note that the elements are separated into two parts, outcomes and processes. **Outcomes** are the expected client outcomes that are predicted along the 8-day continuum, as noted in the "Interval" row across the top of the pathway. Outcomes have four distinct client categories: physiologic, psychologic, functional status/role, and family/community reintegration. **Processes,** also known as *interventions* (bottom section of the clinical pathway), consist of several categories listed along the left column.

Processes reflect the client's needs and the pathway's interdisciplinary focus. Processes are expected to affect the client's identified outcomes in a progressive, timely manner along the pathway continuum. The pathway is, in effect, the client's care plan, the outcome of which is used to evaluate the client's progress on a daily basis. Variances are categorized by either letters or numbers along the bottom of the pathway. In the pathway depicted in this text, two types of variances have been developed: *pathway variances,* which the staff would indicate by writing the codes (P1, P2, etc.) in the interval (days) section across the top of the pathway, and *element variances,* which the staff would indicate by writing the codes (1.1, 2.2, etc.) in the body of the pathway itself, according to where they occur.

Clinical pathways continue to be developed, improved, and implemented in a variety of health care settings. They are expected to reflect the changing trends and complexities of current health care delivery systems. Pathways are useful *communication tools* for nurses during intershift reporting and at other critical times throughout the patient's hospital stay.

IMPLEMENTATION

In this phase of the nursing process the nurse implements the interventions that have been prescribed in the planning phase. Nursing interventions, also termed **nursing orders**

CLINICAL PATHWAY: MANIA

Interval	Day of Admit	Day 2	Day 3	Day 4	Day 5	Day 6	Day 7	Day 8
Location								
Physiologic Pain (1-10) 1-3: mild 4-6: moderate 7-10 severe	*Takes adequate nutrition/fluids with assistance *Complies with lithium level evaluation • Pain___	*Demonstrates increased sleep/rest time *Demonstrates adequate elimination • Pain___	*Takes adequate nutrition/fluids with reminders *Demonstrates adequate elimination • Pain___	*Sleeps 4-6 hrs *Demonstrates adequate elimination • Pain___	*Takes adequate nutrition/fluids *Sleeps 4-6 hrs *Lithium level in therapeutic range *Other drug level in therapeutic range • Pain___	*Sleeps 5-8 hrs *Absence of drug toxicity • Pain___	*Sleep 5-8 hrs • Pain___	*Sleeps 5-8 hrs *Able to manage food and activity requirements independently • Pain___
Psychologic	*Involved in stimulation-reducing activities with staff supervision	*Oriented to person and place	*Demonstrates reduction in: Movement/racing thoughts Grandiosity/euphoria Irritability	*Demonstrates increased attention span *Reality tests with staff *Oriented to person, place, time, and situation	*Demonstrates more reality-based thoughts *Able to focus on one topic × 5-10 min	*Demonstrates euthymic mood *Able to focus on one topic × 5-10 min	*Able to complete activities and unit assignments	*Able to complete activities and unit assignments independently *Able to plan and structure day
Functional Status/Role	*Tolerates orientation to the unit *Refrains with assistance from harming self/others	*Interacting with staff as tolerated *Attends to hygiene/grooming needs with assistance *Refrains with assistance from harming self/others	*Engages in unit activities with staff supervision	*Maintains impulses with reminders *Complies with meds with reminders	*Demonstrates less intrusive behaviors	*Able to interact with peers *Able to make simple decisions	*Demonstrates safe, appropriate activities/behaviors *Independently complies with medical regimen	*Verbalizes need for ongoing med compliance
Family/ Community Reintegration	*Family/significant other aware of treatment program/goals *Family/significant other provide history including meds	*Identifies family/significant other to staff	*Attends community meetings with staff supervision *Communicates with SW for increased understanding of treatment/goals/DC plans	*Family/significant other involved in treatment/goals/DC plans	*Identifies DC needs	*Identifies DC needs	*Identifies DC needs *Able to identify supports and their appropriate use	*Able to utilize supports and list ways to access them *States specific plans to manage symptoms, comply with meds/aftercare

Note: This Clinical Pathway is a tool to assist health care providers in achieving quality patient outcomes by providing appropriate and timely patient care. It is not intended to establish a community standard of care, replace a clinician's medical judgment, establish a protocol for all patients, or exclude alternative therapies. (See Variances at end of figure.)

Abbreviations: *ADLS,* activities of daily living; *CBC,* complete blood count; *DC,* discharge; *ELOS,* estimated length of stay; *eval,* evaluation; *H/O,* history of; *I&O,* intake and output; *IV,* intravenous; *MD,* medical physician; *milieu,* therapeutic patient environment; *OT,* occupational therapist; *Reise writ.* hearing to determine if patient is cognitively able to make a decision to refuse psychotropic medication; *S&R,* seclusion and restraint; *SMAC,* sequential multiple analysis; *SW,* social worker; *UR,* utilization review.

Continued

Fig. 1-4   Clinical pathway example: Mania.

Interval	Day of Admit	Day 2	Day 3	Day 4	Day 5	Day 6	Day 7	Day 8
Location								
Discharge Planning	*SW assessment *Identify DC placement *ELOS, contact family/significant other *Nursing assessment *Identify H/O chronicity *Med compliance, strengths, needs, knowledge deficit	*Team: Involved in DC planning; discuss with MD *UR notify managed care ___	*SW eval completed *Treatment team meeting #1 ___ *Specific DC plans, placement facility identified ___	*Involve family/significant other in DC plans *Review DC plans with patient	*Assist patient/family/significant other DC needs *UR contact managed care as needed ___	*Continue to problem-solve DC needs with patient/family/significant other	*Transition to day treatment if indicated *Assist patient/family/significant other in finalizing DC plans *Treatment team meeting #2 ___	*DC to least restrictive environment completed *UR inform managed care as needed ___
Education	*Orient to unit *Inform of patient's rights *Assess patient's and family's/significant other knowledge of disorder/meds	*Assist with symptom recognition and importance of compliance *Teach family/significant other as needed	*Continue with symptom recognition *Continue teaching patient and family/significant other learning needs	*Assist in linking symptoms with precipitating events	*Teach patient/family/significant other about med effects on symptom management *Instruct in med, diet, exercise regimen	*Emphasize importance of compliance with meds after discharge *Teach about effects of drugs on symptom management	*Develop aftercare plan to manage symptoms and contact supports	*Reinforce aftercare teaching plan with patient/family/significant other as needed
Psychosocial/ Spiritual/Legal	*Assess: Safety Issues ___ Mental status ___ Spiritually ___ *Legal status: Voluntary ___ 72 hour hold ___ Reise writ ___ Payer ___ Conservator ___	*Continue to assess: Safety issues Mental status Spiritual needs Legal status	*Continue to assess: Safety issues Mental status (e.g., racing thoughts, grandiosity, euphoria, irritability) Spiritual/legal needs	*Continue to assess: Safety issues Mental status (e.g., racing thoughts, grandiosity, euphoria, irritability) Spiritual/legal needs	*Continue to assess: Safety issues Mental status Spirituality Voluntary status	*Continue to assess: Safety issues Mental status Spirituality Voluntary status	*Continue to assess: Safety issues Mental status Spirituality Voluntary status	*Complete assessments and confirm: Safety issues Mental status Spirituality Legal status
Consults	*Physical exam within 24 hours *Other consults	*Other consults as needed	*Other consults as needed	*Other consults as needed	*Complete consults as ordered	*Complete consults as ordered	*Complete consults as ordered *Arrange for aftercare consults as ordered	*Complete all consults as ordered
Tests/Procedures	*Lithium level ___ *Tegretol level ___ *Drug screen ___ *Thyroid function ___ CBC/SMAC ___ Other ___	*Tests/procedures as ordered	*Tests/procedures as ordered	*Tests/procedures as ordered	*Check lithium level for therapeutic range *Check other drug levels for therapeutic range as needed *Test procedures as needed	*Check lithium level for therapeutic range *Check other drug levels within therapeutic range as needed *Tests procedures as needed	*Check lithium level for therapeutic range *Check other drug levels within therapeutic range as needed *Test procedures as needed	Confirm lithium level for therapeutic range *Confirm other levels within therapeutic range as needed *Test procedures as ordered aftercare

(Left margin vertical label: P R O C E S S E S)

Fig. 1-4, cont'd For legend see p. 17.

Interval / Location	Day of Admit	Day 2	Day 3	Day 4	Day 5	Day 6	Day 7	Day 8
Treatment	*Monitor: I&O *Sleep/rest patterns *Level of observation 1:1 __; every 15 min __; every 30 min __ *Reduce milieu stimulation *S&R yes __ or no __ *Other	*Monitor: I&O *Sleep/rest patterns *Level of observation 1:1 __; every 15 min __; every 30 min __ *Reduce milieu stimulation *S&R yes __ no __ *Other	*Level of observation 1:1 __; every 15 min __; every 30 min __ *Continue with treatment plan Monitor: I&O Sleep/rest patterns Other	*Continue with treatment plan Monitor: I&O Sleep/rest patterns Other	*Level of observation 1:1 __; every 15 min __; every 30 min __ *Continue with treatment plan Monitor: I&O Sleep/rest patterns Other	*Level of observation 1:1 __; every 15 min __; every 30 min __ *Continue with treatment plan Monitor: I&O Sleep/rest patterns Other	*Level of observation 1:1 __; every 15 min __; every 30 min __ *Aftercare treatment instructions reviewed with patient/family/significant other as needed	*DC with aftercare treatment instructions
Medications (IV & Others)	*Meds as ordered *See relevant protocols: *Lithium *Other *Monitor side effects *Toxicity	*Meds as ordered *Continue to monitor side effects/toxicity	*Meds as ordered *Continue to monitor side effects/toxicity	*Meds as ordered *Continue to monitor side effects/toxicity	*Meds as ordered *Contact managed care if any change in med regimen	*Meds as ordered *Contact managed care if any change in med regimen	*Meds as ordered *Review of meds with patient/family/significant other as needed	*DC with meds and instructions as ordered
Activity	*OT assessment *1:1 brief contacts *Reality orientation *Intervene to manage impulses; prevent harm to self/others	*Engage in stimulation-reducing activities as tolerated *Assist with hygiene, grooming, ADLs *Prevent harm to self/others during activities	*OT eval completed *Encourage hygiene, grooming, ADLs with reminders *Prevent harm to self/others during activities	*Engage in 2 groups per day *Increase group stimulation as tolerated *Prevent harm to self/others during activities	*Encourage: Independent hygiene and grooming Independent ADLs Increased participation in groups	*Engage in all unit activities and groups *Encourage independent decision making	*Reinforce active participation in all unit activities and groups; independent decision making	*Confirm ability to complete activity assignments independently, ability to make decisions independently
Diet/Nutrition	*Nutritional screening *Elicit food preference *Offer adequate nutrition and fluids; normal salt intake *Baseline weight (weekly unless otherwise ordered)	*Provide: Simple meals Finger foods Easy-to-carry drinks	*Encourage meals in patient community as tolerated with staff supervision	*Encourage meals in patient community as tolerated with staff supervision	*Teach family/significant other importance of adequate foods/fluids/salt intake	*Teach family/significant other importance of adequate foods/fluids/salt intake	*Reinforce adequate nutrition/fluids and normal salt intake *Weekly weight	*Confirm patient/significant other/family knowledge of adequate foods/fluids/salt intake

P R O C E S S E S

Clinical Pathway (CP) Variances: P1. CP completed early   P2. Patient of CP   P3. CP completed and patient not discharged   P4. Initial interval not appropriate

Element Variances:

1. Patient/Family
   a. Patient physiologic status
   b. Patient psychologic status
   c. Patient/family refusal
   d. Patient/family unavailable
   e. Patient/family other
   f. Patient/family communication barrier
   g. Element met early

2. Clinician
   a. Order differs from CP
   b. Action differs from CP
   c. Response time
   d. Clinician other
   e. Court/guardianship
   f. Operating unit other

3. Operating Unit
   a. Bed/appointment not available
   b. Lack of data
   c. Supplies/equipment not available
   d. Department over-booked/closed
   e. Court/guardianship

4. Community
   a. Placement not available
   b. Home care not available
   c. Ambulance delay
   d. Transportation not available
   e. Community other

5. Payer
   a. Delayed giving authorization number
   b. Payer limitations
   c. Payer other

Fig. 1-4, cont'd   For legend see p. 17.

or **prescriptions,** are the most powerful component of the nursing process, representing the management and treatment approach to an identified health problem. Interventions are selected to achieve or attain outcomes and prevent or reduce problems.

Criticisms in the literature and in clinical practice say that nursing interventions are often weak, vague, and nonspecific. The interventions listed in this text reflect both actual and typical nursing responses and behaviors derived from research, educational preparation and clinical experience. They are substantive, expressive, and inclusive. In the psychiatric–mental health setting, treatment or therapies frequently constitute verbal communication skills, a major source of psychosocial intervention. Such treatments are intended to effect a change in the client's present condition or circumstance, not merely maintain the problem in its present state. Prescriptions or orders recommend a course of action, not simply support an existing regimen.

Nursing interventions for nursing diagnoses and accompanying etiologies should explicitly describe a plan of therapeutic activity that will help mobilize the client toward a healthier or more functional state. Examples of **therapeutic** interventions follow:

1. Gradually engage the client in interactions with other clients, beginning with one-to-one contacts and progressing toward informal gatherings and eventually structured group activities, occupational therapy first, then recreational therapy.
2. Teach the client and family that therapeutic effects of antidepressant medications may take up to 2 weeks, but that uncomfortable effects may begin immediately, some of which may disappear.

Examples of **nontherapeutic** interventions follow:
1. Assist the client to interact with others.
2. Teach the client and family about medications.

The correct, therapeutic examples demonstrate clarity and substance, as opposed to the weaker, vague, incorrect, nontherapeutic statements. Nursing interventions that simply regurgitate physicians' orders are not substantive enough to treat or manage the health problem effectively and are therefore **nontherapeutic,** as follows:

- "Monitor the client's progress."
- "Check lithium levels."
- "Notify social services."
- "Obtain the client's consent form."

Effective nursing interventions should be able to move the client from a less functional to a more functional health state by virtue of their clarity, substance, and direction.

Impact of Interventions on Etiology

Interventions have the greatest impact when directed toward etiologies (related factors) that accompany the nursing diagnosis. If the problem is a risk nursing diagnosis, interventions are aimed at the risk factors. This suggests that the etiologies of a problem can be modified by nursing. Therefore, to achieve or attain the most successful client outcomes, the nurse should carefully examine each of the etiologic factors and select interventions that would effectively modify each one. For example:

Part 1: *Nursing diagnosis*
- Chronic low self-esteem

Part 2: *Etiology* (related factors)
- Doubt concerning self-worth and abilities
- Perceived rejection by others

Part 3: *Defining characteristics* (signs/symptoms)
- The client verbalizes incompetence, inadequacy, and failure (e.g., "I'm a flop at everything I do").
- Expresses feelings of rejection and disapproval by others (e.g., avoids being part of the group; rarely offers thoughts or suggestions).

Nursing intervention

Help the client become aware of positive aspects of self and abilities.
- "You really helped the other clients in group today, by talking about your own struggles to improve your communication skills."

This intervention is directly aimed at the first etiology (doubt concerning self-worth and abilities) but also addresses the nursing diagnosis (chronic low self-esteem) and the defining characteristics (verbalizes incompetence, inadequacy, and failure).

Nursing intervention

Praise the client whenever attempts are made to communicate and interact with others.
- "I noticed you stayed in the room to chat with others after group. They seemed to enjoy having you join them and share your thoughts."

This intervention is directly aimed at the second etiology (perceived rejection by others) but also addresses the nursing diagnosis (chronic low self-esteem) and the defining characteristics (expresses feelings of rejection and disapproval by others).

Interventions and Medical Actions

Interventions can include medically focused actions, such as the administration of medications, but the major focus of the intervention should emphasize nursing actions, judgments, treatments, and directives. Note the absence of any prescribed nursing actions that would influence the client's health state in the following examples:

1. Administer antipsychotic medication as ordered
2. Observe for extrapyramidal effects.

Although it is important to carry out physician's orders, nursing interventions encompass much more.

Rationale Statements

A *rationale statement* is the reason for the nursing intervention or why it was prescribed and is often included with the intervention statement. This practice often enhances the understanding of the nurse's action or treatment. The authors have liberally used clear and descriptive rationale statements for each intervention throughout this text to foster the reader's overall understanding of the selected intervention, as in the following examples:

Intervention: Actively listen, observe, and respond to the client's verbal and nonverbal expressions.

Rationale: Intervention shows the client that he or she is worthwhile and respected.

Intervention: Initiate brief, frequent contacts with the client throughout the day.

Rationale: Intervention shows the client that he or she is an important part of the therapeutic community.

EVALUATION

Evaluation of achieved or attained expected client outcomes must occur at various intervals as designated in the outcome criteria. The client's health state and capability is of primary consideration when evaluating outcomes. The evaluation phase consists of two steps.

In the **first step** the nurse compares the client's current mental health state or condition with that described in the outcome criteria. For example, is the client's anxiety reduced to a tolerable level? Can the client sit calmly for 10 minutes, attend a simple recreational activity for 10 minutes, and engage in one-to-one interaction with staff for 5 minutes without distractions? Is there a significant reduction in pacing, fidgeting, or scanning the environment? Were these outcomes attained within the times originally projected?

The degree to which client outcomes are attained or not attained is also an evaluation of the effectiveness of nursing.

In the **second step** of the evaluation phase, the nurse considers all the possible reasons why client outcomes were not attained, if this is the case. For example, it may be too soon to evaluate, and the plan of action needs further implementation; or the client needed another 2 days of one-to-one interactions before attending group activities. Also, the interventions may have been too forceful and frequent or too weak and infrequent. Perhaps the outcomes were unattainable, impractical, or just not feasible for this client, or perhaps they were not within the client's scope and capabilities on a developmental or sociocultural level. What about the validity of the nursing diagnosis? Was it developed with a questionable or faulty database? Are more data required? What were the conditions during the assessment phase? Was it too hurried? Were conclusions drawn too quickly? Were there any language or communication barriers?

Based on conclusions drawn from these queries, specific recommendations are then made. These include either continuing implementation of the plan of action or reviewing the previous phases of the nursing process (data collection, nursing diagnosis, planning, or implementation).

The evaluation of a client's progress and the nursing activities involved in the process are critical because they require, even demand, that nursing be accountable for its own standards of care.

Informal evaluation of the client's progress is similar to the nursing process and takes place continuously (see Fig. 1-1).

THE NURSING PROCESS IN COMMUNITY AND HOME SETTINGS

In the past the nursing process and its multistep format have been most associated with the care of *hospitalized* clients. Current trends in health care delivery systems have shifted from inpatient facilities to community and home-based settings and provide yet another vital avenue for use of the nursing process. *Home health care* is the primary alternative to hospitalization, and the nursing process continues to be a major factor in the effective management of home client care.

Psychiatric Home Health Care Case Management System

The changes and demands in the current health care delivery system have resulted in health care reform designed for cost-effective quality care. Although the case management concept has long been used in acute care settings and public health arenas, only recently has the private home health model subscribed to total case management, and only more recently has psychiatric home care been incorporated under the case management umbrella.

Psychiatric home care case management is a method by which a client is identified as a candidate for home care and treated on a health care continuum in the familiar surroundings of the home. The interdisciplinary home care team, facilitated by a registered nurse, coordinates all available resources to meet their goals for treatment and to achieve the client's expected outcomes in a quality and cost-effective manner. At one end of the continuum is the highest degree of independent wellness within the client's capacity. At the other end of the continuum is death. Varying levels of wellness-illness make up the continuum between these two extremes.

Critical to successful utilization of case management is (1) the accurate placement of the client at the entry point on the continuum and (2) a clear understanding of the team's best estimate for the date of cessation of home care services.

NIC and NOC

Nursing-sensitive outcomes classification

Nursing research in the expansion of patient outcomes was developed by the Nursing-Sensitive Outcomes Classification (NOC) research team, formed in August 1991 at the University of Iowa (Iowa Intervention Project, 1996). Its purpose was to conceptualize, label, and classify nursing-sensitive patient outcomes. NOC is complementary to the work of NANDA; both reflect the creation and testing of a professional, standardized language that defines the nursing profession, and both strive to develop patient outcomes that are responsive to nursing interventions. NOC developed the first comprehensive list of standardized outcomes, definitions, and measures to describe patient outcomes that are influenced by nursing practice.

According to the NOC, patient outcomes are considered *neutral* rather than static and reflect patients' ongoing states, such as mobility and hydration *(physiologic),* or coping and grieving *(psychologic).* Such fluid states can be measured on a continuum of care rather than as singular, discrete goals that are either met or not met. Because outcomes are presented by the NOC as neutral concepts, they can be identified and measured in a variety of ways and for different population groups. This is useful in assisting nurses to develop realistic standards that reflect currently achieved outcomes, if the outcomes are satisfactory, or desired higher standards of achievement.

Identifying outcomes responsive to nursing versus depending on the use of interdisciplinary outcomes developed mostly for physician practice is critical for controlling quality patient care and the further development of nursing knowledge, language, and the profession. Agreement on standardizing nursing-sensitive patient outcomes allows nurses to analyze the effects of nursing interventions along a patient care continuum and across health care settings.

Nursing interventions classification

Nursing Interventions Classification (NIC) is the first comprehensive, standardized classification of treatments performed by nurses. NIC works in conjunction with NOC in that patient outcomes need to be identified before an intervention is selected. The classification includes interventions that nurses facilitate for patients, both independently and with other disciplines, for direct and indirect care. NIC interventions include both *physiologic* types (e.g., airway suctioning) and *psychologic* or *psychosocial* types (e.g., anxiety reduction).

As with NANDA and NOC, NIC interventions include a variety of patient populations, settings, groups, and cultures. Although most are geared toward the individual, they also apply to families and entire communities. They can be used for illness prevention, health maintenance, education, environmental management, and health promotion. Although NIC interventions are linked to NANDA diagnoses, there are more possibilities with NIC in that nurses need to know the patient and the patient's condition before selecting the appropriate intervention; therefore the NIC decision-making process is more complex.

Principal investigators/editors Bulechek and McCloskey (1992) have outlined the following three areas in which the nurse must be competent to carry out an intervention:

1. Knowledge of scientific rationale
2. Possession of the necessary psychomotor and interpersonal skills
3. Ability to function within the setting to effectively use health care resources

For more information on NIC and NOC and their relationships to NANDA, refer to current literature on these classification systems.

APPLICATION OF THE NURSING PROCESS

The history and assessment tool (see Fig. 1-3) and the following case study and plan of care are examples of how the care plans in this book can be adapted to an individual client.

CASE STUDY: THE CLIENT WITH ANXIETY

Josh, a 15-year-old high school student, is admitted for the first time to the mental health facility. He is accompanied to the facility voluntarily by his parents, who are noted to be supportive and concerned about their only child. Josh's chief complaint is quoted as: "I suddenly feel I can't cope with schoolwork, friends, or sports; I feel tense, sweaty, and uncomfortable and find it hard to concentrate on my assignments. My heart pounds and I breathe fast even when I'm not moving around, and I find myself wanting to run out of the classroom." He noted that his symptoms have occurred for 10 days and have been increasing in severity and frequency until he now feels they are interfering with his ability to do his school work and perform the activities and sports that he loves.

ASSESSMENT

Problem List

The problems are based on the psychiatric nursing history and assessment (see Fig. 1-3).

Physiologic

1. Shortness of breath at rest
2. Rapid heart rate (greater than 120 beats/min) at rest
3. Sweaty palms when performing schoolwork or sports or talking with peers
4. Feelings of generalized discomfort and tension

Psychologic

1. The client cannot concentrate on schoolwork/assignments, resulting in lower grades.
2. Threatens to quit soccer team due to poor performance.
3. Feels like running away from classroom or peers.
4. Unable to cope with current responsibilities, role, and life circumstances.

Behaviors observed by nurse during assessment and interview are as follows:

1. The client paced back and forth (could not remain seated for more than 1 minute).
2. Burst into tears 3 times during 45-minute interview.
3. Had difficulty in attending interview questions. (Interviewer had to repeat each question at least once.)
4. Spoke in hurried, tense manner (rarely completed a sentence or thought).
5. Stated, "I am worried," at least 3 times during the interview.

Learning Needs Identified

The client needs to learn the following:
- Stressors/stressor events that are precursors to ineffective coping
- Methods/strategies to increase effective coping skills and decrease or minimize anxiety
- Use of healthy, adaptive defense mechanisms
- Cognitive, reframing, and desensitization skills
- Effective ways to cope with stress
- Problem-solving strategies
- Value of support systems and community resources
- Dose, therapeutic, and adverse effects of anxiolytic and antidepressant medications
- Importance of follow-up care/preventive measures

Medical Diagnosis (Based on *DSM-IV-TR* Multiaxial Criteria)

Axis I: Generalized anxiety disorder
Axis II: No noted personality disorder
Axis III: No noted medical condition
Axis IV: Psychosocial/environmental stressors (moderate educational and social stressors noted)
Axis V: Global assessment of functioning: GAF = 55 (current); GAF = 85 (past year)

Nursing Diagnosis: Ineffective Coping

Inability to form a valid appraisal of the stressors, inadequate choices of practiced responses, inability to use available resources.

Etiology (Related Factors)

Anxiety (refer to symptoms/behaviors described previously)
Depletion of usual adaptive/coping methods
Conflicts/stressors that may be associated with current role, relationships, or responsibilities
Perceived threat to physical/psychosocial integrity
Possible feelings of powerlessness or helplessness
Expectations for success exceed actual abilities
Knowledge deficit regarding adaptive coping methods

Defining Characteristics

The client is unable to perform schoolwork, sports, or other activities.
Cries easily for no apparent reason or provocation.
Experiences urge to leave classroom or run away from peers for no apparent reason.

Cannot cope with age-related responsibilities, role, or life circumstances (e.g., schoolwork, sports, activities).
Experiences physiologic symptoms (e.g., rapid heart rate, shortness of breath, sweaty palms) when faced with routine tasks, activities, schoolwork, peers, or sports.
Is unable to attend or concentrate on age-appropriate tasks/roles (e.g., school assignments, activities, sports, friendships).

Outcome Identification and Evaluation

By day 4 of admission, the client demonstrates ability to focus/concentrate on assigned unit task/activity.
By day 4, remains seated throughout individual interactions with staff for 15 minutes.
By day 4, performs slow deep-breathing techniques and muscle tension relaxation exercises (see Appendix B).
By day 5, practices learned cognitive skills, reframing, and desensitization exercises (see Appendix B).
By day 5, completes unit task activities with minimal or absent anxiety symptoms.
By day 6, communicates and relates effectively with peers/staff without hesitation or anxiety responses.
By day 7, adaptively and effectively utilizes (with help of staff) defense mechanisms.
- *Introjection:* role-models calm behavior of staff.
- *Suppression:* consciously attempts to forget anxiety-producing stimuli.
- *Compensation:* practices pleasurable, rewarding activities.
- *Displacement:* transfers energy of anxiety to physical exercises (e.g., jogging, walking, bicycling, volleyball).

Verbalizes ability to perform schoolwork, sports, and other activities effectively without anxiety on day 8 (discharge).
By day 8, exhibits adaptive, healthy coping methods and strategies without supervision.
By day 8, prioritizes and problem-solves appropriate to age, role, and status with absence of anxiety.
- Places schoolwork first on priority list (grades show improvement).
- Makes an effort to interact with peers and support system.
- Participates in sports and other activities (remains with soccer team).
- Attends school functions with peers.
- Engages in meaningful relationships inside and outside school environment.
- Takes prescribed anxiolytic or antidepressant medications as needed.
- Utilizes resources, supports, and strengths effectively.
- Adheres to follow-up treatment plan and prevention.

Verbalizes signs/symptoms of escalating anxiety.
Demonstrates learned skills for interrupting progression of anxiety to panic level.
Functions effectively with level of anxiety that promotes productivity and creativity.

PLANNING AND IMPLEMENTATION

Nursing Intervention	Rationale
Maintain a calm, nonthreatening demeanor while interacting with the client.	Anxiety is transferable, and the client will feel more trusting and secure with a calm, nonthreatening staff member.
Demonstrate active listening, empathy, and understanding as the client verbalizes painful feelings.	The client is more likely to vent feelings in a safe, nurturing environment.
Assure the client of his safety and security by remaining with him and not leaving him alone when he is experiencing symptoms of anxiety, dread, or fear.	The client's anxious symptoms worsen when left alone during such times and may escalate to a panic state.
Use brief, simple messages in a calm, direct manner when speaking with the client, especially during initial stages of hospitalization.	Clients who are highly anxious may be unable to tolerate or comprehend complex, stimulating explanations.
Offer the client simple directives versus asking open-ended questions that require him to respond with lengthy statements, especially in initial hospitalization phase.	Clients experiencing anxiety may become even more anxious when asked to come up with too many answers. The client needs direction to help focus on relevant matters from staff who anticipate his needs.
Decrease environmental stimuli as much as possible. • Keep lights low. • Reduce volume on radio or TV. • Disperse people so they do not all congregate in one area.	A stimulating, busy milieu may increase the client's level of anxiety, whereas a calm environment may reduce anxiety.
Administer prescribed anxiolytic (antianxiety) or antidepressant medications and continue to assess their therapeutic and nontherapeutic effects.	Antianxiety medications may be the most beneficial initial therapeutic modality and should always be closely monitored for effectiveness throughout their use. New-generation antidepressants may also be used to treat anxiety for maintenance therapy and are nonaddictive. Medications do not take the place of a safe, nurturing milieu but may enhance it when necessary.
When the client's anxiety level has been reduced, engage the client in a discussion about identified stressors (school, sports, peers) and their possible connection to his anxiety.	Identification of possible issues that promote anxiety, even if they are not the actual causes of anxiety, is the first step in teaching the client to prevent further escalation of anxiety and to begin to control it.
Encourage the client to talk about the ways that his anxiety has disrupted his role (student, son, and peer) and how this has affected his day-to-day functioning.	Ventilation of feelings in a safe, therapeutic environment helps the client confront painful issues and eventually take steps, with staff help, to resolve them.
Teach the client to identify signs and symptoms of escalating anxiety and methods to interrupt its progression, such as slow deep-breathing exercises, relaxation techniques, physical activities such as walking and jogging (if not contraindicated), meditation, reframing, and visualization (see Appendix B).	Knowledge of impending anxiety and its escalation gives the client the opportunity to use learned physical and cognitive methods to interrupt the negative effects of increasing anxiety and prevent its rise to a panic state.

## chapter 2

Anxiety and Related Disorders

Anxiety disorders are the most prevalent of all mental disorders, and the symptom of anxiety is often identified as a component in other types of mental disorders. Because anxiety is so common in patients receiving medical or nursing care, especially in psychiatric settings, knowledge about its manifestations and treatment is imperative. Awareness can lead to prevention, identification, and treatment of anxiety.

Anxiety is universal among humans. All people become anxious, and although they spend much time, effort, and money trying to avoid or diminish it, anxiety is an unavoidable and inevitable part of the human condition. An important developmental task for people is learning to manage and regulate anxiety in nondestructive, socially acceptable ways.

The term **anxiety** usually has a negative connotation for most people, but it also can be a positive, alerting, and motivating factor that moves an individual toward productivity or to change an otherwise unacceptable situation. Some anxiety is necessary for the student to arise in the early morning and attend class, the nurse to check medications three times before administering them, and the parent to set limits on a child's emerging willful self-system in anticipation of molding character.

Anxiety may be experienced in many ways and at several levels. The *symptom* of anxiety is differentiated from the *syndromes* that constitute anxiety disorders. For example, a symptom of anxiety may manifest as a vague, subjective feeling of apprehension or insecurity that is uncomfortable and moderately stressful for a person during a job interview. On the other hand, anxiety may be excessively severe and overwhelming for persons admitted against their will to a locked psychiatric unit. Table 2-1 presents the levels of anxiety and associated physiologic, perceptual, cognitive, emotional, and behavioral symptoms. Specific symptoms of anxiety disorders are discussed later.

Early recognition of anxiety is imperative for two reasons. First, to be effective, nurses must recognize anxiety in themselves when working with clients and take immediate steps to contain and manage their anxiety. Second, early recognition of anxiety in the client, followed by immediate interventions, often prevents escalation to panic levels and ensures a calmer unit. Anxiety triggered by any source is contagious, and when nurses use keen assessment skills and anxiety reduction strategies, they often prevent the unit from escalating out of control. Strategies and techniques for intervening with anxiety appear in both the treatment section and the care plans later in this chapter.

RESPONSES TO ANXIETY

Stress Versus Anxiety

People often use the word "stress" when they mean anxiety. They also may use "stress" interchangeably for the event or situation that causes the discomfort *(stimulus)*, as well as for the resultant feelings, thoughts, and behaviors evoked *(response)*. Scientifically, the source is the *stressor* (stimulus), and the *reaction* is the response. This distinction is important because stressors are not immediately identifiable in anxiety disorders.

Another distinction arises when comparing **adaptive** and **maladaptive** responses to anxiety. All responses to anxiety could be considered "adaptive" in the broad interpretation because they alleviate the tension and discomfort

Table 2-1	**Stages and Manifestations of Anxiety**		
Stage	Physiologic	Cognitive/Perceptual	Emotional/Behavioral
Mild	Vital signs normal Minimal muscle tension Pupils normal, constricted	Broad perceptual field; awareness of multiple environmental and internal stimuli Thoughts random but controlled	Feelings of relative comfort and safety; relaxed, calm appearance and voice Performance automatic; habitual behaviors
Moderate	Vital signs normal or slightly elevated Tension experienced; may be uncomfortable *or* pleasurable (labeled as "tense" or "excited")	Alert and attentive; perception narrowed and focused Optimum state for problem solving and learning	Feelings of readiness and challenge; energized Engages in competitive activity and new skills Voice and facial expression interested or concerned
Severe	Fight-or-flight response Autonomic nervous system excessively stimulated: vital signs increased, diaphoresis increased, urinary urgency/frequency, diarrhea, dry mouth, appetite decreased, pupils dilated Muscles rigid, tense Senses affected; hearing decreased, pain sensation decreased	Perceptual field greatly narrowed; problem solving difficult *Selective attention*: focuses on one detail *Selective inattention*: block out threatening stimuli Distortion of time, seems faster or slower Dissociative tendencies *Vigilambulism*: automatic behavior	Feels threatened; startles with new stimuli; feels on "overload" Activity may increase or decrease: may pace, run away, wring hands, moan, shake, or stutter; disorganized, withdrawn, or frozen in position, unable to move May seem and feel depressed; may complain of aches or pains; may be agitated or irritable Need for space increased; eyes may dart around room, or gaze may be fixed; may close eyes to shut out environment.
Panic	Above symptoms escalate until sympathetic nervous system release occurs; may pale, decreased blood pressure, hypotension Muscle coordination poor Pain and hearing sensations minimal (see later discussion on panic disorder)	Perception totally scattered or closed; unable to take in stimuli Problem solving and logical thinking highly improbable Perception of unreality about self, environment, or event; dissociation possible	Feels helpless with total loss of control May be angry, terrified; may become combative or totally withdrawn; may cry or run Completely disorganized; behavior extremely active or inactive

that accompany anxiety. An adaptive response, however, is generally considered to be harmless and socially acceptable, whereas a maladaptive response may be harmful or unacceptable.

Anxiety evokes a response that is either adaptive or maladaptive. Over time, people develop characteristic response patterns that become fixed and affect their view of themselves and the environment. These patterns also help to shape a person's personality, choices, interpersonal interactions, relationships, and career outcomes.

Adaptive Responses

If anxiety occurs and the individual is able to regulate and manage it, positive outcomes are possible. All anxiety is not detrimental; it can be a challenging, powerful motivating factor toward problem solving, conflict resolution, and achievement of higher levels of functioning. For example, a person faced with job obsolescence

and the inevitable resultant hardships experiences anxiety that may move the person to return to school to learn new job skills. A student faced with failure on a major examination because of inadequate study may experience the threat of loss of status, self-esteem, identity, and support, and anxiety occurs. This motivator may help the student seek tutoring and make a concentrated effort to pass the test.

Other **adaptive strategies** that people use to manage anxiety are calling a friend or therapist, going for a walk or to the gym, practicing relaxation or meditation techniques, reading a novel, taking a short nap, and crying as a release. These and many other coping methods are used to relieve tension and manage anxiety.

Maladaptive Responses

Automatic relief behaviors that protect the individual from anxiety, defend against threats, and provide alleviation and comfort may also lead to maladaptive response patterns that can result in physical or psychologic symptoms, as well as personal, social, and occupational dysfunction. For example, the ego defense mechanisms of denial, repression, projection, and rationalization serve to protect the person from anxiety but also prevent realistic appraisal of self, other people, situations, or events.

When anxiety is *not* manageable, the individual may resort to coping mechanisms and strategies that are exaggerated and labeled "dysfunctional" or "abnormal" by others. Maladaptive patterns of coping with anxiety include aggressive acting out; withdrawal and isolation; excessive overeating, drinking, gambling, or spending; and drug use or sexual overactivity. Behavior in response to anxiety may become severe enough to be formally labeled an *anxiety disorder.*

Note that the state of uncontrollable anxiety is not restricted to anxiety disorders; clients with other mental or emotional disorders can experience various levels of anxiety. For example, a client with schizophrenia may experience an increase of symptoms because of overstimulation or environmental stressors that exceed his ability to cope. The symptoms occur in response to anxiety and may not necessarily indicate a worsening of the schizophrenic process.

ETIOLOGY

The National Institutes of Mental Health named the 1990s the "Decade of the Brain," with the focus on discovering specific *biologic factors* in the etiology of mental disorders. Although research progress has resulted from the increased biologic focus, economic support, and resultant knowledge, definite genetic markers have not been identified for most mental disorders, including the anxiety disorders. Although specific genes are yet to be identified, some anxiety disorders seem to have a more significant genetic basis (e.g., panic disorder), whereas other anxiety disorders seem more influenced by psychosocial stressors and life altering events (e.g., posttraumatic stress disorder). It may be many years before this complex research identifies definitive causal outcomes. Most likely, a combination of biologic factors coupled with life events generate these disorders. Box 2-1 lists specific etiologic factors of anxiety disorders.

EPIDEMIOLOGY

Anxiety disorders occur in cultures worldwide, not only the United States. Epidemiologic studies throughout the world describe symptoms of panic attack and panic disorder, regardless of culture. Anxiety disorders also are the most common form of mental disorder. In any given year, 28% or more of the U.S. population have mental disorders. Anxiety disorders are the most prevalent of these conditions in age groups: ages 9 to 17 years, 13%;

Box 2-1   Etiology of Anxiety Disorders

BIOLOGIC
Central nervous system dysregulation
- Hippocampus and amygdala
- Locus ceruleus
- Hypothalamic-pituitary-adrenal axis
Sympathetic nervous system activation
- Release of stress hormones (e.g., CRH)
- Adrenal cortex activation (e.g., glucocorticoids)
Hippocampal atrophy
Neurotransmitter alteration
- Gamma-aminobutyric acid (GABA)
- Serotonin
- Norepinephrine
Gonadotrophic hormones

PSYCHODYNAMIC
Anxiety an expression of underlying conflict

PSYCHOLOGIC
Perception of events as traumatic

BEHAVIORAL
Classic stimulus/response
Social learning through observation

COGNITIVE
Negative cognitive interpretations lead to helplessness framework
Loss of control and mastery of life results in anxiety

TRAUMATIC LIFE EVENT(S)
Actual threats (e.g., war, rape)
Loss (e.g., death of mother)
Change (e.g., job)

SOCIOCULTURAL
Societal acceptance (e.g., female demonstration of emotional responses)

CRH, Corticotropin-releasing hormone.

---

ages 18 to 54 years, 16.4%; and ages 55 years and older, 11.4%.

Women have anxiety disorders twice as frequently as men. For example, twice as many women as men have panic disorder without agoraphobia, and three times as many women have panic disorder with agoraphobia. Patients with these disorders have a significant comorbidity rate with substance disorders and mood disorders.

Anxiety is one of the few mental disorders for which an animal model has been developed. Researchers can produce anxiety in animals by introducing stressors.

ASSESSMENT AND DIAGNOSTIC CRITERIA

As shown in *Diagnostic and Statistical Manual of Mental Disorders (DSM-IV-TR)* categories for anxiety disorders, the essential characteristics of these disorders are anxiety symptoms and avoidance behaviors (see box below; see also Appendix A). Anxiety disorders interrupt daily routine functions, as well as occupational and social functioning.

DSM-IV-TR Anxiety Disorders

Panic disorder with agoraphobia
Panic disorder without agoraphobia
Agoraphobia (without history of panic disorder)
Specific phobia
• Specify type
Social phobia
• Generalized
Obsessive-compulsive disorder
• With poor insight
Posttraumatic stress disorder
• Acute/chronic
• With delayed onset
Acute stress disorder
Generalized anxiety disorder
Anxiety disorder due to medical condition
Substance-induced anxiety disorder
Anxiety disorder not otherwise specified

Box 2-2   Symptoms of a Panic Attack

SOMATIC
Heart palpitations
Chest pain
Diaphoresis
Trembling
Difficulty breathing
Choking sensation
Nausea, vomiting
Other gastrointestinal disturbances
Hot flashes or chills
Numbness, tingling sensation
Dizziness, lightheadedness

PSYCHOLOGIC
Fear of losing control
Fear of "going crazy"
Fear of dying
Depersonalization
Derealization

Anxiety disorders take many forms and differ in some aspects, but the symptom of *excessive anxiety* is common to all types. When a person is unable to regulate anxiety, escalation of symptoms may reach the panic stage (see Table 2-1). The occurrence of panic at this level is referred to as a *panic attack,* which may emerge in any anxiety disorder or occur in other mental disorders. To be diagnosed with a panic attack, the person experiences sudden and extreme fear or discomfort in the absence of real danger or threat and has at least four of the symptoms in Box 2-2.

Panic Disorder

The defining characteristic of panic disorder is unexpected, recurrent panic attacks (see Box 2-2). In addition, the person continues to worry for at least 1 month after an attack about another attack occurring, worries about the consequences of an attack, or changes behaviors as a result of the attack (e.g., quits school or job, avoids a freeway). Another criterion for the diagnosis is that the attacks are not caused by a medical condition or the use of substances (toxins, medications, or drugs of abuse). Comorbidity between panic disorder and other mental disorders is common (major depression, substance disorders, other anxiety disorders).

Panic Disorder with Agoraphobia and Agoraphobia without History of Panic Disorder

Agoraphobia is commonly called "fear of the marketplace" but really means the unfounded fears that the "marketplace," or life itself, represents loss of safety or control. The defining characteristic is fear of being in places or situations from which exit might be difficult or embarrassing (e.g., diarrhea) or fear that no help will be available in case of incapacitating symptoms.

This disorder can severely restrict travel or necessitate a constant travel companion. Affected individuals frequently will not leave home because of their extreme discomfort while out of the house alone, in a crowd, or traveling. Most cases of agoraphobia appear to be related to panic disorder; when the latter is treated, agoraphobia usually improves. Avoidance behaviors can greatly interfere with daily functioning. Inability to leave the house to buy groceries, go to a job, or transport children to school can be severely incapacitating to individuals with agoraphobia.

Specific Phobia

The defining characteristic of specific phobia is strong, persistent fear and avoidance of a specific object or situation, such as an animal (dogs, snakes, insects), enclosed places, heights, or the sight of blood. The person usually acknowledges the intense anxiety that results from exposure to the object or situation as excessive and unreasonable, but the avoidance continues (Table 2-2).

Table 2-2	**Common Specific Phobia**
Feared Situation/Object	**Phobia Name**
Heights	Acrophobia
Water	Hydrophobia
Enclosed places	Claustrophobia
Leaving familiar place (home)	Agoraphobia
Animals	Zoophobia
Death	Thanatophobia
Darkness	Nyctophobia
Dirt	Mysophobia
Sex	Genophobia
Venereal disease	Cypridophobia
Being evaluated by others	Social phobia
Women	Gynophobia
Failure	Kakorrhaphiophobia
Homosexuals/homosexuality	Homophobia
Pain	Algophobia

Social Phobia

The defining characteristic of social phobia is strong, persistent fear that while in public and social situations, the individual will do something humiliating or embarrassing. Common examples are fear of choking while eating food with others, fear of saying something foolish in the company of others, and inability to urinate in public rest rooms. These people avoid social phobic situations and usually acknowledge the fear as irrational but seem helpless to eliminate it.

Obsessive-Compulsive Disorder

The defining characteristics of obsessive-compulsive disorder are recurrent thoughts, images, or impulses and behaviors that are extremely distressing to the individual or that interfere with normal functioning.

Obsessions are persistent, intrusive thoughts, ideas, images, or impulses that the person knows are irrational or senseless but that cause excessive anxiety. The most common obsessions are thoughts of *violence* (killing a loved one), *contamination* (touching doorknobs), *orderliness* (continually rearranging closet or desk), *doubt* (worrying about having done something wrong), and *sexual imagery*.

Compulsions are repetitive intentional behaviors performed in a stereotypically routine way or repetitive mental activities (e.g., praying). The act may be carried out in direct response to an obsession as an attempt to suppress or neutralize it. Tension and anxiety are relieved by the act. The most common compulsions are hand washing, counting, checking, and touching.

Obsessions and compulsions can be extremely incapacitating. Individuals may develop complex, involved patterns of ritualistic behavior that interfere with normal living. For example, a multistep morning ritual must be completed before leaving the house, but it takes the entire day to perform and prevents the person from going to work.

Affected individuals usually recognize that the obsessions and compulsions are unreasonable and excessive, but they persist incessantly. More than half of these persons experience acute onset, usually following a stressful event, and depressive symptoms may occur. Suicide is a risk in this disorder because of the relentless and often exhausting symptoms.

Posttraumatic Stress Disorder

The defining characteristic of posttraumatic stress disorder is development of anxiety symptoms following an excessively distressing life event that is experienced with terror, fear, and helplessness. The event is serious, such as seeing a child killed, or involvement in a major earthquake, fire, plane crash, war, rape, or abuse. Symptoms include the following:

- Reexperiencing the traumatic event (recurrent recollections, flashbacks, dreams of the event, or intense distress with events that resemble or represent the event)
- Avoidance of stimuli, thoughts, or feelings associated with trauma (inability to recall aspects of the event, refusal to go to places that are reminders of the event)
- Restricted responsiveness (general numbing, decreased affect, diminished interest, withdrawal from others)

Posttraumatic stress disorder may occur directly after the event or may not be diagnosed until several months or even years later.

Acute Stress Disorder

Symptoms for an acute stress disorder diagnosis are similar to those for posttraumatic stress disorder but develop within the first month after the individual experiences an extremely threatening event or situation. In addition, dissociative symptoms occur in the form of emotional detachment, dazed appearance, depersonalization, derealization, or amnesia in which the person cannot recall parts of the traumatic incident. If symptoms extend past 1 month, the diagnosis of posttraumatic stress disorder is considered.

Generalized Anxiety Disorder

The defining characteristic of generalized anxiety disorder is persistent, chronic (6 months or longer), excessive, unrealistic worry and anxiety over two or more circumstances or situations in the individual's life. For example, a man who makes a generous salary may be anxious and unnecessarily worried about paying his bills each month and worries that his daughter, who consistently achieves high grades, is going to fail college.

Individuals with generalized anxiety disorder are likely to be anxious about things in general. Symptoms of anxiety include the following:

- Apprehensive expectation (worry or fear that something awful will happen)
- Motor tension (restless, tense, sore muscles, easily fatigued)

- Autonomic hyperactivity (shortness of breath, heart palpitations, dizziness, diaphoresis, nausea, frequent urination)
- Vigilance and scanning (feeling on edge, easily startled, irritable, trouble falling asleep, continually looking for something negative to happen)

Somatoform Disorders

The defining characteristics of somatoform disorders are (1) physical symptoms with no evident organic or physiologic findings and (2) concrete or presumptive evidence that symptoms are psychologic in origin and not consciously intentional. The box below lists *DSM-IV-TR* categories for somatoform disorders. Etiology varies.

Somatization disorder

The defining characteristics of somatization disorder is persistent recurrence of multiple physical complaints of many years' duration with no apparent physical explanation. Presentation of symptoms is frequently exaggerated, dramatic, vague, and very involved. The symptom list is extensive and involves various systems. For example, a client consistently describes a stabbing pain that occurs when she swallows, but all examinations are negative.

Conversion disorder

The defining characteristic of conversion disorder is loss or alteration of voluntary motor or sensory function *not* due to pathophysiology (see Appendix A). The symptom usually appears suddenly, at or near the time of a severe conflict or psychosocial stressor (e.g., a soldier poised to shoot the enemy suddenly experiences paralysis of his arm; a child listening to her parents fighting aggressively is suddenly unable to hear).

Symptoms are not feigned and are not intentionally produced. The person may show an apparent lack of concern about the seriousness of the problem *(la belle indifférence)*.

DSM-IV-TR **Somatoform Disorders**

Somatization disorder
Undifferentiated somatoform disorder
Conversion disorder
Pain disorder
- Psychologic factors
- Psychologic factors and medical condition
- Acute/chronic
Hypochondriasis
- With poor insight
Body dysmorphic disorder
Somatoform disorder not otherwise specified

Pain disorder

The defining characteristic of pain disorder is preoccupation with pain that cannot be accounted for through diagnostic evaluation. If there is related organic pathology, the complaints or dysfunctions are grossly excessive. Psychologic factors influence pain onset, maintenance, severity, and recurrence. The person's pain is not feigned.

Hypochondriasis

The defining characteristic of hypochondriasis disorder is preoccupation with a belief or fear that the individual has or will have a serious illness or disease, when no actual physical problem exists. The belief is based on the patient's interpretations of physical signs and sensations as abnormal. It may involve one or a variety of body parts or functions. These individuals usually seek several physicians (go "doctor shopping") in an attempt to gain agreement about the existence of the problem. For example, a woman believes she has bowel cancer and goes from doctor to doctor to substantiate her belief, which is not supported by medical and examination results.

Body dysmorphic disorder

The defining feature of body dysmorphic disorder is preoccupation by a normal-appearing person with imagined bodily flaws or defects or excessive concern over actual minor defects. For example, a woman may constantly look at her face in the mirror and complain of its asymmetry, although it appears normal to all other observers. Anxiety is always present, and the person may avoid social or occupational situations as a result.

Factitious Disorders

The defining characteristics of factitious disorders are intentionally produced symptoms of a psychologic or physical nature that the individual feigns for the purpose of assuming the "sick role." This occurs in the absence of external motivation (e.g., trying to collect disability insurance). The person's behavior is voluntary but presumed to be out of his or her control. For example, a hospital laboratory technician repeatedly injected himself with low doses of contaminated normal saline, became ill, and had to be hospitalized. He received much attention from coworkers and family for his "unusual fevers."

Factitious disorders should not be confused with *malingering,* in which the person fakes symptoms but does so to control the environment, situation, or circumstance. Behavior is voluntary and fully within the control of an individual. For example, a client about to be transferred from the psychiatric unit of a hospital to the less favorable surroundings of a jail suddenly and intentionally develops an acute exacerbation of a gastrointestinal disorder.

Dissociative Disorders

The defining characteristics of dissociative disorders are disturbance of consciousness, memory, or identity.

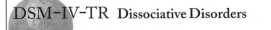

DSM-IV-TR Dissociative Disorders

Dissociative amnesia
Dissociative fugue
Dissociative identity disorder
Depersonalization disorder
Dissociative disorder not otherwise specified

Onset may be sudden or gradual, and the alteration may be transient or chronic. The box above lists *DSM-IV-TR* diagnostic categories for dissociative disorders.

Dissociative identity disorder

Formerly named "multiple personality disorder," the dissociative identity disorder diagnosis reflects the lack of integration of an individual's consciousness, memory, and identity. The defining characteristic is two or more separate and distinct personalities within one individual, with transition from one personality to another (several personalities may exist together). Each personality separately takes full control over the person's behavior. Transitions are usually sudden and occur around psychosocial stressors or conflicts, and the person may or may not have knowledge of all or some of the other personality(ies). Most cases are preceded by physical or sexual abuse or other severe trauma. Dissociative identity disorder is no longer thought to be as rare as it once was.

Dissociative fugue

The defining characteristic of dissociative fugue is that the individual suddenly and unexpectedly leaves the usual home or workplace, travels a distance, assumes a new identity, and is unable to recall all or part of the previous identity. When the person recovers, he or she has no recollection of events leading to the fugue. The disturbance usually occurs at times of severe psychosocial stress and is usually brief, although the fugue may last several months.

Dissociative amnesia

The defining characteristic of dissociative amnesia is the sudden inability to recall information that exceeds mere forgetfulness. Types of amnesia include the following:

1. *Circumscribed amnesia* or *localized amnesia,* the most common form, is the inability to recall events surrounding a specific traumatic or distressful event. For example, the survivor of a house fire cannot remember any of the details until several months later.
2. *Selected amnesia* is the inability to recall parts of a specific event. For example, the survivor remembers calling family and friends about the fire but cannot recall any content of the conversation.

3. *Generalized amnesia* is the complete inability to recall an entire life.
4. *Continuous amnesia* is the inability to recall events from a specific time to the present.

Depersonalization disorder

The defining characteristic of depersonalization disorder is depersonalization that is recurrent or persistent. Symptoms include the sense that one's reality is changed or lost and feelings of detachment from oneself as if "robotlike" or viewing oneself from the outside or in a dream. Reality testing remains intact.

INTERVENTIONS

Therapeutic interventions for anxiety and related disorders focus on counseling, psychotherapy, pharmacotherapy, or some combination of the three. People with anxiety disorders may often avoid seeking treatment because of avoidance aspects of their disorders and their awareness that symptoms are irrational. As a result, clients and families may tolerate the dysfunction, suffering the consequences of the debilitating symptoms and often leading constricted lives. Some clients may frequent the offices of medical physicians seeking diagnoses that have no definable physical cause. When incorrectly diagnosed, clients may spend years in unnecessary treatment, have multiple surgeries, or finally seek unorthodox or even fraudulent cures.

Clients in chronic states of distress from anxiety disorders may also acquire subsequent mental disorders, including major depression, additional anxiety disorders, and substance dependence. When diagnosed correctly, the client can often obtain relief. Appropriate interventions for anxiety symptoms and syndromes are often available and invaluable.

Treatment Settings

Anxiety and related disorders are usually treated in outpatient settings, such as clinics, offices of physicians and licensed therapists, and the client's home. Institutionalization becomes necessary if the client develops complications such as severe depression or suicidal ideation, or if the client requires further intensive assessment and testing to determine exact diagnoses or treatment. When complications of substance abuse become a problem as a result of attempts at self-medication, the client may need to enter a substance-oriented treatment program.

Medications

Medications are often warranted when symptoms are acute. When anxiolytic medications are used, careful monitoring of dose and frequency is necessary because of the risk for substance dependence (see box on p. 32).

Drug treatment is warranted when the severity and duration of anxiety symptoms interfere with a client's daily functions. A combination of pharmacologic and nonpharmacologic approaches is more successful than either therapy alone, and the placebo response is significant, approximately 50%.

The major classes of drugs used to treat anxiety (anxiolytics) are the benzodiazepines, the drug buspirone (BuSpar), and antidepressants. Beta-blockers may be useful as augmentation therapy.

BENZODIAZEPINES

Therapeutic effects with the benzodiazepines, such as alprazolam (Xanax) and lorazepam (Ativan), are usually seen within the first week, with response greater than 70%. Benzodiazepines have anxiolytic properties and are effective in panic disorders. Adverse effects include sedation, drowsiness, and respiratory depression. Alcohol intensifies the central nervous system (CNS) depressant effects. Patients usually develop tolerance to the drug, and higher doses are needed over time to achieve the same relief. Withdrawal may occur even after short-term therapy (4 to 6 weeks). Withdrawal occurs within 24 hours after discontinuation of short-acting agents (mentioned above) and within 3 to 8 days after long-acting agents such as diazepam (Valium). It is therefore necessary to taper the doses, typically decreasing the dose 15% to 25% every 7 to 14 days.

BUSPIRONE

Therapeutic effects with buspirone (BuSpar) therapy are usually seen within 2 to 4 weeks. Buspirone is an agent of choice for patients with a history of substance abuse or with sleep apnea. The initial dose is 7.5 mg twice a day, titrated to 30 mg twice a day. Buspirone has anxiolytic properties but is not effective for panic attacks.

ANTIDEPRESSANTS

Selective serotonin reuptake inhibitors (SSRIs) have anxiolytic properties and are effective in panic disorders. *Venlafaxine (Effexor)* has received U.S. Food and Drug Administration (FDA) approval for the treatment of generalized anxiety disorder. *Tricyclic antidepressants* are effective anxiolytics and useful in panic disorders. Both SSRIs and tricyclic antidepressants may be useful in treating obsessive-compulsive disorder. These drugs are nonaddictive, but side effects include anticholinergic effects and cardiotoxicity. SSRIs generally have fewer side effects and drug interactions than tricyclics.

Therapies

Cognitive-behavioral therapy

Combined cognitive-behavioral therapy has proven to be effective in treating clients with anxiety disorders. This type of therapy is a focused, specific, time-limited approach to cope with anxiety symptoms. Clients are assisted to directly change their thinking and behaviors, which results in altered responses. Cognitive-behavioral therapy has been more successful than long-term insight-oriented therapies, such as psychodynamic or interpersonal models, when treating anxiety disorders. (see Appendix B).

Family therapy

Family therapy is used to reassure and support the family, help reduce environmental stressors, and educate family members about symptoms, interventions, and expected outcomes (see Appendix B).

PROGNOSIS AND DISCHARGE CRITERIA

With early intervention, prognosis is good for most clients with anxiety and related disorders. The avoidance nature of some anxiety disorders may forestall treatment, and the longer a client avoids seeking help, the more fixed the patterns become. A client may refuse all interventions; for instance, clients with obsessive-compulsive disorder refuse to participate in treatment 20% to 25% of the time after being diagnosed. Some anxiety disorders carry a significant risk for suicide, including panic disorder with agoraphobia and severe obsessive-compulsive disorder.

As noted, the client is at risk for substance dependence when taking drugs that relieve anxiety, particularly anxiolytics, alcohol, and "designer" drugs. Self-medication is a common outcome of prolonged or severe anxiety. Substances that relieve anxiety are often readily available, and consequences of long-term use are not known or may be denied by the client who experiences immediate relief after intake. Therapists closely monitor use of these drugs during therapy and in follow-up contacts.

Discharge planning for clients with anxiety disorders and their families uses client goals as general guidelines, including the following:

- The client identifies situations and events that trigger anxiety and ways to prevent or manage them.
- Identifies anxiety symptoms and levels of anxiety.
- Discusses connection between anxiety-provoking situation or event and anxiety symptoms.
- Discusses relief behaviors openly.
- Identifies adaptive, positive techniques and strategies that relieve anxiety.
- Demonstrates behaviors that represent reduced anxiety symptoms.

- Utilizes learned anxiety-reducing strategies.
- Demonstrates ability to problem-solve, concentrate, and make decisions.
- Verbalizes feeling relaxed.
- Sleeps through the night.
- Utilizes appropriate supports from nursing and medical community, family, and friends.

- Acknowledges inevitability of occurrence of anxiety.
- Discusses ability to tolerate manageable levels of anxiety.
- Seeks help when anxiety is not manageable.
- Continues postdischarge anxiety management, including pharmacologic and nonpharmacologic therapy.

The box below provides guidelines for client and family teaching in the management of anxiety disorders.

CLIENT AND FAMILY TEACHING | **Anxiety and Related Disorders**

Nurse Needs to Know

- Anxiety is a universal experience and part of the human condition in both health and illness.
- Anxiety is transferrable from one human to another; therefore nurses need to manage and monitor their own anxiety levels and model the coping behaviors that the client and family are expected to employ.
- Mild forms of anxiety are necessary for people to be productive and creative.
- The more severe forms of anxiety can be maladaptive, causing dysfunctional symptoms and behaviors.
- The symptoms of anxiety may be physiologic, psychologic, cognitive, or behavioral in nature.
- Anxiety is demonstrated in a variety of disorders, such as generalized anxiety disorder, panic, phobias, and obsessive-compulsive disorder.
- Persons with other disorders, such as mood disorders or schizophrenia, can also experience anxiety.
- Recognizing early signs of anxiety and relief behaviors may prevent anxiety from escalating to a panic state.
- It is best to intervene when signs of anxiety first appear to prevent the client from losing control. Reducing stimulation is a useful early intervention.
- Several categories of medications are used to treat anxiety, such as benzodiazepines, buspirone (BuSpar), and antidepressants.
- Many nonpharmacologic techniques are available to manage anxiety, such as cognitive-behavioral, desensitization, deep breathing, relaxation, and guided imagery.
- Foods and beverages containing caffeine tend to exacerbate anxiety.
- Global or vague problems may be overwhelming for the client, and the nurse can help break them down into simple, solvable steps.
- Identify community and personal resources available for the client and family.
- Explore reliable Internet resources for the client and family.

Teach Client and Family

- Explain the diagnosis and obtain feeback to ensure that the client/family understand.
- Teach the client/family to identify stressors and situations that promote or exacerbate anxiety and to avoid them as much as possible.
- Educate the client/family about medications (therapeutic dose, frequency of administration, side effects, untoward effects) and the importance of compliance.
- Help the client/family recognize early symptoms of anxiety to prevent it from escalating (e.g., sweaty palms, racing heart, difficulty concentrating or attending).
- Teach the client/family simple anxiety reduction strategies (e.g., deep-breathing exercises, progressive relaxation) to help prevent escalation of symptoms (see Appendix B).
- Instruct the client to avoid foods and beverages containing caffeine to prevent exacerbation of anxiety symptoms.
- Educate the client/family about phobias and how to reduce urealistic fears; avoid confronting the client with the feared object or situation.
- Explain the technique of *desensitization*, if the physician or therapist has recommended this type of therapeutic intervention to manage phobic behaviors.
- Help the client/family manage the rituals of obsessive-compulsive behaviors; allow the client a set amount of time to perform rituals versus demanding that the client stop.
- Teach the client/family to seek help from available resources when anxious behaviors or medications cannot be managed (e.g., physician, nurse, therapist).
- Teach the client/family how to access community resources and support groups.
- Teach the client/family how to access reliable educational sources on the Internet.

Care Plans

- Anxiety (All Types)
- Phobia
- Obsessive-Compulsive Disorder
- Posttraumatic Stress Disorder/Acute Stress Disorder
- Somatoform Disorder
- Dissociative Disorders

Care Plan
DSM-IV-TR Diagnosis | **Anxiety (All Types)**

NANDA Diagnosis: Anxiety

A vague, uneasy feeling of discomfort or dread, accompanied by an automatic response (the source often nonspecific or unknown to the individual); a feeling of apprehension caused by anticipation of danger. Anxiety is an alerting signal that warns of impending danger and enables the individual to take measures to deal with the threat.

Focus:

For the client who experiences mild, moderate, severe, or panic levels of anxiety that may impede growth potential or exceed the person's ability to cope in a functional manner.

RELATED FACTORS (ETIOLOGY)

Biologic/psychosocial/environmental factors
Threat to biologic, psychologic, and social integrity (illness, injury, actual or perceived loss)
Ineffective use of coping mechanisms/resources
Depletion of coping strategies
Level of stress that exceeds coping abilities
Hopelessness
Powerlessness
Unmet needs/expectations that may be unrealistic or unattainable
Response to long-term illness/hospitalization
Threat to self-esteem
Pain

DEFINING CHARACTERISTICS

Subjective (see Table 2-1)

The client verbalizes the following:
Trouble breathing
Increased muscle tension
Frequent sensation of tingling in hands and feet
Continuous feeling of apprehension
Preoccupation with a sense of impending doom
Inability to identify source/stimulus responsible for emotional/feeling state
Difficulty falling asleep
Concerns about change in health status and outcome of illness/hospitalization
Difficulty concentrating on the task at hand
Gastrointestinal disturbances (decreased appetite, nausea, vomiting, diarrhea, dry mouth)
Urinary symptoms (urgency, frequency, hesitancy)
Narrowed range of perceptions (sight, hearing, pain)
Selective inattention (removal of threatening stimuli from conscious awareness)
Selective enhancement (concentrates on one or few details)
Distortion of environment (objects seem out of proportion to reality)
Need for increased space:
- "Everything is closing in on me."
- "I need to get out of here; I feel trapped."
- "This room is like a closet."
Dissociation (feelings of numbness, separateness, or distancing from the environment)

Objective (see Table 2-1)

The client demonstrates the following:
Psychomotor agitation (fidgeting, jitters, restlessness, shaking leg or foot, pacing back and forth)
Tightened, wrinkled brow
Strained (worried) facial expression
Hypervigilance (scans environment)
Startle response
Distractibility
Fragmented sleep patterns

Continued

Sweaty palms
Diaphoresis
Hyperreflexia
Tachypnea
Tachycardia
Regressive behaviors (crying, biting, curled up in fetal
    position)
Voice change to loud, high pitch
Rapid speech (may be unintelligible)
Inability to move (frozen to spot) or attempts to flee from
    immediate area
Wringing of hands
Decreased cognitive skills (insight, judgment, problem
    solving)
Maladaptive use of ego defense mechanisms (projection,
    displacement, denial)
Avoidance behaviors (withdraws from milieu)
Relief behaviors (pacing, wringing of hands)

OUTCOME IDENTIFICATION AND EVALUATION

Client expresses feeling calm and relaxed, with no muscle
    tension or breathing problems.
Demonstrates significant decrease in physiologic,
    cognitive, behavioral, and emotional symptoms of
    anxiety.

Describes early warning signs of anxiety (increased
    irritability, gastrointestinal upset, increased heart rate).
Identifies levels of anxiety (mild, moderate, severe,
    panic).
Effectively employs learned relaxation techniques.
Identifies anxiety-producing situations when possible.
Utilizes functional coping strategies to assuage anxiety.
Demonstrates decreased use of dysfunctional coping
    mechanisms.
Demonstrates absence of avoidance behaviors (withdrawal
    from milieu, lack of contact with others).
Demonstrates absence of relief behaviors (pacing, wringing
    of hands).
Exhibits ability to make decisions and problem-solve.
Expresses hopeful, positive plans for the future.
Verbalizes control over illness, outcome, and management
    of care.
Seeks support from family, friends, and therapists when
    necessary.
Complies with treatment and medication regimen as
    needed.
Conveys understanding of need to live with mild levels of
    anxiety.
States importance of refraining from caffeine, nicotine, and
    other CNS stimulants.

PLANNING AND IMPLEMENTATION

Nursing Intervention	Rationale
Recognize the client's use of relief behaviors (pacing, wringing of hands) as indicators of anxiety.	Early recognition of anxiety is critical to prevent escalation of symptoms and loss of control.
Observe avoidance behaviors (withdrawal from the milieu).	Withdrawal indicates that the milieu is stress producing to a degree that exceeds the client's ability to cope.
Assess own level of anxiety, and make conscious effort to remain calm.	Anxiety is contagious and easily transferred from person to person.
Approach the client calmly, and help him or her to recognize the anxiety. • "Mr. Jones, I see you pacing back and forth. What are you feeling?"	Asking the client to describe the feeling helps the client to identify it as anxiety.
Client Unable to Describe Feeling as Anxiety	
Assist the client to label the anxiety. • "Mr. Jones, are you feeling anxious?"	Specific labeling helps the client to isolate anxiety as a feeling that the client can begin to understand and manage.
Client with Mild to Moderate Levels of Anxiety	
Assist the client in slow breathing exercises, using appropriate rate and depth; role-model as necessary.	Hyperventilation decreases carbon dioxide (CO_2) symptoms of anxiety. Actual physical symptoms result in addition to "feelings."
Help the client identify the event/situation that preceded the symptoms of anxiety.	The client is assisted to connect the feeling of anxiety with a stimulus or stressor that may have provoked it.

- "What happened just before you had these anxious feelings and began to pace the halls?"

Encourage the client to determine the level of anxiety according to the client's perception (see Table 2-1).

The client's knowledge of his or her typical responses to anxiety-producing stimuli assists the client to begin to manage them.

Inform the client that pacing releases the tension caused by anxiety and that pacing usually represents relief behaviors.

The client is calmed by the knowledge that relief behaviors reduce anxiety and that the nurse understands and does not criticize or ridicule the behaviors.

Walk with the client while you both discuss the anxiety.

The physical exercise of walking tends to reduce the tension associated with anxiety. A low-key discussion may calm the client by allowing ventilation. Remaining with the client is critical because persons who are anxious feel out of control, and the presence of a confident, therapeutic nurse offers control and safety.

Help the client associate feelings of anxiety with possible unmet needs or expectations that may represent a threat to the self-system.
- "So you're saying you expected to be discharged by 5 o'clock, and now it's 7 o'clock, and you're feeling anxious."

The client's knowledge that unmet needs and expectations can precipitate anxiety may also bring relief.

Help the client recognize that desired outcomes may differ from actual outcomes, especially if the client does not consider all the facts.
- "I know you hoped to be discharged by 5 o'clock, but the exact time of your discharge has not been established yet."

The client's understanding that expectations may not always be fulfilled, and that unmet expectations may be caused by a misperception rather than punitive action, may decrease the anxiety that often stems from anger, frustration, low self-esteem, and unmet needs.

Suggest to the client alternate steps that may achieve desired outcomes (if feasible).
- "Let's telephone your doctor to find out if you can get a tentative discharge time."

Helping the client to meet needs when possible builds trust, acknowledges the client's worth, and reduces anxiety.

Assist the client to accept delayed need gratification while acknowledging the client's anxiety.
- "I realize you are anxious about not going home when you planned, but it may be a few more days before you will be ready for discharge."

Offering the client factual information while recognizing feelings helps to promote trust and decreases the anxiety that generally accompanies uncertainty and disappointment.

Discuss with the client activities that may be initiated to help ease the tension until desired outcomes can be achieved.
- "What kinds of activities will best help you pass the time until your doctor can give you a firm discharge date?"

Demonstrating that staff members are willing to help ease the client's disappointment by problem solving with the client is in itself anxiety reducing. Engaging in meaningful activities will redirect anxiety-producing energy and occupy the client so that less time will be spent on concerns about discharge.

Help the client bear the burden of anxiety that stems from unmet needs by pointing out alternative outcomes that can be realistically achieved.
- "It's difficult for you to accept the fact that you will be living in a residential treatment center instead of your parents' home, but you can visit your parents every week as planned."

Softening disappointing facts with some positive information offers the client hope and decreases the impact of anxiety.

Client with Escalating Anxiety or Sudden, Severe to Panic Levels of Anxiety

Accompany the client to a smaller, quieter area away from others, using direct, gentle reassurance.

A quiet unstimulating environment with only the client and a reassuring nurse helps the client gain control over anxiety that threatens to be overwhelming.

Continued

PLANNING AND IMPLEMENTATION—cont'd

Nursing Intervention	Rationale
Client with Escalating Anxiety or Sudden, Severe to Panic Levels of Anxiety—cont'd	
• "I'll go with you to a quieter place where we can talk if you like."	
Remain with the client, continuing with a calm approach.	Persons who demonstrate high levels of anxiety tend to experience feelings of fright, dread, awe, or terror. The nurse's calm presence offers safety, support, and control at a time when the client's self-system is threatened and coping mechanisms are depleted. A client who is left alone during such times may experience serious physical or psychologic complications.
Reduce all environmental stimulation (noise from radio or television, bright lights, people moving and talking).	Increased stimulation tends to increase anxiety; decreased stimulation tends to decrease anxiety.
Consider administration of prescribed anxiolytic or other appropriate medication as needed.	Medication may be the most therapeutic and least restrictive measure to decrease severe or panic levels of anxiety.
Consider seclusion/restraint for clients who may be a danger to self or others as a result of high anxiety.	Seclusion/restraint may be the method of choice for the client's and others' immediate safety if all other interventions fail. The client may agree that seclusion is an appropriate intervention before anxiety escalates to a point at which it is a safety threat. Medication may also be used as part of the client's treatment plan (see section on pharmacotherapy).
Client Able to Focus and Discuss Anxiety Experience and Problem-Solve Strategies to Prevent or Reduce Anxiety	
Actively listen to and accept the client's concerns regarding subjective feelings of anxiety and the threat they pose to that patient's self-system.	Active listening and unconditional acceptance of the client's experience of anxiety convey respect, validate the client's self-worth, assure the client that concerns will be addressed, and provide an avenue for ventilation, all of which reduce anxiety.
Assist the client to build on previously successful coping methods to manage anxiety symptoms, illness, and treatment and to integrate them with newly learned strategies. • "What methods have helped you get through difficult times like this in the past?" • "How can we help you to use those methods now?" • "Let's discuss some new alternative strategies that may fit into your particular situation."	Use of previously successful coping methods in conjunction with newly learned techniques equips the client with multiple skills to manage anxiety.
Help the client identify support persons who can help him or her take care of personal/business details while he or she is hospitalized.	Significant supportive individuals can help to reduce the client's anxiety by reassuring the client that matters of concern will be attended to in a safe, reliable manner.
Inform the client frequently of status and progress made during hospitalization. • "You were able to sit calmly through most of the meeting today, Bob." • "You seldom interrupted during group this afternoon, Kate."	Clients who are well informed of their condition are better able to control illness, outcome, and treatment regimen, which tends to reduce anxiety generated from helplessness and loss of control.
Encourage the client to use coping mechanisms such as *suppression* and *displacement* when the client is unable to do so through more direct methods. **Suppression:** postponing anxiety-producing issues. • "It's perfectly OK to think about those things at a time when you feel less anxious."	When client is not ready to face troubling issues, use of adaptive coping mechanisms may successfully manage anxiety that cannot be averted through confronting techniques.

- "Let's talk about a less troubling topic for a while; we can discuss this subject later."

Displacement: converting anxiety to harmless activities.

- "Some exercise or activity may help you feel more relaxed."
- "Perhaps a game of Ping-Pong will help expend your energy."

Instruct the client in the following anxiety-reducing strategies. Individualize according to the client's preference and ability.

- *Progressive relaxation:* tense and relax all muscles progressively from toes to head (see Appendix B).

  Progressive relaxation relieves stress-related muscular tension and reduces the physiologic effects of anxiety.

- *Slow, deep-breathing exercises:* practice slow, rhythmic, controlled breathing (see Appendix B).

  Breathing exercises slow the heart rate by supplying oxygen to the heart and lungs, which relaxes and distracts the client, thus decreasing feelings of anxiety.

- Focusing on a single object or person in the room.

  Focusing helps the client to disengage from all other visual stimuli and promotes control and relaxation.

- Listening to soothing music or relaxation tapes (client may prefer to close eyes).

  Soothing music or tapes reduce anxiety by providing relaxing effects and an overall tranquil environment.

- *Visual imagery:* visualization of an image that evokes a soothing, peaceful sensation (ocean, waterfall, field of flowers).*

  Visual imagery provides the client with a mental representation that inhibits anxiety and invokes an opposing, peaceful image.

Provide simple clarification of environmental events or stimuli that are not related to the client's illness and management of care but that may still elicit anxiety.

- "The nurse is preparing medication for another client."
- "That client is concerned because visitors are late."
- "Staff are not upset with you; they're busy giving a report."

Clarification of events or stimuli that are unrelated to the client helps the client to disengage from external anxiety-provoking situations, which decreases apprehension and anxiety.

Teach the client to distinguish between anxiety that can be connected to identifiable objects or sources (illness, prognosis, hospitalization) and anxiety for which there is no immediate identifiable object or source.

- "The shortness of breath you're experiencing is not unusual during times of anxiety."
- "Frequently it is difficult to determine exact causes of anxious symptoms."
- "It's OK to feel upset when people you expect don't visit you."
- "It's understandable to feel anxious about being in a hospital with people you hardly know."

A client who is informed and reassured about expected symptoms of anxiety coming from a recognizable stressor is better able to control anxiety and maintain a realistic perspective of illness, prognosis, and hospitalization. Awareness that anxiety cannot always be traced to a specific source or object reduces the threat of anxiety and allows the client to concentrate on anxiety-reducing strategies.

Inform the client of the importance of abstaining from caffeine, nicotine, and other CNS stimulants.

Avoidance of stimulating substances helps reduce symptoms of anxiety.

Teach the client to tolerate mild levels of anxiety and to channel anxiety toward constructive behaviors and activities, such as arts and crafts, Ping-Pong, and other games and sports.

Anxiety is an integral part of human existence that can be accepted and tolerated in its mild to moderate states and may be used to motivate productive, satisfying behaviors.

Continue to support and monitor prescribed medical and psychosocial treatment plans.

Close observation and support help prevent anxiety from escalating to unmanageable levels.

Visual imagery employs the concept of reciprocal inhibition, a behavioral approach used for clients with phobic disorder who experience panic when exposed to a feared object or situation. With this method, anxiety-producing stimuli are paired with stimuli associated with an opposite feeling strong enough to diminish the anxiety. Other behavioral techniques, such as systematic desensitization, flooding, aversive methods, hypnosis, biofeedback, and yoga, are also used to treat anxiety and related disorders (see Appendix B).

Care Plan
DSM-IV-TR Diagnosis   **Phobia**

NANDA Diagnosis: Ineffective Coping
Inability to form a valid appraisal of the stressors; inadequate choices of practiced responses; inability to use available resources.

Focus:

For the client with a persistent, irrational, or excessive fear* of a specific object, situation, or event, which may induce a panic anxiety state when the client is exposed to such stimuli. The client may fear being harmed or out of control, and resultant avoidance behaviors often interfere with personal growth, adaptive coping, and social and occupational functioning.

RELATED FACTORS (ETIOLOGY)

Biologic/psychologic/environmental factors
Phobic response (see Table 2-1)
Fear of subsequent phobic response (anticipatory state)
Life-style of avoidant behaviors secondary to fear of phobic stimulus
Perceived threat of feared object, situation, or event
Powerlessness secondary to phobic disorder
Knowledge deficit regarding adaptive methods of coping
Depletion of adaptive coping mechanisms/strategies
Unidentified conflicts/stressors

DEFINING CHARACTERISTICS

Client persistently avoids other clients, eating in the dining room, and group activities or outings.
Continuously avoids public places such as shopping malls, movie theaters, restaurants, bathrooms, and open spaces.
Refuses to use elevators or to be enclosed in small areas.
Demonstrates increased anxiety or panic symptoms when exposed to specific feared object or situation (animals, heights, freeways, restaurants) (see Table 2-1).
Verbalizes dread of eating in public places for fear of uncontrolled episodes of choking, urination, defecation, or other embarrassing occurrences.
Expresses excessive fear of speaking in public or of giving a prepared speech.
Remains housebound for an excessive length of time (months or years).
States fear of being out of control when outside an enclosed building or house.

Repeatedly avoids driving on busy freeways, even when late for work or appointments.
Enlists family or friends to run errands such as grocery shopping and transporting children to school, appointments, and activities.
Verbalizes inability to meet the demands of everyday life.
- "I need my prescription, but I can't cope with the crowds in the drugstore."
- "My kids missed their bus, and I'm afraid to drive them to school."
- "I can't go to Jane's house; she has cats."
- "I can't accept that job; it means I'll have to use the elevator every day."
- "I won't go on the client outing; there are bugs and animals in the woods."
- "I can't attend group meetings; I could get germs or others will laugh at me."
- "I won't eat in the dining room; I might choke or wet my pants."
- "I'm afraid to go to sleep tonight; I might die."

OUTCOME IDENTIFICATION AND EVALUATION

Client verbalizes significant decrease in phobic response during progressive exposure to feared objects, events, and situations (decreased physiologic and emotional symptoms of severe to panic anxiety states).
Demonstrates significant reduction in avoidance behaviors when threatened with exposure to feared stimuli: remains in dining room despite fear of crowds and eating in public; remains in area with small pets; refrains from going to room during visiting hours or other peak times.
Tolerates feared objects, events, or situations commensurate with level of progress: attends outings; visits shoping malls; eats in the dining room or public restaurants; verbalizes in groups; confronts small animals.
Relates increase in understanding of phobic disorder and behaviors needed to manage phobic response.
Limits intake of caffeine, nicotine, and other CNS stimulants that produce physiologic symptoms of anxiety.
Participates actively in prescribed treatment plan and learned therapeutic strategies to reduce phobic responses: deep breathing, relaxation exercises, visual imagery, reframing, desensitization (see Appendix B).

Psychoanalytic theory differentiates fear from anxiety in that fear *emanates from a known source and* anxiety *evolves from an unknown, unresolved conflict.*

PLANNING AND IMPLEMENTATION

Nursing Intervention	Rationale
Environment	
Be aware of own level of anxiety (see Table 2-1). Use appropriate strategies (deep breathing, relaxation, cognitive techniques) to decrease anxiety to a tolerable level before approaching client (see Appendix B).	Anxiety is readily transferred from person to person.
Approach the client in a calm, direct, nonauthoritarian manner using a soft tone of voice.	A calm, direct approach helps the client gain control, decreases apprehension and anxiety, and fosters security. A nonauthoritarian manner decreases powerlessness.
To Establish Trust Early in Nurse-Client Relationship	
Listen actively to the client's fears and concerns, regardless of how irrational they may seem.	Active listening signifies unconditional respect and acceptance for the client as a worthwhile individual. Listening builds trust and rapport, guides the nurse toward problem areas, encourages the client to vent concerns without fear of ridicule or reproach, and sets the stage for management of phobic responses.
Acknowledge the client's feelings, concerns, and limitations in a simple, matter-of-fact manner. • "It sounds as if you're frustrated with your responses." • "It is difficult to avoid certain situations and objects." • "It's OK right now to do only those things you can handle."	Acknowledgment of the client's feelings and concerns regarding the limitations induced by the phobic disorder shows that the staff understands and will be supportive.
Refrain from exposing the client to the identified feared object or situation. • If the client adamantly refuses to attend an outing with the rest of the clients for fear of exposure to small animals, snakes, or bugs, it is best not to insist that the client comply at this time. • If the client is afraid to eat in the dining room with others, allow the client to eat in an uncrowded area.	Exposure to feared stimuli without adaptive coping strategies could escalate the client's anxiety to a panic state. Forced compliance increases powerlessness and loss of control and decreases the client's trust in the staff and treatment regimen.
Schedule an alternative, less threatening activity for the client (chess, checkers, occupational/recreational activities) while the group attends the outing.	Participation in milieu activities increases the client's confidence, self-esteem, and control.
Inform the client that the staff understands the client's refusal to attend the group outing is not caused by resistance to treatment but rather by the phobic disorder for which the client is seeking treatment.	Acknowledgment of the client's diagnosis minimizes a sense of failure and conveys hope.
Client Able to Discuss Phobic Responses without Experiencing Incapacitating Anxiety	
Assist the client to describe physiologic responses to identified feared objects, situations, or events (see Table 2-1).	Teaching the client to identify autonomic nervous system responses to anxiety in the early stages helps the client to acknowledge the feelings rather than deny or avoid them. This sets the stage for symptom management.
Assist the client in identifying factors that increase or decrease phobic responses. • Size of object (small or large bug or animal) • Texture of object (perceived "sliminess" of snake, furry or hairy bugs or animals) • Movement (wiggling worms, crawling spiders, flying bugs or birds)	Helping the client differentiate between most feared and least feared objects gives the client some control and decreases feelings of powerlessness. It also sets the stage for therapeutic strategies. • *Desensitization technique:* The client is exposed to feared objects, beginning with the most feared and ending with the least feared, until the client's anxiety symptoms are under control (see Appendix B).

Continued

PLANNING AND IMPLEMENTATION—cont'd

Nursing Intervention	Rationale
### Client Able to Discuss Phobic Responses without Experiencing Incapacitating Anxiety—cont'd	
Assist the client to determine other factors associated with feared stimuli that may precipitate a phobic response. • "What else bothers you about this situation?" • "You were able to eat with the group yesterday. What is different about today?"	The client's recognition that factors such as increased noise or fatigue may contribute to the client's vulnerability may encourage the client to modify those situations or elements that can be controlled.
Teach the client about the effects of caffeine, nicotine, and other CNS stimulants.	Caffeine and nicotine produce physiologic effects of anxiety (increased heart rate, jitteriness).
Explore with the client previously successful coping methods. • "What methods have helped you handle your reactions in the past?" • "How can we help you use those methods now?"	Use of previously successful coping strategies in conjunction with newly learned skills better prepares the client to deal with the anxiety of the phobic disorder and promotes more control over the feared situation, object, or event.
Discuss with the client why usual coping methods no longer seem to work. • Usual support systems, persons, or situations are no longer available. • New stressors have emerged. • The client can no longer avoid feared stimuli.	Identification of possible reasons why usual coping methods have failed is the first step toward helping the client manage the phobic response.
Help the client identify alternative adaptive coping techniques (relaxation exercises, deep breathing, visual imagery, cognitive techniques) to manage anxiety from excessive or irrational fears instead of using avoidance behaviors (see Appendix B).	The client may need help in activating adaptive coping strategies because energy and motivation are depleted in times of anxiety.
Practice with the client alternative adaptive coping strategies commensurate with the client's life-style and capabilities.	Role playing therapeutic techniques when in a calm state enables the client to activate such strategies more readily in times of anxiety.
### For the Client Who Is Able to Use Cognitive-Perceptual Skills	
Utilize relabeling or reframing techniques to change the client's perceptions of feared objects, situations, or events. *Client:* "I feel so nervous when I think about going into that crowded activity room." *Nurse:* "When you feel that way, relabel the word 'nervous' with a less-threatening word like 'excited' and note the change in symptoms."	Reframing or relabeling volatile words with less-threatening terms helps the client place thoughts and feelings in a different perspective and tends to decrease anxiety.
Teach the client to combine reframing techniques with another learned strategy when necessary. *Client:* "I feel so anxious and begin to breathe very fast whenever I go off the unit to a store or on a pass." *Nurse:* "When you get that feeling, relabel the word 'anxious' with 'overactive' and begin the deep-breathing exercises we practiced."	Combining a newly learned skill with a previously learned strategy provides the client with more than one technique to cope adaptively with anxiety because each strategy reinforces the other.
Teach the client thought substitution and behavioral substitution strategies. Refer to Appendix B for thought and behavioral substitution therapies. *Client:* "I'm afraid to go for a walk; a snake might crawl out of the bushes." *Nurse:* "When you think about snakes crawling out of the bushes, focus your thoughts on the bush, on the color of	Replacing the fearful thought or image with a pleasant one and performing concomitant relaxation techniques tends to diminish anxiety.

the foliage or flowers on the bush. Then, use our learned relaxation technique."

For the Client Who Has Successfully Practiced the Preceding Strategies

Assist the client to confront the feared object under safe conditions, if the client is willing and able. Refer to Appendix B for desensitization technique.
Client: "I'd like to go to Jane's party, but when I'm in her house I'm preoccupied with avoiding her cat and I can't enjoy myself."
Nurse: "It sounds like you're using a lot of energy with your concern about the cat. Would you be willing to locate the cat as soon as you enter Jane's house and perhaps even stroke it once?"

Confronting the feared object in a familiar setting diminishes the phobic responses and the anticipatory anxiety that precedes it.

Expose the client progressively to feared stimuli. Example for the client who fears dining with crowds: The nurse can initially dine alone with client, then one or two familiar persons may be added. Next, the client can progress to a secluded or quiet area of the dining room. Finally, the client can sit in a more populated area of the dining room with significant reduction in phobic responses.

Exposing the client to feared situations in a gradual manner helps lessen the anxiety-provoking impact.

For the Client Who Refuses to Go on Outings Because of a Fear of Small Animals

Go with the client on a short group outing where small animals will be seen and stay with the client throughout. Next, take the client on a longer outing, leaving him or her with familiar persons. Continue exposing the client to longer outings with more frequency until the client can tolerate exposure to small animals with a significant reduction in phobic responses. Refer to Appendix B for desensitization technique.

Clients who are gradually and serially exposed to anxiety-provoking situations (predetermined by the client's treatment planning team) and graded from least to most anxiety-provoking, are eventually desensitized to the feared stimulus.

Offer positive reinforcement whenever the client demonstrates a decrease in avoidance behaviors or an increase in socialization skills and other milieu activities.
- "It showed strength to stay in the dining room, John."
- "It was a sign of real progress to stroke the cat, Sara."
- "Attending the group outing was a fine effort, Sam."

Positive statements convey confidence and hope and reinforce the client's adaptive coping skills.

Care Plan
DSM-IV-TR Diagnosis **Obsessive-Compulsive Disorder**

NANDA Diagnosis: Impaired Social Interaction
Insufficient or excess quantity or ineffective quality of social exchange.

Focus:
For the client with *obsessions* (thoughts, images, impulses), involuntarily produced, persistent, and recurring, that invade consciousness and are generally perceived as intrusive, repetitive, senseless, and anxiety-producing AND *compulsions* (repetitive, seemingly purposeful actions or behaviors) per-

formed in a stereotypical, ritualistic fashion in an attempt to ignore, suppress, negate, or neutralize anxiety. Obsessive-compulsive behaviors occur together and inhibit the client's interpersonal social interactions and relationships.

RELATED FACTORS (ETIOLOGY)
Neurobiologic/psychologic/environmental factors
Overwhelming anxiety (exceeds ability to cope adaptively)

Continued

RELATED FACTORS (ETIOLOGY)—cont'd

Altered thought processes (intrusive and recurrent)

Inability to control thoughts, images, and impulses in a purposeful, voluntary manner

Repetitive, ritualistic behavior patterns that interfere with social interactions

Ambivalence, indecisiveness

Inflexible thought and behavior patterns

Guilt, shame, or doubt

Depletion of effective coping mechanisms/strategies

Knowledge deficit regarding adaptive measures to manage anxiety

Impaired judgment and insight

Perceptual-cognitive impairment

Unidentified early life conflicts/stressors

Unresolved/misdirected anger

Powerlessness

Decreased psychologic and physical energy/endurance secondary to obsessive-compulsive behavior

DEFINING CHARACTERISTICS

Client verbalizes irrational, recurrent thoughts of violence, contamination, or doubt.

- "I keep thinking and worrying that I'm going to kill my baby."
- "I can't even go into my best friend's bathroom; I'm afraid the toilet is contaminated."
- "After I stop driving, I constantly worry that I've caused an accident."

Expresses awareness that thoughts images impulses are alien to self-perception and self-concept.

- "I know my thoughts are foolish and absurd and have nothing to do with my life."

States inability to prevent intrusion of repetitive thoughts images impulses.

- "I can't stop these thoughts from occurring, and I can't stop them once they begin."

Demonstrates repetitive, stereotypical rituals (compulsive acts) in response to anxiety produced by the obsessions that may or may not be related to the obsessions: cleans room several times a day; checks doors and windows throughout the night; dresses and undresses many times during the day and evening; washes hands continuously until skin is red, cracked, or bleeding.

Repeats same story or belief automatically, generally related to doubt, violence, or contamination.

- "I know it's foolish, but I keep thinking I won't wake up tomorrow."
- "I continually think about death and dying."
- "I never go to the movies because the theater is full of germs."

Demonstrates difficulty completing routine activities of daily life. (Much of client's time is spent in compulsive ritualistic behaviors.)

Reports diminished satisfactory interpersonal relationships.

OUTCOME IDENTIFICATION AND EVALUATION

Client verbalizes understanding that thoughts impulses images are involuntary and may worsen with stress.

Expresses understanding that involuntary, automatic obsessions may be related to biochemical factors and repressed conflicts.

Relates knowledge that ritualistic behaviors may be an attempt to decrease the anxiety produced by the obsessions.

Verbalizes awareness that early conflicts may remain repressed, but obsessions and compulsions can be reduced or eliminated by more adaptive management of anxiety and stress.

Participates actively in learned therapeutic strategies to manage anxiety and decrease obsessive-compulsive behaviors.

States significant reduction in obsessive thoughts images impulses.

Verbalizes reduction of intrusive, involuntary thoughts.

Demonstrates significant reduction in compulsive ritualistic acts and behaviors (pacing, cleaning, checking, hand washing).

Demonstrates absence of suicidal ideation, gestures, or attempts.

Verbalizes significant increase in control over involuntary thoughts and repetitive behaviors.

Uses majority of time to complete basic tasks and activities of daily life (nutrition, hygiene, grooming, socialization, occupation).

Participates in milieu activities without being interrupted by compulsive acts and rituals.

Continues to participate in planned psychosocial and medical treatment regimens.

PLANNING AND IMPLEMENTATION

Nursing Intervention	Rationale
Be aware of own level of anxiety (see Table 2-1). Use appropriate strategies (deep breathing, relaxation exercises, cognitive techniques) to decrease anxiety to a tolerable level before approaching the client (see Appendix B).	Anxiety is readily transferred from person to person.

Approach the client in a calm, direct, nonauthoritarian manner, using a soft tone of voice.	A calm, direct approach decreases anxiety and allows the client to regain some control. A nonauthoritarian manner decreases powerlessness and agitation. These clients are generally proud and knowledgeable, and an autocratic approach may be demeaning.
Actively listen to the client's obsessive themes no matter how absurd or incongruent they seem, without focusing too intently on the rituals.	Active listening signifies respect for the client as a worthwhile person and helps the nurse elicit the client's feelings and intent (violence, guilt, powerlessness, ambivalence) to individualize care. The less focus placed on the rituals, the less anxiety will occur, with a possible decreased need for the compulsive act.
Acknowledge the effects that automatic thoughts and ritualistic acts have on the client by demonstrating empathy rather than disapproval.	

Therapeutic Responses

• "I know these thoughts and behaviors are troubling; our staff notices that they are difficult to control." • "I saw you undress several times today; that must be tiring for you." • "I realize that thoughts of death are very troubling. The staff will be available when you want to talk about it."	Reflecting the client's feelings in an empathetic manner reduces the intensity of the ritualistic behavior and promotes trust and rapport, which encourages compliance with the treatment plan.

Nontherapeutic Responses

"I know these thoughts and behaviors are annoying. They bother me, too." "Try to dress only once a day, and you won't be so tired."	Implying that the client's behaviors are annoying or bothersome to others gives the client a sense of disapproval by staff that may inhibit trust and rapport, increase anxiety, and promote dysfunctional behaviors. The client may become more resistant to the treatment plan.
Assist the client to gain control of overwhelming feelings and impulses through verbal interactions. • "You seem upset about going to the activity; let's walk together, and you can tell me what's troubling you" (nurse to client who is pacing the hall and wringing hands with a worried facial expression just before an activity).	Anxiety is relieved by expressing thoughts and feelings, being understood by another person, and actively walking and talking. The client therefore feels more in control. Concern of staff builds trust and rapport.

Client Who May Be Danger to Self or Others

Assess the client for suicidal or self-destructive thoughts or impulses regularly by directly asking the client if he or she is feeling suicidal and by observing self-destructive acts or gestures.	Clients with obsessive-compulsive disorder may be at risk for suicide as a result of depressive or destructive obsessive thoughts.
Protect the client who is at risk for suicide or self-destructive acts using the suicide precautions practiced at individual facilities.	Initiating suicidal precautions when necessary helps prevent harm, injury, or death to the client.
Assess the client for homicidal ideation or impulses.	Clients with obsessive-compulsive disorder may experience violent thoughts toward others.
Protect others in the environment from the client who is potentially violent.	Protecting other clients when warranted helps prevent harm, injury, or death to others.
Protect the client as much as possible from the curiosity of other clients or visitors.	The client may feel embarrassed or undignified if others seem offended or amused by the compulsive acts. All clients deserve as much privacy as possible when their behavior is out of control.

Continued

PLANNING AND IMPLEMENTATION—cont'd

Nursing Intervention	Rationale
### Client with Ritualistic Hand-Washing Behaviors That Threaten Skin Integrity and Quality of Life	
Interact verbally with the client to encourage protection of skin until rituals can be better managed through learned strategies. • "I noticed that your hands are becoming raw from too many hand washings. There are several things you can do to protect them. Apply petroleum jelly to your hands before washing them; apply hand lotion to your hands after washing them; begin to wash your hands once every 15 minutes instead of once every 5 minutes; begin to wash your hands for 10 seconds instead of 30 seconds. Staff will remind you."	Verbal interventions help protect the client from pain or damage to skin integrity while giving the client the opportunity to reduce ritualistic behaviors. The nurse can also assess the client's ability to use problem-solving methods to control the compulsive acts, which can be used as a guide in treatment planning.
### Client Whose Excessive Rituals Promote Activity Intolerance	
Assist the client in planning rest periods between planned activities and rituals. Rest periods may become progressively longer as the client learns strategies that reduce anxiety and decrease ritualistic behaviors.	Rest periods help the client conserve energy and strength for leisure activities and activities of daily living (hygiene, grooming, socializing).
### Client Performing Ritualistic Act	
Allow the client to complete the ritualistic act initially, knowing that it comes from the anxiety produced by the troubling, automatic thoughts, images, or impulses (unless it poses a threat or danger to the client or others). Assess the client's ability to control the compulsive act, the level of intensity during the rituals, frequency and duration of the behaviors, and stage of the client's involvement in the treatment regimen. • Is the client newly admitted? • Has trust been established? • Which strategies have been taught, if any? • Is medication also needed to decrease anxiety?	The client may not yet possess adaptive means to reduce anxiety because obsessions are initially beyond the client's control. Anxiety may escalate to a panic state if rituals are abruptly interrupted. The level of the client's progress is a critical factor in determining and structuring psychosocial interventions. A client who is forced to control compulsive acts when anxiety exceeds the client's ability to focus on strategies, or a client who has not yet mastered strategies, may fail and become discouraged.
### Client with Whom Trust Has Been Established	
Work with the client to arrange the schedule to satisfy both the client's and the facility's routines. • "You have been missing breakfast every morning because it takes an hour to clean your room and get dressed. What do you think about getting up at 6 o'clock instead of 7 o'clock so you can make it to breakfast?"	Setting up directives for the client in a collaborative manner provides the structure and relief the client needs when impulses and functions are out of control. A nonauthoritarian approach preserves the client's dignity. Obsessive-compulsive clients are generally proud, knowledgeable, overly perfectionistic individuals who may feel anger, shame, or guilt if they are reprimanded.
### Client Ready and Able to Focus on Strategies	
Suggest activities that will reduce stress or anxiety (warm bath, listening to music, taking walk, performing simple exercises). Assist the client to learn stress reduction strategies, including deep breathing, relaxation exercises, visual imagery, cognitive techniques, and behavior modification (see Appendix B).	Simple, familiar activities can have a calming effect on the client and also interrupt obsessive themes and ritualistic behaviors. Stress management strategies reduce and channel anxiety in an adaptive, functional manner and interrupt automatic thoughts and substitute for ritualistic acts.

Engage the client in constructive activities when able, such as quiet games (chess, checkers, dominoes) and arts/crafts (needlepoint, ceramics, painting, leatherwork).	Planned activities offer the client less time for obsessive thoughts and compulsive behaviors and help the client focus on adaptive and creative endeavors that offer positive feedback.

Client Able to Tolerate Limit Setting

Help the client to schedule activities at least 1 hour apart to provide a reasonable, but not excessive, amount of time for ritualistic behaviors.	Planned activities offer the client structure and meaning and substitute for ritualistic behaviors. At the same time, the client's anxiety could escalate to a panic state if initially there is not sufficient time for compulsive acts.
Allow the client eventually to choose the amount and frequency of time needed for ritualistic behaviors while encouraging the client to perform anxiety-reducing strategies when necessary.	This choice provides the client with some control over the obsessive-compulsive sequence, supported by learned therapeutic techniques.
Offer praise and positive reinforcement (your time, attention, interactions) when the client engages in meaningful activities or attempts to manage ritualistic behaviors through learned strategies.	Praise and reinforcement increase the client's self-esteem and promote continued adaptive behaviors. A behavioral therapy called *exposure and response prevention* may be effective in reducing anxiety and decreasing obsessive and ritualistic behaviors (see Appendix B).

Client Receptive to Learning about Disorder

Teach the client and family about the obsessive-compulsive disorder (the meaning and purpose of the behaviors) in accordance with the treatment plan, their level of understanding, and their readiness to learn. • "One theory states that a biochemical disruption in the brain has a role in your disorder. Another theory states that early conflicts and life stressors may have some influence. These troubling behaviors may be the body's way of managing anxiety that comes from the intrusive thoughts." • "Often a combination of medication and stress-reducing strategies can decrease anxiety, which in turn may reduce your troubling thoughts and behaviors."	Information and knowledge help to uncover the mystery that generally surrounds mental health disorders and decreases the client's powerlessness, while increasing hope for successful symptom management.

Client and Family Preparing for Client's Discharge

Summarize with the client and family the meaning and purpose of the behaviors. • The behaviors occur to reduce the thoughts, impulses, and images. • The feelings that emerge with the behaviors include guilt, shame, and anger. • The identifiable stressors that may precipitate the rituals include loss of job, status, loved ones, and finances.	Reinforcing learned knowledge before discharge gives the client control over the disorder and the confidence to manage it.
Review with the client the learned cognitive-behavioral strategies used to manage anxiety and reduce the symptoms of obsessive-compulsive disorder.	Reviewing therapeutic strategies before discharge reminds the client that successful methods are available to manage anxiety and reduce obsessive-compulsive behaviors. The client will then approach discharge with confidence and hope.
Teach the client's family and close friends (with the client's permission) about obsessive-compulsive disorder and how they can assist the client to manage anxiety and ritualistic acts. Support and monitor the client's prescribed psychologic and medical treatment plans.	Significant others add support and understanding and are critical adjuncts to the success of the client's overall treatment plan. Postdischarge support helps to maintain the client's physiologic and psychosocial integrity.

Care Plan

NANDA Diagnosis: Posttrauma Syndrome

Sustained maladaptive response to a traumatic, overwhelming event.

Focus:

For the client who develops fear, terror, dread, or helplessness following exposure to a traumatic event (rape, war, natural disaster, abuse, experiencing or witnessing serious trauma or violence). Symptoms range from emotional "numbness" to vivid nightmares in which the traumatic event is recalled.

RELATED FACTORS (ETIOLOGY)

Overwhelming anxiety secondary to:

War experiences/military combat

Natural disasters (earthquake, hurricane, tornado, flood)

Personal assaults (rape, incest, molestation, beatings, abuse)

Kidnap of self or significant others

Catastrophic illness or accident

Prisoner of war death camp hostage experiences

Learning of a loved one's serious accident, injury, or maiming

Destruction of home or valued resources

Witnessing a serious accident or act(s) of violence (car crash, building collapse, mother being beaten, killing of family member)

Viewing a scene in which there are dead and/or maimed bodies (aftermath of war, plane or train crash, earthquake)

Threat to physical and emotional integrity (all of the above)

DEFINING CHARACTERISTICS

Client relates frequent intrusive recollections of past traumatic experience.

States that recollections are accompanied by feelings of dread, terror, helplessness, powerlessness, cardiac palpitations, shortness of breath, and other symptoms of emotional physical reactivity (see Table 2-1).

- "I feel out of control and terrified when I recall the event."
- "I get out of breath and my heart beats faster and faster."
- "I have a sense of doom, as if something terrible is going to happen."

Describes recurrent dreams or nightmares in which vivid details of traumatic event are relived or reenacted.

- "I had another horrible nightmare last night and went through the same trauma and anxiety all over again."

Expresses feelings of "numbness," detachment, or loss of interest toward people and the environment (generally occurs immediately after the traumatic event).

Demonstrates avoidance or lack of responsiveness toward stimuli associated with the traumatic event (in rare instances, may experience psychogenic amnesia).

- A war veteran avoids hospitals, injured persons, bandages, and blood.
- An accident victim demonstrates a flat affect while listening to a news report describing a traumatic event.

Demonstrates symptoms of physiologic reactivity (anxiety symptoms) when exposed to events that resemble or symbolize the original trauma.

- A young woman develops fear, dread, or terror when she attempts sexual intimacy with her partner because it reminds her of when she was raped.
- A prison camp victim experiences sympathetic nervous system stimulation (rapid heart rate, shortness of breath, nausea, diarrhea) while sitting in a cell-sized room.
- A war veteran who fought in a hot, humid climate experiences dread and terror when exposed to similar weather many years later.

Demonstrates symptoms of increased arousal (inability to fall asleep or remain asleep, hypervigilance, exaggerated startle response).

Manifests unpredictable episodes of explosive anger or aggression.

Verbalizes inability to concentrate or complete tasks.

- "I'm too distracted to make my bed or go to an activity."
- "I can't concentrate on my crafts."
- "I can barely shower and groom myself."

Relates inability to express angry feelings.

- "I feel as if I might explode, but I can't let it out."
- "I can't begin to express my anger."

Expresses thoughts of self-blame and guilt regarding a traumatic event.

- "If only I had locked the door, it wouldn't have happened."
- "If I had been there on time, it wouldn't have occurred."

Verbalizes anger at others for perceived role in traumatic event.

- "If they had helped more, he would have lived."
- "If they had called for help right away, I wouldn't be so badly injured."

OUTCOME IDENTIFICATION AND EVALUATION

Client verbalizes awareness of psychologic and physiologic symptoms of anxiety that accompany recollections of a past traumatic event.

Identifies situations/events/images that trigger recollections and accompanying responses of a past traumatic experience (small or enclosed spaces, hot or cold climate, arguments or fights, sexual intimacy).

Communicates and interacts within the milieu to control and manage anger and relieve thoughts of self-blame and guilt.

- Communicates thoughts/feelings to a trusted person.
- Problem-solves source of thoughts/feelings.
- Participates in group activities.

- Engages in physical activities/exercise.
Utilizes learned adaptive cognitive-behavioral therapeutic strategies to manage symptoms of emotional and physical reactivity.
- Attends process groups for group therapy (see Appendix B).
- Slow, deep-breathing techniques
- Progressive relaxation exercises
- Thought, image, and memory substitution
- Cognitive restructuring
- Systematic desensitization
- Behavior modification
- Assertive behaviors (see Appendix B)
Relates understanding that anger, self-blame, and guilt are common in persons who have experienced or witnessed traumatic events in which others were injured, assaulted, or threatened.
- "I realize others who have gone through this have had similar reactions."
Verbalizes ability to control or manage symptoms of emotional and physical reactivity that tend to occur during recollections of the traumatic event.
- "I can deal with my anxiety much better now."
- "My symptoms are much less troubling now."
- "I feel more in control of my reactions."
Demonstrates ability to remain significantly calmer when exposed to situations or events that symbolize or are

similar to the original traumatic event (displays relaxed affect and facial expression; smooth, nonagitated psychomotor movements).
Expresses relief from anger, self-blame, or guilt related to the traumatic event.
- "I'm not so hard on myself anymore; I realize things happen that we can't control or change."
- "I'm not overcome with anger anymore."
Verbalizes realistic hopes and plans for the future with absence of suicidal thoughts.
- "I'm going back to my old job; I have a lot of reasons to live; my family needs me."
Identifies significant support systems (family, friends, community groups).
Identifies the normal progression of grief symptoms that may be a part of the traumatic event (shock, denial, awareness, anger, restitution, acceptance).
Verbalizes self-forgiveness and forgiveness of others for actions or nonactions perceived by the client to have influenced the traumatic event.
- "I can finally forgive myself for being human."
- "They did what they could to help at the time."
- "It's time to forgive and get on with my life."

PLANNING AND IMPLEMENTATION

Nursing Intervention	Rationale
Listen actively to the client's details and ruminations about the recollections surrounding the traumatic event.	Active listening builds trust, allows the client to vent, decreases feelings of isolation, and guides the nurse toward significant problem areas (guilt, self-blame, anger).
If part of the client's treatment plan, encourage the client to identify and describe specific areas surrounding the traumatic event that are most troubling and that elicit powerlessness or loss of control.	"Talking it out" with a trusted person helps the client bring the details of the event into the open during a safe, nonthreatening time. It gives the client an opportunity to gain some influence over the traumatic event and decreases apprehension about intrusive recollections.
Determine the client's readiness to discuss traumatic events. Determine whether this approach is therapeutic or may result in increased anxiety.	If the client is not ready to vent or is being asked to repeat the "story" by too many staff members, this approach may not be therapeutic, and the client may need more time. Keen assessment is key.
Assist the client in structuring time for basic needs (hygiene, grooming, rest, nutrition).	Good hygiene and grooming increase self-esteem, promote health and safety, and provide fewer opportunities for painful recollections of the traumatic event.
Conduct a suicide assessment by observing the client for self-destructive behaviors or questioning the client directly for possible suicidal thoughts and feelings (see Suicide Assessment Tool, Box 3-6).	A suicide assessment provides for the client's safety; clients with posttrauma syndrome may become depressed and suicidal.
Assess the client's anxiety level (see Table 2-1).	Observing the client's anxiety level prevents escalation of symptoms through early interventions.

Continued

PLANNING AND IMPLEMENTATION—cont'd

Nursing Intervention	Rationale
Encourage the client to communicate and interact within the milieu according to the client's level of tolerance, as follows: • Engage in frequent one-to-one interactions with assigned staff. • Eat all meals in the clients' dining room. • Participate in recreational activities. • Attend community meetings.	The client's interaction within the milieu provides the following therapeutic benefits: • Prevents or decreases feelings of isolation and detachment from others and the environment. • Enhances socialization. • Uses energy in rewarding here-and-now activities. • Decreases opportunities for painful recollections of the traumatic event.
Avoid statements that dictate to the client what to feel, think, and do. **Nontherapeutic Responses** "You really have to stop blaming yourself and get on with your life." "Don't feel that way; it's self-destructive." "If I were you, I would break off with your old war buddies."	The client's behaviors and decisions are best influenced by the client's needs, desires, and life-style, not by the singular opinions of others. Preaching to the client will elicit resistance and delay the therapeutic process.
Teach the client adaptive cognitive-behavioral strategies to manage symptoms of emotional and physical reactivity (dread, terror, helplessness, sense of doom, cardiac palpitations, shortness of breath) that accompany intrusive recollections of the traumatic event. • Slow, deep-breathing techniques • Relaxation exercises • Cognitive therapy • Desensitization • Assertive techniques (see Appendix B)	*Deep-breathing/relaxation exercises* provide slow, rhythmic, controlled patterns that decrease physical and emotional tension, which reduces the effects of anxiety and the threat of painful recollections. *Cognitive therapy* helps the client substitute irrational thoughts, beliefs, or images for more realistic ones and thus promotes a greater understanding of the client's actual role in the traumatic event, which may decrease guilt and self-blame. *Systematic desensitization* helps the client gain mastery and control over the past traumatic event by progressive exposures to situations and experiences that resemble the original event, which eventually desensitizes the client and reduces painful effects. *Assertive behaviors* enable the client to manage anger and self-doubt by choosing to respond to painful recollections through adaptive strategies rather than being controlled by painful consequences.
Assist the client to develop objectivity in perceptions of the traumatic event by providing a fresh perspective. • "Rape is not a mutual sexual act; it is an act of violence that cannot be anticipated or prevented." • "No one could have predicted the accident; it just happened."	This objectivity may help promote a greater understanding of the client's actual versus perceived role in the event and may reduce feelings of self-blame and guilt.
Problem-solve with the client in areas in which some control is possible versus areas beyond control. • "No one can control who lives and who dies in a war, but the survivors can be helped to deal with the memories." • "It's hard to know if the robbery would have occurred if your door was locked, but anyone can forget to lock a door." • "The past can't be changed, but the impact can be lessened in time."	Problem solving helps the client begin to "let go" of aspects that are impossible to resolve (death, loss, injury) and begin to focus on areas that *can* be influenced (attitudes, coping methods).
Involve the client in decisions about the client's care and treatment. • "What are some of the behaviors and coping methods you use to decrease anxiety and control intrusive memories?"	This involvement helps foster feelings of empowerment, control, and confidence in the client rather than feelings of being a helpless victim of external effects.

- "I notice the methods you've been using seem to reduce your symptoms effectively. What do you think?"

Engage the client in group therapy sessions with other clients with posttraumatic stress disorder when the client is ready for the group process (see Appendix B).

The group process provides additional support and understanding through involvement with others who may have similar problems. Also, seeing the success of others gives hope to the client.

Promote the client's awareness of his or her own avoidance of experiences similar to the traumatic event.

Awareness gives the client the opportunity to integrate the past traumatic event into present and future life experiences without fear or apprehension.

Provide realistic feedback and praise whenever the client attempts to use learned strategies to manage anxiety and reduce posttraumatic stress response.
- "The staff has noticed you practicing the relaxation exercises."
- "You handled your anger well in the assertiveness training class today."
- "Your thoughts about yourself have become more realistic."

Positive reinforcement promotes self-esteem and gives the client the confidence to continue working on the treatment plan.

Assist the client and family to develop realistic life goals (school, work, community, and leisure activities).

The client and family will be better prepared for a hopeful future that will absorb and alleviate the posttraumatic stress response.

Care Plan
DSM-IV-TR Diagnosis **Somatoform Disorder**

NANDA Diagnosis: Ineffective Coping
The state in which an individual demonstrates impaired adaptive behaviors and problem-solving abilities in meeting life's demands and roles

Focus:
For the client who manifests physical symptoms or loss of physical functions as a means of coping with anxiety. The anxiety generally arises from unresolved conflicts/stressors that are too painful to be exposed to the conscious mind.

RELATED FACTORS (ETIOLOGY)

Psychologic conflicts/stressors
Severe anxiety, repressed
Fear of responsibility/failure/loss
Value-belief system
Psychosocial stressors
Past experience with true organic disease (self or others)
Exposure to persons with actual physical symptoms
Ineffective use of adaptive coping mechanisms/
    strategies
Dependent personality traits/disorder
Histrionic personality traits/disorder
Narcissistic personality traits/disorder
Obsessive-compulsive personality traits

Depressed mood state (secondary to dysthymic or major
    depressive disorder)
Negative self-concept (low self-esteem)

DEFINING CHARACTERISTICS

Client has preoccupation with body functions, such as
    heartbeat, sweating, or peristalsis, or with minor
    problems, such as mild cough or sore throat.
- "I can't seem to stop concentrating on my heartbeat."
- "I can't get my mind off my physical problems."
Interprets body functions or sensations as evidence of a
    serious disease.
- "I'm sure I have cancer somewhere in my body; I can feel
    it."
- "I just know I'm going to have a heart attack soon."
Verbalizes continued need to seek medical assistance for
    perceived physical symptom(s) despite physician's
    reassurance of no demonstrable organic pathology
    ("doctor-shopping").
- "If I don't get any satisfaction, I'll just see another
    doctor."
- "I'll keep going for checkups until they find out what's
    wrong with me."
Relates history of excessive visits to physicians, clinics,
    and emergency departments and possibly multiple
    surgeries.

Continued

Presents elaborate or detailed lengthy history of perceived physical symptomatology.

Demonstrates anger and frustration toward physicians when perceived physical symptoms are not diagnosed or treated.

- "I'm frustrated and upset at those doctors who refuse to give my symptoms a name."
- "How can they treat me if they can't figure out what I have?"

Promotes anger and frustration in health care providers who cannot find a physiologic basis for the client's perceived symptoms.

Denies correlation between physical symptoms and psychologic conflicts/stressors.

- "I'm so fed up with everyone who thinks it's all in my head."

Experiences continuing deterioration of health care provider relationships as a result of mutual anger and frustration.

- "I'm very upset that I can't find a doctor who will stay with me."
- "My doctor is avoiding me like all the others did after a while."

Relates family's frustration regarding inability of medical profession to diagnose and treat perceived symptomatology.

- "My family is so upset about this; sometimes I think they blame me."
- "My husband says we may need counseling to get through this."

Relates history of family members with similar symptoms as client, some of whom are deceased.

- "My great-aunt died, and she suffered from the same symptoms that I have."
- "My dad had trouble swallowing before he died, and I always feel as if I have a lump in my throat."

Demonstrates excessive dramatic or histrionic behavior when describing perceived physical signs and symptoms.

Demonstrates intermittent symptoms of anxiety that rapidly decrease as physical symptoms emerge.

Focuses on self and physical symptoms during interactions and group activities with clients and staff.

- Persistently discusses physical symptoms in all conversations, no matter what the original topic.
- Demonstrates exaggerated physical dysfunctions or alterations during group meetings and activities.
- Refuses to attend recreational activities because of perceived limitations rendered by physical symptoms or dysfunctions.

"You know I can't play Ping-Pong; I can't stand or walk."

"How can I play bingo? I can't see the numbers with my double vision."

Relates history of dependency on significant family members.

- "My father always protected me when I was a young girl."

- "I don't know what I'd do without my husband; he does everything for me."
- "I have wonderful kids; they take care of the house and do all the cooking."

Manifests depressed mood states that occasionally require hospitalization.

- "I've been treated for depression, but they still couldn't find the cause of my physical symptoms."

Relates history of prescription drug use for perceived physical pain, dysfunction, or other symptomatology.

Verbalizes progressive reduction in social activities that client directly attributes to perceived physical deterioration.

- "I hardly see my friends anymore; I'm too sick to socialize."
- "My physical problems have really limited my social life."

Relates prolonged history of job absences directly related to long-standing symptoms or problems for which there are no demonstrable organic findings or pathology (e.g., back pain, nausea and vomiting, muscle weakness or paralysis, painful menstruation, fainting, dizziness, blurred vision).

OR

Relates work history that began early in life and involved strenuous work with rare breaks or vacations (workaholic).

- "I never missed a day of work in my life; now my back hurts so much, I can't work."
- "I used to work overtime for years, but since my head injury I have blurred vision."

Attributes present perceived physical symptoms to an old injury.

- "My back pain is due to bending over the wrong way many years ago."
- "This hip pain is due to an old auto accident."
- "These headaches are the result of bumping into an open door during childhood."

Refuses persistently to attribute perceived physical symptoms to possible psychologic or emotional factors or influences.

- "They're trying to tell me that psychotherapy might help my pain; I can't believe it!"
- "My problems are physical, so how could they be caused by anything emotional or psychologic?"
- "How could some emotional problem that happened long ago have anything to do with these physical symptoms?"

Demonstrates a loss of or alteration in physical functioning of a body part or system that generally suggests, but is not limited to, a neurologic disease (e.g., paralysis, aphonia, seizures, blindness, anesthesia, coordination disturbance), which is an expression of a psychologic conflict or need.

- To prevent his wife from deserting him, a man who is dependent on her claims he cannot stand or walk when she threatens to divorce him.
- A woman is unable to speak after becoming enraged during an argument (rather than expressing anger outwardly), but no organic pathology exists.

Demonstrates markedly decreased anxiety concomitant with the manifestations of perceived physical symptoms, dysfunctions, or alterations. Primary gain: conflict is kept out of conscious awareness as anxiety is converted to a physical symptom.

Avoids particular activities or behaviors as a result of physical dysfunction or alteration. Secondary gain: Support is obtained from the environment that may not be forthcoming if the client functions normally.

- A man who thinks he is unable to stand or walk can relinquish responsibility and remain dependent on the environment.
- A woman who believes she is "blind" gains support and sympathy from others.

OUTCOME IDENTIFICATION AND EVALUATION

Client verbalizes absence or significant reduction of physical symptoms, dysfunctions, or alterations.

- Feels normal sensations in previously "numbed" arm.
- Stands and walks on legs that were once "paralyzed."
- Experiences significant decrease in duration and frequency of "gastrointestinal distress."

Demonstrates a significant decrease in anxiety in the absence of physical symptoms/dysfunction/alterations. This indicates that anxiety is being managed through adaptive coping mechanisms/methods rather than being converted to a physical symptom/dysfunction/alteration.

Verbalizes awareness of correlation between physical symptoms and psychologic conflicts/stressors.

- "Perhaps my early troubled childhood did influence my physical problems."
- "I can see how my combat experience may have played a part in my physical symptoms."
- "I was always afraid I would get sick and die like my brother did; maybe that did affect my body."

Explains body structure and functions in realistic terms.

- "I can tell the difference between a normal heartbeat and a racing one."
- "I know it's OK for my stomach to feel fluttery when I'm excited or nervous."

Communicates and interacts with others in the milieu.

- Seeks out staff for one-on-one interactions.
- Discusses thoughts and feelings with concerned clients.
- Problem-solves source of thoughts and feelings.
- Participates in community/didactic groups.
- Engages in physical activities/exercises.
- Shares information in process groups.

Uses learned adaptive cognitive-behavioral therapeutic strategies to manage and reduce anxiety.

- Slow, deep-breathing techniques
- Relaxation exercises
- Thought, image, and memory substitution
- Cognitive restructuring
- Desensitization
- Behavior modification
- Assertive behaviors (see Appendix B)

Recognizes the need to grieve normally for actual loss or impairment of body structure/function/integrity.

- "It's OK to feel bad that my arm will never be totally normal, as long as I don't dwell on it."
- "I want to be able to get angry about all those surgeries I've had and then get on with my life."
- "I need to have a good cry about my back injury and then try to make the best of it."

Accepts laboratory tests and clinical diagnostic results as valid criteria for health status.

- "I realize that repeated laboratory tests indicate accurate results of my condition."
- "Several doctors have examined me, and all of them agree that they could find nothing significantly wrong."

Refrains from discussing perceived physical symptoms/dysfunction/alterations with clients/staff/family.

Functions independently and assertively in social and personal situations.

- Takes care of basic needs without asking for help.
- Interacts as mature role model in milieu.
- Facilitates adult role with spouse and children.
- Initiates work or school role with positive attitude.

Demonstrates absence of physical symptoms/dysfunction/alterations, unless there is actual residual impairment.

Verbalizes absence of physical pain or discomfort, unless there is actual residual discomfort.

PLANNING AND IMPLEMENTATION

Nursing Intervention	Rationale
Review all current laboratory and diagnostic results with the client in clear terms according to the client's level of comprehension. • "Mrs. Jones, your test results are all normal." • "Mr. Smith, your test results indicate no physical disorder."	The client has the right to knowledge about health status. Anxiety can inhibit learning, so clear, concise terms are helpful. It is also important to offer information that will assist the client to accept facts regarding his or her health status.
Ensure that the client's treatment team members are equally informed of the latest relevant test results.	It is imperative that the client be given consistent, accurate information to decrease anxiety about health status and promote trust.

Continued

PLANNING AND IMPLEMENTATION—cont'd

Nursing Intervention	Rationale
Convey your understanding that, although the symptom is real to the client, no organic pathology has been found. • "Mrs. Jones, I know you feel the pain in your arm. Exams and tests have been taken, and no physical cause has been found." • "Mr. Brown, I realize you still have trouble standing and walking. X-rays and lab studies have shown no physical cause." • "Ms. Smith, I understand you feel no sensation in your hand. Test results did not show any physical cause."	Denial of the client's feelings could inhibit trust and decrease the client's self-esteem. Reassurance that no organic pathology has been found presents facts that are incongruent with the client's symptoms and difficult to challenge.
Assist the client in basic needs, routines, and activities in the initial stages of the therapeutic relationship, with the realization that prolonged help may result in secondary gains (e.g., client may use physical symptoms to preserve dependency and relinquish milieu responsibilities). • "Ms. Dale, staff will help you organize your daily routine for the first 2 days." • "Mr. Brown, staff will show you the shower and laundry rooms so you'll be able to bathe and to wash your clothes tomorrow." • "Mrs. Jones, I'll let you know when activities are today, and I'll give you a written schedule for the rest of the week."	The client needs some assistance during times of vulnerability. Denying the client's vulnerability when trust is being established could result in increased anxiety and intensification of physical symptoms and other maladaptive behaviors.
Gradually decrease the time and assistance given to the client according to the client's level of progress and level of trust. • "Mr. Brown, if you get to the dining room early, you can finish dinner and still have time to wash and dry your shirt before visiting hours." • "Ms. Dale, your clothes and makeup look nice today. It seems you can manage those well now." • "Mrs. Jones, I didn't call you for group because yesterday I gave you a schedule for all activities. You were on time for everything else, so I know you can do it."	Fostering the client's independence at the appropriate time enhances self-esteem, promotes adaptive coping and continuity of independent behaviors (organizational and problem-solving skills), and distracts the client from dwelling on physical symptoms and impairment.
Listen actively to the client's verbalizations of fears and anxieties without encouraging or focusing on the physical symptoms or dysfunction.	Expression of feelings with a trusted person enables the client to vent pent-up emotions, which in itself decreases anxiety. Verbalization also helps the client clarify unresolved issues or conflicts and guides the nurse toward problem areas. Not drawing attention to the client's physical symptoms discourages repetition of maladaptive behaviors.
Redirect the focus of communication whenever the client begins to ruminate about physical symptoms and impairments. • "Bob, you were talking about baseball a few minutes ago, and then you got off track. Let's talk more about baseball. What is your favorite team?" • "Sue, let's go back and continue our talk about your relationship with your sister." • "Steve, I'd like to hear more about what happened on the group outing."	Redirection toward more therapeutic topics helps the client focus on areas of communication that are more beneficial to recovery.
Inform the client whenever physical abilities and behaviors are incongruent with the client's verbal statements about physical symptoms and impairments.	This helps to point out the contradictions between the client's verbal statements and actual behavior in a therapeutic, nonthreatening manner.

- "Joe, I noticed you moving your legs and crossing them more often today. You may be able to stand and walk, too."
- "Jackie, that was a good game of Ping-Pong. Your arm seems to be stronger today."

Assist the client to connect the onset of physical symptoms with stressful events by exploring past experiences that can be recalled. (If this is too distressing for the client, postpone until client is able to tolerate.)

Connecting stressful situations with the onset of physical symptoms can eliminate maladaptive denial and prevent the client from using physical symptoms to manage anxiety.

Discuss with the client alternative coping strategies to reduce anxiety commensurate with the client's capabilities and life-style (see Appendix B).
- Deep-breathing techniques
- Relaxation exercises
- Physical activities (walking, running, exercising)
- Milieu activities (checkers, chess, cards, Ping-Pong, bingo)

As the client's denial decreases and the client no longer relies on physical symptoms to manage anxiety, adaptive coping techniques become meaningful ways to reduce anxiety and to prevent anxiety from escalating.

Teach the client therapeutic cognitive-behavioral strategies to manage anxiety and reduce the need to rely on physical symptoms (see Appendix B).
- Cognitive therapy
- Desensitization
- Reframing-relabeling
- Assertive behaviors

As the client becomes more aware that physical symptoms may be influenced by psychologic and emotional stressors, cognitive-behavioral skills can be used to effect a more positive change in attitude and to reduce or eliminate ineffective coping behaviors (see posttraumatic stress disorder).

Praise the client realistically for using adaptive coping behaviors to manage anxiety rather than resorting to physical symptoms, dysfunction, or impairment to reduce anxiety.
- "Jane, your use of deep breathing has helped slow down your heartbeat."
- "John, you have made a real effort to concentrate on your thoughts and not on your physical problem."
- "Jim, I've noticed that you can be calm now without focusing on your leg pain."
- "Sue, it seems the relaxation techniques have helped reduce your anxiety. You haven't discussed your stomachache in 3 days."

Positive feedback increases the client's self-esteem, offers hope for recovery, and encourages repetition of functional behavior.

Care Plan
DSM-IV-TR Diagnosis | **Dissociative Disorder**

NANDA Diagnosis: Ineffective Coping
Inability to form a valid appraisal of the stressors, inadequate choices of practiced responses, and/or inability to use available resources.

Focus:
For the client whose disturbances or alterations in normally integrative functions of identity, memory, or consciousness (dissociative identity disorder, dissociative amnesia, dissociative fugue, depersonalization disorder) are a result of ineffective coping (e.g., denial) related to painful, unresolved conflicts and can lead to inability to cope with subsequent stressors, as noted by impaired problem-solving/decision-making skills, relationships, and independent functioning.

RELATED FACTORS (ETIOLOGY)
Personal or psychosocial vulnerability
Overwhelming stressors that exceed the ability to cope
- Childhood: sexual abuse, trauma
- Adulthood: accident, trauma, military combat
Inadequate or ineffective support systems (family, early role models)
Anxiety, fear, or doubt
Anger, guilt, or shame
Threat to self-concept or physical integrity
Ineffective denial
Depressed mood

Continued

DEFINING CHARACTERISTICS

Dissociative Behavior in General

Client demonstrates inappropriate use of defense
mechanisms (e.g., maladaptive denial).

- Amnesic episodes
- Presence of alternate personalities
- Loss of perception and experience of self
- Loss of sense of external reality

Verbalizes inability to recall selected events or experiences
related to dissociative states.

Expresses confusion/disorientation about sense of self and
purpose or direction in life.

Relates altered perception or experience of self, ego
boundaries, and sense of external reality.

Reports lost or distorted periods with episodes of
confabulation in an attempt to "fill in" the memory gaps
(common in alcoholic amnesic states).

Verbalizes history of ineffective coping since childhood,
with specific symptoms emerging at various stages of
growth and development.

Demonstrates inability to meet role expectations in stages
of growth and development subsequent to traumatic
events.

Dissociative Identity Disorder

Client experiences two or more distinct personalities or
personality states that interfere with goal-directed
activities; personalities may or may not be aware of one
another.

Demonstrates changes in physiologic and psychologic
characteristics from one personality to another.

- One personality experiences physical symptoms
  (generally allergic in nature), and another personality is
  asymptomatic.
- Different personalities have different eyeglass
  prescriptions.
- Different personalities respond differently to psychologic
  tests or intelligence (IQ) tests.
- One or more of the personalities report being of the
  opposite gender or a different age or race.

Manifests discrepancies in attitude, behavior, self-image,
and problem-solving abilities from one personality to
another.

- A person alternates between one personality who is shy,
  quiet, and retiring and another personality who is
  flamboyant and promiscuous.
- A person has one personality who responds to aggression
  with childlike fright, a second personality who responds
  with submission, and a third personality who responds
  with counterattack.
- A person has one personality who is reasonably functional
  or adaptive (e.g., gainfully employed) and another
  personality who is clearly dysfunctional or appears to have
  a specific mental disorder.

Relates history of destructive behavior directed at self or
others, alcohol/drug abuse, or sex-related crimes.

Demonstrates anger, fear, confusion, guilt, shame, or
frustration associated with inability to cope with
unresolved early conflicts and subsequent stressors; may
also be a symptom of other dissociative states.

Addresses each identified personality by own proper name
or symbolic meaning, which usually differs from the
person's birth name.

- "Melody" is a personality that expresses herself through
  music.
- The "protector" presents a function given to a personality
  whose role is to protect the individual or group of
  alternate personalities.

Psychogenic Fugue

Client experiences episodes of sudden, unexpected travel
away from home or work with assumption of a new
identity.

Demonstrates inability to recall previous identity when
questioned, with concomitant episodes of confusion and
disorientation (rule out mental disorder).

Exhibits completely different behavioral characteristics
during fugue periods than those manifested in the
original identity.

- An individual who is usually quiet and passive becomes
  more gregarious and uninhibited during a fugue
  period.
- A person changes names or residences and engages in
  functional, complex social activities that do not reflect the
  existence of a mental disorder.

Note: The travel and behavior noted in psychogenic fugue are
generally more purposeful than the confused wandering
observed in clients with psychogenic amnesia.

Psychogenic Amnesia

Client exhibits sudden inability to recall important personal
information to a greater extent than ordinary
forgetfulness, generally associated with a circumscribed
period of time (e.g., first few hours after a profoundly
traumatic event or accident).

Demonstrates perplexity, disorientation, and purposeless
wandering during amnesic experience (generally
reported by others).

Displays an indifferent attitude toward memory
impairment during amnesic period *(la belle indifference).*

Depersonalization

Client demonstrates persistent, recurrent episodes of
altered perception or experience of the self in which the
usual sense of reality is lost or changed.

Expresses feelings of detachment or of being an "outside
observer" of own body or mental processes or as if in a
dream.

Verbalizes feelings like an "automated" robot or as if out of
control of actions and speech, with various types of
sensory "numbness." Experiences are *ego dystonic,* and
the client maintains intact reality testing.

Perceives bizarre alterations in surroundings so that sense of external reality is lost *(derealization)*.
- Objects may appear to have altered sizes or shapes
- People may seem mechanical or "dead"
- Sense of time may be distorted
- Anxiety
- Depression
- Obsessive-compulsive ruminations
- Fear of going insane
- Somatic concerns

OUTCOME IDENTIFICATION AND EVALUATION

Client identifies ineffective coping behaviors (fugue states, depersonalization, alternative personalities) and their negative effects on life functions, relationships, and activities.

Expresses feelings appropriately in an attempt to cope with and more effectively manage anxiety, fear, anger, confusion, guilt, or shame.

Identifies stressful situations that may trigger fugue states, depersonalization, transition from one personality to another, and other dissociative states, and develops methods to avoid them.
- Seeks out staff for support interaction medication.

- Alters stress-producing environment.
- Leaves stressful area or situation.

Demonstrates use of effective coping methods.
- Verbally expresses fear, anger, confusion, guilt, or embarrassment with trusted staff person.
- Writes thoughts and feelings in a diary or log.
- Engages in milieu activities and exercises.

Engages in ongoing, insight-oriented therapy with specialist in dissociative disorders.

Exhibits significant reduction in or absence of fugue states, amnesic episodes, and depersonalization.

Demonstrates progress toward integration of identified personalities or personality states.

Identifies helpful resources and support systems available on discharge.
- Relatives or friends who replace dysfunctional family
- Employer who is willing to learn about the problem and work with the client
- Day-treatment team (nurses, health care personnel)
- Psychotherapist
- Social services
- Community services

PLANNING AND IMPLEMENTATION

Nursing Intervention	Rationale
Be aware of own feelings, thoughts, doubts, and beliefs regarding dissociative disorders, especially *dissociative identity disorder,* before coming in contact with these patients.	The diagnosis must be accepted and understood by staff because any doubts or misinterpretations will be transferred to the client as anxiety or fear and pose a barrier to treatment.
Discuss concerns about the dissociative disorder with qualified staff or therapist.	Information from a specialist increases knowledge about these disorders and lessens own doubts and confusion, because these clients generally fear being doubted or questioned about the validity of their disorder.
Assure the client that he or she is not to blame for behaviors that occur during dissociative states.	This assurance will reduce the client's fears, guilt, and embarrassment when the client is vulnerable and unable to cope effectively with internal conflict.
Assure the client that staff will remain with the client during times of overwhelming anxiety, dissociation, or transition from one personality to another.	This assurance will promote feelings of trust, support, and psychologic safety during stressful times when the client is too frightened and confused to cope effectively.
Demonstrate to the client that staff will intervene to help the client cope more effectively during times of dissociation, depersonalization, or personality transition. • Remain calm and accepting of the client's behavior. • Assess the type of dissociative behavior being experienced. • Listen actively to the client and try to identify which personality is currently dominant (if dissociative identity disorder). • Arrange protection if a violent personality dominates.	A reliable, confident staff, using a consistent team approach, helps to assure the client that someone is in control when the client is unable to cope and may fear "going insane" or "falling apart."

Continued

PLANNING AND IMPLEMENTATION—cont'd

Nursing Intervention	Rationale

- Direct *primary personality* to monitor and control the behaviors of the potentially violent personality; usually one primary personality can be called on to prevent violence.
- Consult with treatment team as necessary.

Verbalize to the client the importance of discussing stressful situations and exploring associated feelings. (Treatment team should consult and agree on intervention strategies.)

Ventilation of feelings in a nonthreatening environment may help the client come to terms with serious issues that may be associated with the dissociative process.

Help the client understand that confusion, fear, and disequilibrium are normal during disclosure of painful experiences, when integration occurs and adaptive coping methods return.

The client who is aware of what to expect during disclosure of feelings and resolution of dissociative state is more apt to engage in treatment with less apprehension and a greater sense of trust.

Demonstrate acceptance of whatever experiences are disclosed by the client, making certain that your nonverbal behavior does not reveal disapproval, shock, or surprise.

Clients with dissociative disorders find it difficult to disclose experiences, even in a trusting relationship, because of fear of being criticized. They should be assured that the experience will be treated tactfully.

Structure the environment to reduce stimulation, such as loud noises, bright lights, or extraneous movement.

A less stressful external environment generally helps to calm the client's internal state and prevents or minimizes dissociative symptoms.

Protect the client from harm or injury during dissociative episodes (amnesia, loss of external reality, altered self-perception, poorly defined ego boundaries, distorted sense of time, emergence of alternate personality).
- Accompany client to assigned areas in the milieu.
- Move furniture against the wall.
- Distinguish boundaries through explanation and touch.
- Prevent others from injury caused by client's confused state.
- Initiate seclusion/restraint, if necessary.

Client may become confused, disoriented, or frightened during dissociative episodes and may require safety measures by an alert staff.

Help the client identify effective coping methods used in the past during stressful situations or experiences.

The client is helped to recall prior successful coping strategies whenever anxiety is overwhelming.

Assist the client to utilize new alternative coping methods.
- Provide opportunities for the client to vent anger, fears, frustration, shame, or doubt in a trusted environment.
- Engage the client in physical activities that require energy and concentration.
- Encourage the client to write thoughts, feelings, and fears in a diary or log.

The client is encouraged to deal with painful feelings, thoughts, and conflicts in a healthy, effective manner rather than using maladaptive denial.

Assist the client to evaluate the benefits of each coping strategy and its consequence.

The client is encouraged to problem-solve and develop a plan of action for future anxiety-provoking incidents, and autonomy is promoted.

Praise the client for using effective coping strategies.

Praise reinforces repetition of adaptive behaviors.

Assess the client for possible substance use/abuse.

A significant number of clients with dissociative identity disorder and other dissociative behaviors use alcohol or drugs as a means of coping, masking symptoms, or interfering with treatment and progress.

Assess the client for the presence and degree of depression, depletion of coping methods, and suicidal ideation (threats, gestures, plans), especially clients with dissociative disorders in whom one or more personalities may be suicidal. (Consult with treatment as needed.)

Clients with dissociative disorders may become discouraged and depressed because treatment is a long-term process (possibly 10 years or more), and the client needs protection against self-destructive acts.

Engage the client in appropriate therapies, such as *insight-oriented therapy*. (Refer to specialist in this type of analytical therapy, as necessary.)

Specialized therapy promotes expression of anxieties, fear, guilt, anger, or shame. Dissociative symptoms arise from internal conflicts and serve to protect the client from psychic pain. Subsequent stressors can produce similar reactions. Insight-oriented therapy with a knowledgeable therapist in a supportive setting allows the client to explore past and painful conflicts and eventually resolve them.

Discuss with the client feelings and problems related to lengthy treatment.

Feelings of frustration and discouragement will occur because of the long-term treatment regimen, and the client may resort to past, ineffective coping methods and destructive behaviors.

Help the client identify support systems that will assist in coping with early conflicts that cannot be completely resolved, such as childhood incidents of sexual abuse or trauma
- Trusted therapist
- Treatment team (inpatient and day treatment)
- Identified significant persons (may need to replace dysfunctional family members with newer, healthier friends)
- Social services
- Community resources

A strong support system will provide a network of support to strengthen the client's coping abilities and ease the pain that stems from memories that continue to interfere with the client's life functions.

Educate the client and significant others about available information regarding dissociative disorders, particularly dissociative identity disorder.

Obtaining current knowledge from professionals helps to dispel confusion and fear surrounding these disorders, reinforces continued treatment, and offers hope.

Care Plan
DSM-IV-TR Diagnosis   **Dissociative Disorders**

NANDA Diagnosis: Risk for Self-Directed Violence; Risk for Other-Directed Violence

At risk for behaviors in which an individual demonstrates that he or she can be physically, emotionally, and sexually harmful to self and others.

Focus:

For the client whose normally integrative functions of identity, memory, or consciousness (dissociative identity disorder, dissociative amnesia, dissociative fugue, depersonalization disorder) are a result of ineffective coping related to early life conflicts and can lead to inability to manage subsequent stressors, resulting in destructive acts toward self or others.

RELATED FACTORS (ETIOLOGY)

Risk Factors

Anger/frustration/rage related to amnesic episodes
Anger/frustration/rage reaction of one or more personalities (dissociative identity disorder)
Perceived threat to self-concept or physical integrity

Panic anxiety state
Overwhelming stressors that exceed the ability to cope in a reasonable manner
Conflicts between personalities (dissociative identity disorder)
Depressed mood
History of suicidal threats/behaviors
History of loss of control/violence toward others
Low self-esteem

OUTCOME IDENTIFICATION AND EVALUATION

Client demonstrates nonviolent behavior.
- Absence of suicidal threats/gestures
- Absence of aggressive acts toward others
- Absence of panic/rage reactions

Uses assertive behaviors to meet needs.
- Maintains relaxed, nonthreatening posture.
- Uses calm, matter-of-fact manner.

Uses resources and support systems effectively to help maintain self-control and prevent violence.
- Releases anger through verbal expression.
- Writes volatile feelings in diary or log.

Continued

- Seeks out trusted individuals for help when over-whelmed with anger.
- Engages in physical activities to release angry feelings.

Verbalizes understanding that disorder requires long-term treatment and that strategies to reduce anger and elimi-nate violence are continuous.

Engages in appropriate insight-oriented therapies in the hospital and after discharge to reduce the risk of suicide and violence toward others.

Demonstrates self-confidence and increased self-esteem as integration of personalities takes place, minimizing risk of violence.

PLANNING AND IMPLEMENTATION

Nursing Intervention	Rationale
Assure the client that staff will protect the client and others from harm or injury during dissociative episodes (amnesia, loss of external reality, altered self-perception, poorly defined ego boundaries, distorted sense of time, emergence of alternate personalities).	Clients may demonstrate fear, anger, panic, anxiety, or rage during dissociative episodes and need help to control behaviors they cannot yet manage alone. Knowing that qualified staff will be there to prevent violent episodes is in itself anxiety reducing.
Be aware of behavioral changes that are clues to destructive acts. Clients with dissociative disorders, especially *dissociative identity disorder*, can switch behaviors dramatically from calm to violent because different personalities have different behaviors. • Voice tone changes from calm and passive to loud and harsh. • Facial expressions change from blunted or smiling to troubled or scowling. • Movements change from smooth and relaxed to erratic with possible pacing. • Verbal expressions change from benign or friendly to hostile and threatening.	Behavioral changes that are clues to a risk for violence are important for staff to anticipate to ensure the client's and others' safety and protection.
Take immediate and decisive action when violence to client or others is imminent, according to severity of threat and history of previous violence. • Seclude/restrain if necessary. • If the client has dissociative identity disorder, direct the *primary personality* to monitor and control the behaviors of the potentially violent personality (e.g., tell the personality to "stop" until the personality calms down). Usually, one primary personality or "protector" can be called on to prevent violence. • Offer appropriate as-needed (prn) medication.	Quick decisive action prevents harm or injury to client and others in the environment.
Refrain from passing judgment on the client; instead, let the client know he or she is a worthwhile individual with strengths and is not responsible for early childhood trauma and sexual abuse.	The client is relieved from blame, which decreases guilt and shame and builds self-esteem.
Structure the environment to reduce external stimulation. • Reduce noise, lights, and extraneous movement. • Assist the client to avoid stressful environment when practical.	Calm surroundings precipitate a less stressful internal state within the client and reduce the risk for violence.
Assess presence and degree of depression and evidence of suicidal ideation in any of the client's personalities who emerge.	Client may become discouraged and depressed because treatment is a long-term process (may be 10 years or more), and the client needs protection against self-destructive behavior.
Examine the client's behaviors closely for abrupt changes that may signal a risk for suicide (threats, gestures, plans).	Close observation allows staff to intervene early and interrupt self-destructive act; also provides opportunity to interact with the client rather than resorting to physical interventions.

Assist the client to identify alternatives to aggression or violence.
- Verbalize feelings in a safe setting.
- Engage in physical activities.
- Write thoughts and feelings in a diary.

These activities will divert overwhelming impulses of anger and hostility toward constructive behaviors.

Engage the client in appropriate, insight-oriented therapy with a specialist in dissociative disorders, specifically dissociative identity disorder.

A knowledgeable therapist can help to bring painful conflicts and feelings into the consciousness and reduce the risk for dysfunctional coping, suicide, and violence toward self or others.

Educate the client and family about the most current information regarding dissociative disorders, especially dissociative identity disorder.

Increased knowledge will help to dispel the myths surrounding these disorders, reduce fear and confusion, and reinforce continued treatment with a specialized therapist.

Praise the client for attempts to control anger and rage and for participation in ongoing therapeutic regimen.

Praise and positive feedback increase self-esteem and reinforce continued treatment. Because treatment for dissociative disorders is a long-term process (may be 10 years or more), positive reinforcement is necessary.

## chapter 3

Mood Disorders

Mood disorders manifested by depression or mania are among the top 10 major causes of disability worldwide and are the second most prevalent type of all mental disorders. Mood disorders take a huge toll in terms of personal loss of hope, disturbed or fractured relationships, loss of productivity, cost of treatment, and deaths by suicide. Mood disruption is often an underlying component, if not a primary cause, of acting out against self and others.

Individuals with debilitating mood disorders definitely suffer, but they are not alone on the journey. Parents, siblings, spouses, children, friends, employers, co-workers, and others in the client's social circle are often caught in a web of mixed emotions as they live and interact with the client who has a chronic mood disorder. Family or significant others contend with feeling frustrated, sad, helpless, or inadequate because they cannot "fix" the client, make the client feel better, or change circumstances that invariably surround recurrent mood disorders. When the disorder is severe, disruptive symptoms often prevent clients from attaining or maintaining employment. As a result, added financial burden may be placed on others, leaving caregivers resigned, resentful, or angry.

A nurse beginning work in a psychiatric setting may have difficulty grasping the magnitude of mood disorder symptoms and the their impact on clients' lives. Nurses may have insufficient personal experience with severe disorders, although they assume that everyone experiences "highs and lows" of mood. Mental health personnel,

however, must distinguish normal moods of sadness or elation from the symptom extremes that can manifest in mood disorders. Students and new nurses say, "My life has many more stressors, so why is this client in the hospital?" Because clients with depression or mania may be unable to verbalize the severity of their feelings, nurses cannot effectively ensure client safety and well-being until nurses develop a keen awareness of how clients feel *and* have a plan for active intervention.

Mood refers to the state of how or what a person feels. Mood is the internal, subjective, usually sustained, and pervasive emotion that influences the way a person thinks, behaves, and perceives self and the world around him or her . . . the environment. A mood may be happy, sad, anxious, elated, frightened, or *mixed* when several mood states exist together. When moods change or "swing" suddenly or frequently, the mood is referred to as being **labile.**

Affect is the external, observable manifestation of a person's mood and may appear flat, blunted, expansive, or constricted. Affect is what the nurse observes and objectively reports. Clients sometimes report a mood that is incongruent with their apparent affect (e.g., reports "happy" while slumped dejectedly in a chair).

The nurse needs good assessment skills and therapeutic communication techniques to help clients learn to identify their feelings and regulate moods. Multiple interactive skills that assist the nurse to intervene with clients who have mood disorders are discussed in this chapter's care plans.

ETIOLOGY

Since the early 1990s, the "Decade of the Brain," biologically based theoretic and clinical research has shed light on the etiology of mental disorders, including mood disorders. To date, however, definitive causes for mood disorders are still undetermined because of the complex, dynamic involvement of each person's unique internal (biologic) and external (psychosocial/environmental) factors *(heterogeneity)*.

Just as each person's biologic makeup is unique, so is the development of adaptive or maladaptive coping skills. Presence or absence of adaptive support networks is a major influencing factor. In addition, the role of altered brain chemistry or function in depression or mania is not clearly defined. These brain alterations may be a cause, but they also may be a correlating factor or a consequence of the mood disorder (Box 3-1). The etiology of mood disorders is probably a combination of internal biologic and external factors and influences.

EPIDEMIOLOGY

Depression

Although 15% of the general population have major depression, fewer than one third are accurately diagnosed or treated. Some fail to be identified or treated because they are unaware of the severity of their symptoms and do not seek help. They and their families endure symptoms, placing clients at risk for disrupted daily function or even suicide. Of persons with major depression, 15% commit suicide, making *risk of suicide* a significant factor in mood disorders (see later discussion). Some clients may finally seek help for related symptoms from practitioners of general medicine, who may misdiagnose and prolong appropriate treatment. Clients with depressive disorders often have somatic complaints that make the correct diagnosis more difficult. Depressive symptoms also may be noted in other mental and organic conditions (Box 3-2).

Depression may occur in the absence of a traumatic event but often is preceded by a severe psychosocial stressor, such as the death of a loved one, divorce, or loss of a job. Substance abuse is common as the person attempts self-medication in an effort to feel better. The risk for recurrence of a depressive episode is high: 50% after the first episode, 70% after the second episode, and 90% after the third episode. A severe first episode is a predictor that the disorder will recur.

Major depressive disorder may begin at any age, even in early childhood, with a median age in the mid-20s to 30s. A few decades ago the average age was in the 40s, but the age of onset has decreased for those born more recently. Left untreated, symptoms of depression often

---

Box **3-1**   Etiology of Mood Disorders

BIOLOGIC
Neurotransmitter dysregulation
- Monoamine hypotheses: catecholamines, indolemines
- (GABA) acetylcholine systems
Reduction of neurotrophic factors in hippocampus
Genetic predisposition
Structural defects: birth trauma/stress related
Neuroendocrine dysfunction

STRESS RELATED
Mobilization of sympathetic nervous system
Hypothalamic-pituitary-adrenal axis overactivation
CRH hypersecretion

COGNITIVE-BEHAVIORAL
Learned helplessness
Distorted interpretations of situations/events
Hopeless outlook and worldview

PERSONALITY
Personality disorder mediating stress and depression
Temperament predisposing to depression and anxiety
Personality correlates of mood disorders
- Avoidance
- Dependence
- Reactivity
- Impulsivity

GENDER RELATED
More women with depression than men
Correlation with life events for women

PSYCHOSOCIAL
Death of loved one
Divorce
Major losses
- Affection
- Social status
- Employment
- Severe illness/disability
Past or current parental neglect or abuse
- Physical
- Sexual
- Psychologic
Inadequate parent-child bonding
Absent or inadequate support system
Intergenerational care burden: caring for elderly parents and children

GABA, Gamma-aminobutyric acid; *CRH*, corticotropin-releasing hormone.

Box 3-2 **Depressive Symptoms in Conditions Other Than Depression**

Substance use/abuse
Organic disorders
- Alzheimer's disease
- Multiinfarct dementia

Prescription/over-the-counter drug use/abuse
Dysfunctional grief
Personality disorders
Anxiety disorders
Schizoaffective disorder
Schizophrenia (all types)

Box 3-3 **Manic Symptoms in Conditions Other Than Bipolar Disorder**

Substance use/abuse
Prescription/over-the-counter use/abuse
Attention deficit/hyperactivity disorder (ADHD)
Anxiety disorders
Physiologic impairment of central nervous system
Schizophrenia
Schizoaffective disorder

improve within 9 months if there are no complications, but symptoms usually abate more quickly when treated.

Unlike "catching a cold," having depression is usually not completely cured with medical intervention. Studies show that up to 40% of those diagnosed with a major depressive episode will continue to have symptoms after 1 year that are severe enough to constitute major depression. About 20% continue to have some symptoms but do not meet full diagnostic criteria, and 40% have no mood disorder.

There are significant familial patterns for major depression, which occur up to three times more often in first-degree biologic relatives (parents, siblings) as in the general population. First-degree relatives also have a higher incidence of alcohol dependence, anxiety disorders, and attention deficit/hyperactivity disorder. Twice as many women as men have depression.

Bipolar Disorder

Unlike major depression, the incidence of bipolar disorder (commonly referred to as manic depression) is equal in both genders. Also, race and ethnicity are not significant factors. People with bipolar disorder commit suicide at a high rate, and suicide usually occurs during a *depressive episode*. As with depression, *risk of suicide* is a major factor in bipolar disorders. Other problems or disruptive behaviors associated with a *manic episode* include spousal or child abuse, violence, school or occupational failures, divorce, substance abuse, gambling binges, spending sprees, and sexual indulgence.

Average age of onset for bipolar disorder is 20 years. More than 90% of people who have a single manic episode go on to experience future episodes. An average of four major manic episodes occur in a 10-year period. Intervals between manic episodes decrease as the person ages, however, resulting in more frequent occurrences, often with more severe symptoms. Manic symptoms may also be noted in the other mental and organic conditions (Box 3-3).

ASSESSMENT AND DIAGNOSTIC CRITERIA

The defining characteristic of all mood disorders is *disturbance of mood*. Various categories of mood disorders have been identified based on *Diagnostic and Statistical Manual of Mental Disorders (DSM-IV-TR)* criteria and include depressive and bipolar disorders (see box below and Appendix A).

Episodes of Mood Disorders

The periods of symptom disturbance that represent mood disorders are called **episodes.** Each disorder includes one or more specific episodes.

Major depressive episode

The defining characteristic of a major depressive episode is 2 weeks or more of either (1) *depressed mood* that lasts most or all of each day or (2) *anhedonia* (loss of interest or pleasure in nearly all activities). In addition, at least four of the following symptoms are present:

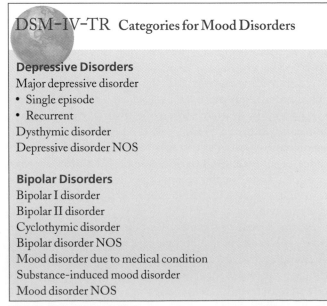

DSM–IV–TR Categories for Mood Disorders

Depressive Disorders
Major depressive disorder
- Single episode
- Recurrent
Dysthymic disorder
Depressive disorder NOS

Bipolar Disorders
Bipolar I disorder
Bipolar II disorder
Cyclothymic disorder
Bipolar disorder NOS
Mood disorder due to medical condition
Substance-induced mood disorder
Mood disorder NOS

NOS, Not otherwise specified.

- Marked change in appetite
- Significant weight loss or gain
- Insomnia or hypersomnia
- Psychomotor retardation or agitation
- Fatigue, lack of energy
- Lack of libido
- Feelings of hopelessness, worthlessness, guilt
- Decreased ability to think or concentrate
- Recurrent thoughts of death or suicide

Severely depressed clients may appear extremely despondent, a mood that is distinctly different from the normal mood of sadness or "the blues." These clients (1) express loss of capacity to enjoy life, family, friends, activities, or events that previously brought pleasure; (2) complain of low energy; (3) often resist or refuse others' efforts to help them or encourage them to help themselves; and (4) describe themselves or their situation as "hopeless."

Clients may cry often, or they may be unable to cry or express feelings of sadness but continue to withdraw and isolate themselves. It is often painfully difficult for them to engage with others, even concerned staff. They feel worthless and are unable to accept praise and approval. Other manifestations of major depression are guilt, helplessness, and indecisiveness. Ruminations of negative feelings and experiences may be prevalent. Low self-esteem, negative self-concept, and poor self-image seem pervasive.

Physiologic systems are slowed, and neurovegetative symptoms may occur. Most clients lose their appetite, with resultant weight loss, but some overeat and gain weight, often with the explanation that eating "fills the emptiness." The sleep-wake cycle is disturbed, and clients may experience *hypersomnia* (sleeping most of the day and night) or *hyposomnia* (decreased ability to sleep), difficulty falling asleep, or multiple awakenings. Constipation is common and is worsened by antidepressant medications. Clients with major depression have decreased or no desire for sex (frigidity in women, impotence in men), and amenorrhea may occur in depressed women.

Manic episode

The defining characteristic of a manic episode is at least 1 week of persistent mood that is excessively elevated, expansive, or irritable. In addition, at least three of the following symptoms must be present:

- Inflated self-esteem
- Grandiosity
- Decreased need for sleep
- Pressured or excessive speech
- Flight of ideas
- Psychomotor agitation
- Distractability
- Increase in goal-directed activity with frequent decreased purposefulness and completions
- Increase in activities for pleasure and socialization (with potential for danger, disappointment, or other painful consequences)

The client's insight and judgment are poor in the manic phase. Before hospital admission the client may have been engaged in excessive activities such as gambling or spending sprees, sexual indulgence, phoning family and friends in the middle of the night to "party," and engaging in ill-fated business ventures that the individual is not prepared to handle.

When admitted to the hospital, the client with mania may be hyperactive, pacing or running up and down the halls, intruding in others' activities, sleeping and eating little, and changing clothing several times a day. Clothing, jewelry, and makeup may be excessive, with unusually bright, garish combinations.

During this acute phase, the manic client is hyperverbal, demonstrates pressured speech, and talks constantly and rapidly to anyone who will listen. The client says whatever comes to mind and rapidly changes topics *(flight of ideas)*, described by the client as "racing" thoughts. The client may frequently insult staff and other clients, often with foul or sexually explicit language. The client tests unit rules and limits, insists on having own way, is often manipulative, and may become hostile and combative when thwarted, exploding in an angry tirade. Some manic clients exploit the weakness of other clients and staff, dividing staff and causing management problems. The client may be seductive, flaunt sexuality, or invite other clients and staff to engage in sexual acts.

The client with mania may describe the euphoric mood as feeling "high" and may elect to stop taking medications to achieve this state. Manic clients are frequently preoccupied with religious, political, sexual, or financial ideas that may reach delusional proportions.

Mixed episode

The defining characteristic for a mixed episode is at least 1 week during which criteria for depressed episode and manic episode occur each day. Moods rapidly alternate (irritable, elated, frustrated, sad). Other symptoms that usually accompany a mixed episode include the following:

- Agitation
- Insomnia
- Disturbed appetite
- Suicidal thinking, attempts
- Psychosis

Hypomanic episode

The defining characteristic for hypomanic episode is at least 4 days of persistent exaggerated mood that is expansive, elevated, or irritable. Hypomania closely resembles the manic episode in associated features as well, but the hypomanic client has no or minimal impairment of judgment or performance.

Additional Criteria for Episodes

Rapid cycling of mood episodes and psychosis during episodes are other symptom criteria that can develop in mood disorders.

Rapid cycling

Rapid cycling refers to four or more major mood episodes occurring in a 12-month period. The symptoms meet criteria for major depressive, mixed-manic, or hypomanic episodes, with remission intervals between episodes or a switch from depressive to manic, and vice versa. Rapid cycling occurs in 10% to 20% of people with mood disorders, 70% to 90% of whom are women.

Psychotic features

Psychotic symptoms may occur in episodes of depression or mania in mood disorders. **Psychosis** is a severe mental disturbance defined as the impaired ability to recognize reality. Perception, thoughts, mood, affect, and behavior are disturbed in psychosis, with resultant major disturbances in social and occupational function. Psychosis is demonstrated by the presence of either **delusions** (fixed thoughts or beliefs that are not real), **hallucinations** (sensory-perceptual alterations), or both delusions and hallucinations. When psychotic symptoms present in mood disorders, differential diagnosis is necessary to distinguish the mood disorder from schizoaffective disorder, substance-induced disorder, disorder caused by medical condition, or other disorders.

Delusions and hallucinations are usually consistent with the type of mood disorder. In depression, for example, delusions follow themes of poverty and nihilism, as in the following examples:

- A man refuses to eat, saying that there is no need to eat because the world has ended (*nihilistic* type).
- A woman believes her body is rotting away, her heart is made of stone, and she doesn't deserve to live (*somatic* type).

Hallucinations may be *visual* (e.g., seeing a deceased loved one), or *auditory* (e.g., hearing the voice of someone that the client believes he or she deceived). Hallucinations may also occur in any of the other senses, but less frequently. Occasionally clients experience hallucinations and delusions at the same time, such as the following client:

- A woman hears her dead husband's voice, sees his image, and tells him she caused his cancer and resultant death.

If the person has mania with psychosis, delusions are usually grandiose or persecutory. Examples of *grandiose delusions* include the following:

- A man believes he is God and rules the universe (is someone special).
- A woman believes she is married to the hospital chief administrator, so staff should follow her directions (knows someone important or famous).
- A client has the formula for cloning brilliant minds (knows something extraordinary).

    Persecutory delusions include the following:

- A man believes the staff belongs to a cult and is afraid to go to sleep for fear of what staff might do.

- A client's neighbors are plotting to have her evicted from her apartment now that she has been "locked up in this foreign prison" against her will.

The essential characteristic of bipolar disorder is one or more manic episodes that may or may not be accompanied by depressive episodes. Diagnosis depends on the symptoms of the *current* episode. Clients may have rapid cycling of moods, or moods may fluctuate between manic and depressed states with periods of normal mood between these extremes. Episodes of mania in bipolar disorder have a more rapid onset and are of shorter duration than depressed episodes in major depressive disorder.

Major Depressive Disorder

- Single episode
- Recurrent episodes

In addition to one (single) episode or more than one (recurrent) episode of major depression, diagnosis of major depressive disorder includes that the client has never had a manic episode, mixed episode, or hypomanic episode. Depression is also noted as either mild, moderate, or severe. Other features may be added to this diagnosis:

- **Catatonia.** (Presence of two or more criteria), motor immobility *(stupor)*, mutism, inappropriate or bizarre posturing or grimacing, purposeless excessive activity with no external stimulus, negativism (e.g., resists attempts to move or be moved).
- **Melancholia.** Severe anhedonia and three of the following: severe depressed mood; mood worsens in morning; early-morning awakening (2 hours before regular time); marked agitation or retardation of movement (psychomotor retardation); excessive guilt; extreme anorexia or weight loss.
- **Postpartum onset.** Onset occurs within 4 weeks of childbirth. Symptoms are the same as those in major depressive, bipolar, or mixed episodes.
- **Postpartum psychosis.** Incidence: 1 in 500 to 1000 deliveries. Psychotic features may be present; if infanticide occurs, it is usually during a psychotic state. Women are at higher risk if they have (1) prior postpartum mood episodes, (2) prior history of mood disorder, or (3) familial history of bipolar disorder. The risk of recurrence in subsequent deliveries is 30% to 50%. In postpartum major depressive episodes, anxiety *(panic attacks)* frequently occur.

The more severe postpartum depression just described must be distinguished from the normal "baby blues" that occurs within 10 days of delivery in 70% of women. These postpartum symptoms are transient and do not radically impede function. The dramatic postpartum neuroendocrine changes and the many necessary, unanticipated readjustments trigger this milder condition.

- **Seasonal pattern.** Onset and remission, usually of major depressive episodes, occur at specific times of the year. Most clients have a *winter* seasonal pattern; depression begins in fall or winter and remits in spring. Symptoms include lack of energy, overeating with weight gain, carbohydrate craving, and hypersomnia. Onset of manic or hypomanic episodes may be linked to increased light. Light therapy may trigger manic or hypomanic episodes in some depressed individuals.

Dysthymic Disorder

The defining characteristic for dysthymic disorder is a chronically depressed mood for the major part of most days over a 2-year period for adults, or 1 year for children and adolescents. Dysthymic disorder differs from episodic major depression, and two or more of the following symptoms are present:

- Appetite disturbance (lack of appetite/overeating)
- Sleep disturbance (insomnia/hypersomnia)
- Fatigue/general lack of energy
- Difficulty concentrating/decision making
- Self-esteem disturbance (lowered)
- Hopelessness

The client with dysthymia must not have had a previous manic or mixed episode, and the disorder must not have been caused by other mental disorders, medical conditions, or substance use.

Bipolar I and II Disorders

The defining characteristic for **bipolar I disorder** is either a manic or a mixed episode. Usually the person has had one or more prior major depressive episodes.

The defining characteristic for **bipolar II disorder** is the presence or history of one or more major depressive episodes and at least one hypomanic episode. Both bipolar I and bipolar II disorders may also have the following specifiers:

- Mild/moderate/severe
- Single/recurrent episode
- Features of catatonia/melancholia/postpartum onset/rapid cycling/seasonal pattern

Cyclothymic Disorder

The defining characteristic for cyclothymic disorder is chronic course (2 years for adults; 1 year for children or adolescents) of mood fluctuations that include several hypomanic and depressed periods without a 2-month period of symptom relief during that time. The symptoms do not meet the full criteria for manic or depressive episodes, and psychotic features are absent.

Mood Disorder Due to Medical Condition

The defining characteristic of physiologic mood disorder is depressed, manic, or mixed symptoms, as described earlier, with the disturbance the direct physiologic result of a medical condition. Several general medical conditions have been identified and correlated with mood disturbances (Box 3-4).

Substance-Induced Mood Disorder

The defining characteristic of substance-induced mood disorder is the presence of mood disorder symptoms previ-

Box 3-4   Related Medical/Mood Disturbances

Parkinson's desease
Huntington's disease
Alzheimer's disease
Cerebrovascular accident (stroke)
Multiple sclerosis
Cushing's disease
Metabolic dysfunction (thyroid, adrenal)
Autoimmune disorders (lupus)
Some cancers (degree of involvement/stage)
Viral (HIV, hepatitis)
Postsurgical conditions (organ transplants, disfiguring types)

Box 3-5   Substances of Abuse That May Cause Mood Disorders

INTOXICATION	WITHDRAWAL
Alcohol	Alcohol
Amphetamines	Cocaine
Cocaine	Amphetamines
Anxiolytics	Sedatives/hypnotics
Sedatives/hypnotics	Anxiolytics
Opioids	
Phencyclidine (PCP)	
Inhalants	
Hallucinogens	

ously described, developing within a month of substance intoxication or substance withdrawal. Besides substances of abuse (Box 3-5) other substances (medications, toxins) may be involved in mood disorders. Somatic treatments, such as light therapy and electroconvulsive therapy, can also alter moods dramatically.

COMPLICATIONS

Suicide

Depressed clients often have recurrent or persistent thoughts of death and suicide, for which nurses continually assess (Box 3-6). Because clients may withhold this information, nurses use empathy, but also skillful, open, honest confrontation, to help clients through this difficult time, always keeping in mind that the client's safety is paramount. Staff is aware that clients frequently make gestures or attempts at suicide when the depression appears to be lifting. Brighter affect may actually signify relief from ambivalent feelings that surround opposing desires to live or die, instead of the misinterpretation that the client "feels better." Novice staff may think this change in client affect

---

Box 3-6   Suicide Assessment Tool for Inpatient Setting***

	Yes	No
1. Is the client hopeless?	—	—
• Does the client see no prospects for the future?	—	—
• Does the client see no solutions to his or her problems?	—	—
2. Has the client made a recent suicide attempt?	—	—
• Are the client's suicide attempts severe or multiple?	—	—
• Does the client show impulsivity?	—	—
3. Are suicide attempts increasing in frequency or lethality?	—	—
• Is the client obsessing or fantasizing about suicide or death?	—	—
4. Does the client have insomnia with suicidal ruminations at night that continue into the early-morning hours?	—	—
5. Along with depression, is the client anxious?	—	—
• Are there any symptoms of panic or posttraumatic stress disorder (PTSD)?	—	—
6. Does the client have bipolar disorder, postpartum psychosis, or psychotic depression?	—	—
• Is the client experiencing pathologic grief, especially with command hallucinations, guilt, or other comorbid conditions (chemical dependency, alcoholism, personality disorder)?	—	—
7. Does the client have a history of suicide by a relative or close friend?	—	—
• Is the client isolated?	—	—
• Does the client lack resources and available family?	—	—
8. Does the client have detailed suicidal plans?	—	—
• Are lethal means available to the client for suicide, such as a gun or other weapon?	—	—
9. Did the client leave a suicide note or give away valued possessions?	—	—
10. Is the client becoming increasingly frustrated with therapy, illness, or problems?	—	—
• Is the client feeling powerless and unable to learn how to cope?	—	—
11. Has the patient been offered electroconvulsive therapy (ECT) and demonstrated ambivalence over it?	—	—
• Has the client interpreted the recommendation as an admission of failure and hopelessness versus a positive solution?	—	—

*A combination of depression and a "Yes" answer to any one of these questions suggests that the client must be assessed carefully by the treatment team for possible admission to a locked facility, with suicide precautions instituted as per policy.
Courtesy Raymond A. Fidaleo, MD, Clinical Director, Sharp Mesa Vista Hospital, San Diego, California.

---

is a sign that the client is less depressed, and they may lower their guard. Also during this time, the client's energy starts to return, and those who are seriously suicidal are more capable of planning and attempting or completing the suicide.

The *risk for suicide* is high for clients with mood disorders, diagnosed in 15% of clients with depression and 10% to 15% of those with bipolar disorder (Box 3-7). More than 30,000 people commit suicide annually. Four times more women than men attempt suicide, but four times more men actually succeed, usually by more violent means. Death by suicide for children and adolescents has increased alarmingly in the last half century. Although the number has fluctuated slightly over the last 2 decades, suicide at an early age continues to be a major problem in the United States.

Suicide attempts and completions occur more often when the client has the following:

- Severe symptoms
- Psychosis
- Coexisting mental disorders
- Coexisting substance abuse
- Late-onset disorder

Box 3-7   Risk Factors for Suicide

Male/adolescent/over 40 years old
Divorced/widowed/separated
Elderly/infirm
Impulsive/seclusive style
History of previous attempt, with or without injury
Attempts that have been unsuccessful in changing behavior of others
Lack or perceived lack of support systems
Giving away possessions
When mood begins to lift following depression
Major medical/psychiatric illness
Alcoholism/drug abuse
Bipolar disorder
Major depression

| PHARMACOTHERAPY | **Bipolar Disorder** |

LITHIUM

Lithium, a natural element and mood stabilizer, is the first-line medication for acute episodes of mania and depression typically seen in bipolar disorder. Lithium is also effective as maintenance therapy for bipolar disorder. Therapeutic effects are seen in 1 to 2 weeks. Therefore for a quick response, an anxiolytic such as a benzodiazepine or an antipsychotic medication may be needed initially. Therapeutic blood levels for acute mania are 0.8 to 1.2 mEq/L, whereas maintenance levels are 0.8 to 1.0 mEq/L. Lithium levels need to be monitored initially every 5 to 6 days and with a change in dosage, then regularly every 6 months for maintenance doses.

LABORATORY WORKUP

Before lithium therapy is initiated, laboratory workup should include thyroid function tests, urinalysis, renal function tests, electrolytes, and a complete blood cell count (CBC). Lithium is excreted through the kidneys and parathyroid glands and has a narrow therapeutic range, so both the initial workup and the routine monitoring of lithium blood levels are critical. Clients taking lithium should use normal amounts of salt in their diet, or lithium could be taken up by the body in place of sodium, resulting in *lithium toxicity,* which could be serious. Physical exercise and perspiration due to hot weather could also deplete the body of salt and water, which could lead to lithium toxicity. These clients are advised to drink large quantities of water to prevent dehydration and lithium toxicity.

VALPROATE

Valproate (Depakote) is also considered a first-line agent in both acute and maintenance therapy for bipolar disorder and is preferred over lithium for rapid cycling and dysphoria (depressed mood). Therapeutic blood levels are 50 to 125 μg/ml. Liver toxicity is a risk, especially for young children, and liver function should be monitored carefully.

CARBAMAZEPINE

Carbamazepine (Tegretol) appears to be effective in both acute and maintenance therapy for bipolar disorder. Therapeutic levels are 8 to 12 mg/L. Carbamazepine has many drug interactions. Adverse effects include rash and Stevens-Johnson syndrome; both require a discontinuance of drug therapy because Stevens-Johnson syndrome may prove fatal and also presents with a rash. Because of the small risk of agranulocytopenia (low white blood cell count), clients taking carbamazepine require close monitoring of CBC, as well as liver function tests.

GABAPENTIN

Gabapentin (Neurontin) is an anticonvulsant used as adjunct therapy for manic and depressive episodes of bipolar disorder. Dosage ranges from 900 to 3600 mg.

LAMOTRIGINE

Lamotrigine (Lamictal) is an anticonvulsant used as adjunct therapy for manic and depressive episodes of bipolar disorder. Lamotrigine requires a titration schedule to 300 to 500 mg daily in divided doses. Adverse effects include a rare but life-threatening rash (Stevens-Johnson syndrome), especially in young children, in whom lamotrigine is discontinued immediately.

TOPIRAMATE

Topiramate (Topamax) is an anticonvulsant that is also considered an adjunct therapy in the treatment of bipolar disorder. The dosage used to treat bipolar disorder is lower than when used as an anticonvulsant.

CALCIUM CHANNEL BLOCKERS

Verapamil (Calan) and other calcium channel blockers may be useful in the treatment of bipolar disorder.

OXACARBAZEPINE

Oxacarbazepine (Trileptal) is as effective as carbamazepine in the treatment of bipolar disorder but is better tolerated with less liver toxicity. Routine blood level monitoring is not necessary with oxycarbazepine, but its cost is high.

- Medical illnesses
- Stressful life events
- Family history of suicide

Prevention is paramount because studies reveal that people who survive the crisis of suicide attempts are thankful. When suicide attempts are thwarted, clients are invariably appreciative that someone intervened on their behalf when they were unable to provide for their own safety. During acute, severe symptoms of mental pain and hopelessness, individuals fully believe there is "no end to what they are feeling," "no way out," or "no future." This thinking is erroneous, so nurses are present to prevent acts of suicide. The first care plan in this chapter offers nurses and other mental health personnel practical interventions and rationale for preventing suicide and assisting clients to rekindle hope for the future.

Comorbidity

Clients with mood disorders typically have coexisting mental disorders or physical illnesses *(comorbidity).* Anxiety disorders occur in half the major depressive disorders. Substance use disorders are present in up to 40% of clients with mood disorders, and mood disorders worsen unless substance abuse or dependence is treated. A high correlation exists between mood disorders and personality disorders. Several medical conditions also are often identified in people with mood disorders, including coronary artery disease, hypertension, and arthritis.

TRICYCLIC ANTIDEPRESSANTS

The first-generation tricyclic antidepressants have continued to be effective. The disadvantage is these drugs' significant side effects, such as anticholinergic symptoms, cardiotoxicity, and sedation. Medication may be taken at bedtime to prevent or modify the effects of sedation during the day. Also, overdose of tricyclics can be fatal, so medications should be dispensed with care.

SELECTIVE SEROTONIN REUPTAKE INHIBITORS

The selective serotonin reuptake inhibitors (SSRIs), such as flu-oxetine (Prozac), paroxetine (Paxil), and sertraline (Zoloft), have become the first-line antidepressants because they have fewer side effects than the tricyclics, with no cardiotoxicity and less sedation. This advantage makes them more readily accepted. The disadvantage is that the SSRIs may lead to sexual dysfunction in both men and women.

MONOAMINE OXIDASE INHIBITORS

The monoamine oxidase inhibitors (MAOIs) are generally indicated for atypical or refractory depression. MAOIs have significant side effects and drug-to-drug interactions (including over-the-counter cold remedies) and drug-to-food interactions (avoid tyramine-rich foods) that could result in a hypertensive crisis and subsequent cerebrovascular injury.

VENLAFAXINE

The selective serotonin-norepinephrine reuptake inhibitor (SSNRI) venlafaxine (Effexor) has quick action as its main advantage. Side effects include gastric intolerance; an H_2-receptor antagonist such as famotidine or ranitidine may help, as well as taking venlafaxine with food. Another side effect of venlafaxine is increased diastolic blood pressure; blood pressure monitoring is important.

TRAZODONE

Because of its sedating effect, trazodone (Desyrel) is not only used as an antidepressant but also as a sleep inducer. Trazodone is especially effective for older adults with sundown sydrome and sleep disturbances. An advantage of trazodone is that it is rarely fatal in overdose. Trazodone can cause priapism (painful sustained erection), a rare but serious medical condition that requires medical attention.

NEFAZODONE

The serotonin antagonist reuptake inhibitor (SARI) nefazodone (Serzone) is chemically similar to trazodone but is much less sedating. Because of its relatively short half-life, nefazodone is given in divided doses.

BUPROPION

The dopamine/norepinephrine reuptake inhibitor (DNRI) bupropion (Wellbutrin), besides its antidepressant effect, is useful for smoking cessation because it reduces nicotine craving. An important side effect is that bupropion increases the seizure threshold.

MIRTAZAPINE

The primary effect of mirtazapine (Remeron) appears to be antagonism of presynaptic autoreceptors and heteroreceptors, which prevents release of norepinephrine and serotonin. Mirtazapine is more sedating at a lower dose (15 mg) than doses above 45 mg. Remeron also increases appetite and is a good alternative medication for older adults.

▌ INTERVENTIONS

Treatment Settings

Although outpatient treatment for mood disorders is common (home, physician/therapist office, clinic), persons with severe depression or mania often require hospitalization. Suicide or homicide risk or an inability to meet the needs for food, clothing, and shelter is a direct indication for hospitalization. Other indications for hospitalization of clients with depression or mania include severity of symptoms, rapid escalation of symptoms, and lack of availability or capability of an individual's support systems. Frequently, persons with mood disorders resist suggestions for hospitalization because of the very nature of the disorders. Severely depressed people are unable to make decisions because of slowed and impaired cognitive functions, a hopeless outlook on life, or feelings of unworthiness. Clients with mania may believe that hospitalization is absurd because of delusional systems that significantly impair their perception, judgment, and insight.

Medications

Bipolar disorder

Most studies reveal a higher rate of treatment success for clients with mood disorders when psychopharmacologic and other psychotherapeutic interventions are combined. See pharmacotherapy box on p. 69.

Major depression

Efficacy among the different classes of antidepressants is similar, with about a 60% to 70% response rate to drug therapy. The choice of a particular antidepressant depends on the drug profile, drug interactions, and patient acceptance. See pharmacotherapy box above.

To minimize side effects and adverse reactions, initial doses should be divided. The target dose should be achieved as quickly as possible. Improvement is generally seen in 3 to 4 weeks, with a maximum response in 8 weeks. If the client is not responsive, another antidepressant should be tried. Side effects are usually more severe initially, then taper off over time. It is important to educate the client and family about medication side effects to promote compliance.

Electroconvulsive Therapy

Electroconvulsive therapy (ECT), also referred to as **electroshock therapy (EST),** is an effective biologic intervention for major depression, the disorder for which it is most commonly administered. ECT remains a subject of much controversy. Some data indicate that ECT may be beneficial for acute manic states and some cases of schizophrenia, particularly schizoaffective disorder, in which mood is disrupted.

Therapies

Research indicates bimodal therapy that combines use of medications with interactive therapies is more effective than either one alone. Interactive therapies that have proven effective in treating mood disorders include but are not limited to nurse-client relationship principles, cognitive-behavioral therapies, group therapies, family therapies, and activity (adjunctive) therapies.

This chapter's care plans provide practical techniques that nurses can use to focus these therapies in treating clients with mood disorders.

Nurse-client therapeutic relationship

The relationship that develops between nurse and client, the *therapeutic alliance,* is a vehicle for client change and wellness (see Chapter 1). This alliance is most valuable when working with clients who have mood disorders. The alliance is based on trust and rapport. The nurse uses basic therapeutic communication techniques and multiple skills specifically directed toward client symptoms and behaviors associated with mood disorders.

Activity therapy

Activity therapies provide diversion and respite from the serious verbal processing that occurs during insight-oriented sessions in groups and individually. Activity therapy, however, is not considered "play." Each modality uses techniques that encourage the client's awareness to minimize pathology and promote healthy thoughts, feelings, and behaviors.

Cognitive-behavioral therapy

Cognitive theorists believe that depression is the consequence of a person's negative thoughts about self and circumstances. Cognitive therapy involves helping the individual identify, modify, and eventually change negative thought patterns by practicing thinking realistically about self and situation. Emphasis is on immediate issues and interpersonal relationships, not on past intrapsychic phenomena.

Behavioral theory proponents state that the most effective way to alleviate depression is to change the behavior. Reinforcement of negative behaviors is a principal element of depression. Behavioral therapies vary in focus and specific techniques that identify goals, methods for attaining the goals, and reinforcers for goal attainment (see Appendix B).

Family therapy

Family therapy can be an effective treatment modality for clients with mood disorders. The focus is on the family unit and its role in perpetuating depression. Family therapy also evaluates the effect depression has on the family as a whole. Marriages and family functions are frequently imperiled, and divorce rates are high in families of mood-disordered clients. Symptoms result in impaired relationships in families of clients with mood disorders, which often leads to psychosocial dysfunction.

Secondary gain (attention from others and relief from responsibility as a result of the sick role) may reinforce dysfunction. Families benefit from learning about the disorder, which is often out of client's control. Blame decreases as understanding and empathy increase.

Group therapy

Group therapy represents a microcosm of a larger society in which clients can interact and express themselves safely. If clients are able to tolerate the interpersonal process, groups are therapeutic for mood-disordered clients. Groups enhance therapeutic communication and socialization, both of which are essential goals for manic and depressed clients. Group modalities include recreational/occupational/projects, art, dance/movement, and psychodrama. Clients with depression or mania who are unable to verbalize their problems often find freedom of expression in one of these modalities.

PROGNOSIS AND DISCHARGE CRITERIA

Prognosis for the client with a mood disorder depends on the following factors:
1. Level of symptom severity: mild/moderate/severe
2. Whether episode is the first (single episode) or a subsequent (recurrent episode) occurrence
3. Presence or absence of additional features (e.g., psychosis)
4. Personal resilience based on multiple unique internal and external factors: biologic makeup, personality type, cognitive style, support system, situational circumstances

For example, if person experiences a first episode that is mild, without complications, and unencumbered with multiple psychosocial stressors, prognosis is usually more favorable. Conversely, if the individual has had several previous episodes and currently has suicidal ideation or has made gestures and attempts, the prognosis is more guarded.

Discharge planning is based on the following factors:

1. The client's level of recovery at discharge: complete or partial remission
2. Presence or absence of a willing and capable support network: family, significant others, medical/nonmedical individuals/agencies
3. Access to treatment

The nurse keeps individual client and family needs and problems in mind when developing a plan. The following client goals for discharge planning are considered general guidelines:

- The client verbalizes plans for future, with absence of suicidal thoughts or behavior.
- Verbalizes realistic perceptions of self and abilities.
- Relates realistic expectations for self and others.
- Sets realistic attainable goals.
- Identifies psychosocial stressors that may have negative influences, and begins to modify them.
- Describes methods for minimizing stressors.
- States positive methods to cope with threats and stressors.
- Identifies signs and symptoms of disorder.
- Contacts appropriate sources for validation/intervention when necessary.
- Uses learned techniques and strategies to prevent or minimize symptoms.
- Verbalizes knowledge of food-drug and drug-drug interactions and potential problems.
- States therapeutic effects, dose, frequency, untoward effects, and contraindications of medications.
- Makes and keeps follow-up appointments.
- Expresses guilt and anger openly, directly, and appropriately.
- Engages family or significant others as sources of support.
- Structures life to include healthy activities and diversions.

The following boxes provide guidelines for client and family teaching in the management of depression and mania.

CLIENT AND FAMILY TEACHING   Depression

Nurse Needs to Know

- Depression is among the most common psychiatric disorders in adults and can affect all ages.
- Suicide is a fatal outcome of depressed individuals, especially if depression is accompanied by ongoing hopelessness, insomnia, panic disorder, posttraumatic stress disorder (PTSD), bipolar disorder, or alcoholism.
- Most people who are depressed and suicidal are ambivalent about wanting to die and are amenable to nursing interventions that can prevent suicide.
- A brightened affect following a suicide attempt may be a warning that the person's ambivalence has lifted and that the client has made the decision to attempt suicide again.
- Suicidal clients require one-to-one observation by staff until the danger has lifted. The environment must be free of sharps and other harmful objects.
- Onset of depression develops from days to weeks, unlike Alzheimer's disease, which is insidious.
- The most distinguishing symptoms of depression are depressed mood, hopelessness, and loss of interest or pleasure (anhedonia), specifically in things previously enjoyed.
- Symptoms of major depression are physiologic, psychomotor, cognitive, and psychosocial in nature. In general, these systems function at reduced levels during depression.
- Strong neurobiologic and genetic components are connected to depression.
- Psychotic symptoms may be a part of depression, especially delusions and hallucinations, and are usually negative and self-deprecating.
- Antidepressant medications are generally the first method of treatment for major depression, with a 60% to 70%

Teach Client and Family

- Teach the client/family how to identify symptoms of major depression.
- Teach the family to recognize symptoms of suicidal ideation and how to conduct a suicide assessment.
  - Make sure the family has a plan before discharge to contact help.
- Instruct the family not to leave the client alone when he or she is suicidal and to call the physician, hospital, or suicide crisis center immediately because the client may need hospitalization.
- Describe the side effects of antidepressant medications, which begin immediately. Symptom relief takes 3 to 4 weeks, and maximum response is in 8 weeks.
- Emphasize that antidepressants can cause constipation, which may be prevented with a good bowel regimen, adding fiber to the diet, and drinking water.
- Instruct the client/family to check blood pressure periodically because antidepressants may lower the blood pressure. Assure them that some side effects will disappear in time.
- Educate the client/family on specific client behaviors, as appropriate.
  - Clients with sleeping problems may need medication for insomnia.
  - Clients with depressed thoughts may develop suicidal ideation.
  - Clients with major depression may experience early-morning wakening with depressed mood that may lift as the day progresses, possibly a result of biologic disruption in the sleep-wake cycle.
  - In less severe forms of depression, such as dysthymia, clients generally wake up feeling fine but become more depressed throughout the day because of stressors that affect them during the day.

response to drug therapy. Improvement is seen in 3 to 4 weeks.

- Anticholinergic and cardiovascular side effects of antidepressants usually begin immediately.
- Clients may need a bowel regimen, including a high-fiber diet, to prevent constipation.
- Blood pressure must be monitored because many antidepressants have a hypotensive effect.
- Studies reveal a higher rate of treatment success when drugs are combined with psychosocial therapies, such as cognitive-behavioral, family, and group therapies.
- Antipsychotics are given to treat psychotic symptoms in the depressed client with psychotic characteristics.
- Electroconvulsive therapy (ECT) is an effective biologic treatment for major depression but is controversial.
  - Clients and families should be instructed in ECT before its administration. A professional video presentation approved by the client's physician is a useful educational tool.
- Clients with depression generally have a positive outcome and prognosis when treated early and effectively.
- Medication compliance is critical to a positive client outcome.
- Community and personal resources are available for the client and family.
  - Internet resources should be current and accurate.

- Teach the client/family about postpartum depression and its recurring nature, especially if the client is pregnant and has experienced postpartum depression in the past.
- Instruct the family not to take over all aspects of client care after discharge because this may reinforce the client's feelings of inadequacy.
- Tell the family to offer the client some household responsibilities, within the client's level of capability, to promote self-esteem.
- Explain the risks and benefits of other medications if prescribed, such as anxiolytics, antipsychotics, and benzodiazepines.
- Teach the client/family about the benefits and nontherapeutic effects of ECT.
  - Explain the ECT procedure in basic, accurate terms in collaboration with the psychiatrist.
- Explain that good nutrition and exercise are important in the client's overall well-being.
  - Some studies show that exercise improves mood but is not a substitute for treatment.
- Avoid making life changes while the client is experiencing or recovering from depression.
- Inform the client that couples therapy and family counseling can be effective when recovering from depression, and request that a psychiatrist be consulted.
- Emphasize that a depressed person should not be isolated for long periods. Postdischarge plans should include a balance between social activities and solitary pursuits.
- Instruct the client/family that the client should gradually resume normal activities because rushing into activities can result in relapse.
- Teach the client about domestic violence or physical abuse, if warranted, so that immediate help and a safe environment can be arranged. (Follow the domestic violence guidelines in your facility.)
- Teach the client/family how to access community resources and support groups.
- Teach the client/family how to access current educational resources on the Internet.

CLIENT AND FAMILY TEACHING | **Mania**

Nurse Needs to Know
- Prominent symptoms of mania are euphoric, expansive, and irritable mood.
- The defining characteristic of bipolar disorder is one or more manic episodes that may or may not be accompanied by depression.
- Mania may also be accompanied by psychotic symptoms, such as delusions of grandeur, omnipotence, or persecution, which can result in injury or death.

Teach Client and Family
- Teach the client/family how to identify symptoms of mania and hypomania.
- Teach the family how to recognize behaviors that are a danger to the client or others.
  - Make sure the family has a plan before client discharge to contact help.
- Emphasize the importance of medication compliance.

Continued

CLIENT AND FAMILY TEACHING   Mania—cont'd

- Clients with mania often need close monitoring because they may become suicidal or homicidal as a result of their psychosis.
- Episodes of mania in bipolar disorder have a more rapid onset and shorter duration than depressed episodes in major depressive disorders.
- Clients with mania often experience flight of ideas or racing thoughts, which are manifested by rapidly changing topics that may become unintelligible.
- Clients with mania may become angry, insulting, manipulative, sexually explicit, or combative and may need to be secluded/restrained to maintain safety.
- Clients may overspend, gamble, accumulate credit card debts, and place serious financial burden on the family.
- During a manic episode the client may wear inappropriate, bright, garish clothing and excessive makeup and jewelry that may draw ridicule from other clients.
- Hypomania is not a diagnosis but has many of the features of mania, only less severe. The client may not require hospitalization unless the hypomania escalates to a manic state.
- Conversations should be brief because clients in the manic phase may have difficulty concentrating.
- Avoid sensitive, volatile topics that could anger or frustrate the client.
- Serve finger foods or sandwiches that clients can carry with them while moving about the milieu because they may find it difficult to sit down to a meal.
- Serve frequent drinks, especially water, to prevent dehydration because the client's constant motion can lead to perspiration and dehydration.
- Lithium is the drug of choice for mania. It is a natural element and mood stabilizer and requires laboratory workup before administration.
  - Therapeutic effects of lithium are seen in 1 to 2 weeks; therefore other medications (anxiolytics, antipsychotics) may be given initially for a quick response.
  - Lithium has a narrow therapeutic range; therefore it is critical to monitor lithium levels initially every 5 to 6 days and every 6 months for maintenance.
  - Therapeutic lithium levels for acute mania are 0.8 to 1.2 mEq/L, and maintenance levels are 0.8 to 1.0 mEq/L.
  - Lithium is mainly excreted through the kidneys. Clients taking lithium need normal amounts of salt, or the body could take up lithium, resulting in lithium toxicity.
- Valproate (Depakote) is also used as a first-line agent for acute and maintenance treatment of mania.
  - Therapeutic valproate levels are 50 to 125 µg/mg.
  - Valproate carries the risk of liver toxicity.
- Carbamazepine (Tegretol) appears to be effective in both acute and maintenance treatment of mania.

- Explain that the therapeutic effects of lithium will begin in 1 to 2 weeks and that other medications may help control agitation initially.
  - Reinforce the warning that mixing alcohol or other drugs with lithium may worsen the condition and may even be fatal.
- Tell the family that mania often feels good to the client, which may prevent the client from taking medication or seeking treatment.
  - Instruct the client/family about the narrow therapeutic range of lithium/and the importance of having blood drawn regularly to check lithium levels.
  - Discuss the common side effects of lithium, signs of lithium toxicity, and signs that the client is not taking lithium.
- Encourage the family to talk to the client when he or she is not experiencing mania about effective ways to manage mania when it occurs and how to seek help.
- Advise the family that the client may attempt to spend money recklessly and use credit cards during manic episodes so that the family has an opportunity to protect funds.
- Tell the family it is important that the client be given some responsibility to make financial decisions while not in the manic phase so that the client feels empowered.
- Advise the family to keep conversations brief while the client is hypomanic or manic to minimize confusion and frustration for both the client and family.
- Inform the client/family that physical exercise and perspiration due to hot weather could deplete the body of salt and water, leading to lithium toxicity.
  - Explain that drinking large quantities of water can help avoid dehydration and lithium toxicity.
  - Emphasize the use of normal amounts of salt in the client's diet.
- Advise the family to avoid sensitive or volatile topics while the client is in the manic phase to avoid anger or possible violence.
- Help the family to understand that anger directed at them by the client is likely to be transitory and will improve as mania subsides.
- Help the family to understand that the client's superficial, bright mood is often transitory and does not necessarily mean that the client is improving.
- Help the family deal with the client's hyperverbal symptoms.
  - Interrupt in a gentle yet firm manner.
  - Walk away, letting the client know you will return.
- Teach the client/family about alternate medications that may be prescribed to treat mania, including their therapeutic and adverse effects.
- Emphasize the importance of aftercare treatment.
- Teach the client/family how to use available community resources.

- Therapeutic carbamazepine levels are 8 to 12 mg/L.
- Serious adverse effects are associated with carbamazepine therapy.
- Several anticonvulsants are used to treat mania, and some can have serious or even life-threatening effects, especially the rash of Stevens-Johnson syndrome.
- Investigate community/educational/Internet resources for the client and family.

- Teach the client/family how to access reliable Internet resources.

Care Plans

Depression (All Types)
- Risk for Suicide
- Impaired Social Interaction
- Chronic Low Self-Esteem
- Ineffective Coping
- Hopelessness
- Powerlessness
- Self-Care Deficit

Care Plan
DSM-IV-TR Diagnosis **Depression (All Types)**

NANDA Diagnosis: Risk for Suicide
At risk for self-inflicted, life-threatening injury.

Focus:
For the client who is severely depressed, with suicidal ideation, and who threatens suicide and demonstrates suicidal gestures and attempts.

RISK FACTORS

The client has a history of attempts to harm self during depressed episodes.

Demonstrates overt attempts to harm self.
- "Cheeks" and hoards medications.
- Self-mutilates.
- Attempts to hang self.

Verbalizes suicidal ideation or plan.
- "I don't want to live anymore. I'm going to take an overdose of medication."

Expresses sadness, dejection, hopelessness, or loss of pleasure or purpose in life.
- "Nothing gives me any joy. Life just isn't worth living anymore."
- "Everything is hopeless."

Refuses to eat.

Resists or refuses medication and treatments.

Relates inability to see any future for self.

Suddenly gives or wills away possessions.

Frequently tearful, agitated, or morose.

Progressive withdrawal from milieu.

Affect does not brighten as day goes on.

Potentially positive situations, events, or interactions fail to change the client's ideation.

Refuses to sign a "no self-harm" contract or to verbally agree not to harm self.

Expresses loss of self-esteem.
- *Subjective:* "I'm just not worth anything. I don't deserve to live."
- *Objective:* self-care deficit, with impaired grooming, hygiene, and appearance; isolation; and withdrawal.

Shows *ambivalence:* experiencing two opposing feelings, thoughts, drives, or intentions at the same time (wanting to live and wanting to die).

Displays *sudden* mood elevation or calmer, more peaceful manner, with more energy.
- Elevated mood may indicate relief from ambivalent thoughts and feelings about killing self, which is a signal to staff that suicide attempt may be imminent.

OUTCOME IDENTIFICATION AND EVALUATION

The client verbalizes absence of suicidal ideation or plans.
- "I want to live."
- "I no longer think about dying."

Expresses desire to live and lists several reasons for wanting to live.
- "I want to get on with my life."
- "My kids need me and count on me."
- "I have lots of things I want to do for myself and my family."

Displays consistent, optimistic, hopeful attitude.
- Affect appears brighter.
- May smile appropriately.
- Conversation focuses on present activities or future-oriented plans of positive nature.

Makes plans for the future that include follow-up care and medication compliance.
- "My first priority is to go back to work part-time."
- "I'll definitely keep my appointments and take my medications without fail."

Continued

PLANNING AND IMPLEMENTATION

Nursing Intervention	Rationale
Check the client and the client's room for potentially destructive implements: sharp objects, belts, shoelaces, socks, chemicals, hoarded medications.	The nurse's first priority is to provide for the client's safety and protect the client from self-inflicted life-threatening injury or death.
Assess the client's risk for suicide through careful observation of behaviors and direct questioning (asking for suicidal intent and plans). Initiate suicide precautions as needed, according to policy and regulatory standards.	There is always a chance that clients at risk for suicide will act on their thoughts, and studies show that the more detailed the plans, the greater the risk for suicide. A comprehensive assessment helps to identify clients at risk for suicide.
Refrain from judging or preaching to the client or having a shocked facial expression at the client's verbalization of suicidal thoughts, feelings, or intentions. Instead, demonstrate a calm, empathetic, confident attitude.	A judgmental or chastising response may embarrass or humiliate the client and block further disclosure of suicidal thoughts or intent. A calm, caring, confident approach reassures the client that he or she will be helped and protected, and it promotes trust and further communication.
Listen actively to the client's story as to how the client came to the point of suicide, using therapeutic skills such as reflection, clarification, and validation, and indicate acceptance of the client's thoughts and feelings.	Allowing the client to verbalize helps the client relieve pent-up thoughts/feelings/emotions related to suicide and is in itself therapeutic. It also gives the nurse information about the critical events that influenced the client's current level of hopelessness and despair. Acceptance of the client's story promotes trust and instills hope.
Listen to your "gut" feelings, as well as the client's account, in determining suicide ideation. Approach the client in a "neutral" state by managing your own stress and anxiety before attempting to assess the client.	Instinct and experience are often essential elements in assessing a client at risk for suicide. If staff approach the client in a "neutral" or stress-free state, they can better detect distress signals from the client that may indicate suicidal ideation. Then staff can follow through with a treatment plan that provides the necessary elements of safety and protection.
Observe the client for behaviors that are precursors to suicide: threats, gestures, giving away possessions, making a will, leaving a suicide note, obsessing or fantasizing about death, self-deprecating or command hallucinations, delusions of persecution, insomnia with recurring thoughts of suicide, hopelessness.	These behaviors are strong indicators of a client's suicidal ideation and cue the staff to take steps to prevent the client from acting on suicidal thoughts and feelings and to secure the therapeutic environment.
Develop a comprehensive treatment plan consisting of suicide precautions, frequent therapeutic interactions, psychosocial therapies, medication, and continuous reassessment of the client's risk factors and level of hopelessness.	A comprehensive treatment plan that involves all disciplines reassures the client that everything is being done to help and protect the client during times in the illness when the client is feeling out of control and vulnerable.

Client Receiving Electroconvulsive Therapy (ECT)

Inform and educate the client about the benefits and possible side effects of ECT, using current literature that has been approved by the physician and facility and meets regulatory standards.	Suicidal or depressed clients may view ECT as a failure of their responses to other therapeutic interventions. They may also interpret ECT as a "last ditch" effort to become healthy, which may increase their hopelessness. The client may also fear ECT effects; education about ECT dispels myths and allays the client's and family's fears.
An ECT video/disc presentation may be used in the presence of a nurse. It should be approved by the physician and facility and should meet current treatment standards. The client may want the family to view the video/disc as well.	A quality, tasteful ECT video/disc presentation in the presence of a nurse encourages the client and family to ask questions in a safe setting and better prepares them for the procedure.

Client Requiring Seclusion/Restraint (SR)

SR may be used as a least restrictive therapeutic intervention.

SR is used (1) to help clients gain control when suicidal or self-destructive behaviors cannot be helped by other therapeutic interventions and (2) to intervene when clients need immediate protection.

Help the client solve or manage actual and perceived problems one step at a time; *do not give the client false hope.*
- Tell the client you will help the client sort out problems that can be immediately solved: disruptive roommates, completing activities of daily living, arriving at group therapy on time.
- Assist the client to cope with problems that cannot be solved immediately: effects of illness and medications, destructive family environment, long-time issue with a board and care home.
- Inform the client that some problems are temporary (feelings of depression, suicidal ideation) and that with treatment, the client may not always experience such feelings.

A client who is depressed and suicidal may experience increased hopelessness and isolation when problems become overwhelming, which may increase the risk for suicide.
Helping the client sort out problems in a step-by-step manner reduces feelings of aloneness and hopelessness as the client begins to see "light at the end of the tunnel."
Genuine efforts by a caring staff along with education about depression and suicide instill hope in the client that problems can be solved and that the client may not always have the present feelings.
Such powerful interventions may decrease the client's risk for suicide.

Tell the client that staff will protect the client from acting on suicidal thoughts and impulses.
Tell the client to come to staff whenever the client experiences such thoughts or feelings.

Knowing that protection from suicidal thoughts or feelings is always present helps the client gain control over suicidal impulses that may change in intensity throughout the day.
Constant staff support and protection reduce the client's fear of suicidal impulses and offer hope for survival.

Help the client see that suicide is not an alternative to life's problems but is rather a temporary experience often brought about by an actual illness and exacerbated by life stressors.
- Tell the client, "Time is on your side."

Educating the client about the temporary nature/experience of suicide and depression promotes the client's insight about the treatability of the disease process and offers hope for the future.

Structure the client's day hour by hour, adjusting the time to meet the client's needs or level of tolerance.

Structuring the client's day helps to manage the anxiety resulting from overwhelming impulses and assures the client that staff are present, caring, and protective. This also gives staff the opportunity to observe the patient throughout the day.

Client with Paranoid Thoughts and Obsessing/Fantasizing about Suicide/Death

Do not become caught up in the client's paranoia. For example, if the client believes that he or she is being poisoned by some outside force, and that death by suicide is the only answer, it is best to sidestep the paranoid content and focus on the client's fear and anxiety.
Client: "I know they're mixing my medications with poison gas. I'll just have to die to get away from them."
Nurse: "I see how concerned you are; I know you're trying very hard to get through this. Let us help you deal with this, and you won't feel so alone."

Focusing on the client's feelings or intent tells the client that he or she is being understood and valued and that the client does not need to be ashamed or embarrassed by the paranoid thoughts.

Be genuine, empathetic, and caring in discussing the client's feelings about suicidal ideation.
Client: "But Chris killed himself, and he must have known that death was the only escape. He found the answer."

An open, genuine discussion about the client's feelings regarding another client's suicide informs the client that he or she can talk to staff about these topics without fear of being ridiculed or chastised.

Continued

PLANNING AND IMPLEMENTATION—cont'd

Nursing Intervention	Rationale

Client with Paranoid Thoughts and Obsessing/Fantasizing about Suicide/Death—cont'd

Nurse: "Chris killed himself because he was going through a bad time in his depression. We all cared for him, and we care for you, too, and don't want you to die. We'll help you get through this, and we'll keep you safe."	Offering help/support/protection to the client relieves the fear/anxiety related to intrusive thoughts and helps move the client from an unrealistic belief system to a more rational "safe place" with nurturing caregivers who can be trusted.
	Talking openly about the client's fears of "copying" the suicidal behavior of a client who successfully completed suicide defuses such feelings, because the client knows staff are present to listen and give help and protection when needed.

Education and Discharge

Assist the client in maintaining nutritional needs/hygiene/grooming/appearance.	Helping the client with activities of daily living promotes health/safety/dignity/self-esteem when the client is overwhelmed and preoccupied with suicidal thoughts/feelings/impulses.
Praise the client for attempts at positive self-evaluation, self-control, and realistic goal setting. • "Staff agrees with those positive qualities you listed about yourself." • "Your statements in group today were appreciated. We're all glad you are doing better."	Realistic praise promotes the client's self-esteem and provides continued hope for change. This approach also increases the client's focus on the benefits of living.
Educate the client and family about the importance of medication and treatment, and elicit their feedback.	Education promotes client/family treatment, compliance, follow-up care, and safety and helps to prevent rehospitalization.
Continue to assess the client's continuing or decreasing risk for suicide. • Shows improved appetite/hygiene/grooming. • Demonstrates ability to cope with greater stress. • Shows stable medication management. • Sleeps through the night. • Demonstrates reduction/cessation of suicidal talk/obsessions or self-destructive behaviors. • Shows motivation to participate in groups and other milieu activities. • Helps and supports other clients. • Solves problems within capacity, and tolerates unchangeable situations. • Expresses hope for the future. • Defines real plans for the future. • Identifies a support network.	Reassessment of suicidal risk includes keen observations of the client's appearance, talk, and behaviors, which offer clues to suicidal feelings and perceptions. Improvement in all these areas indicates to staff that (1) the client has hope for the future, (2) suicidal ideation is lessening or may be dissolved, and (3) there is a genuine move by the client toward health and recovery.
Contact the client's support system before discharge, including the family, significant others, outpatient program, board and care home, or Independent Living managers, in collaboration with social services and other case managers.	Aftercare support and care are critical to the client's continued feelings of well-being and self-worth. A strong support network lessens feelings of alienation that may be precursors to the client's suicidal ideation. This system acts as a buffer to protect the client from recurring suicidal thoughts and behaviors and may prevent readmission or suicide.
Continue to support and monitor prescribed medical and psychosocial treatment plans.	Postdischarge support helps to maintain the client's safety.

Care Plan
DSM-IV-TR Diagnosis **Depression (All Types)**

NANDA Diagnosis: Impaired Social Interaction
Insufficient or excessive quantity or ineffective quality of social exchange.

Focus:
For the severely depressed client who often finds it difficult to communicate, to attain and maintain relationships, or to engage in a therapeutic alliance.

RELATED FACTORS (ETIOLOGY)

Self-concept disturbance (low self-esteem and self-image)
Depletion of coping skills
Hopelessness
Powerlessness
Negative cognitive patterns: mistrust, ambivalence, delusions of persecution
Knowledge deficit regarding social skills
History of traumatic or unsatisfactory relationships
Insufficient energy to initiate social skills (secondary to depression)
Actual or perceived losses or stressors: breakup of a relationship, change or loss of job/status, death of significant other, altered body image/integrity, financial loss
Recent traumatic event: life-threatening illness
Absence of significant other or peers
Dissatisfaction or change in role or relationship
Social isolation

DEFINING CHARACTERISTICS

The client demonstrates decreased or no participation in activities.
Fails to engage other clients or staff in conversation.
Is unresponsive to others' attempts to initiate communication or to engage the client in activities.
Remains in room most of the day and evening.
Expresses discomfort in social interactions.
- "I'd rather stay in my room than go to group."
- "Don't bother me; I want to be alone."
Shows discomfort in social situations: slumped posture, head down, avoids eye contact, fidgety, restless.
Refuses/resists visits from significant others.
Other clients do not seek the client's company.
Other clients reject the client.
States he or she is unworthy of anyone else's time and company.
Cites lack of energy as reason for nonparticipation.
Claims that attempts at social interactions bring unsatisfactory results.
- "I didn't enjoy the activities at all."
- "The community meeting was a waste of time."
- "I shouldn't have gone bowling in the first place."
Verbalizes inability to achieve a mutual sense of acceptance, caring, or understanding through social interactions.
- "We just didn't get along at all."
- "There was no understanding between us."
- "Our talk was a waste of time."
Resists engaging in a therapeutic alliance with staff.
Demonstrates discomfort and resistance when interacting with staff.

OUTCOME IDENTIFICATION AND EVALUATION

The client engages in therapeutic alliance with staff.
Initiates social interactions with peers and staff.
Participates actively in all milieu and group activities.
Verbalizes satisfaction with social interactions.
- "I really enjoyed our talk."
- "The activity was fun, and everyone got along OK."
Demonstrates comfort and enjoyment during interactions: eye contact, brighter affect, alert responses.
Expresses awareness of some of the problems that precipitated impaired social interactions.
- "I do so much better in group once my medication begins to take effect."
- "I should do my one-to-one talks with my nurse later in the day, when I feel better."

PLANNING AND IMPLEMENTATION

Nursing Intervention	Rationale
Continue to engage client in interactions.	Clients with depression resist becoming involved in a therapeutic alliance, which necessitates acceptance and persistence.
Actively listen, observe, and respond to the client's verbal and nonverbal expressions.	Active listening lets clients know they are worthwhile and respected. The client will be encouraged to continue seeking out others.
Initiate brief, frequent contacts with the client throughout the day.	Frequent contact tells the client that he or she is an important part of the milieu and encourages the client to participate, at whatever level. Brief contacts are better tolerated by clients with depression.

Continued

PLANNING AND IMPLEMENTATION—cont'd

Nursing Intervention	Rationale
Remain with the client even if he or she does not engage in conversation, and offer brief, accepting comments. • "Good morning. I see you are unable to participate today." • "I'll just sit here with you for 15 minutes."	The client who is severely depressed and energy depleted may be unable to engage in conversation. The presence of a concerned caregiver offers the client comfort and security and increases self-worth.
Use a low-key, matter-of-fact approach when offering the client simple choices.	A nondemanding approach avoids threatening clients with expectations they cannot meet.
Therapeutic Response • "Good morning. It's 8 o'clock, and breakfast stops being served in the dining room at 8:30."	Offering choices gives clients a sense of having some control over the situation.
Nontherapeutic Response "It's 8 o'clock. You should be up and dressed by now. Everyone in the dining room is waiting for you."	Critical statements can promote feelings of failure and inadequacy by blaming clients for the inability to exercise control over their behavior.
Encourage the client to ask for assistance when necessary.	Clients need to understand that they must interact with nurse and staff to have their needs met.
Refrain from overzealous behaviors. • Lifting up window shades or pulling back curtains to "let the sunshine in the room." • Delivering excessively cheerful greetings, such as "Time to rise and shine." or "It's a beautiful day."	Clients become overwhelmed in the presence of such cheery behavior and feel more despondent when they cannot meet or match the nurse's affect and demeanor.
Initially comment on neutral topics or subjects of common interest (items in the room, daily news topics, the menu).	Usually, social conversation initially helps establish rapport and aids the client in making the transition toward therapeutic communication.
Gradually engage the client in interactions with other clients, beginning with one-to-one contacts, progressing toward informal gatherings, and eventually participating in structured group activities, with occupational therapy first, then recreational therapy.	Clients experience success when social interactions are pursued in relation to their level of tolerance (simple to complex or structured to less structured).
Suggest journal writing as a means to recount successful social interactions when they occur and feelings provoked by social experiences.	Writing about interactive experiences in a log or journal reinforces repetition of successful behaviors, promotes awareness of feelings, and gives the client more opportunity to manage social encounters because responses are expected and less traumatic.
Encourage phone calls and visits with supportive significant persons.	Social contact reinforces rewarding, supportive relationships.
Help the client identify the value of attendance at meals, activities, group outings, and other social situations.	Efforts toward human contact are important, even though enjoyment cannot yet be attained.
Make available those activities that the client finds rewarding and satisfying.	Activities that interest the client are more apt to provide enjoyment, which acts as a catalyst for future social interactions.
Explore with the client alternative social interactions that may be more appropriate and effective.	Often, clients continue to utilize ineffective methods of interacting because change is difficult and results are uncertain.
Practice with the client alternative interactive techniques in a safe setting, while offering tactful but honest feedback.	Role playing and constructive criticism in a safe setting provide the client with the confidence to try learned skills with others in the environment.
Discuss with the client the responses of other clients to the client's interactions (when client is ready for such feedback).	Such discussion allows clients to evaluate realistically and accept the effects of their behaviors on others, whether negative or positive.

Help the client set realistic goals and limits in interactions with others.

Inform the client that all needs will NOT be met through interactions.

Encourage the client to set specific times for interactions with staff.

Encourage the client to give and accept appropriate praise and compliments during social exchanges.

Teach the client to challenge irrational beliefs about self and capabilities and to replace them with a more realistic view of self and abilities. (see cognitive and rational-emotive therapies, Appendix B).

Develop a written or verbal contract with the client, emphasizing interactive goals.

Emphasize the importance of group involvement, such as psychosocial therapies, outings, and group activities (see Appendix B).

Conduct a suicide assessment as necessary.

Teach the client and family that the therapeutic effects of antidepressant medications may take up to 2 weeks but that uncomfortable effects may begin immediately.

Continue to support and monitor prescribed medical and psychosocial treatment plans.

Limit setting helps the client develop more realistic expectations of self and others.

Such information helps to promote realistic expectations and outcomes.

Setting times for staff contact helps the client to accomplish positive self-generated interactions.

Giving and accepting positive feedback helps to ensure mutually satisfying social interactions.

A more realistic view of self gives the client more confidence in social interactions.

A goal-directed contact reminds the client of basic expectations for interacting in the milieu.

A variety of social situations helps the client gain support from others, learn social skills vicariously, and see that the client's problems and concerns are similar to those of others.

An effective suicide assessment may prevent harm, injury, or death (see suicide risk care plan on p. 77).

The client and family need to know that the mood will not lift immediately and that adverse effects may initially be troublesome for the client.

Support after discharge promotes the client's self-confidence and hope for the future.

Care Plan
DSM-IV-TR Diagnosis | **Depression (All Types)**

NANDA Diagnosis: Chronic Low Self-Esteem
Long-standing negative self-evaluation/feelings about self or self-capabilities.

Focus:
For the client with pervasive low self-esteem derived from negative, unrealistic values that the individual ascribes to self-concept (idea, belief, or mental image a person has of self, based on perceived strengths, weaknesses, and status). The person with low self-esteem thinks, feels, and behaves as if unworthy and incapable of achieving or performing at a level consistent with own expectations or those of others.

RELATED FACTORS (ETIOLOGY)
Long-standing unrealistic perceptions and irrational assumptions about self or situations
Neglectful, abusive, domineering, overprotective relationships
Identity problems (self, sexual)

Negative body image, actual or perceived
Doubt concerning self-worth and abilities
Consistent rejection by others
Unresolved losses, actual or perceived
Role dissatisfaction
Situational crises
Goal obstacles
Psychosocial stressors
Biologic factors (neurophysiologic, genetic, structural)

DEFINING CHARACTERISTICS
The client fails to attend to appearance/hygiene.
Has weight problems.
Demonstrates difficulty communicating or interacting with others: poor eye contact, reticent, paucity of speech, soft or inaudible voice.
Ruminates and repeats statements about negative thoughts/situations/experiences.

Continued

Expresses incompetence/inadequacy/failure/inability to deal with situations.
- "I'm a flop at everything I try to do."
- "I can't do anything right."
- "I'm a failure at life."
- "I can't handle anything."

Expresses shame or guilt.
- "I'm so ashamed of myself for being such a failure."
- "I'm responsible for all this misfortune."

Displays excessive shyness.

Rejects positive comments and attention from others.

Exaggerates negative feedback about self.

Demonstrates inability to make decisions.

Fears trying new things or situations.

Demonstrates anxious behaviors.

Is overly sensitive to critical appraisal.

Continually asks for approval from others concerning self or capabilities.

OR

Completely avoids interactions regarding self-context.

Delusional thinking and expressions (see Glossary for examples).

Expresses/shows suicidal ideation.

OUTCOME IDENTIFICATION AND EVALUATION

The client demonstrates self-care (appearance/hygiene) appropriate for age and status.

Initiates conversation with staff and others.

Demonstrates absence of self-deprecating statements.

Verbalizes realistic positive statements about self and others.
- "I've always gotten along well with people."
- "Everyone here is nice to me."

Stands and walks with a self-assured demeanor.

Begins projects and activities without encouragement.

Discusses negative mind-set, irrational beliefs, and values with staff.

Uses techniques (deep-breathing relaxation exercises) to decrease anxiety (see Appendix B).

Acknowledges encouragement from others.

Accepts suggestions for strategies to increase esteem and assertiveness.
- Attends assertiveness training and cognitive therapy sessions.

Practices techniques for increasing esteem and assertiveness.
- Asks for assistance when necessary.
- Asserts self to have needs met.
- Speaks in clear audible tones.
- Replaces negative self-deprecating thoughts with realistic thinking.

Demonstrates absence of delusions.

Verbalizes will to live/reasons for living/plans for future.

PLANNING AND IMPLEMENTATION

Nursing Intervention	Rationale
Encourage the client to wash, dress, comb hair, and use appropriate toiletries.	The act of attending to grooming and the results increase confidence and esteem.
Praise the client for all attempts at engaging staff appropriately.	Positively rewarded behavior tends to be perpetuated, which helps the client to distinguish between self-defeating and self-enhancing socialization.
Engage the family in plans to give genuine praise to the client when warranted.	Some families need reminders to support one another. Positive strokes from significant others greatly increase the client's self-worth/esteem.
Keep all appointments with the client.	Keeping appointments increases the client's sense of importance/worth/esteem.
Teach the client assertiveness skills, such as use of "I" messages, how to say "no," and how to have needs met in an appropriate way. (see assertiveness training, Appendix B).	Becoming assertive helps the client have needs met, gives the client a sense of control over life, and brings respectful regard from others.
Encourage the client to identify positive aspects of self by different methods (verbalize, write, draw). • "You have talked about some of the things you like about yourself today. Sometimes making lists helps in thinking of more positive qualities. If you make a list or write about your good qualities in a daily journal or log, we can discuss it during our meeting tomorrow."	The more the client expresses positive aspects of self, the less likely the client is to focus on negative aspects.

Irrational Belief System	
Listen to the client's expression of beliefs.	The client will let go of irrational beliefs and behaviors
Allow the client to vent feelings.	when a more realistic awareness of self is established.
Accept the client's feelings without judging or shutting out	The client's realistic self-awareness develops gradually
the client because of your discomfort.	through talking with a therapeutic listener who is
Encourage the client to explore alternatives and other	knowledgeable about cognitive-behavioral skills.
perspectives about self.	
Respectfully confront persistent irrational convictions.	
Encourage thought-stopping and thought-substituting	
techniques (see Appendix B).	
Replace irrational thoughts with realistic ones.	

Client with Delusions	
State your reality, giving accurate information.	Discussing interpretations of reality and focusing on
Do not ask for detailed explanations regarding the delusion;	the client's *feelings* about the delusion help the client
focus on feelings engendered by the delusion, *not* the content.	correct distorted perceptions.
Do not argue with the client about the delusion, regardless	These approaches present reality to the client in a
of its absurdity.	nonthreatening way.
Discuss realistic interpretations or possible alternatives to	
perceptions.	
Present realistic activities and projects in which the client	Graded activities that allow success raise the client's
can succeed.	confidence and esteem.
Recognize the client's anxiety, and encourage techniques to	Anxiety-reducing strategies calm the client and better
control anxiety, such as deep-breathing/relaxation	prepare the client to accomplish tasks that will build
exercises (see Appendix B).	self-esteem.
Praise the client's acceptance of compliments and	Praise and encouragement from others reinforce
encouragement from others.	self-esteem.
Encourage participation in group activities and therapies	The client experiences the curative factors of groups: altruism,
(see Appendix B).	unconditional acceptance, catharsis, instillation of hope.
	The client sees that he or she is not the only person with a
	problem.

Statements of Suicide	
Encourage the client to discuss thoughts and feelings about	Openly discussing suicidal thoughts and feelings with a
wanting to die.	caring staff helps the client feel valued and accepted,
Discuss the client's plan, if any.	which is a major step toward increasing hope and
Explore alternatives.	self-worth (see suicide risk care plan on p. 77).
Reinforce statements regarding will to live and plans for future.	
Continue to support and monitor prescribed medical and	Continued support reinforces the client's progress toward
psychosocial treatment plans.	reestablishing self-esteem.

Care Plan
DSM-IV-TR Diagnosis **Depression (All Types)**

NANDA Diagnosis: Ineffective Coping
Inability to form a valid appraisal of the stressors; inadequate choices of practiced responses; or inability to use available resources.

Focus:
For the client who is depressed and has decreased energy, for whom the tasks of coping with the disorder and meeting the requirements of daily living exceed capabilities. Therefore the individual may resort to coping methods that are maladaptive.

RELATED FACTORS (ETIOLOGY)
Situational crisis
Personal vulnerability

Continued

RELATED FACTORS (ETIOLOGY)—cont'd

Ineffective support system, actual or perceived
- Absent, neglectful, or overprotective parents

Dysfunctional family system
- Alcoholic parents or spouse
- Domineering or abusive role models
- History of sexual molestation

Unresolved grief or anger

Negative cognitive patterns: self-deprecating or
    self-persecutory thoughts

Unrealistic or irrational self-perception

Unmet or unrealistic goals

Disturbance in self-concept: feelings of worthlessness or
    inadequacy

History of multiple stressors over time
- Job or financial loss
- Breakup of relationship
- Death of significant other

Decisional conflict

Hopelessness

Powerlessness

Role dysfunction

DEFINING CHARACTERISTICS

The client expresses an inability to cope or to ask for help.
- "I don't know how I'll get through this."
- "I can't take the stress any more."
- "Who can I turn to?"

Frequently cries with no obvious provocation.

Demonstrates depletion of coping resources.
- "I'd be better off dead."

Expresses suicidal ideation or makes gestures and
    attempts.

Exhibits problem grouping (stating several problems
    together).
- "I can't hold a job."
- "My wife and kids have left me."
- "There's nowhere for me to live."
- "My doctor is fed up with me."

Ineffective use of coping methods.
- Is unable to express or resolve anger or grief.
- Directs feelings toward self.
- Blames others for illness and hospitalization.
- Regresses to earlier stages of development.
- Seeks help for simple tasks.
- Fails to meet basic grooming and hygiene needs.

Verbalizes delusions.
- "I'm going to die soon because I don't deserve to
    live."
- "There's no need to eat because I don't have any
    insides."

Verbalizes self-deprecating thoughts.
- "I'm a failure at everything I do."
- "I'm a terrible person."
- "I'm a bad parent."

- "I'm no good to anyone anymore."

Displays social isolation and withdrawal.
- Spends most of the time in bed or room.
- Resists interacting with staff or clients.
- Refuses to attend meetings and activities.

Fails to assert self to meet own needs.

Demonstrates ineffective problem-solving and decision-
    making skills.

Fails to make decisions regarding care and treatment.
- "I can't decide if I should stay with my family or move into
    a board and care home."
- "I can't decide what to do first: get a job or begin day
    treatment."

Shows impaired judgment and insight.
- "I stopped taking my antidepressants because I felt
    drowsy."
- "I was doing OK before I came in here."

OUTCOME IDENTIFICATION AND EVALUATION

The client verbalizes ability to cope in accordance with age
    and status.
- "I think I'll be able to handle my responsibilities when I
    go back home."

Demonstrates effective problem-solving and decision-
    making skills.
- "I've made up my mind to see my kids once every 2 weeks
    instead of every week for now."
- "I've decided to walk every morning before breakfast for
    my daily exercise."

Verbalizes increased insight and judgment.
- "I tend to get sick when I do too much, so I'll take one day
    at a time."
- "I know if I continue to take my medicine, I will do
    better."

Demonstrates effective coping strategies.
- Does not blame or accuse others for own
    problems.
- Does not become angry or make hostile remarks.
- Displaces feelings appropriately (talking,
    exercising).

Exhibits self-restraint and control in situations that
    previously invoked crying spells.

Demonstrates effective prioritizing of problems.
- "I think I'll get back on my feet before I take on
    parenthood."

Expresses sense of self-worth.
- "I deserve the love of my family and friends."
- "I'm worth being helped."

Verbalizes realistic thoughts and situations about
    self.
- "Everything hasn't been perfect, but my family is still
    together and love one another."
- "I didn't get to be supervisor, but at least I'll have time to
    pursue that poetry I'm writing."

Demonstrates absence of delusions.

Verbalizes feelings of hopefulness.

- "Things seem to be getting better each day."
- "I can't wait to see my new grandchild."

Verbalizes sense of power and control.

- "I know now I can do many things to prevent becoming so depressed."

Demonstrates absence of suicidal thoughts and actions.

PLANNING AND IMPLEMENTATION

Nursing Intervention	Rationale
Encourage the client to focus on strengths rather than weaknesses.	The client becomes aware of positive qualities and capabilities that have helped the client cope in the past.
Help the client identify individuals who help the client to cope and who support the client's strengths. • "I notice you seem more relaxed during your sister's visits." • "You seem upset each time your friend calls. I'm here if you want to talk about it."	The client becomes more aware of the positive effect of supportive individuals in the client's life, increasing the client's confidence in own coping abilities.
Assist the client to learn strategies that promote more positive thinking, such as cognitive-behavioral techniques or guided imagery (see Appendix B).	Therapeutic modalities can help the client replace or substitute irrational self-deprecating thoughts/images with more rational beliefs/images.
Help the client to prioritize problems. • Assist the client to list problems from most urgent to least urgent. • Assist the client to find immediate solutions for the most troubling problems. • Postpone problems that can be addressed later. • Delegate some problems to significant others. • Acknowledge problems beyond the client's control.	Listing problems in priority helps to reduce their overwhelming effects and breaks them into more manageable increments. The ability to manage problems is a major step toward effective coping.
Respond to the client's persistent self-deprecation with realistic, nonchallenging evidence. • "Your children phone you every day." • "I enjoyed reading your poems." • "I like the color of your shirt."	Pointing out contradictions to the client's self-deprecation in a calm, nonchallenging way encourages the client to focus on positive aspects of self and minimizes self-deprecation.
Respond to delusional statements by stating your reality of the situation without arguing about the client's reality.	The client may not be able to cope with reality at this time, and challenging the delusion may decrease the client's self-esteem and increase self-doubt.
Praise the client for adaptive coping: making rational decisions based on accurate judgment, solving own problems, and demonstrating independence.	Genuine praise emphasizes the client's adaptive behaviors and encourages their continuance through positive reinforcement.
Teach the client basic assertiveness skills (see Appendix B).	The use of healthy assertiveness assists the client in having needs met, coping with demands of the environment, and building confidence.
Encourage the client to describe his or her role performance (family member, student, employee) and the satisfaction it brings the client and significant others.	Discussing the client's role performance and resulting satisfaction promotes more functional role adaptation.
Encourage the client to discuss feelings generated by ineffective coping (frustration, anger, inadequacy). • "It's OK to talk about your feelings. It helps you work through your problems."	Acceptance of feelings without judgment or retaliation helps the client externalize emotions that may be a source of depression.
Teach family and friends that the client may direct anger toward them but that the client is learning more constructive methods to deal with feelings.	Family members who are well informed are better able to use their energies to support the client rather than focus on their own reactions.

Continued

PLANNING AND IMPLEMENTATION—cont'd

Nursing Intervention	Rationale
Help family members cope with the client's troubling behaviors by including them in those areas of the treatment plan that are relevant to them.	Families who are aware of effective coping methods are more empowered and better able to manage family-client interactions.
Assist the client to increase socialization and involvement in activities according to level of tolerance.	Socialization provides opportunities to practice coping skills while reducing isolation.
Conduct a suicide assessment as needed.	An effective suicide assessment can prevent harm, injury, or death (see suicide risk care plan on p. 77).
Continue to support the client and monitor prescribed medical/psychosocial treatment plans.	Support after discharge builds hope and may prevent rehospitalization or suicide.

Care Plan

DSM-IV-TR Diagnosis | **Depression (All Types)**

NANDA Diagnosis: Hopelessness

Subjective state in which an individual sees limited or no alternatives or personal choices available and is unable to mobilize energy on own behalf.

Focus:

For the client who experiences a sense of futility about his or her situation and the environment and thus perceives that life holds no meaning.

RELATED FACTORS (ETIOLOGY)

Illness progression despite compliance with therapy
Long-term stressors
Illness-related regimen
Abandonment/isolation
Ineffective individual coping
Chronic low self-esteem
Fear/anxiety regarding illness/outcome of illness

DEFINING CHARACTERISTICS

The client verbalizes that life situation status seems hopeless or futile.
• "There's no sense in even trying."
• "I can't do anything about it."
Demonstrates frequent sighing and despondent content.
Demonstrates decreased or absent verbalizations.
Displays decreased saddened, flat, or blunted affect.
Withdraws from the environment.
Engages in behavioral demonstrations (turning away from speaker, closed eyes, lack of eye contact, shrugging shoulders).

Displays persistent despondent or "blue" mood or sense of impending doom.
Has physiologic symptoms of anxiety (tachycardia, tachypnea).
Displays decreased or absent appetite.
Increases sleep time.
Demonstrates lack of involvement in care.
Is passively receptive to care.
Demonstrates lack of involvement or interest in significant others.

OUTCOME IDENTIFICATION AND EVALUATION

The client expresses hopeful thoughts and feelings.
• "My future looks brighter now."
• "I feel more positive about my life."
Demonstrates hopeful, enthusiastic attitude and behaviors (erect posture, good eye contact, cheerful voice tone).
Participates willingly in daily activities and self-care.
Exhibits brightened affect with broad range of expressions (smiles/laughs appropriately).
Engages in positive relationships with significant others or identified support persons.
Sets attainable goals that indicate hope for the immediate future.
Uses effective coping methods to counteract feelings of hopelessness.
• Talks out feelings with staff.
• Exercises daily.
• Shares concerns with other clients in group meetings.

PLANNING AND IMPLEMENTATION

Nursing Intervention	Rationale
Conduct a suicide assessment, asking the client for plans, method, and access to method (see suicide risk care plan on p. 77).	Hopelessness, especially if more pronounced, is a major risk factor in suicidal ideation and must be addressed.
Encourage the client to verbalize feelings of hopelessness/despondency/aloneness.	The client has the opportunity to vent and explore feelings realistically.
Identify positive aspects in the client's world. • "Your family phones the hospital every day to ask about you." • "I see you washed your hair today, and you're wearing a new shirt." • "The clients in group responded favorably to your comments."	Reflecting appreciation of the client's progress and participative efforts by staff/family/supportive peers conveys hope and reduces alienation.
Assist the client to identify behaviors that promote hopelessness: morbid conversations, dwelling on negative ideas, avoiding interactions with staff, decreased participation in activities, procrastination.	This type of explanation helps the client develop an awareness of experiences that perpetuate negative themes.
Teach the client to construct pleasant thoughts and images to combat hopelessness (see Appendix B). • Being with a supportive person. • Recalling a previous successful experience. • Setting a future attainable goal.	Pleasant and positive thoughts/ideas/images tend to inhibit or reduce the intensity of unpleasant negative experiences and to offer hope.
Encourage the client to engage in experiences that promote positive thoughts and feelings. • Communicate with staff. • Participate in activities. • Share experiences in supportive groups. • Phone concerned family members.	These types of supportive activities tend to discourage and interrupt hopelessness and alienation.
Offer genuine praise for the client's efforts toward setting goals, initiating self-care, and participating in activities.	Praise promotes continuance of positive behaviors and decreases hopelessness and alienation.
Inform the family that the client needs unconditional love, support, and encouragement.	Families have the power to give clients hope and strength through their unconditional love and acceptance.
Continue to support and monitor prescribed medical and psychosocial treatment plans.	Continued support, especially after discharge, builds hope and may prevent rehospitalization or suicide.

Care Plan
DSM-IV-TR Diagnosis **Depression (All Types)**

NANDA Diagnosis: Powerlessness
Perception that one's own actions will not significantly affect an outcome; a perceived lack of control over a current situation or immediate happening.

Focus:
For the client who perceives that he or she can do nothing to change negative thoughts, feelings, behaviors, or circumstances.

RELATED FACTORS (ETIOLOGY)

Lifestyle of learned helplessness
Reaction to chronic recurrent illness

Illness progression despite compliance with treatment
Health care environment despite therapeutic value
Hopelessness
Ineffective coping
Impaired internal locus of control
Unmet role expectations, perceived or actual

DEFINING CHARACTERISTICS

The client makes verbal expressions of having no control or influence over a situation or outcome.
• "Nothing I do will improve my situation."
• "I can't do one thing that will make my life better."

Continued

Demonstrates behaviors that reflect a loss of control over self and environment.
- Is apathetic toward staff/other clients/environment.
- Fails to assert self to have needs met.
- Allows other clients to dominate/intimidate self.
- Allows staff to make basic decisions, (e.g., when to dress, what to wear, what to eat).

Expresses despair over illness and inability to see a way out of it or to help self become healthy despite compliance with treatment.

Fails to participate in activities or meetings despite staff support and coaxing.

Verbalizes dissatisfaction and disgust over inability to perform previous tasks, skills, or activities.
- "I used to be so good at sports. Now I don't have the energy to play Ping-Pong."

Expresses serious doubts regarding role and role performance.
- "I'm not sure what my function is or what purpose I serve."
- "My kids always turned to me for help. Now I'm useless to them."
- "I've been a big disappointment to my friends."

Demonstrates dependence on others that may result in irritability/resentment/anger/guilt.

Accepts without resistance decisions made for the client by staff and significant others.

Fails to defend self/ideas/opinions in favor of others when challenged.

Demonstrates apathy or indifference about decreased energy level.

OUTCOME IDENTIFICATION AND EVALUATION

The client verbalizes feeling in control of self and situations.
- "I was a help to my team in the volleyball game."
- "It was tense in group when John got upset, but I handled it OK."

Questions or challenges decisions being made on his or her behalf.
- "I'm sure I want to go back to live in that place."
- "I want to know more about this medication."

Makes choices regarding management of care.
- "I can do my own laundry."
- "I prefer to attend the assertiveness training class today."

Verbalizes more realistic role expectations and goals for meeting them.
- "I think I'll see my kids once a week instead of every day, and try not to do so much."
- "I'm ready for a part-time job, but I can't manage full-time work right now."

Demonstrates internal locus of control by taking responsibility for care/situation/outcome.
- "I know I can help myself by taking my medications regularly."
- "I think I can keep a part-time job if I get help as soon as I begin to feel bad."

PLANNING AND IMPLEMENTATION

Nursing Intervention	Rationale
Observe for behaviors that indicate the client's sense of futility: shrugging shoulders, slouched posture, head lowered, lack of eye contact, isolating self from others and activities.	Early observations of cues to powerlessness give the nurse an opportunity to intervene in the process before the client's sense of powerlessness becomes overwhelming.
Identify situations and events that contribute to the client's sense of powerlessness.	Early identification helps the nurse to avoid or minimize situations and events that are out of the client's control.
Accept the client's expressions of powerlessness without indicating that the perceptions are correct. • "I understand that you think you have nothing to say in group, but your attendance is still wanted." • "You're saying you can't play volleyball, but I noticed you got the ball over the net several times."	Acceptance of the client's feelings and thoughts while focusing on behavior and capabilities builds trust and helps the client develop awareness of his or her strengths.
Assess the client's response to the treatment plan. • Is the client passively compliant? • Is the client willingly compliant and knowledgeable about the purpose of treatment?	Passive compliance indicates powerlessness. Clients who are involved in their care and attempt to understand the reasons behind it are seeking more control over their illness and outcome.
Identify factors that may contribute to the client's loss of control: new environment, rules/regulations, sharing space, uncertainty about outcomes.	If the nurse knows the factors that provoke the client's powerlessness, a plan can be formulated to reduce or minimize contributing factors.

Help the client identify aspects of life that the client can control and to cope more effectively with aspects the client cannot change.	Realistic appraisal helps the client better understand how to achieve successful outcomes, and it reduces frustration and powerlessness.
Explore with the client areas in life that the client has mastered successfully.	Recalling past successes encourages future attempts to gain or regain control in a positive way.
Provide opportunities for the client to exercise control in situations that the client can manage. • Allow the client to decide placement of items in room. • Give the client choices of food. • Allow the client to decide where to sit at meetings.	Positive reinforcement promotes healthy feelings of power and control.
Do not offer choices where none exists (whether to take medications/engage in therapeutic activities).	Choices should not include opportunities that interfere with the client's treatment plan.
Reduce or eliminate unnecessary restrictions whenever possible and safe.	Having fewer unnecessary restrictions promotes the client's sense of control.
Identify the client's use of manipulative behavior, and note its effect on other clients.	Clients may resort to manipulative methods to manage powerlessness because of distrust of others or fear of interpersonal closeness.
Encourage the client to express needs openly. Discuss ways needs can be met without using manipulation (see assertiveness training, Appendix B).	Giving the client permission to express needs openly teaches the client to use positive strategies to promote control rather than manipulation.
Discuss with interdisciplinary staff the importance of giving the client control.	A team effort to give the client as much control as possible over treatment provides a consistent approach to care and enhances the client's power.
Assist the family with ideas and methods that empower the client in the home environment.	Family involvement promotes consistency in the treatment plan and assures the client that he or she has control over specific aspects of life.
Recognize when the client begins to take responsibility for self and outcome ("I could prevent this by taking my medication regularly") rather than seeing self as a victim of circumstances ("Everything happens to me").	Such admissions indicate that the client is developing an internal locus of control rather than attributing experiences to external sources.
Add responsibilities as the client progresses in self-care (assign one or two tasks per week).	Added responsibilities further develop the client's internal locus of control.
Provide the client with a daily written schedule of activities in which the client is expected to participate.	The client's contribution in the milieu increases feelings of power over the situation and outcome.
Assist the client to set attainable short-term goals. • Attend a meeting once a day for 1 week. • Be on time for each meal for 1 week.	Short-term goals ensure achievement and promote a sense of control.
Continue to support and monitor prescribed medical and psychosocial treatment plans.	Postdischarge monitoring supports the client's efforts to regain control over life.

Care Plan
DSM-IV-TR Diagnosis | **Depression (All Types)**

NANDA Diagnosis: Self-Care Deficit
Impaired ability to perform or complete feeding/bathing/toileting/dressing/grooming activities for self.

Focus:

For the client whose emotional or mental health is compromised to the extent that the client cannot provide for basic self-care needs.

Continued

RELATED FACTORS (ETIOLOGY)

Depressed mood
Hyperactivity/distractibility (e.g., as in mania)
Decreased activity/energy
Apathy/withdrawal
Extreme/continuous anxiety
Perceptual/cognitive impairment
Developmental lag

DEFINING CHARACTERISTICS

The client demonstrates inability to maintain appearance at satisfactory, age-appropriate level: unkempt hair/clothing/appearance.
Displays inadequate personal hygiene: foul body/mouth odor.

Demonstrates infrequent, ineffective bathing/showering.
Displays inadequate toileting (urine/stool stains found on undergarments).
Fails to launder clothing.
Repeatedly wears soiled clothing.
Has unshaven facial hair (male).
No longer uses makeup (female).

OUTCOME IDENTIFICATION AND EVALUATION

The client consistently performs self-care activities consistent with ability/health status/developmental stage.
- Bathes/dresses/grooms/brushes teeth/toilets/launders clothes.

PLANNING AND IMPLEMENTATION

Nursing Intervention	Rationale
Continue to assess the extent to which self-care deficits interfere with the client's functions.	Ongoing assessment of the client's functional abilities helps to determine the client's strengths, as well as areas that require assistance.
Assist with personal hygiene, appropriate dress, grooming, and laundering until the client can function independently.	Personal hygiene assistance helps to preserve the client's dignity and self-esteem.
Reduce environmental stimulation such as noise, lights, bright colors, and people during self-care activity times, especially for clients with hyperactivity, mania, anxiety, and perceptual-cognitive impairments.	A quieter environment is more soothing to the senses and tends to decrease the client's anxiety to allow better concentration on tasks.
Make available only the clothing that the client will wear; add more clothing as the client's judgment and attention span improve.	Reducing the number of choices minimizes the client's confusion and simplifies the selection process.
Provide clean clothing/grooming/toileting supplies as needed; obtain the client's own clothing and supplies as quickly as possible.	The client feels more comfortable and less confused if personal supplies are available.
Establish routine goals for self-care: bathe or shower each day, brush teeth twice daily, comb hair every morning, wash clothes twice a week. Add more complex tasks and increase frequency as the client's condition improves.	Routine and structure organize the client's chaotic world and promote success.
Initiate grooming and hygiene tasks when the client is best able to comply.	Depressed clients have more energy and brighter affect later in the day, and clients with anxiety and hyperactive behaviors are more attentive to self-care after taking medication.
Encourage the client to initiate the activity of grooming even when unwilling.	The act of grooming and its results can influence the client's attitude in a positive way.
Provide privacy during self-care consistent with safety factors.	Providing as much privacy as possible helps to preserve the client's dignity.
Ensure that the client is clean and well groomed.	A neat appearance prevents the embarrassment and emotional/physical trauma that result from being an object of ridicule.

Praise the client for attempts at self-care and each successfully completed task.	Positive reinforcement increases feelings of self-worth and promotes continuity of functional behaviors.
Teach the family the importance of promoting the client's self-care abilities.	Family involvement provides continuity between the hospital and home environment and ensures the client's progress while decreasing dependency.
Continue to support and monitor prescribed medical and psychosocial treatment plans.	Supporting ongoing therapies encourages the client to maintain self-care routines.

Care Plans

Mania (All Types)
- Risk for Self-Directed/Other-Directed Violence
- Risk for Injury
- Impaired Social Interaction
- Disturbed Thought Processes
- Defensive Coping
- Imbalanced Nutrition: Less than Body Requirements

Care Plan
DSM-IV-TR Diagnosis | **Mania (All Types)**

NANDA Diagnosis: Risk for Self-Directed/Other-Directed Violence

At risk for behaviors in which an individual demonstrates that he or she can be physically/emotionally/sexually harmful to self or others.

Focus:

For the client with mania whose negative, uncontrolled thoughts/feelings/behaviors pose a threat or danger to self or others.

RISK FACTORS

The client has history of attempts to harm self or assault others during manic phase.

Has history of another's death as a result of client's abuse.

Has history of substance use/abuse.

Makes overt attempts to harm self or assault others.

Verbalizes intent to harm self or assault others.

Demonstrates aggressive behaviors and mannerisms: hits/kicks objects, clenched fists, rigid posture, taut facial muscles.

Exhibits increasing motor activity with agitation: paces back and forth, bumps into furniture/objects/people.

Scans environment with angry/startled/frightened facial expression.

States that others in the environment are threatening or planning to harm or kill self.

Verbalizes that he or she is omnipotent or destructive.

Demonstrates inability to exercise self-control.

States feeling threatened/closed in/crowded.

OUTCOME IDENTIFICATION AND EVALUATION

Verbalizes ability to recognize and describe early symptoms of escalating anxiety/agitation that may lead to violence, and takes necessary steps to interrupt them.

Demonstrates absence of verbal intentions to harm self or assault others.

Demonstrates absence of violent or aggressive behaviors.

PLANNING AND IMPLEMENTATION

Nursing Intervention	Rationale
Conduct an assault risk and self-harm assessment.	An early comprehensive assessment of self-harm or assault risk behaviors may prevent harm or injury.
Listen for verbal threats or hostile remarks directed toward self or others. • "I hate you. I could just kill you." • "Maybe we would be better off dead." • "Mark is terrible. I wish he would die." Look for aggressive gestures toward self or others. • Client clenches fists. • Strikes out as if to hurt someone. • Bangs fist or head against a wall. Observe for any physical contact that is unwanted by others. • Client slaps another person on the back in a hurtful way.	The client's verbal threats, physical contact, and acting out may be precursors or cues to impending violence.

Continued

PLANNING AND IMPLEMENTATION—cont'd

Nursing Intervention	Rationale

- Hugs others in the milieu in a manic frenzy.
- Puts arm around another client's shoulder.
- Sits too close to staff member in a personal or a sexual way.

Help the client manage angry, inappropriate, or intrusive behaviors in a therapeutic but firm, direct manner. Offer medications as necessary.
- "It sounds like you're angry, Julie. There are other ways to deal with your anger. Let's go over your anger management program."
- "Tom, we can't let you hurt yourself or anyone here. We've tried talking and exercising. Let's try a prn medication."
- "Touching others is not appropriate behavior and is not acceptable, Mark. When you have these feelings, contact the staff to help redirect you."

Helping the client manage angry, inappropriate, or intrusive behaviors early in the escalation phase may prevent assault or violence.
Redirecting the client with alternative therapeutic activities helps the client reorganize negative energy toward more socially acceptable behaviors.
Medication may be used to help calm the client before behaviors reach a full-blown manic state and before violence erupts, harming the client and others.

Reduce milieu noise and stimulation, or accompany client to a calmer, quieter environment at early signs of anger, agitation, or frustration.

A calm external environment often helps to promote a relaxed internal state within the client and may lessen agitation and prevent violence.

For the client whose behavior is out of control and who poses a danger to self or others in the milieu, use seclusion/restraint when warranted as a least restrictive therapeutic intervention.

Seclusion/restraint is used to help a client gain control when threats of violence or actual physical violence cannot be managed by other therapeutic means, and when the client and others in the milieu need protection.

For the client with excess physical energy who experiences hyperactivity or hypomania, engage the client in gross motor activities (running, jogging, swimming) on a regular basis if the client's medical history does not contraindicate physical exertion.

Physical activity is a healthy way to expend excess energy and can assist the client to gain more control and organization over disorganized and disruptive behaviors that can result in physical violence.

Suggest journal writing (*journaling*) for the client who is constantly engaged in intellectual conversations that often lead to anger or frustration.

Writing about angry thoughts/feelings helps the client connect negative thoughts/feelings with events/situations that may provoke them. The client can learn to avoid/manage anger-provoking situations and also benefits from intellectual exercise.

Remind the client to continue seeking staff when *first* experiencing frustration, anger, hostility, or suspiciousness, rather than waiting until negative thoughts and feelings are out of control, which can lead to violence.

Staff can help the client prevent negative feelings from reaching destructive levels if they know the client's state in advance. Staff can engage the client in therapeutic activities/exercises and can offer medication when necessary (see Medication section in this chapter).

Praise the client for efforts made to control anger or hostility directed at self or others.

Positive feedback reinforces repetition of positive, functional behaviors.

Teach the client and family to recognize early signs and symptoms of escalating agitation or hypomanic behaviors (yelling, cursing, threatening, pacing, intrusiveness, suspiciousness) that can lead to full-blown mania, self-harm, assault, or violence.
Instruct the family to seek out appropriate resources, such as physician, support network, or professional staff, and to use appropriate interventions, such as medications, learned therapeutic strategies, and hospitalization, as necessary.

It is important to equip the client and family effectively with resources and interventions when the client's behavior threatens the safety of self or others and the integrity of the environment. The knowledgeable client and family can accurately identify escalating or hypomanic activity and are better prepared to intervene before the client's behaviors result in injury or death.

Care Plan
DSM-IV-TR Diagnosis **Mania (All Types)**

NANDA Diagnosis: Risk for Injury
At risk for injury as a result of environmental conditions interacting with the individual's adaptive and defensive resources.

Focus:
For the client who is susceptible to injury as a result of excessive interaction or collision with environmental obstacles due to impulsive/hyperactive/intrusive behaviors.

RISK FACTORS
Increased internal stimulation secondary to neurobiologic alterations
Environmental stressors that exceed coping abilities
History of injury during manic phase
Hyperactivity/distractibility
Impulsivity/intrusiveness

Inattentive to environmental obstacles
Grandiosity: attempts feats beyond capabilities (jogging, jumping, tumbling, lifting heavy objects, punching hard objects with bare fists)

OUTCOME IDENTIFICATION AND EVALUATION
The client maintains physical integrity.
Demonstrates awareness of physical environment in proximity to body boundaries.
Exhibits decreased hyperactivity.
• Walks around environment more slowly.
Manifests reduced impulsivity.
• Reacts more slowly/appropriately to internal and external stimuli.
Avoids obstacles when moving around environment.
Attempts activities within physical capabilities.

PLANNING AND IMPLEMENTATION

Nursing Intervention	Rationale
Reduce or minimize environmental stimulation, or accompany the client to a quiet, calm area.	A soothing external environment helps to calm the client's internal state, reduces hyperactivity, and prevents accident or injury.
Remove furniture with sharp edges from the client's environment, and place furniture/obstructing objects as close to the wall as possible.	An open, uncluttered space is more likely to prevent accident or injury.
Accompany the client on walks, and provide other gross motor activities in an open, secure area.	Walking and exercising help the client expend and redirect chaotic energy toward safe, healthy activities.
Praise the client for efforts made to use physical energy productively and avoid accident or injury.	Positive feedback reinforces safe, adaptive behaviors and increases the client's self-esteem.
Continue to support and monitor the client's prescribed medical and psychosocial treatment plan.	Effective, consistent treatment helps to prevent escalating agitation and subsequent accident or injury related to mania or hypomania.

Care Plan
DSM-IV-TR Diagnosis **Mania (All Types)**

NANDA Diagnosis: Impaired Social Interaction
Insufficient or excessive quantity or ineffective quality of social exchange.

Focus:
For the client who demonstrates hyperactive behavior that is incompatible with effective interpersonal interactions.

RELATED FACTORS (ETIOLOGY)
Neurobiologic alterations
Expansive, irritable/euphoric mood

Hyperactivity (motor/verbal)
Impaired judgment
Impulsivity
Altered thought processes (paranoia/grandiosity)

DEFINING CHARACTERISTICS
The client invades others' personal space/property.
Interrupts others' conversations/activities.
Uses critical/sarcastic/insulting/sexually provocative dialogue.
Engages in sexually provocative behavior in the presence of staff and clients:

Continued

- Wears seductive, inappropriate clothing.
- Tells lewd stories or jokes.
- Makes obscene remarks about others' attributes.

Damages/steals other people's possessions.

Demonstrates inability to sit through or participate in group activities.

Blames others without substantiation.

Uses incomprehensible, rapid, forced speech pattern.

Claims to be omnipotent or famous.

- "I'm God/Superman/the devil/the president."

Demonstrates flamboyant, excessively gregarious behavior.

Changes clothes several times a day.

- Often dresses in bizarre, garish clothing with loud, bright colors that are mismatched or uncoordinated.

States that he or she has "racing" thoughts.

OUTCOME IDENTIFICATION AND EVALUATION

The client identifies self accurately to others.

Listens to others converse without interrupting.

Communicates with others by using appropriate language/tone/speech pattern.

Maintains adequate distance from others when interacting.

Refrains from violating/damaging others' property.

Dresses/grooms appropriately for age/status.

Participates in individual/milieu/group activities without outbursts/disruptions.

Identifies escalating behaviors and takes steps to circumvent them.

Acknowledges reasons for and necessity of compliance with medication regimen.

PLANNING AND IMPLEMENTATION

Nursing Intervention	Rationale
Actively listen, observe, and respond to the client's verbal and nonverbal expressions.	Active listening signifies unconditional respect and regard for the client. It builds trust and rapport, guides the nurse toward problem areas, and encourages the client to express concerns and continue in the interactive process.
Redirect negative behaviors in a calm, firm, nondefensive manner. • Suggest a walk, physical activity, or quiet time.	Redirection provides the client with a healthier avenue to direct energy and prevents further escalation of behavior.
Provide activities suitable to the client's level of tolerance/capability that are noncompetitive (e.g., brisk walk, physical exercise, stationary bicycle).	Tolerable activities help the client avoid frustration and resultant outbursts and prevent a sense of failure.
Initiate a verbal or written contract, if warranted, that clearly describes appropriate social behaviors.	A written agreement assists the client to comply with unit and milieu rules and to avoid disruptions that affect other clients and their attitude toward the client with mania.
Protect other clients from the impact of negative, intrusive behaviors. • Increase staff/patient ratio as necessary.	Safe, protective measures can help to prevent emotional and physical trauma for all clients and staff.
Set limits on the client's intrusive, interruptive behavior. • "When you keep interrupting, it is difficult to stay on the topic, so please wait for your turn." • "It's Sam's turn to speak now. When your turn comes, no one will interrupt you."	Setting appropriate limits with simple, direct instructions helps the client develop awareness and attain/maintain control and helps others to tolerate the client's presence.
Demonstrate appropriate role modeling during one-to-one and group activities.	Role modeling of appropriate social behaviors helps to promote change by example.
When the client is able to be receptive, offer feedback concerning the effect of negative behaviors on others. • "Others leave the area when you interrupt them and behave in a disruptive manner."	Awareness of how others view the client helps the client attain/maintain control and helps others to tolerate the client's presence.
Assist the client to develop more productive ways to meet needs and achieve goals (e.g., activities, games, physical exercise).	This type of assistance helps the client use healthier methods to meet needs and not to rely on dysfunctional, nonproductive strategies.

Assist the client with eating/grooming/hygiene.

A neat appearance prevents ridicule from other clients and preserves dignity and self-esteem.

Praise the client for attempting and using socially appropriate behaviors.
- "You spoke up in group more appropriately today; other clients responded very well."

Praising the client for effective social behaviors provides positive feedback, promotes subsequent appropriateness, and increases self-esteem.

Help the client achieve effective, independent problem-solving skills.

The ability to solve problems independently fosters independence and decreases regression.

Encourage the client to verbalize feelings rather than acting them out in socially inappropriate or destructive ways.

The client's verbalization defuses hostile feelings, promotes impulse control, and prevents negative consequences.

Initiate frequent, brief contacts with the client throughout the day.

Brief contact allows continual monitoring of social and communication capabilities.
The client with impaired social interaction generally cannot tolerate extended contact.

Gradually engage the client in interactions with other clients, beginning with one-to-one contacts and progressing toward more formalized groups.

The client's level of tolerance must be considered for the client to succeed in socialization skills.
Gradual exposure from simple to more complex social situations is most effective.

Include the family as appropriate in those aspects of the client's treatment plan that relate to socialization and interactive skills.

Families who are aware of the client's problems with social skills are better equipped to respond in a more effective way and are more willing to learn the social skills necessary for more successful family-client interactions.

Assist the client in identifying escalating behaviors.
- "What do you feel just before you begin to act in a disruptive manner?"
- "What are some cues that let you know you're angry enough to act aggressively?"

Helping the client to connect feelings or cues to disruptive behavior gives the client the opportunity to seek help from staff or engage in acceptable activity before losing control.

Set constructive limits on manipulative behavior in accordance with the client's ability to comply.

Setting constructive limits and guidelines help clients with manipulative behavior maintain control.

Administer routine and as-needed (prn) medications judiciously.

Maintaining an effective medication regimen helps to reduce and minimize manic symptoms.

Seclude/restrain the client and administer medication when the client is unable to maintain control and poses a danger to self or others (see care plan for risk for self-directed/other-directed violence on p. 95).

Seclusion/restraint helps the client to regain control and composure and prevents harm to the client and others.

Continue to support and monitor prescribed medical and psychosocial treatment plans.

Postdischarge support helps to maintain the client's physiologic and psychosocial integrity.

Care Plan
DSM-IV-TR Diagnosis **Mania (All Types)**

NANDA Diagnosis: Disturbed Thought Processes
Disruption in cognitive operations and activities.

Focus:
For the client who has impaired judgment/insight/comprehension/perception/problem-solving abilities and who may experience flight of ideas/delusions/ideas of reference.

RELATED FACTORS (ETIOLOGY)

Ineffective processing and synthesis of internal environmental stimuli
Neurobiologic alterations
Anxiety secondary to the manic state
Low self-esteem
Psychosocial stressors

Continued

DEFINING CHARACTERISTICS

The client demonstrates inaccurate interpretation of environmental events and incoming information.

- Mistakes a friendly gesture as a potentially harmful or violent act.

Demonstrates inaccurate belief about self or others.

- Believes he or she was sent by God to save humankind.

This is a *delusion of grandeur*, to compensate for feelings of low self-esteem.

Believes others in the milieu are planning to kill or harm him or her.

- *Delusion of persecution*, representing fear or threat to the self-system; may present as hypervigilence.

Displays exaggerated/inappropriate/disruptive behaviors/reactions directed toward environment/others

- Laughs or talks too loudly.
- Uses foul or sexually explicit language.

Demonstrates inability to follow/comprehend others' directions, unrelated to language/cultural differences.

Expresses confusion about circumstances surrounding admission to the mental health facility.

Demonstrates inability to see self as ill and in need of treatment.

- "I'm only here to have my ankle checked. It's swollen." (Client is unaware that the ankle was injured during manic episode.)

Impaired judgment or decision-making/problem-solving abilities.

- Attempts activities or feats beyond capabilities.
- Wears loud, garish, bizarre clothing combinations.
- Displays careless hygiene/bathing/grooming habits.

Projects suspiciousness/anger/fear toward environment/others.

Describes thoughts as "racing" (flight of ideas).

Rapidly shifts from topic to topic (flight of ideas).

Uses *pressured speech* (cannot express thoughts quickly enough).

Demonstrates preoccupation with sexual/religious/political/financial ideas; may be delusional.

Refuses to eat/drink/take medication; may reflect persecutory thoughts that someone wants to poison the client.

OUTCOME IDENTIFICATION AND EVALUATION

The client expresses logical, goal-directed thoughts/ideas with absence of delusions.

Solves problems and makes decisions appropriate for age and status.

Demonstrates socially appropriate behaviors.

PLANNING AND IMPLEMENTATION

Nursing Intervention	Rationale
Listen actively to the client's conversation, focusing on key themes (most frequently discussed topics), meaning of content, feelings, and reality-oriented words or phases.	Active listening helps to build trust between the client and nurse, assists in comparing the client's content with the underlying meaning or intent, and identifies key themes that are important or disturbing to the client. It also encourages the client to relate to others, because many clients with thought disturbances resist becoming involved in a therapeutic alliance.
Assist the client to correct any misinterpretations about environment/self/experiences by recalling events and problem solving. • "Let's go back and discuss what happened, one step at a time."	Exploring events with the client step-by-step encourages reality orientation.
Convey acceptance of the client's need to hold onto the false belief while not agreeing with the delusion. • "I'm a powerful, important person. Other people are jealous of me and are out to get me." **Therapeutic Response** • "I know you believe that now. These people, including me, are hospital staff and want to help you."	Acceptance of the client and the client's needs and condition builds trust and maintains the client's dignity and self-esteem. Presenting reality and offering help lessens the client's fear and anxiety and provides hope. It also lets the client know that he or she is not alone and that staff want to help.

Nontherapeutic Response

"If you say so. I won't disagree with you. Let's not worry about that now."

Agreeing, even to pacify the client, implies the belief is real and may further confuse and frighten the client. Telling the client not to worry negates the client's need and may decrease self-esteem.

Focus on the meaning/feeling/intent of the client's delusion rather than only the words or content.

Focusing on intent and feelings versus content helps to better meet the client's needs, reinforces reality, and discourages false beliefs.

Therapeutic Responses

- "It sounds like you're feeling threatened. How can staff help you?"
- "I want to understand how you feel. Are you feeling sad or lonely?"

Nontherapeutic Response

"Describe those people you say are out to get you."
"I don't believe anyone is out to get you, and no one else does either."
"Powerful people don't end up here."

Validating the delusion only confuses the client further and reinforces the false belief.

Avoid challenging the client's delusional system or arguing with the client.

Arguing or challenging the client who is experiencing a delusion can diminish trust, provoke a volatile response, or force the client to cling even more to the false belief to preserve dignity and self-esteem.

Distract the client from the delusion at the first sign of anxiety or escalating behaviors by introducing a less volatile topic or suggesting an activity.
- "Let's talk about today's activities for awhile."
- "I think a walk around the unit would be helpful now."
- "It might be a good time to finish our Ping-Pong game. We can talk again this afternoon."

Distracting the client from troubling delusions that threaten loss of control interrupts the client's volatile agitated state and allows the client to focus energies toward productive, less provocative activities. Discussion can resume when the client is less agitated.

Gradually encourage the client to discuss experiences before the onset of the delusion.
- "What happened just before you started thinking that your roommate was stealing your clothes?"
- "When your wife phoned to say she wouldn't visit you today, how did it make you feel?"

This approach helps the client identify threatening thoughts and feelings and connect them to real situations rather than to delusional content.

Focus on real topics and events to which all persons can relate (e.g., weather, movies, music), and avoid volatile subjects (e.g., sex, politics, religion).

A nonthreatening reality-based discussion distracts the client from focusing on delusional content and brings the client closer to a shared reality.

Offer praise as soon as the client begins to differentiate between reality-based and non–reality-based thinking.
- "What you're saying now is clear and makes sense."
- "The group's response to your statements showed that they understand your meaning."

Positive reinforcement increases self-esteem and encourages continued reality-based thoughts and behaviors. Clients know they are improving and responding to treatment when others validate their positive responses.

Teach the client to interrupt irrational thoughts or replace them with rational ones and to notify staff when irrational thoughts begin (see thought stopping/substitution, Appendix B).

This approach helps the client break the pattern of illogical thinking and prevents further impairment of thought processes. Participating in treatment provides the client with more control.

Refrain from the use of touch with delusional clients, especially if thoughts reflect ideas of persecution.

Clients who are suspicious or paranoid may perceive touch as threatening and may misinterpret intentions and respond with aggression.

Continued

PLANNING AND IMPLEMENTATION—cont'd

Nursing Intervention	Rationale
Give simple, concrete explanations, and avoid abstractions or metaphors.	Clients with disturbed thought processes interpret abstractions are likely to concretely and will misunderstand the message.

Therapeutic Response (Concrete)
- "It's time to get out of bed."

Nontherapeutic Response (Abstract)
"Time to rise and shine."

Assist the client with hygiene/bathing/grooming until a decision is made based on an evaluation of the client's basic needs.	Helping the client with basic needs preserves dignity and self-esteem and prevents the client from becoming an object of ridicule by other clients.
For the client who believes that food or medication is being poisoned, allow the client to select own food and drink, read the labels, and open own unit-dose medication packets.	These actions offer the client more control when the client cannot be dissuaded from the belief that his or her food or medicine may be "contaminated" or "poisoned."

Therapeutic Responses
- "I don't believe your food is poisoned, but you may get yourself another tray of food today."
- "This is the medication you've been taking all along. Read the name and open the packet yourself."

This is not an unspoken agreement that the delusion is factual but rather an attempt to provide the client with the nutrition needed to sustain life and the medication needed to encourage reality-based thoughts.

Nontherapeutic Responses
"Of course the food isn't contaminated. Would we serve bad food to clients?"
"If you refuse your medication, I'll have to call your doctor and you'll probably get a shot."

This response is defensive and challenges the client's belief system.
This statement threatens the client, which can increase fear and decrease self-worth.

Correct, with simple factual information, the client's misinterpretation of others in the environment as being threatening or dangerous.	Such clarifying statements serve to allay the client's fears and suspicions about others in the environment and bring the client relief and security.

- "Those two clients are Tom and Joe, and they're talking about baseball."
- "That's Dr. Smith, who is here to see your roommate."

Clarify the client's identity and status and that of the caregiver.	This type of clarification helps to counteract the belief that client and staff have other identities and purposes.

- "You're William Brown, and you're a client here at Hillview Hospital."
- "I'm Sara Sloan, the nurse assigned to this unit today."

Inform the client when behavior is not acceptable. Direct the client, in a firm but nonthreatening manner, toward activities or solutions that encourage more appropriate behaviors.	Firm, nonthreatening directives guide the client whose thoughts and actions are out of control toward more appropriate methods by which to gain control.

Therapeutic Responses
- "Harassing other clients in the group activity is not acceptable here. I'll go with you for a walk around the patio, which will release some of that energy."
- "Other clients are disturbed when you curse and talk about sex so much. This might be a good time to play that game of Ping-Pong on the patio."

Therapeutic responses inform the client that although the behavior is not acceptable, the client is still worthy of help. The client relies on the nurse and other caregivers to intervene in such circumstances and provide safety and security.
Note: Irrational thoughts can invoke inappropriate behavior. If behavior escalates, the client may require seclusion/restraint.

Nontherapeutic Responses

"You're behaving badly and need to control yourself, or someone is going to get hurt."	Nontherapeutic responses indicate that the client has the power to control behavior and, if not, that the client is threatened with painful, frightening consequences.
"If you continue to talk like that, no one here will want to be around you."	
Teach the family about the dynamics underlying the client's altered thoughts and how best to respond to the client.	Families empowered with knowledge (within their capabilities) are better able to manage family-client interactions and are less fearful toward the client.
Continue to support and monitor the client's prescribed medical and psychosocial treatment plans.	Ongoing support helps the client and family to manage anxiety and delusions and increases reality-based thoughts.

Care Plan
DSM-IV-TR Diagnosis **Mania (All Types)**

NANDA Diagnosis: Defensive Coping

Repeated projection of falsely positive self-evaluation based on a self-protective pattern that defends against underlying perceived threats to positive self-regard.

Focus:

For the client with mania who defends against feelings of inadequacy/insecurity/anger/fear/anxiety by using coping mechanisms in a maladaptive way in an effort to increase self-esteem and raise self-concept/image.

RELATED FACTORS (ETIOLOGY)

Irrational beliefs and assumptions (long-standing)
Unrealistic perceptions of self/situation (long-standing)
Disturbed relationships (neglectful, domineering, overprotective, abusive)
Identity problems (self, sexual)
Goal obstacles (unrealistic/unattainable goals)
Social learning patterns
Impaired self-concept/esteem/image
Low impulse control
Knowledge deficit regarding coping methods
Stressors that exceed coping abilities

DEFINING CHARACTERISTICS

The client displays excessive use of makeup/jewelry/toiletries/color of clothing.
Changes clothes several times a day.
Demonstrates restlessness/hyperalertness.
Is hyperverbal.
Is confrontational/ "testy" with staff/other clients.
Blames others for unsubstantiated acts.
Rationalizes when explaining behaviors/situations/ideas.
Swears/shouts.
Becomes angry when intentions or activities are thwarted.

Is nonparticipative in activities with others (short attention span).
Demonstrates difficulty interacting/communicating (boisterous/intrusive/boastful).
Is delusional, grandiose, and boastful regarding identity/ importance/knowledge, *or* may be delusionally paranoid.
• "I'm God/Superman/the devil/the President."
• "I know the secrets of the universe."
• "Everyone wants to rob me of my powers."

OUTCOME IDENTIFICATION AND EVALUATION

The client dresses appropriately in relation to status/situation, with minimal changes of clothing.
Uses moderate makeup/jewelry/other accessories.
Waits turn to speak.
Refrains from interrupting groups/conversations/ activities.
Uses nonoffensive, moderate speech (tone/amount/ frequency).
Refrains from hyperactivity; able to sit still and engage in group and one-to-one conversation.
Uses defense mechanisms more adaptively.
Explores beliefs/problems/values with staff.
Discusses perceived threats to self-system with staff.
Ceases to "split" staff when feeling threatened or vulnerable; relies on staff for appropriate support.
Recognizes when he or she has gained control and discusses this with staff.
Expresses recognition of attempts by staff/other clients to help support the client.
Decreases manipulation of staff/clients.
Adheres to prescribed facility regimen.
Absence of delusional/boastful behaviors.

PLANNING AND IMPLEMENTATION

Nursing Intervention	Rationale
Protect the client from embarrassment and ridicule that may occur during uninhibited behavior, such as undressing in public, sexually explicit acting out, and threats to others.	Uninhibited behaviors may embarrass the client after a manic phase. Staff awareness can intercept or prevent embarrassment, preserve dignity, and promote self-esteem by intervening on the client's behalf.
State and restate (when necessary) in a calm, matter-of-fact way all unit rules and dress/makeup codes.	Repetition of rules may be necessary during a manic phase, when the client has difficulty concentrating and is impulsive.

Therapeutic Responses

• "The television hours are from 6 to 10 PM, Tom. It's 11 PM, and the TV will be off so that others can sleep." • "Here are two outfits, Sally. Select one, and I'll put the other one away."	Nonthreatening, consistent repetition can serve as a stable external source of structure for the client.

Nontherapeutic Response

"I've told you a dozen times why you can't watch TV, so turn it off now and get to bed."	Authoritarian statements may antagonize the client because clients with mania have a low tolerance for authority.
Present a unified approach as a staff when interacting with the client, enforcing unit rules, and meeting the client's needs.	A unified staff promotes structure and consistency for the client and diminishes confusion. It also reduces imposed isolation that individual staff may experience when not working as a team.
Provide mature role modeling for the client through self-assessment and staff discipline.	Acting-out behaviors decrease when the client learns adaptive coping skills by identifying with positive, consistent staff behaviors.
Inform the client that staff believe the client is capable of meeting own needs and that staff will help the client accomplish this. • "I know you want me to make your bed, but I think you can do it. I'll stay with you until you're through."	Staff expressions of support and belief in the client's ability increase the client's confidence, self-esteem, and sense of security.
Praise the client for attempts to achieve realistic goals. • "You were able to sit for 15 minutes in group today; that's a real improvement." • "You were able to get dressed and make your own bed before breakfast. That's a big accomplishment."	Praise serves as a guide for expected behavior and promotes repetition of positive behavior. Rewarding a client for progress also increases self-esteem.
Encourage the client to express feelings and explore false self-assumptions and beliefs. • "You said you felt more important when you were telling others you were a hospital administrator." • "Let's discuss important aspects of going to college as you were doing earlier."	Through discussions with therapeutic staff members, the client gains insight, becomes more realistic, and is able to modify maladaptive responses.
Praise the client for statements of realistic self-appraisal and insights. • "I'm glad you're aware that the symptoms recurred when you stopped taking the medication and that you see that relief of symptoms helps you manage your life."	Positive reinforcement strengthens and perpetuates the client's insight and judgment.
Provide activities and opportunities for the client to interact with others in appropriate ways.	Interaction allows the client to gain support, learn vicariously, and expend energy adaptively, while encouraging reality-based thinking.
Support the family members in their efforts to interact effectively with the client in light of the client's defensive coping style.	Families need continued encouragement in maintaining appropriate family-client interactions during such challenging times.

Set limits, in a nonpunitive way, on behavior that is unacceptable or threatening to staff and client (blaming swearing, confronting).

Limiting the setting helps the client regain control, prevents the client from alienating others, and preserves self-esteem over time.

Continue to support and monitor prescribed medical and psychosocial treatment plans.

Supporting ongoing therapies encourages the client to use healthy, adaptive coping strategies.

Care Plan
DSM-IV-TR Diagnosis   **Mania (All Types)**

NANDA DIAGNOSIS: Imbalanced Nutrition: Less Than Body Requirements
Intake of nutrients insufficient to meet metabolic needs.

Focus:
For the client whose nutritional state may be compromised because of hyperactive behaviors that distract the client from the social and physical functions of eating. There is also a danger of decreased salt intake, which could lead to lithium retention and subsequent toxicity (body will use lithium if blood sodium is insufficient).

RELATED FACTORS (ETIOLOGY)

Inadequate intake and hypermetabolic need secondary to the manic state

Loss of appetite secondary to constipation/urinary retention

Diarrhea/excessive perspiration

Paranoid delusion (belief that food is poisoned or contaminated)

Grandiose delusion (belief that food is unnecessary because of the client's omnipotent state)

DEFINING CHARACTERISTICS

The client is at least 20% less than ideal body weight.

Is distracted from task of eating/drinking.

Demonstrates inability to sit through routine meals.

Reports food/fluid intake less than recommended daily allowance.

Appears wary/frightened when offered food.

Frequently refuses to eat or drink.

Has dry mouth.

Displays sore, inflamed buccal cavity.

Has pale mucous membranes/conjunctivae.

Displays capillary fragility.

Loose dry skin/turgor/decreased subcutaneous fat.

Has poor muscle tone.

Fluid/electrolytes are below normal levels.

Has hyperactive bowel sounds.

Develops shakiness/tremulousness secondary to increased lithium level.

Develops nausea/gastrointestinal upset secondary to increased lithium level.

OUTCOME IDENTIFICATION AND EVALUATION

The client consumes adequate daily calories per kilogram of body weight.

Eats adequate amounts of different food groups.

Shows fluid intake equal to output.

Demonstrates/maintains ideal body weight.

Has fluid and electrolyte levels within normal range.

Exhibits no signs of lithium toxicity.

Skin turgor/muscle tone reveal nutritional state commensurate with physiologic and metabolic needs.

PLANNING AND IMPLEMENTATION

Nursing Intervention	Rationale
Offer the client frequent carbohydrate and protein snacks.	Protein is necessary for building and repairing body cells and tissues. Carbohydrates are needed for energy.
Offer the client nutritious finger foods and sandwiches.	This strategy provides convenient methods for eating and maintaining nutritional integrity.
Offer the client easy-to-carry drinks that are high in vitamins, minerals, and electrolytes.	Convenient methods of hydration and nutrition help to maintain fluid and electrolyte levels.
Regularly assess the client's fluid/electrolyte status, especially sodium and lithium levels.	Lithium toxicity may result from a decrease in sodium and electrolyte imbalance.

Continued

PLANNING AND IMPLEMENTATION—cont'd

Nursing Intervention	Rationale
Continually assess the client's urine output.	Polyuria (excessive urination) is a common side effect of lithium because of polydipsia (excessive thirst), and clients need to be kept well hydrated.
Check time/frequency/consistency of bowel movements.	Regular assessment of the client's bowel functions is crucial. Liquid/diarrheal/tarry stools may indicate impaction/dehydration/ulcerative condition.
Assess for abdominal pain or discomfort.	The client may be constipated or obstructed.
If warranted, examine abdomen for firmness.	A firm abdomen may indicate constipation.
If warranted, auscultate abdomen in all four quadrants	Auscultation is used to assess bowel sounds because hypoactive or absent bowel sounds may indicate serious pathology.
Administer high-fiber foods unless contraindicated, more liquids, and prescribed stool softeners.	High-fiber foods and increased fluids prevent or relieve constipation and increase appetite/hydration.
Examine the urinary bladder for firmness and pain.	Examination assesses for urinary retention and need for increased fluids or catheterization.
For the client who refuses to eat or drink, assess for a possible delusion.	The client may believe the food is poisoned or contaminated, which is the reason for avoiding nourishment. Therapeutic response reflects the nurse's understanding of the client's avoidance of food.

Therapeutic Response
- "You're not eating and seem troubled."

By not agreeing with the client's delusion, the nurse also presents reality in a nonchallenging way and allows the client to maintain control and dignity. The nurse also acknowledges the client's feelings, which builds trust.

Nontherapeutic Response
"You can trust the food here. You know you have to eat."

Nontherapeutic response, although well meaning, does not acknowledge the delusional beliefs that the food may be poisoned. It challenges the client's false belief and suggests that no alternative exists. The client is thus likely to cling to the delusion to preserve control and self-esteem.

Nursing Intervention	Rationale
Offer alternative selections of foods and fluids in a direct, calm manner versus an authoritarian, threatening approach.	Offering several choices of food provides variety and promotes the client's interest in eating without resistance. The client is less likely to believe that the food selected is poisoned.
Reduce stimulation (noise, lights) when the client is ready to resume meals in the dining room.	This environment promotes a more relaxing atmosphere that is conducive to eating.
Praise the client for any attempts to eat or drink.	Positive reinforcement promotes continuity of functional behaviors.
Educate the client/family/significant others about the need for adequate nutritional intake	Knowledge and education help to maintain the client's physiologic integrity and bowel/bladder function.
Teach the client and significant others about the need for adequate sodium intake. Inform them that lithium is a salt and that reduced sodium intake can result in lithium retention with subsequent toxicity	Adequate sodium in the body prevents lithium toxicity. Salt should not be eliminated from the client's regular diet.
Educate client/family/significant others about the signs of lithium toxicity and elicit their feedback.	Education and feedback promotes the ability to differentiate between expected effects and toxic effects of lithium.
Continue to support and monitor prescribed medical, psychosocial, and dietary treatment plans.	Postdischarge support helps to maintain the client's physiologic and psychosocial integrity.

## chapter 4

Schizophrenia and Other Psychotic Disorders

Schizophrenia, a psychotic disorder, is one of the most serious and persistent of all mental disorders. In some types of schizophrenia, symptoms occur that may seem strange or bizarre and frightening for the client and witnesses. Although only a small percentage of clients with this disorder are aggressive or dangerous, they are most often sensationalized in the media. These isolated incidents of violence increase the stigma and bias prevalent in many countries of the world, resulting in ostracism and alienation of the clients and families who struggle with schizophrenia.

Treatment has progressed remarkably in the last few decades and has allowed many clients with schizophrenia to rejoin society, giving them hope and a will to continue living and functioning in meaningful ways when not struggling with acute episodes. The use of antipsychotic medications to alleviate symptoms has proven effective for many clients. However, complete recovery from schizophrenia is the exception rather than the rule. Regardless of the type, symptoms of schizophrenia are not curable as in, for example, the common cold. Instead, the disorder typically persists or recurs many times over a client's lifetime. Schizophrenia interferes with personal, social, and occupational functions of the client and significant others during these episodes.

Schizophrenia usually makes an untimely debut. The first episode most often occurs in late adolescence or early adulthood. As a result, it dramatically affects important milestones of this period, including education, employment, and relationships. Like a tumbling house of cards, all aspects of the person's well-being are often disrupted and disconnected at a time when the maturing individual would otherwise be involved in one of the most productive times of his or her life.

Clients and families have candidly revealed their first experiences and subsequent recurrences of schizophrenia, as in the following remarks:

- "It pulled the plug out of life."
- "Just like getting hit by a tornado that doesn't stop."
- "A dark cloud descended over our lives, and sometimes we get a glimpse of the sun."
- "Our life together as we knew it ended, and chaos took its place."
- "He/she became an entirely different person."
- "Initially we felt possessed . . . it was as if a demon took over our lives."

These statements help nurses to begin understanding the impact of schizophrenia on individuals and families.

ETIOLOGY

The definitive etiology of schizophrenia is yet to be determined. Current research, however, favors the *diathesis-stress model*, which states that the disorder is caused by constitutional/genetic predisposition or vulnerability, coupled with biologic, environmental, and psychosocial stressors. Despite evidence for genetic etiology, specific genes responsible for schizophrenia have not yet been identified; multiple genes are thought to be involved. Several inherent anatomic physiologic abnormalities and changes have been discovered in the brains of individuals with schizophrenia. Likewise, many external factors that may influence onset have also been identified.

Schizophrenia is most likely caused by a convergence and interaction of genetic and environmental factors (Box 4-1). Questions remain about whether the brain changes are the cause versus the consequence of the disorder, or in some cases the result of treatment with medications.

EPIDEMIOLOGY

Schizophrenia is present in approximately 1% of the world's population. In the United States and United Kingdom, some Asian-American and African-American groups are diagnosed more often as having schizophrenia than other races. It is uncertain whether this results from actual racial differences, clinical interviewer bias, or insensitivity to cultural differences. Cultural variations may be part of the explanation because normal behavior in one culture may be a disorder in another culture. For example, seeing or hearing the voice of a dead loved one is not considered abnormal in some areas of the world but would probably be considered psychotic symptoms in the general population of the United States. When a clinician interviews clients from a different culture and lacks comprehensive understanding of that culture's differences, the clinician may have difficulty avoiding influences from personal, cultural, and social standards. Such influences may affect assessment outcomes.

Biologic first-born relatives of individuals with schizophrenia have a 10 times greater risk than the general population for developing the disorder. Studies of twins, adoptees, and families strongly support this finding. (Fig. 4-1). Some relatives of people with schizophrenia are also at risk for related mental disorders, including schizoaffective disorder and schizotypal, paranoid, schizoid, and avoidant personality disorders.

Onset of Schizophrenia

Schizophrenia usually occurs in late adolescence to the mid-30s. In one pattern of onset, the first psychotic episode may occur abruptly in a person previously considered normal by most standards. This onset is often associated with recent major psychosocial stressors (death of a loved one, leaving home for college or the military, breakup of relationship). A prodromal period usually precedes the disorder, in which the person begins to behave in unusual ways that contrast with the individual's typical behavior. This behavior worries family members, who frequently say the person has "changed." Symptoms show a decline in normal function, and behaviors unusual for the person include the following:

- Increasing isolation
- Withdrawal from usual contacts
- Loss of interest in previously enjoyed activities
- Neglected hygiene/grooming
- Expression of beliefs/experiences
- Unprovoked anger

Some or all of these symptoms may precede a psychotic episode.

Another pattern of onset consists of a lifelong history of marginal functioning and unusual behaviors and perceptions, as reported by the client, family, and teachers. This history includes the following:

- Problems with family relationships
- Few if any friends ("loner")/few social contacts
- School truancy/low grades
- Trouble with the law
- Lack of interest in school or work
- Neglected hygiene/dress/grooming
- Excessive interest/participation in unusual topics/activities (cults, outlying spiritual attractions, the paranormal, vampires, either in person or through virtual participation in video games/computer access).

Within this time the eruption of one or more psychotic episodes occurs. This long-standing second pattern for schizophrenia may be associated more with significant neurodevelopmental/neurophysiologic deficits or changes.

Schizophrenia affects both genders equally, but usually at different times of life for men and women. Age of onset in most cases is earlier for men (18 to 25 years) than women (25 to 35 years). Childhood schizophrenia is rare. Also once thought to be rare, late-onset cases (over 50 years)

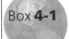

Box 4-1   **Etiology of Schizophrenia**

Genetic Factors (Fig. 4-1)
Neurodevelopmental factors: brain abnormalities
- Enlarged ventricles
- Cortex laterality (left localized)
- Temporal lobe dysfunction
- Phospholipid metabolism
- Frontal lobe dysfunction
- Brain circuitry dysfunction
- Neuronal density

Neurotransmitter systems
- Dopaminergic dysregulation (excess)
- Serotonin (2A receptor gene variant)

Prenatal stressors
- Depression
- Influenza
- Poverty
- Rh-factor incompatibility
- Physical injury

Development/birth-related findings
- Short gestation
- Low birth weight
- Delivery complications
- Disrupted fetal development

Environmental pollutants
Multiple/varied psychosocial stressors
Viral infections of central nervous system

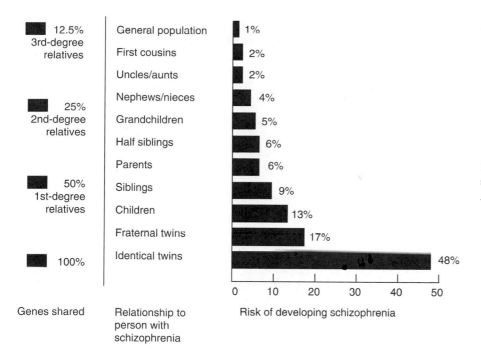

Fig. 4-1 Risk for developing schizophrenia. (From *Surgeon General Report*, 1999.)

occur more often in women than men. One theory holds that women are protected by female hormones, which diminish with menopause, leaving them more vulnerable to the disorder.

Course of Schizophrenia

The course of schizophrenia varies. Some clients experience periods of exacerbations and remissions, whereas others have severe and persistent symptoms, in some cases the positive symptoms abate, but the negative symptoms often persist. Both positive and negative symptoms are described in the next section. Clients seldom return to their normal, premorbid level of functioning. The course for schizophrenia is influenced by many factors (Box 4-2).

Box 4-2   **Factors Influencing the Course of Schizophrenia**

Severity of symptoms
Access to treatment
Client response to therapies
Client awareness of condition/situation
Motivation to improve
Accepting support network
• Family
• Treatment sites/staff
• Economic aspects
• Appropriate social diversions
• Skills retraining/rehabilitation facilities

Drug Use

Comorbidity rates of schizophrenia with substance-related disorders is high. Nicotine dependence is a particular problem, with 80% to 90% of clients with schizophrenia being dependent smokers who also choose high-nicotine brands. Several other drugs, often illegal ones, are frequently used by individuals with this diagnosis. The dual diagnosis of schizophrenia and a drug abuse or drug-dependent diagnosis is now common.

Clients with schizophrenia, who have compromised insight and judgment from the disorder, often are victims of ruthless drug peddlers who use the clients to meet their own needs. For example, clients may spend their meager income on drugs instead of psychotropic medications, rent, or food, or they may become involved in selling sexual favors in exchange for drugs. In all cases the clients are abused emotionally, psychologically, socially, morally, and often physically. In some individuals, the first psychotic episode is triggered by drug experimentation or use; however, the reader is cautioned not to confuse every drug induced psychosis with schizophrenia. Specific criteria constitute the diagnosis of schizophrenia and are discussed in this chapter under Types of Schizophrenia.

Mortality and Suicide

The mortality rate in schizophrenia is high. Many of these clients are at higher risk for some diseases and conditions because of their life-style, which leaves them uninformed and unprotected.

The suicide rate among clients with schizophrenia is also high. They may commit suicide during episodes of active psychosis, when they are delusional or hallucinating, or during periods when they are more lucid and able to examine their quality of life, then choose not to continue the struggle.

ASSESSMENT AND DIAGNOSTIC CRITERIA

One criterion included in all types of schizophrenia is **psychosis**, which is the defining characteristic of this disorder and which must be present to make the diagnosis of schizophrenia. Other categories of mental disorders (major depression with psychotic features, Alzheimer's disease with psychotic features) may include psychotic symptoms as a component, but these are not considered psychotic disorders.

Symptoms of Schizophrenia

The term *psychosis* has been defined and described in many ways over the decades. Multiple definitions have found favor at different times in the history of the reporting and recording of psychiatric disorders. No single definition of psychosis receives total acceptance.

One effective way to understand the psychosis of schizophrenia is to refer to the description of *positive* and *negative* symptoms. Both types of symptoms refer to function, as follows:
- **Positive symptoms** represent a distortion or excess of normal function and include delusions, hallucinations, disorganized thinking/speech, and grossly disorganized or catatonic behavior.
- **Negative symptoms** represent a decrease, loss, or absence of normal function and include flat affect, alogia, and avolition (Box 4-3).

In addition to the positive and negative symptoms (see Box 4-3), other symptoms are evident in schizophrenia, as described next. Note that each type of the disorder includes specific criteria and that all of the following symptoms will not be demonstrated in every type of schizophrenia.

Box 4-3   Positive and Negative Symptoms of Schizophrenia

POSITIVE SYMPTOMS

Delusions are firmly held erroneous beliefs caused by distortions/exaggerations of reasoning and misinterpretations of perceptions/experiences. Delusions of being followed or watched are common, as are beliefs that comments, radio/TV programs, and other sources are directing special messages directly to the client.

Hallucinations are distortions/exaggerations of perception in any of the senses, although *auditory* hallucinations ("hearing voices" within, distinct from one's own thoughts) are the most common, followed by visual hallucinations.

Disorganized speech/thinking, also described as *thought disorder* or *loosening of associations*, is a key aspect of schizophrenia. Disorganized thinking is usually assessed primarily based on the client's speech. Therefore tangential, loosely associated, or incoherent speech severe enough to substantially impair effective communication is used as an indicator of thought disorder by the *DSM-IV-TR*.

Grossly disorganized behavior includes difficulty in goal-directed behavior (leading to difficulties in activities of daily living), unpredictable agitation or silliness, social disinhibition, or behaviors that are bizarre to onlookers. Their purposelessness distinguishes them from unusual behavior prompted by delusional beliefs.

Catatonic behaviors are characterized by a marked decrease in reaction to the immediate surrounding environment, sometimes taking the form of motionless and apparent unawareness, rigid or bizarre postures, or aimless excess motor activity.

Other symptoms in schizophrenia are not common enough to be definitional alone.
- Affect inappropriate to the situation or stimuli
- Unusual motor behavior (pacing, rocking)
- Depersonalization
- Derealization/somatic preoccupations

NEGATIVE SYMPTOMS

Affective flattening is the reduction in the range and intensity of emotional expression, including facial expression, voice tone, eye contact, and body language.

Alogia, or poverty of speech, is the lessening of speech fluency and productivity, thought to reflect slowing or blocked thoughts, and often manifested as laconic, empty replies to questions.

Avolition is the reduction, difficulty, or inability to initiate and persist in goal-directed behavior; it is often mistaken for apparent disinterest.

Modified from *DSM-IV-TR, Diagnostic and statistical manual of mental disorders,* ed 4, revised.

Duration of symptoms

Another criterion that defines schizophrenia is duration of symptoms. Before the diagnosis of schizophrenia is made, at least 6 months of persistent disturbance exists, with 1 month of active-phase symptoms (see Box 4-3). When treated with medications and relevant psychosocial therapy, clients with schizophrenia have a variable active phase.

Acute Phase of Schizophrenia

Symptoms of the active, or *acute,* phase of schizophrenia vary. Disturbances occur in multiple psychologic and psychosocial areas, including thought, affect, perception, and behavior.

Thought disturbance

Thought disturbance may be manifested in many ways. *Disturbed content* refers to dysfunctional beliefs, ideas, and interpretations of actual internal and external stimuli. *Delusions* are examples of disturbed thought content; some common types of delusions in schizophrenia are persecutory, grandiose, religious, and somatic, as follows:

- The client believes that stereo speakers, TV, or computers are controlling her thoughts.
- Intergalactic electrical waves are beaming on the world, ready to destroy the client.
- The client has the power to change the seasons.
- The client believes he is the messenger from God.
- The client has a demon in the stomach that causes sounds.

Other symptoms include thought *broadcasting* (thoughts or ideas are being transmitted to others), *thought insertion* (others can put thoughts into the client's mind), and *thought withdrawal* (thoughts can be taken from the client's mind).

Content disturbance is also noted by *ideas of reference,* which are beliefs that other people or messages from the media (TV, radio, newspaper) are directly referring to the client as follows:

- Two strangers may be across the room holding a conversation about the weather, and the client believes they are talking about her.
- The president of the United States gives a speech on TV about the space program, and the individual believes it is a message for him to become an astronaut.

The client's preoccupation with particular thoughts or ideas that are persistent and cannot be eliminated *(obsessional thinking)* also represents content disturbance. Frequently, such thoughts are accompanied by ritualistic behavior. Clients with schizophrenia often make symbolic references to actual persons, objects, or events. For example, the color red may symbolize anger, death, or blood to the client.

Incoherence, loose associations, tangentiality, circumstantiality, neologisms, "word salad," echolalia, perseveration, verbigeration, and autistic and dereistic thinking may be noted by staff as the client speaks, writes, or draws.

Disturbed thought process includes thought blocking, poor memory, symbolic or idiosyncratic association, illogical flow of ideas, vagueness, poverty of speech, and impaired ability to abstract *(concrete thinking)*/reason/calculate/use judgment.

Affective disturbance

Affective disturbance may be characteristically evidenced by flat (blunted) or inappropriate affect. The person with **flat affect** demonstrates little or no emotional responsivity. Facial expression is immobile, voice is monotonous, and the client describes not being able to feel as intensely as he or she once did or not being able to feel at all. **Inappropriate affect** is manifested by emotional expression that is incongruent with verbalizations, situation, or event; client's ideation and description do not match the affective display. For example, the individual may describe the death of a parent and laugh. Other affective manifestations may appear as sudden, unprovoked demonstrations of angry or overly anxious behavior, silliness, or giddiness. The person may be responding to internal stimuli at such times (hallucinations).

Persons with schizophrenia may demonstrate or express a wide range of emotions and say they feel terrified, perplexed, ambivalent, ecstatic, omnipotent, or overwhelmingly alone, or that they do not feel anything at all. These clients are frequently not in touch with their feelings or have difficulty expressing them.

Note: Staff's knowledge of the action and adverse effects of antipsychotic medications is essential because affective displays may represent the manifestations of schizophrenia or may be a reaction to the medications. Interventions depend on the nurse's correct assessment to avoid overmedication or undermedication of the client.

Perceptual disturbance

Perceptual disturbances may include hallucinations, illusions, and boundary and identity problems.

Hallucinations

A common perceptual dysfunction in schizophrenia is the hallucination, a sensory perception by an individual that is not associated with actual external stimuli. Although hallucinations may occur in any of the senses (hearing, sight, taste, touch, smell), the most common are *auditory hallucinations.* The voices that clients hear carry messages of various types but are usually derogatory, accusatory, obscene, or threatening.

It is important for staff to thoroughly assess the **auditory command type** of hallucination, in which voices tell the client to harm self or others, so that staff can initiate protective interventions. Some clients describe their auditory hallucinations as thoughts or sounds rather than voices.

Visual, gustatory, tactile, and olfactory hallucinations are less common in schizophrenia. Delusions may or may not accompany hallucinations. Delusional content usually parallels or incorporates the hallucination, as if the client is attempting to "make sense" of the hallucination.

Illusions

Occasionally the client may experience illusions, which are misinterpretations of actual external environmental or sensory stimuli. For example, as the sun is setting, the patient looks out a window and tells staff that the bush he sees is instead his grandfather. Differentiation between illusions and hallucinations by staff is often difficult and requires keen assessment.

Boundary and identity problems

The client with schizophrenia may seem confused and lack a clear sense of self-awareness. The client is not sure of personal boundaries and sometimes cannot differentiate self from others or from inanimate objects in the environment. This is often frightening for the client. The client may also describe **depersonalization** or **derealization** phenomena. In depersonalization, individuals have the sense that their own bodies are unreal, as if they are estranged and unattached to the world or the situation at hand. Derealization is the experience that external environmental objects are strange or unreal.

A client with schizophrenia may perceive a loss of sexual identity and doubt his or her own gender or sexual orientation. This may be frightening for the client and should not be interpreted as homosexuality by the staff.

Behavioral disturbance

Behavioral disturbances may be demonstrated by impaired interpersonal relationships. Because of these clients' difficulties with communication and interaction, the individual is frequently emotionally detached, socially inept, and withdrawn and has difficulty relating to others. Forming a therapeutic relationship with these clients is a challenge because of the detached affective responses, illogical thinking, egocentrism, lack of trust, and other problems described previously. A concerted effort must be made to engage the client with schizophrenia because the usual encouraging cues to continue interaction are often absent. The nurse is aware that during acute episodes the client may be more isolative and restricted in thought and speech production (alogia), so initiation of contacts by the nurse is imperative.

Psychomotor disturbances such as grimacing, bizarre posturing, unpredictable and unprovoked wild activity, odd mannerisms, and compulsive stereotypical or ritualistic behavior may be present, or the patient may stare into space, seem totally out of touch with the external surroundings or persons in it, and show little or no emotional response, spontaneous speech, or movement. Clients may appear stiff or clumsy, be socially unaware of their appearance and habits, and fail to bathe or wash their clothes. They may spit on the floor and in extreme cases may regressively play with or smear feces. Clients frequently demonstrate anxious, agitated, fearful, or aggressive behavior.

After an acute episode, clients almost always lack energy and initiative to engage in goal-directed activity. Interest and drive seem absent *(impaired volition)*.

Another characteristic manifested in schizophrenia is **ambivalence,** or opposing thoughts, ideas, feelings, drives or impulses occurring in the same person at the same time. For example, when asked to come to the group meeting, the client may step out of and reenter his or her room dozens of times, unable to make a decision. *Negativistic behavior* is usually demonstrated as frequent oppositions and resistance to suggestions.

DSM-IV-TR Criteria

A diagnosis of schizophrenia depends on the symptoms demonstrated by the client and is assigned for the purposes of treatment focus. Various types of schizophrenia have been identified according to the *Diagnostic and Statistical Manual of Mental Disorders (DSM-IV-TR)* criteria (see box below; see also Appendix A).

■ TYPES OF SCHIZOPHRENIA

Paranoid Type

Distinguishing characteristics of paranoid schizophrenia are (1) persistent delusions with a single or closely associated, tightly organized theme usually of persecution or grandeur and (2) auditory hallucinations about single or closely associated themes. Clients are guarded, suspicious, hostile, angry, and possibly violent. Anxiety is pervasive in the paranoid disorder. Social interactions are intense, reserved, and controlled. Onset is later in life than with other types. Paranoid schizophrenia has a more favorable prognosis as a rule, particularly in regard to independent living and occupational function.

DSM-IV-TR   Schizophrenia and Other Psychotic Disorders

Schizophrenia subtypes
- Paranoid
- Disorganized
- Catatonic
- Undifferentiated
- Residual

Schizophreniform disorder

Schizoaffective disorder

Delusional disorder

Brief psychotic disorder

Shared psychotic disorder

Schizophrenia from other causes
- Medical conditions
- Medications/drugs/other substances

Disorganized Type

The distinguishing characteristics of disorganized schizophrenia are grossly inappropriate or flat affect, incoherence, and grossly disorganized primitive and uninhibited behavior. These clients appear very odd or silly. They have unusual mannerisms, may giggle or cry out, distort facial expressions, complain of multiple physical problems (hypochondriasis), and are extremely withdrawn and socially inept. Invariably the onset is early, and the prepsychotic period is marked by impaired adjustment, which continues after the acute episode. Clients may hallucinate and have delusions, but the themes are fragmented and loosely organized. Other classifications name this type *hebephrenic*.

Catatonic Type

The distinguishing characteristic of catatonic schizophrenia is marked disturbance of psychomotor activity. The behavior of the catatonic client is manifested as either motor immobility or psychomotor excitation, or the client can alternate between the two states.

The client may be immobile (stuporous) or exhibit excited, purposeless activity. The client may be out of touch with the environment and display negativism, mutism, and posturing. These individuals can be placed in bizarre positions *(waxy flexibility)*, which they may rigidly maintain until moved by a staff member. It is as if they do not even feel their bodies. Careful supervision is required to prevent injury, promote nutrition, and support physiologic/psychologic functions.

Undifferentiated Type

Clients with a diagnosis of undifferentiated schizophrenia display florid psychotic symptoms (delusions, hallucinations, incoherence, disorganized behavior) that do not clearly fit under any other category.

Residual Type

The residual category is used when a client has had at least one acute episode of schizophrenia and is free of psychotic symptoms at present but continues to exhibit persistent signs of social withdrawal, emotional blunting, illogical thinking, or eccentric behavior.

Schizophreniform Disorder

Diagnostic criteria for schizophreniform disorder meet those for schizophrenia except for two factors: (1) duration of the illness is at least 1 month but less than 6 months, and (2) social/occupational function may not be impaired.

Schizoaffective Disorder

Defining characteristics of schizoaffective disorder are demonstration of symptoms of both schizophrenia (delusions and/or hallucinations, disorganized speech/behavior, negative symptoms) and a mood disorder (major depressive, manic, mixed). The episode must last for 1 month.

OTHER PSYCHOTIC DISORDERS

Delusional Disorder

The presence of one or more nonbizarre delusions that persist for 1 month or more defines delusional disorder. *Bizarre* delusions are composed of strange and markedly unusual or incredible content. For example, a person believes his brain was removed by alien beings and replaced by a computer that controls his life. *Nonbizarre* delusions, however, are plausible and could possibly exist in the individual's life. For example, a student believes there is a conspiracy to keep her from graduating from college. Subtypes of delusional disorder are identified by their delusional themes, as follows:

- **Erotomanic.** The theme centers around belief and conviction that another person is in love with the client, which in fact is untrue. The individual may go to great lengths to communicate with the loved object (stalking, phoning, spying).
- **Jealous.** The theme is that the individual's lover or spouse is unfaithful without real evidence to support the belief. Incorrect inferences are made about the spouse's clothes or bed sheets, and efforts are made to follow or "catch" the partner in "the act."
- **Grandiose.** The theme focuses on the individual having an extraordinary or important undiscovered talent or special knowledge, that the individual knows an important or famous person, or less frequently, that the individual *is* a famous person.
- **Persecutory.** The theme centers on the belief that the individual is a victim of conspiracy, poisoning, spying, harassment, or cheating. The person frequently is angry or resentful or may be violent.
- **Somatic.** The belief focuses on bodily sensations or functions. Most frequent somatic delusions include belief that the person has a foul odor emanating from a body part (mouth, vagina, skin), that insects or parasites are on or in the body, or that a body part (bowel) is nonfunctional.

Brief Psychotic Disorder

The defining characteristic of brief psychotric disorder is at least one of the following symptoms: hallucinations, delusions, disorganized speech, or behavior disturbance (disorganized or catatonic). Symptoms last at least 1 day but less than 1 month. The person returns to premorbid level of function following the episode.

Shared Psychotic Disorder

Shared psychotic disorder, a delusional disorder also known as *folie à deux*, develops in a person who is involved in a relationship with another individual who already has a psychotic disorder with prominent delusions.

Psychotic Disorder due to Medical Condition

Defining characteristics are prominent hallucinations and/or delusions due to physiologic effects of a medical condition.

Substance-Induced Psychotic Disorder

Defining characteristics are prominent hallucinations or delusions due to physiologic effects of a substance (drugs of abuse, medication, or toxin). The disorder first occurs during intoxication or withdrawal stages but can last for weeks thereafter.

▮ INTERVENTIONS

There are three distinct treatment phases for schizophrenia: (1) active phase, (2) maintenance phase, and (3) rehabilitation phase. Treatment is aimed at alleviation of symptoms, improvement in quality of life, and restoration of productivity within the client's capacity. In each treatment stage, evidence indicates that a combination of modalities, including psychopharmacology, psychosocial therapy, and psychoeducation of client and family, is most effective.

Frequently, intensive forms of therapy and case management involving interdisciplinary teams are necessary for clients whose symptoms severely disrupt their lives and the lives of family members, especially when symptoms are persistent. Clients and significant others are encouraged to become familiar with recognizing symptom changes and to report them to designated members of the treatment team to prevent more serious episodes whenever possible.

The following modalities are recognized forms of intervention for clients who are diagnosed with schizophrenia. In addition, the care plans provide specific nursing interventions and rationale for therapeutic interactions with these clients.

Medications

Although schizophrenia often is not curable, it is treatable, and current methods of treatment are effective. Schizophrenia became more managable with the advent of antipsychotic medications, also referred to as *neuroleptics*. The first-generation, conventional antipsychotics relieved the positive symptoms, which was a milestone but did little to target the *negative* symptoms (Boxes 4-4 and 4-5). Even though the clients' delusions, hallucinations, and incoherence that define psychosis subsided, their lack of motivation and decreased desire to engage in activities persisted, leaving them uninvolved, seclusive, and isolated. Newer types of neuroleptics produced over the past decade, however, act on the positive symptoms and are often effective in alleviating negative symptoms as well. Also, fewer adverse side effects are seen with the newer generation antipsychotics (see Pharmacotherapy box).

Therapeutic Nurse-Client Relationship

The nurse-client relationship is a therapeutic vehicle for the person with schizophrenia to attain a sense of acceptance and self-worth. Within the trusting relationship the client can learn and practice new skills, receive nonjudgmental feedback about progress, and gain support and encouragement in the process. Focus is on interpersonal communication, socialization skills, independence, and survival skills for

---

> ### Box 4-4 Extrapyramidal Symptoms (EPS)
>
> Extrapyramidal symptoms (EPS) are a variety of motor-related side effects that result from the dopamine-blocking effects of antipsychotic medications (most commonly the typical group).
>
> **DYSTONIA**
> Occurs in 10% of clients treated. Spasms affecting various muscle groups may be frightening and result in difficulty swallowing, jeopardizing the person's airway.
>
> *Treatment*
> - Mild cases: oral anticholinergic drugs
> - Severe or unresolved cases: benztropine (Cogentin) 2 mg IM and diphenhydramine (Benadryl) 50 mg IM
>
> **PSEUDOPARKINSONISM**
> Occurs in 15% of clients treated. A variety of symptoms including tremors, slowed or absent movement, muscle jerks (cogwheel rigidity), shuffling gait, loss of facial muscle movement (masked facies), and drooling.
>
> *Treatment*
> - Anticholinergic drugs or dopamine agonists.
>
> **AKATHISIA**
> Literally means "not sitting." Occurs in 25% of clients treated. Motor restlessness, pacing, rocking, foot-tapping, inability to lie down or sit still. Can be confused with anxiety, so keen assessment is critical.
>
> *Treatment*
> - Reduction in antipsychotics (may not be practical if psychosis is responding well to antipsychotics).
> - Beta blockers and benzodiazepines are the most common adjunctive treatment.
> - Occasionally benztropine if client is able to tolerate.
>
> **TARDIVE DYSKINESIA**
> Literally means late-occurring abnormal movements. Occurs in 4% of clients treated; may be irreversible in 50% of those clients. Classically described as oral, buccal, lingual, and masticatory, these rapid, jerky movements can occur anywhere in the body.
>
> *Treatment*
> - Prevention by monitoring the client every 6 months during treatment.
> - Withdrawing antipsychotics over time may cause temporary increase in symptoms.
> - Benzodiazepines can be used, although relief generally lasts only several months.
> - Clozapine (Clozaril) has been beneficial in treating severe tardive dyskinesia.
> - Vitamin E has been used with inconsistent and modest results.

Box **4-5**   Neuroleptic Malignant Syndrome (NMS)

A potentially fatal but rare consequence of drug therapy, neuroleptic malignant syndrome (NMS) has a mortality rate of about 10%.

RISK FACTORS (for NMS)
- High-potency, conventional antipsychotics
- High doses of antipsychotics
- Rapid increase in dosage

SYMPTOMS
- Decreased level of consciousness
- Greatly increased muscle tone (rigidity)
- Autonomic dysfunction (hyperthermia, labile hypertension, tachycardia, diaphoresis, drooling)

NMS is believed to result from dopamine blockade in the hypothalamus. Muscle necrosis can be so severe as to cause myoglobinuric renal failure. Laboratory abnormalities include greatly elevated creatine phosphokinase levels and leukocytosis.

TREATMENT
- Discontinue antipsychotic medications.
- Keep patient well hydrated.
- Administer antipyretics and provide cooling blankets if hyperthermia exists.
- Treat arrhythmias.
- Administer low doses of heparin to decrease the risk of pulmonary emboli.
- Administer bromocriptine mesylate (dopamine agonist) and dantrolene (direct-acting skeletal muscle relaxant) to reduce muscle spasm.

Note: Other medications may be added to the antipsychotic regimen. Often clients will be prescribed antianxiety medications and mood stabilizers. Choice of medications depends on symptoms.

Group Therapy

Group therapies that focus on assisting clients and families in practical life skills are much more effective than psychodynamic types of therapy aimed at gaining insight. Because clients with schizophrenia have cognitive dysfunction such as loose associations and disorganized thinking, the insight-oriented therapies often prove to be nontherapeutic or harmful for clients who are unable to participate.

Individuals who may be psychotic are more successful in a low-stress group whose members receive positive reinforcement for even minimal functioning. The goals of these focus groups are realistic, meet the needs of the members, and address such issues as identification and support of strengths, hygiene/grooming, activities of daily living, socialization skills, motivation, self-esteem problems, and stress and anxiety reduction. Anxiety-reducing strategies include deep-breathing and relaxation exercises (see Appendix B).

Psychosocial Therapy

Psychosocial therapy is a necessary component in comprehensive care of clients with schizophrenia. Psychopharmacology coupled with support therapies has proven more effective than either form of therapy alone. During all stages of schizophrenia the medications either relieve symptoms or help to prevent symptoms from returning, thereby enabling the client to be more receptive to other types of psychosocial therapy. Because a major characteristic of schizophrenia is the impaired ability to form and maintain interpersonal relationships, a major focus of interventions centers on helping the client enter into and maintain meaningful socialization consistent with the client's ability.

Family Therapy

Because the value of family support for the person with schizophrenia is immeasurable, family therapy is imperative whenever available. In therapy the families learn about schizophrenia and how to (1) prevent or reduce relapses, (2) give and gain support from others, (3) receive direction and resource aids in crises, (4) avoid crises, and (5) gain

posthospitalization (skills and confidence gained from the one-to-one relationship to begin new social connections).

PHARMACOTHERAPY   Antipsychotic Medications

Antipsychotic medications are classified as *typical* and *atypical* and are the primary drugs used for schizophrenia and other psychotic disorders. Atypical antipsychotics are thought to be more beneficial than typical antipsychotics, such as haliperidol (Haldol) and chlorpromazine (Thorazine), especially for the treatment of negative symptoms, such as anhedonia, flat affect, alogia, poverty of speech, poor eye contact, poor grooming, apathy, lack of volition, disturbed family relationships, decreased spontaneity, and gestures. The atypical antipsychotics include olanzapine (Zyprexa),

risperidone (Risperdal), ziprasidone (Geodon), and quetiapine (Seroquel). Clozapine (Clozaril) is reserved for refractory psychosis due to the risk of agranulocytosis, a critical reduction in leukocytes in 2% of the population who takes clozapine. The atypical antipsychotics have fewer side effects than the typical antipsychotics, fewer extrapyramidal side effects, less cardiovascular toxicity, and less risk for tardive dyskinesia. Consequently, the atypical antipsychotics are now considered first-line treatment, despite significantly higher cost.

skills for problem solving, communicating, daily living competencies, and behavior modification.

Long-term studies have consistently found that family intervention improves client and family function, increases feelings of well-being, and prevents or delays symptom relapse. In most areas of the United States, groups of families of the clients with severe mental impairment such as schizophrenia meet to learn from each other, provide support for each other, and show strength in numbers when addressing governing bodies to improve legislation for the mentally disordered population.

Community-Based Treatment

Severe and persistent mental disorders such as schizophrenia require intervention on several levels. *Inpatient services* focus on symptom amelioration, reduction of risk for danger to self and others, reintegration, and discharge planning for the client's return to the community. Because of the type and severity of symptoms, clients with schizophrenia frequently are unable to function independently day to day when discharged from the inpatient setting back into the community. These clients are often placed in ongoing *outpatient day treatment* programs, where they benefit from daily contact with skilled staff and other clients. Staff assess and monitor the client's mental status and medications and provide opportunities for socialization with staff and others. Clients are encouraged to participate in scheduled meetings, groups, and activities consistent with their ability. An interdisciplinary treatment team is usually involved in the client's care and is composed of nurses, physicians, social workers, and other therapists as budget and policy allow.

Support and education groups for clients and families are usually available in the community after clients are discharged. A comprehensive treatment focus usually includes rehabilitation and inclusion in vocational training or jobs if the client is able. A large perentage of the homeless population have mental disorders, and often their needs are minimally met or unmet. This is a harsh reality that remains open for improvement by U.S. cities, the states, and the federal government.

PROGNOSIS AND DISCHARGE CRITERIA

Complete remission is uncommon in clients with schizophrenia, but several factors have been associated with a better prognosis (Box 4-6). Some types of schizophrenia also have a better prognosis (paranoid type) than others (undifferentiated type).

Discharge criteria are tailored to meet each client's needs and problem areas, with a focus on reintegration into the family and the community. The following basic list of criteria may be modified and expanded to fit the client's discharge plan:

- The client verbalizes absence or reduction of hallucinations and other sensory alterations (see following text).
- Identifies psychosocial stressors/situations/events that trigger hallucinations.
- Recognizes/discusses connections between increased anxiety and occurrence of hallucinations.
- Describes several techniques for decreasing anxiety and managing stress.
- Identifies family/significant others as support network.
- States methods for contacting physician/therapist/agencies to meet needs.
- Describes importance of continuing use of medication, including dose, frequency, and expected/adverse effects.
- Discusses vulnerability in social situations and realistic ways to avoid problems.
- Verbalizes knowledge of responsibility for own actions and wellness.
- Describes plans to attend ongoing social support groups and rehabilitation/vocational training within limits.
- States alignment with aftercare facilities (e.g., home, board and care, halfway house).

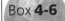 Box **4-6**   Prognosis for Schizophrenia

FAVORABLE COURSE/PROGNOSIS

1. Good premorbid social, sexual, and work/school history
2. Preceded by definable major psychosocial stressors or event
3. Late onset
4. Acute onset
5. Treatment soon after episode onset
6. Brief duration of active phases
7. Adequate support systems
8. Paranoid/catatonic features
9. Family history of mood disorders

UNFAVORABLE COURSE/PROGNOSIS

1. Poor premorbid history of socialization
2. Early onset
3. Insidious onset
4. No clear precipitating factors
5. Withdrawn/isolative behaviors
6. Undifferentiated/disorganized features
7. Few if any support systems
8. Chronic course with many relapses and few remissions

Clients with chronic schizophrenia may never be entirely free of hallucinations but can learn to control them. Individuals who chronically experience hallucinations require closer supervision. The box below provides guidelines for client and family teaching in the management of schizophrenia and other psychotic disorders.

CLIENT AND FAMILY TEACHING	Schizophrenia

Nurse Needs To Know

- Schizophrenia is a long-standing disorder with debilitating symptoms that challenges the client, family, health care workers, and the community.
- The client periodically experiences psychosis such as delusions and hallucinations, which may be frightening to the client and others.
- The client and others may need protection if hallucination is a command type that orders the client to harm or kill self or others.
- Do not argue with the client about the reality of the delusion or hallucination, but be honest in sharing your perception of reality.
- Be aware that the client's verbal response may be inconsistent with mood or affect, and further exploration may be warranted.
- Involve the client in hospital activities with the realization that poor motivation and low energy levels may be caused by illness and sedative effects of medication, not laziness.
- Engage the client/family in medication administration and monitoring side effects.
- Learn about the therapeutic/nontherapeutic effects of typical and atypical antipsychotic medication and the benefits of the atypical drugs.
- Observe the client for side effects and dangerous adverse effects of antipsychotic medication (e.g., anticholinergic/extrapyramidal effects, tardive dyskinesia, neuroleptic malignant syndrome).
- Review current treatment and prevention for adverse medication effects.
- Learn about state and federal laws regarding involuntary treatment, seclusion/restraint, and patient rights.
- Be aware that high amounts of stress and expectations can exacerbate symptoms and that very low stress and lack of challenge are also harmful.
- The client/family should focus on goals that are meaningful and realistic.
- The client with a dual diagnosis of schizophrenia and substance abuse needs to have both issues addressed in treatment.
- Recognize that the client with schizophrenia is more likely to be a victim of crime than a perpetrator, and that the family needs assistance to plan for client safety without being overly restrictive.
- Identify institutional/psychosocial/family stressors that may exacerbate the client's symptoms, and learn how to manage/prevent them.

Teach Client and Family

- Explain to the client/family that schizophrenia is a chronic disorder with symptoms that affect the person's thought processes, mood, emotions, and social functions throughout the person's lifetime
- Teach the client/family about the primary symptoms of schizophrenia, delusions and hallucinations, and how to determine if they pose a threat or danger to the client or others.
- Explain to the client/family that although it is part of schizophrenia, *psychosis* (loss of reality) is not always present, and the client functions better in the absence of psychosis.
- Assist the family in developing a plan for dealing with the client during early signs of acute illness, which may prevent hospitalization.
- Instruct the client/family to recognize impending symptom exacerbation and to notify physician/hospital/emergency support services when the client poses a threat or danger to self or others and requires hospitalization.
- Teach the client/family about the importance of medication compliance and the therapeutic/nontherapeutic effects of antipsychotic medications.
- Tell the family that the client may not always have the energy or motivation to engage in family/social activities, which may be caused by the nature of the illness and the sedative effects of the medication.
- Instruct the family to have patience when interacting with the client, especially during times of stress/thought disturbances/fatigue.
- Inform the family that the client will be more responsive during more functional periods, such as when medications are working and the client is well rested.
- Explain the state laws regarding involuntary treatment, patient rights, and seclusion/restraint to the client/family, as warranted.
- Ask the client/family to repeat what you have taught so that you will know what they have learned and what needs to be reinforced.
- Use different methods of teaching, because some clients may have more cognitive deficits than others and may benefit from alternative techniques.
- Teach the client/family to identify psychosocial/family stressors that may exacerbate symptoms of the disorder, as well as methods to prevent them.
- Instruct the client/family on the importance of continuing medication after discharge and to report any adverse/life-threatening effects.

Continued

CLIENT AND FAMILY TEACHING	Schizophrenia—cont'd

- Recognize that schizophrenia is a chronic illness that can exhaust and frustrate a family and that members need help in managing the client and illness.
- Be aware that the family may need assistance with the client's living arrangements, job placement (if capable), and managing day-to-day affairs.
- Reinforce the importance of taking medication after discharge and notifying physician/emergency support services if serious side effects occur.
- Investigate local chapters of mental health organizations, such as the National Alliance of the Mentally III (NAMI), that can provide education, advocacy, and social support for the family.
- Investigate group homes, community groups, and other resources to help the client/family after discharge; include social work in this effort.
- Investigate current educational resources available on the Internet and in local libraries.

- Help family members recognize that there are limits to what they can do for the client. Aspects of schizophrenia can be frustrating and exhausting to the family, and organizations can assist them.
- Educate the family about the educational and support services of the NAMI, and refer the family to the local chapter.
- Inform the client/family about local community groups and resources that can help the client manage daily affairs, find a job (if capable), and investigate living arrangements; include social work in this effort.
- Teach the client/family how to access current educational/therapeutic resources on the Internet and in the community.

Care Plans

Schizophrenia (All Types)
- Disturbed Sensory Perception
- Disturbed Thought Processes
- Social Isolation
- Impaired Verbal Communication
- Defensive Coping
- Disabled Family Coping
- Self-Care Deficit (see Chapter 3)

Care Plan
DSM-IV-TR Diagnosis | **Schizophrenia (All Types)**

NANDA Diagnosis: Disturbed Sensory Perception

Change in the amount or patterning of incoming stimuli accompanied by a diminished/exaggerated/distorted/impaired response to such stimuli.

Focus:

For the client who experiences sensory perceptions that are incongruent with actual stimuli, as demonstrated by hallucinations, illusions, or impaired awareness of self/environment.

RELATED FACTORS (ETIOLOGY)

Neurobiologic factors (neurophysiologic, genetic, structural)

Psychosocial stressors that are intolerable for the client and that threaten the client's integrity and self-esteem

Disintegration of boundaries between self and others and self and the environment

Altered thought processes

Severe/panic anxiety states

Loneliness and isolation, perceived or actual

Powerlessness

Withdrawal from environment

Lack of adequate support persons

Inability to relate to others

Critical/derogatory nonaccepting environment

Low self-esteem

Negative self-image/concept

Chronic illness/institutionalization

Disorientation

Derealization/depersonalization

Ambivalence

DEFINING CHARACTERISTICS

The client is inattentive to surroundings (preoccupied with hallucination).

Startles when approached and spoken to by others.

Talks to self (lips move as if conversing with unseen presence).

Appears to be listening to voices or sounds when neither is present; cocks head to side as if concentrating on sounds that are inaudible to others.

May act on "voices"/commands.
- Attempts multilating gesture to self or others that could be injurious.

Describes hallucinatory experience.
- "It's my father's voice, and he's telling me I'm no good" *(auditory)*.
- "My mother just walked by the patio, and I saw her go behind that tree" *(visual)*.
- "There's an awful taste in my mouth . . . like rotten eggs" *(gustatory)*.
- "I can feel my brain moving around inside my head." *(somatic).* "It's turning into a transmitter" (coupled with a delusion).
- "There are things crawling under my skin" *(tactile).*

Has false perceptions hallucination when falling asleep *(hypnogogic)* or waking from sleep *(hypnopompic).*

Misinterprets environment *(illusion).*
- Perceives roommate's teddy bear as own dog.
- Interprets a statue in the yard as brother.

Describes feelings of unreality.
- "I feel like I'm outside looking in, watching myself" *(depersonalization).*
- "Everything around me became really strange just now" *(derealization).*

Continued

May voice concern over normalcy of genitals/breasts/other body parts.
- "My breasts are distorted."
- "My penis is abnormal."

Misinterprets actions of others.
- "Sarah is coming at me with her tray; she wants to kill me."

Leaves area suddenly without explanation; may perceive environment as hostile or threatening.

Has difficulty maintaining conversations; cannot attend to staff member's responses and own hallucinatory stimuli at same time (confused/preoccupied).

Interrupts group meetings with own experience, which is irrelevant to the situation/event and has symbolic, idiosyncratic meaning only for the client.

Demonstrates inability to make simple decisions.
- Cannot decide which socks to wear or what foods to eat.
- Uncertain whether to sit or stand during a group session (may indicate ambivalence or suspicion).

OUTCOME IDENTIFICATION AND EVALUATION

The following criteria depend on severity of symptoms, client diagnosis, and prognosis. In some cases, staff expectations may be for modification of symptoms rather than for complete change of behavior.

The client demonstrates the ability to focus relevantly on conversations with others on the unit.

Ceases to startle when approached.

Ceases to talk to self.

Seeks staff when feeling anxious or when hallucinations begin.

Seeks staff or other clients for conversation as an alternative to autistic preoccupation.

Refrains from harming self and others.

Relates decrease/absence of obsessions.

No longer expresses feelings of self/environment as being unreal or strange.

Describes body parts as being normal and functional.

Demonstrates ability to hold conversation without hallucinating.

Remains in group activities.

Attends to the task at hand (group process, recreational/occupational therapy activity).

States that hallucinations are under control.
- "The voices don't bother me anymore."
- "I don't hear the voices anymore."

Utilizes learned techniques for managing stress and anxiety (see deep-breathing/relaxation exercises, Appendix B).

States realistic expectations for self and future.
- "I plan to live in a good board and care home and take one college class this semester."

PLANNING AND IMPLEMENTATION

Nursing Intervention	Rationale
Establish rapport and build trust with the client.	The client must trust the nurse before talking about hallucinations/other sensory-perceptual alterations.
Continuously orient the client to actual environmental events or activities in a nonchallenging way.	Brief, frequent orientation helps to present reality to the client with sensory-perceptual disturbance.
Call the client and staff members by their names. • "Pam, I'm Kathi, your staff person for today." • "These people are other hospital staff members, like me, and they are other clients, like you." • "This is Mark; he's a client, too."	Using correct names of staff and clients reinforces reality and reduces the impact of hallucinations.
Use clear, concrete (versus abstract or global) statements. **Therapeutic Concrete Message** • "Mark, it's time to get out of bed." **Nontherapeutic Abstract Message** "Mark, it's time to rise and shine."	Because of misperceptions, altered thinking, and idiosyncratic symbolization, the client may not understand or may misinterpret an abstract message. Also, not addressing the client by name may cause the client to confuse your statement with an ongoing hallucination.
Use clear, direct verbal communication rather than unclear or nonverbal gestures (do *not* shake your head yes or no, do *not* point to indicate directions).	Unclear directions or instructions can confuse the client and promote distorted perceptions or misinterpretation of reality.
Refrain from judgmental or flippant comments about hallucinations. • "Don't worry about the voices, as long as they don't belong to anyone real."	Telling the client not to worry, even with good intentions, indicates a lack of concern about the client's problem and could compromise trust.

Help the client focus on real events/activities in the environment.	Focusing on actual events helps to reinforce reality and diverts the client from a hallucinatory experience.
Reassure the client (frequently if necessary) that the client is safe and will not be harmed. • "Pam, you're in Haven Hospital, and you're safe. The staff is here to help you."	Alleviation of fear is necessary for the client to begin to trust the environment and to feel safe.
Observe for verbal/nonverbal behaviors associated with hallucinations (statement content, talking to self, scanning, eyes averted, staring, bolting and running from the room).	Early recognition of sensory-perceptual disturbance promotes timely interventions and alleviation of the client's symptoms.
Describe the hallucinatory behaviors to the client. • "Sue, you seem to be distracted while we're talking. Are you hearing voices?" • "You're staring at the ceiling, Sam. What do you see?"	The client may be unable to disclose perceptions, and the nurse can openly facilitate disclosure by reflecting on observations of the client's behaviors, which helps the client engage in more open discussion with the nurse, which in itself brings relief.
Attempt to determine *precipitants* of the sensory alteration (stressors that may trigger the hallucination). • "Jim, what happened just before you heard the voices?"	The hallucination may occur after an anxiety-provoking situation. When such situations are identified, the client understands the connection and can begin learning to manage, avoid, reduce, or eliminate the hallucination.
Identify, wherever possible, the need fulfilled by the hallucinations (loneliness, dependency, rejection, or lack of interpersonal intimacy).	Hallucinations may fill the void created by the lack of satisfying human contact. Once the client's need is elicited, the nurse can begin to replace the hallucinations with a therapeutic interpersonal relationship and activities that meet unfulfilled needs. The client who feels understood is likely to experience decreased anxiety, which in itself reduces hallucinations.
Modify the client's environment to decrease situations that provoke anxiety (excessively competitive, noisy, challenging activities). • "That was a loud basketball game, Don. I know you're upset because you say you're hearing voices again. I'll go with you to work on your model." • "You left the group, Bob. It was pretty hectic today. Let's go for a walk outside."	Decreased anxiety can reduce the occurrence of hallucinations.
Explore the content of auditory hallucinations to determine the possibility of harm to self, others, or the environment *(auditory command hallucination)*. • "You seem frightened, Bob, and you say you're hearing voices. What do the voices that you hear say?"	Exploring the content of the hallucination helps the nurse identify if the sensory-perceptual disturbance is threatening or dangerous to the client, such as a command type of hallucination that may be telling the client to harm or kill the client or others. The nurse can then reinforce treatment and safety precautions.
When danger or violence is imminent, protect the client and others by following facility procedures and policies for seclusion, medication, or behavioral restraint. *Note:* These procedures are used only when less restrictive verbal and behavioral methods are unsuccessful.	Seclusion/restraint and medication are used as therapeutic methods to help the client control behavior that may be harmful to the client or others.

If Client Is Not Harmful to Self or Others, Proceed as Follows

Recognize and acknowledge the feelings underlying the hallucination or other sensory experience rather than focusing on the content. • "You look sad, Nancy. You say the voices you hear keep telling you bad things about yourself. The staff is here to help you get relief from the voices." • "You seem frightened, Tom. Are you hearing voices now?"	When the client feels understood, anxiety and the sense of being alone are diminished, thus decreasing the hallucinatory experience. The knowledge that staff will bring relief and are willing to share the client's burden promotes trust and reduces the client's fear.

Continued

PLANNING AND IMPLEMENTATION—cont'd

Nursing Intervention	Rationale
If Client Is Not Harmful to Self or Others, Proceed as Follows—cont'd	

Nursing Intervention	Rationale
State your reality about the client's hallucinatory experience.	The client is helped to distinguish the actual voices, which promotes reality.
Therapeutic Responses • "I don't hear the voices you describe, Tom. I know you hear voices, but with time they may go away." • Do not deny the existence of the client's experience. • "I hear your voice and my voice, Tom, as we talk with one another." • Present the reality of your experience.	Continuous reality orientation by staff helps to convince the client that the hallucinations (and accompanying delusion, if present) are not real. The client may then begin to let go of the importance attached to the experience.
Nontherapeutic Response "There aren't any voices. Your father isn't here. You're making them up yourself." Refrain from arguing or having lengthy discussions about the content of the client's hallucination.	Nontherapeutic responses negate the client's hallucination and accuse the client of lying, which can destroy trust and decrease client's self-esteem. Arguing with the client or having long discussions only increases anxiety, which may increase hallucinations.
Therapeutic Response • "We talked about the voices earlier, Tom. I'll walk to the activity room with you so you can continue with the project you started."	This therapeutic response effectively diverts and redirects the client, who may need a break from the hallucinations.
Nontherapeutic Response "Tom, this is Lori Jenkins, a new nurse on our unit. Tell her what the voices say to you and what they tell you to do."	This nontherapeutic response encourages the client to focus on and defend the experience, which reinforces it for the client. The client also becomes an object of curiosity, which is demeaning.
Teach the client techniques that will help to interrupt the hallucinations. • Nurse tells the voices to "go away." • Nurse describes disbelief in derogatory or negative messages that the voices carry. "I don't believe you're the devil, Tom." • Client sings, whistles, or plays music over voices. • Client seeks person in milieu for conversation. • Client tells staff when voices are bothersome. • Client engages in an activity, exercise, or project when the voices begin.	Such techniques distract the client from the hallucination, provide alternative competition for the hallucination, and give the client some control. Activities can be healthy alternatives and distractions to hallucinations.
Accept and support the client's feelings (sadness, fear, anger) underlying the hallucination. • "I know the voices that you hear make you feel frightened, Sue. Staff is here for you."	Acceptance and support convey empathy and understanding and reduce the client's fear and anxiety.
Accept, within limits, hostile, quarrelsome outbursts without becoming personally offended.	The client's actions represent the client's own discomfort and do not reflect feelings toward staff.
Set limits on behavior when necessary. • "Your cursing is interrupting the activity, Sarah. Take a 10-minute quiet time in your room."	Helping the client take a respite may prevent violence and keeps the environment safe and comfortable for clients and staff.
Praise the client's efforts to use learned techniques to distract from or manage hallucinations (joining activities, using techniques described previously).	Positive feedback increases the client's self-esteem and promotes repetition of successful behavioral strategies.
Encourage the client to take prescribed medications.	Medication compliance helps to control psychotic symptoms.

Teach the client/family about the therapeutic effects of medications and the important role medications play in reducing psychotic symptoms.	Knowledge and understanding may increase compliance.
Educate the client/family about the adverse effects of medications and how to manage them according to the client's treatment plan (see Pharmacotherapy box).	Education helps to ensure the client's/family's understanding of the effects of medication and provides comfort.
Provide environmental opportunities to expand the client's social network. • Start with one-to-one sessions, then add group activities as appropriate and tolerated by the client.	Satisfying experiences with others tend to decrease/replace hallucinations.
Provide a consistent, structured milieu for the client.	Constancy and a dependable environment promote trust, safety, and a sense of well-being for disorganized clients.
Discuss realistic plans and goals with the client/family for the prevention/management of sensory-perceptual alterations.	The client begins to practice and use available personal skills and resources while in a safe environment.
Provide group situations in which the client can learn and practice activities of daily living, communication skills, and social skills, as well as improve interpersonal relatedness/independence.	Group interaction increases feelings of adequacy, satisfaction, and self-esteem, which decreases negative sensory-perceptual experiences and promotes reality.

Care Plan
DSM-IV-TR Diagnosis **Schizophrenia (All Types)**

NANDA Diagnosis: Disturbed Thought Processes
Disruption in cognitive operations and activities.

Focus:
For the client with thought disorders and inability to test reality who experiences delusions, magical thinking, loose associations, ideas of reference, thought broadcasting, thought insertion, thought withdrawal, and impaired judgment/comprehension/perception/problem solving.

RELATED FACTORS (ETIOLOGY)

Impaired ability to process/synthesize internal/external stimuli
Disintegration of boundaries between self and others and self and the environment
Biologic factors (neurophysiologic, genetic, structural)
Sensory-perceptual alterations
Psychosocial/environmental stressors

DEFINING CHARACTERISTICS

The client inaccurately interprets incoming information.
• Thinks others in the environment are spies or demons.
• Believes the psychiatric intensive care unit is a prison.
• Perceives others' benign statements or gestures as hostile or sexual overtures.
Demonstrates inability to distinguish internally stimulated *(autistic)* thoughts from facts or actual events; the client's statements reflect combined segments of reality and fantasy.

• "The president is our leader. He is the ruler of the universal life and death."
Perceives that others in the environment can hear the client's thoughts *(thought broadcasting)*.
Demonstrates neologisms, "word salad," thought blocking, thought insertion, thought withdrawal, poverty of speech, or mutism (see Glossary).
Believes that his or her thoughts are responsible for world events or disasters *(magical thinking, delusion)*.
• "My thoughts are causing all those fires; they're burning up the world."
Thinks that he or she is omnipotent and capable of superhuman powers *(delusion of grandeur)*.
• "I'm a messenger for the devil and can destroy the universe."
Believes that others in the environment are plotting evil deeds against the client *(delusion of persecution)*.
• "I know they're planning to capture me and use my brain for science."
Inappropriate reactions to others' communication, behavior, and environmental events.
• Laughs in response to sad or despondent content
Incites fear or confusion in other clients.
Demonstrates inability to follow or comprehend others' communication or simple instructions, unrelated to language or cultural differences.
Demonstrates impaired ability to abstract, conceptualize, reason, or calculate.
• Interprets the proverb "A stitch in time saves nine" as "It takes nine stitches to save time" (paralogical, concrete thinking).

Continued

Directs suspiciousness, anger, or fear toward the environment or others.

- Demonstrates hypervigilance or scanning with angry, frightened, or confused facial expression.
- Withdraws from activities and others in the milieu.
- Has outbursts of rage or fear.
- Makes statements that reveal mistrust or hostility without apparent external basis.

Shows distractibility, decreased attention span, or difficulty concentrating on simple activities or events.

Disorganized, incoherent, fragmented, illogical speech patterns (looseness of associations; tangential, circumstantial references; see Glossary).

- "The sea is the water hole of life, the sea of life; I want to marry in the sea."

Attachment of symbolic or idiosyncratic meanings to environmental events, objects, persons, or colors.

- The color purple symbolizes death.
- Blondes represent goodness.
- A particular film star is revered as a savior.

Has preoccupation with religious or sexual ideas, manifested by chanting, preaching, praying, condemning, or making erotic references and gestures.

Makes generalizations from specific or isolated events or persons.

- "My mother has blue eyes and she's an alcoholic, so all blue-eyed women are alcoholics."

Demonstrates ambivalence through statements and behaviors.

- "I want to kill my brother so he could live."
- "I love everyone here so much, I want to leave right now."

Makes a violent gesture while verbalizing pleasant statements.

States that the major influences in life are God and the devil.

Believes that information coming from the media or immediate environment refer to the client (*ideas of reference*).

- "The president was referring to me when he spoke about the space program."
- "The food trays are late because I wasn't ready to eat."

Demonstrates interrupted sleep patterns or inability to fall asleep related to delusions or frightening thoughts.

OUTCOME IDENTIFICATION AND EVALUATION

The client demonstrates reality-based thinking in verbal and nonverbal behavior.

Demonstrates absence of psychosis: delusions; incoherent, illogical speech; magical thinking; ideas of references; thought blocking; thought insertions; thought broadcasting.

Demonstrates the ability to abstract, conceptualize, reason, and calculate consistent with developmental stage.

Exhibits judgment, insight, coping skills, and problem-solving abilities consistent with developmental stage.

Distinguishes boundaries between self and others and self and the environment.

PLANNING AND IMPLEMENTATION

Nursing Intervention	Rationale
Assess own level of anxiety, and use anxiety-reducing strategies to reduce anxiety to tolerable level (see Appendix B).	Anxiety is transferable, and clients experiencing psychosis are extremely sensitive to external stimuli. The nurse's anxiety can increase the client's anxiety and foster disturbed thought processes.
Approach the client in a slow, calm, matter-of-fact manner.	A calm approach helps to avoid distorting the client's sensory-perceptual field, which could promote disturbed thoughts and perceptions.
Maintain facial expressions and behaviors that are consistent with verbal statements.	The client with disturbed thought processes may have difficulty interpreting correct meanings if the nurse misrepresents intent with a conflicting or "double" message.

Nontherapeutic or "Double" Messages

The nurse smiles while discussing a serious matter with the client.

The nurse frowns and appears impatient while telling the client that the nurse accepts and understands the client's behavior.

Continue to assess the client's ability to think logically and to utilize realistic judgment and problem-solving abilities.	Reassessment of the client's functioning helps to determine the extent of cognitive impairment and progress made in use of logical thinking.
Listen attentively for key themes and reality-oriented phrases or thoughts in the client's communication with staff and other clients.	Keen listening helps to elicit problem areas, promotes the client's willingness to relate to another person, and helps meet the client's needs.

Interpret the client's misconceptions and misperceived environmental events in a calm, matter-of-fact manner.
- "That's John, your new roommate. You met him this morning."
- "Those clients are discussing the lunch menu. We're having chicken today."
- "The president is talking about the budget. He is being televised from Washington, D.C."

Presenting reality in a matter-of-fact manner assists the client in correcting misconceptions or ideas of reference without challenging the client's belief system.

Instruct the client to approach staff when frightening thoughts occur.

Knowing staff is available to protect the client helps to reduce fear and anxiety when the client is experiencing "scary" cognitive disturbances.

If the client is capable, teach cognitive replacement strategies, such as interrupting irrational thoughts with realistic thoughts (see Appendix B).

This exercise may be one method of bringing the client closer to reality, although it may not be appropriate for all clients.

Refrain from touching a client who is experiencing a delusion, especially if it is persecutory type.

Clients who are suspicious, hostile, or paranoid may perceive touch as a threatening gesture and react aggressively.

Use simple, concrete, or literal explanations, and avoid use of abstractions or metaphors.

Clients with disturbed thought processes interpret abstractions concretely and may misunderstand or misinterpret the meaning of the message.

Therapeutic Response (Concrete)
- "It's 10 o'clock and time for you to go to bed."

Nontherapeutic Response (Abstract)
"It's 10 o'clock and time to hit the hay."

Avoid challenging the client's delusional system or arguing with the client.

Delusions cannot be changed through logic, and challenging the belief, no matter how irrational, may force the client to cling to it and defend it.

Distract the client from the delusion by engaging the client in a less threatening or more comforting topic or activity at the first sign of anxiety or discomfort.
- "This subject seems troubling for you. Let's work on your jigsaw puzzle."
- "You seem uncomfortable with this topic. Let's walk out to the patio."

Dwelling on delusional content may increase the client's anxiety, aggression, or other dysfunctional behaviors.

Focus on the meaning, feeling, or intent provoked by the delusion rather than the delusional content.

Focusing on the intent or feeling versus the content or words helps meet the client's needs, reinforce reality, and discourage the false belief without challenging the client.

Therapeutic Response
- "I know that's troubling for you. I'm not frightened because I don't believe the end of the world is here."

Nontherapeutic Response
"Describe those people who are out to get you. What do they look like?"

This nontherapeutic response feeds into the client's delusion by reinforcing the belief that "these people" are real, which could further confuse the client.

Gradually encourage the client to discuss experiences that occurred before the onset of the delusion.
- "What happened just before you felt this way?"
- "I noticed when you received the phone call that you became anxious and began to think those troubling thoughts."

Discussing predelusional experiences helps the client identify threatening thoughts, feelings, or events and associate them with reality rather than with the delusional content.

Continued

PLANNING AND IMPLEMENTATION—cont'd

Nursing Intervention	Rationale
Avoid pursuing the details of the client's delusion.	Persistence of delusional details may reinforce the client's false belief and further distance the client from reality.
Offer praise as soon as the client begins to differentiate reality-based and non–reality-based thoughts and behaviors.	Positive reinforcement increases self-esteem and encourages the client to identify and continue reality-based thoughts and behaviors.
Respond to the client's delusions of persecution with calm, realistic statements.	Delusions of persecution represent the client's fears or threats to the self-system in an environment he or she perceives as hostile. Focusing on the client's concerns, fears, and insecurity rather than on the content of the delusion promotes the client's trust and willingness to be helped.

Therapeutic Responses
- "At this time, you may believe your food is poisoned, Pam."
- "I don't think your food is poisoned, but it sounds like you have some concerns, and the staff is here to help."

Nontherapeutic Response

"Mark, do you really believe a hospital would serve the clients poisoned food? There's no reason to be afraid to eat the food."

This nontherapeutic statement challenges the client's belief by focusing on the delusional content (whether or not the food is poisoned) and forces the client to cling to the delusion in an attempt to justify it and protect self-esteem. The client's feelings and concerns are negated, which disrupts trust, blocks communication, and increases the client's fear, insecurity, and sense of isolation.

| Respond to the client's delusions of grandeur or omnipotence in a calm, nonchallenging manner, focusing on the client's need to retain or regain control over own status or situation. | Challenging a client with delusions of grandeur will promote defending behaviors and reduce self-esteem. |

Therapeutic Responses
- "Jim, when you say you are God and can change the world, it sounds like you're unhappy about being a client in the hospital and would like to change your situation."
- "You're John Smith, a client in this hospital. It must be scary to think you're a messenger for the devil. In time you may not believe this."

These types of responses present reality without challenging the client's belief system, focus on the client's intent and meaning behind the delusions (helplessness, powerlessness), and express the staff's desire to understand and help the client maintain safety, control, dignity, and hope at a time of vulnerability.

Nontherapeutic Responses

"Jim, you know you're not God and can't change the world."
"There's no such thing as the devil, so you can't possibly be his messenger, John."

These nontherapeutic responses, although truthful, tactlessly challenge the client's belief system, threaten the client's self-esteem, overlook the meaning and intent behind the delusions (powerlessness, helplessness, fear, frustration), and negate the client's feelings, all of which inhibit the client's trust and block communication.

| Use simple declarative statements when talking to the client who demonstrates fragmented, disconnected, incoherent, or tangential speech patterns that reflect loose associations. | Simple statements tend to enhance the meaning of the message, which is important for a client struggling to interpret and express reality. |

Therapeutic Responses
- "I want to understand you better. Tell me again."
- "I'm having trouble understanding you now. Let's get a snack, and we'll talk some more."
- "It sounds as if you may be upset because your mom isn't here yet. It's 7 o'clock now; visiting hours aren't over until 8 o'clock."

These responses let the client know that the nurse wants to understand the message and meet the client's needs. This reduces anxiety and helps the client to collect thoughts and engage in more goal-directed communication. The responses do not place blame on the client but rather focus on the nurse's desire to pursue the meaning and intent of the client's communication and to help the client communicate more clearly.
Occasionally, the client may be able to write the message or make gestures to convey needs.

Nontherapeutic Responses

"You're just not making any sense at all. Try to concentrate harder on what you want to say."

"I can't understand one word you're saying. Go lie down and clear up your thoughts."

These nontherapeutic responses reflect the nurse's frustration in trying to understand the client's message, place the blame for the behavior on the client, and challenge the client's message. The effort to meet the client's needs is absent, which may increase the client's anxiety and perpetuate dysfunction.

Offer the client clear, simple explanations of environmental events, activities, and the behaviors of other clients, when necessary.

- "That remark was not meant for you. It was directed to all of us in the community meeting."
- "That noise is coming from the patio. The clients are playing volleyball."
- "John got a little upset in the group meeting, so he raised his voice, but everything is OK now."
- "You will not be harmed here."
- "Those people are clients, not spies. They are deciding on an activity."

Clear, direct explanations of environmental events help to lessen the client's suspiciousness and fear or mistrust of the surroundings and others and can prevent aggressive behavior.

Remain silently and patiently with the client who demonstrates mutism or poverty of speech, without demanding a response.

Quiet company helps the client to feel worthy even though the client is unable to participate at the time.

Therapeutic Responses

- "I know your thoughts are troubling you now. Let's wait a while, and then continue our talk. I'll sit here with you."
- "We don't need to talk now. But I'd like to stay here with you."

These responses illustrate the nurse's understanding and acceptance of the client's inability to engage in a meaningful, goal-directed interaction at this time. The nurse shows willingness to help meet the client's needs while offering comfort, safety, and companionship.

Nontherapeutic Responses

"I can't understand a word you say. I'll come back later after you've had a chance to rest."

"I know your thoughts are affecting your speech. Try to concentrate on what you really want to say."

These nontherapeutic responses focus on the client's inability to express thoughts. Leaving the client at this time may increase anxiety and decrease self-worth, which could perpetuate symptoms.

Asking the client to rest or concentrate places the responsibility to "fix the problem" on the client through unrealistic means.

Assess the client's nonverbal behavior, such as gestures, facial expression, and posture.

This assessment may help to meet the client's needs that cannot be conveyed through speech.

Continue to support and monitor prescribed medical and psychosocial treatment plans.

Postdischarge support helps maintain the client's ability to accurately interpret and respond to the environment.

Care Plan
DSM-IV-TR Diagnosis   Schizophrenia (All Types)

NANDA Diagnosis: Social Isolation
Aloneness experienced by the individual and perceived as imposed by others and as a negative or threatening state.

Focus:
For the client who is isolated because of mental or emotional impairment. This isolation does not refer to the voluntary solitude that one seeks for personal rejuvenation, the aloneness needed for creativity, or the loneliness experienced after a major loss.

RELATED FACTORS (ETIOLOGY)
Altered sensory perception (hallucinations, illusions; may result in mistrust of or rejection by other clients in the environment)

Continued

Altered thought processes (delusions, magical thinking, ideas of reference, thought blocking, thought insertion; see Glossary).

Impaired verbal communication (neologisms, "word salad," loose associations, tangentiality, incoherence, poverty of speech, mutism)

Long-term illness, hospitalization, or environmental deprivation

Ineffective support systems (e.g., family, friends, work, school)

Unsatisfying or ineffective role/relationships

Unaccepted social values (may result in behavior inconsistent with accepted social norms)

Impaired developmental stage (may be socially inept and unable to perform age-appropriate tasks)

Decreased energy level

Fear or anxiety

Impaired volition

Impaired social interactions

DEFINING CHARACTERISTICS

The client withdraws from the environment and from others in the environment.

Isolates self in room or bed for most of the day and night.

Has difficulty in establishing bonds or relationships with others in the environment; fails to seek out or respond to others.

Makes statements that indicate feelings of rejection from others in the environment.
- "I guess I'm not wanted by the other clients in the group."
- "The staff never seem to be available for me."
- "No one ever seems to notice me."
- "My family never visits me. They don't know I exist."
- "I just wish people liked me more."

Demonstrates inability to engage in social interactions or milieu activities.

Demonstrates inability to share or express feelings with others in groups or one to one.

Verbalizes difficulty in engaging in social conversations.
- "I have trouble talking to others on any subject."
- "I'm really uncomfortable socializing with strangers."
- "I don't have anything of interest to add to a discussion."

Relates history of inadequate or unsatisfactory relationships.
- "I was never involved in a happy relationship."
- "I could never seem to find anyone who really cared about me."
- "My parents never approved of me."

Expresses a lack of purpose in life.
- "Life holds no meaning for me."
- "The days seem to drag by endlessly without meaning."
- "I have no real plans or desires for my life."

Demonstrates inappropriate/immature interests or activities for developmental level.

Is noncommunicative, with flat/dull affect and minimal or absent eye contact.

Is preoccupied with dysfunctional thoughts, activities, or rituals; may be responding to obsessions, hallucinations, or delusions.
- Remains in room, rearranging clothes.
- "I'm not really a client; I'm here to meditate for all mankind."

Demonstrates inability to concentrate or make decisions.

Expresses feeling "useless" or "worthless."
- "I'm no good to anyone."
- "I just don't seem to matter."
- "I'm not worth talking to."

Demonstrates physical inactivity.

Verbalizes decreased or lack of energy.
- "I don't feel like getting involved in groups or discussions."
- "I don't have the strength to get out of bed just to talk to people."

Demonstrates changes in appetite or eating habits (overeats or undereats).

OUTCOME IDENTIFICATION AND EVALUATION

The client verbalizes willingness to engage in social interactions and activities with others in the environment.
- "I plan to come to community meeting this afternoon."
- "I'm going to contact my staff person for a one-to-one discussion after lunch."

Engages in social activities with others in the milieu (e.g., meals, exercises, crafts, games, outings).

Expresses pleasure derived from social conversations and activities with other clients, staff, and significant others.
- "I liked talking to my roommate today."
- "I got a lot out of my meeting with my staff person."
- "Bowling yesterday was fun."
- "It was good to see my family."

Spends most of time out of room, involved with others in the environment.

Expresses belief that he or she can make meaningful contributions to social discussions and activities.
- "The group seemed to like my input."
- "I helped my bowling team win last night."

PLANNING AND IMPLEMENTATION

Nursing Intervention	Rationale
Assess the extent of the client's self-imposed isolation.	Assessment of the client's isolative behaviors helps the nurse plan strategies to break the pattern of withdrawal with interactions and activities.
Assist the client to meet basic needs (e.g., sleep, nutrition, personal hygiene) during times of social withdrawal.	Meeting basic needs helps to promote the client's physical health and well-being.

Structure each day to include planned times for brief interactions and activities with the client.

Structure helps the client organize times to engage with others and tells the client that participation is expected and that the client is a worthwhile member of the community.

Spend brief intervals with the client each day, engaging in meaningful, nonchallenging interactions.

Brief interactions help to ease the client into the community by first developing trust, rapport, and respect.

Discuss with the client anything of interest to the client (e.g., items in room, favorite activities/hobbies).

Discussing the client's interests encourages social skills and decreases social isolation.

Identify the client's significant support persons, and encourage them to contact the client for interactions, phone conversations, activities, and visits.

A strong supportive network increases the client's social contact, enhances social skills, promotes self-esteem, and facilitates positive relationships.

Help the client compare the difference between social isolation and a desire for solitude or privacy.

The client may occasionally choose to be alone at appropriate times and should be given the opportunity.

Assess the client's self-concept (sense of worth, self-esteem) and coping abilities and their relationship to social isolation.

Low self-esteem and maladaptive coping strategies may result from and perpetuate social isolation.

Act as a role model for social behaviors in one-to-one and group interactions.
• Maintain good eye contact, appropriate distance, calm demeanor, and moderate voice tone.

Effective role modeling by staff helps the client identify appropriate social skills for age and status.

Engage other clients and significant others in social interactions and activities with the client (e.g., card games, meals, sing-alongs).

Encouraging social activities and interactions between client, peers, and family helps promote social skills in a safe setting.

Help the client seek out other clients to socialize with who have similar interests.

Shared or common interests promote more enjoyable socialization, which is likely to be repeated.

Praise the client for attempts to seek out others for interactions and activities and to respond to others' attempts to engage the client.
• "Your participation in group was helpful, Amy."
• "Your consent to go with Karen and Paul to lunch was a positive step, Greg."

Praise given for attempts at socialization and successful initiation of social situations promotes repeated positive social behaviors.

Provide the client with stimulation from recreational and other milieu activities.

These activities expose the client to social situations and increase opportunities to practice socialization and improve social skills.

Provide the client with progressive activities according to level of tolerance and cognitive and affective functioning: (1) meal planning, (2) simple game with one staff member, (3) simple group activities, (4) process group interaction.

Gradual exposure of the client to more complex interactive exercises and activities increases the client's level of tolerance and acceptance of social activities and situations.

Provide the client with outings (e.g., shopping malls, grocery stores, day care centers, pet shops, museums, the zoo).

Outings encourage a variety of interactive experiences for the client outside the hospital community and reduce social isolation.

For the Client Demonstrating Compulsive Acts, Hallucinations, Delusions, and So On

Intervene with the client demonstrating compulsive acts, hallucinations, delusions, or impaired verbal communication.
• Remain with the client during acute phases.
• Engage in brief, calm social contacts with the client throughout the day.

Caring, empathetic behaviors demonstrate the nurse's understanding of the client's limitations and help to fill the client's social void during vulnerable times.

Keep all appointments for interactions with the client. If unable to keep an appointment, make sure client is told ahead of time by a trusted source.

Promptness and reliability promote the client's trust and self-esteem, which enhance socialization.

Continued

PLANNING AND IMPLEMENTATION—cont'd

Nursing Intervention	Rationale
For the Client Demonstrating Compulsive Acts, Hallucinations, Delusions, and So On—cont'd	
Encourage the client to engage in social activities that are within the client's physical capabilities and tolerance level.	Activities provide the client with successful social experiences likely to be repeated and demonstrate understanding and consideration of the client.
Continue to support and monitor prescribed medical and psychosocial treatment plan.	Postdischarge support helps maintain the client's learned social skills.

Care Plan
DSM-IV-TR Diagnosis **Schizophrenia (All Types)**

NANDA Diagnosis: Impaired Verbal Communication
Decreased, delayed, or absent ability to receive, process, transmit, and use a system of symbols.

Focus:
For the client whose altered thought content and withdrawal from reality often result in misinterpretations that affect the ability to communicate verbally or to use language in a meaningful way. The client's comprehension of others' communication is also compromised.

RELATED FACTORS (ETIOLOGY)
Disturbances in form of thinking (autistic)
Altered thought processes (delusions, magical thinking; see Glossary)
Poverty of speech/mutism
Sensory-perceptual alterations (hallucinations)
Disturbances in structure of associations (neologisms, "word salad," perseveration; see Glossary)
Obsessive thoughts (sexual, religious)
Inability to reason/abstract/calculate/problem-solve
Impaired insight/judgment
Inability to distinguish self from environment or from others in the environment
Panic or anxiety state
Inability to distinguish internally stimulated thoughts from actual environmental events or common knowledge
Withdrawal from environment into self/lack of external stimulation
Regression to earlier developmental level

DEFINING CHARACTERISTICS
The client uses distorted verbal communication.
- "It's 5 o'clock in the morning and I am the dawn of the new age" *(loose/tangential association)*.
- "There are no *cornerfrocks* here, only *doppel skirts*" *(neologisms)*.
- "Sit to seagreen underwear;" "Jump out winter sludge" *("word salad")*.

Uses words that may rhyme or are similar in sound but not meaning (clang associations; "ping-a-long," "the man can," "ding-dong").
Uses, vague, obscure speech that gives little information and may be repetitious.
Repeats words that are heard (echolalia; may reflect inability to distinguish boundaries).
Uses symbolic references or idiosyncratic meanings (attributed to names, objects, events, people, or shapes).
- States that the color red means *dead* or *blood*.
- All blue-eyed people are relatives.
- Cross-shaped objects have magical powers.
- "My name is Dawn Eve, dawn of the universe, Eve of the garden where Adam is waiting."
Verbalizes concrete or literal interpretations in relation to abstract terms.
- Interprets the proverb "People who live in glass houses shouldn't throw stones" as "houses made of glass will break if they're struck with stones."
Uses impaired verbal techniques.
- *Circumstantiality:* digression of inappropriate thoughts into ideas.
- *Perseveration:* repetition of same word/idea in response to different questions.
- *Stereotype:* continuous repetition of speech/activities.
- *Verbigeration:* meaningless repetitions of speech.
- *Circumlocution:* roundabout way of speaking to reach desired goal.
Demonstrates repetitious, ritualistic verbalization of religious or sexual topics that are socially inappropriate.
- Chants or preaches endlessly from the Bible or other holy book.
Addresses others in the environment with odd or idiosyncratic phrases, titles, or identifications that hold meaning only for the client ("Lily Pureface," "Green Goddess," "Funny Man," "Mary from the Sanctuary").
Accuses staff and other clients of plotting or planning to harm or kill the client.
- "I know Liz has poisoned my food."
Accuses others in the environment of reading the client's thoughts.

- "I'm sure Tim knows what I'm thinking right now."

Claims to be able to read the thoughts of others.

- "I have telepathic powers and can read minds."

Introduces self to others as an omnipotent figure with superhuman powers.

- "I'm king of the universe and have been sent here to heal the world."

Speaks minimally or not at all for long periods (poverty of speech, mutism).

Uses speech that is vague and obscure and gives little or no information (poverty of content).

Responds inappropriately/irrationally to rational statements/questions posed by others.

Nurse: What would you like for lunch?

Client: Bricks and sticks on white copper sand; *or* Delicious turmoil of life's bread and guts (loose associations).

Claims that thoughts are responsible for events, cause events to occur, or can prevent an occurrence via magical means.

- "I willed those wars to happen, and they did."
- "The menu was changed to chicken because of my thoughts."

Converses with voices emanating from radio/television. Talks/perseverates/mumbles incoherently to self with no apparent external stimuli.

Frequently interrupts group sessions with verbal outbursts that may/may not be reality based.

OUTCOME IDENTIFICATION AND EVALUATION

The client communicates thoughts and feelings in a coherent, goal-directed manner.

Demonstrates reality-based thought processes in verbal communication.

Displays meaningful and understandable verbal communication.

Demonstrates verbal communication that is congruent with affect and other nonverbal expressions.

Recognizes that increased anxiety states exacerbate impaired verbal communication.

Identifies psychosocial stressors that increase anxiety and perpetuate impaired verbal communication.

Initiates strategies to decrease anxiety and promote coherent, meaningful verbal communication.

Responds coherently in group sessions without frequent, inappropriate verbal interruptions.

PLANNING AND IMPLEMENTATION

Nursing Intervention	Rationale
Assess the extent to which impaired verbal communication interferes with the client's ability to convey to others the meaning behind the client's verbal message. • Note reaction of other clients to client's communication attempts. Do they appear puzzled, frightened, shocked, or offended?	Assessment of the client's communicative ability serves as a guideline for helping the client and peers learn alternate methods of communication, develop trust and patience, and better meet each other's needs.
Demonstrate a calm, patient demeanor rather than attempting to force the client to speak coherently.	A calm approach helps to decrease the client's fears and anxieties about the inability to communicate needs and demonstrates acceptance of the client.
Actively listen to and observe verbal/nonverbal cues and behaviors during the communication process	Active listening and keen observations help to understand the meaning of the client's message and demonstrate a willingness to meet the client's needs.
Use communication strategies such as restatement, clarification, and consensual validation (see Box 1-6). • "When you say (this), do you mean (that)?" • "I'm not sure what you mean by that. Tell me again." • "Are you saying. . . ?" • "Please explain that again."	Effective therapeutic communication strategies help to reveal the intent of the client's message.
Acknowledge the client's inability to use the spoken word while encouraging alternative methods to convey messages (e.g., gestures, writing, drawing). • "I know you find it difficult to speak now. Maybe you can tell me with a gesture or sign."	Acknowledgment and understanding of the client's limitations and strengths demonstrate empathy, develop trust, and encourage the total communication process.

Continued

PLANNING AND IMPLEMENTATION—cont'd

Nursing Intervention	Rationale
• "Although you're not able to speak now, you may be able to write your thoughts." • "If you're having trouble expressing yourself now, you can try again in a few minutes. I'll still be here."	
Instruct the client to seek assistance from staff when experiencing communication problems.	Staff can help facilitate the communication process in a variety of ways, as noted previously.
Anticipate the client's needs until the client can communicate coherently and meaningfully.	Anticipating the client's needs in times of vulnerability provides safety, comfort, and support.
Act as a liaison between the client and the client's peers while the client is unable to speak coherently.	The liaison role facilitates the communication process and decreases alienation from other clients.
Assign staff persons who are familiar with the client's methods of verbal/nonverbal communication, and encourage clear intershift reports. • The client has a delusional system with the persistent theme of achieving world peace, which reflects the client's fear of war and death. The nurse communicates this to other caregivers so that staff can consistently provide a calm, low-stimulation environment in a collaborative effort to meet the client's needs.	Intershift communication facilitates consistency and increases opportunities to understand the meaning behind the client's actions and expressions.
Encourage the client to approach other clients for conversations.	Encouragement assists the client to practice communication skills in a safe setting.
Assist the client to listen and engage in actual conversations (one-to-one interactions with staff and peers, group meetings/activities).	Interaction encourages the client to respond to reality rather than to own inner (autistic) thoughts.
Assess the effects of the client's cultural and spiritual background on dysfunctional speech patterns to individualize client care. • The client speaks to deceased relatives more frequently as anxiety escalates, but during periods of higher functioning, some behaviors are culturally appropriate and provide comfort.	Religious/spiritual discussions may be appropriate depending on the client's condition, situation, or culture.
Teach the client strategies to use whenever the client initially experiences impaired verbal communication (see Appendix B). • The client practices deep-breathing exercises and progressive relaxation. • Replaces/interrupts irrational, negative thoughts with realistic ones. • Takes periods of quiet time. • Seeks out a supportive person. • Engages in a simple exercise or activity.	Therapeutic strategies help the client decrease anxiety, which may exacerbate symptoms, and promote more functional speech patterns.
Praise the client's attempts to speak more coherently and to engage in more meaningful conversations with others.	Positive reinforcement increases the client's self-esteem and promotes continued functional speech patterns.
Continue to support and monitor prescribed medical and psychosocial treatment plans.	Postdischarge support helps maintain the client's ability to understand and express verbal communication.

Care Plan
DSM-IV-TR Diagnosis **Schizophrenia (All Types)**

NANDA Diagnosis: Defensive Coping
Repeated projection of falsely positive self-evaluation based on a self-protective pattern that defends against underlying perceived threats to positive self-regard.

Focus:
For the client who copes by defending against perceived threats to the self-system (e.g., persistently blaming, accusing, or threatening others, generally in a hostile manner). Underlying this behavior is often a negative self-concept.

RELATED FACTORS (ETIOLOGY)

Depletion of adaptive coping strategies
Moderate to severe anxiety states
Altered thought processes
Perceived threats to self-system (integrity, self-esteem)
Low self-esteem
Sensory-perceptual alterations
Developmental impairment secondary to personality disorder
Suspicion and mistrust of persons and situations in the environment secondary to schizophrenic process
Misinterpretations of actual environmental events and activities
Inability to interpret or express emotions
Inability to displace angry/hostile feelings constructively
Inability to have needs met through direct communication channels
Impaired reality testing
Ambivalent/mistrustful family dynamics

DEFINING CHARACTERISTICS

The client projects blame/hostility/responsibility on others.
- "You made me late for group today."
- "It was all your fault that I got caught smoking."
Displays hypersensitivity to slightest criticism.
- Leaves group in middle of discussion; angers easily when confronted.
Demonstrates grandiosity; may be delusional.
- "I'm the smartest person in this room."
- "I'm the nephew of the president of the United States."

Displays superior attitude toward others.
- "I shouldn't be here, I'm not sick."
- "I know more about psychiatry than my doctor does."
Has difficulty establishing and maintaining relationships.
- Makes no friends on the unit.
- Other clients leave when client enters room.
Uses hostile laughter and ridicules others.
Takes other clients' cigarettes or other belongings, then denies it or projects behavior to others.
Sabotages own treatment and therapy with overt defensive behaviors.
- Fails to attend groups or acts out during group activities to elicit negative attention.
Demonstrates feelings of being persecuted; may be delusional.
- "I feel as if everyone here is against me."
- "I just know my roommate wishes I was dead."
Displays paranoid ideation and uses ideas of reference.
- "Those clients are always whispering. I'm sure it's about me."
- "Everyone I see on TV is talking about me."
Abuses drugs/alcohol during unit passes, and brags about behavior to other patients.

OUTCOME IDENTIFICATION AND EVALUATION

The client uses coping strategies in a functional, adaptive manner in appropriate situations.
Demonstrates trust in staff and other clients in the environment.
- Seeks out staff for one-to-one interactions.
- Participates with clients in groups and activities.
Expresses feelings appropriately through verbal interactions with staff and other clients.
Displaces the energy of anxiety toward physical exercise and group activities.
Accurately interprets environmental events and behavior of others in the environment.
Meets own needs through clear, direct methods of communication.
Demonstrates absence of hypersensitivity, suspiciousness, or paranoia during interactions with others.
Demonstrates absence of verbal abuse, threats, or ridicule or physically aggressive behavior directed at others.

PLANNING AND IMPLEMENTATION

Nursing Intervention	Rationale
Accept hypersensitivity, ideas of reference, and paranoia as part of the client's impaired delusional system and altered reality testing.	Acceptance helps to establish trust, which begins the groundwork for a therapeutic nurse-client relationship that also involves other professionals.
Demonstrate calm, nonjudgmental, nonthreatening demeanor in all interactions.	Nonthreatening approaches help to diminish the client's perceived threats to the delusional system and encourage more adaptive coping.
Assure the client who exhibits mistrust, suspicion, or paranoia that the environment is safe. • "You're in the hospital, and you're safe here." • "Those people are clients. They're discussing an arts and crafts activity."	Reassuring the client that the environment is safe and secure helps to decrease the client's anxiety, build trust, and identify reality.
Refrain from attacking or challenging the client's delusional system.	Attacks can alienate the client, diminish trust, and force the client to defend the delusion in an effort to justify the belief and thereby preserve self-esteem.
Engage the client in frequent, brief contacts. • Avoid whispering or laughing. • Refrain from arguing. • Inform the client about schedule changes. • Gently question irrational grandiosity/paranoia. • Speak in a calm, clear, concise manner.	These measures help to establish a therapeutic, trusting nurse-client relationship that includes other disciplines and to reduce ambivalence, suspicion, and other defensive behaviors.
Inform the client gently but firmly when you do not share the client's interpretation of an event, even though you acknowledge the client's feelings. • "The group is not against you, although you think so now. Your cursing upsets them." • "Sam didn't take your cigarettes. You gave the last one to Jeff last night." • "It's OK to feel bad about not getting your pass. The staff is not to blame."	Pointing out factual situations in a nonchallenging, matter-of-fact way helps the client focus on actual versus perceived situations.
Refocus conversations to realistic topics when the client begins to misinterpret events and the behaviors of others. • "I know your thoughts are upsetting. Let's talk about the group activity this afternoon."	It is therapeutic to encourage reality-based thinking and minimize defensive behaviors when the client's misinterpretations are troubling to the client. Redirecting the client may prevent escalation of unrealistic thoughts and prevent anger/aggression.
Offer feedback when the client resorts to defensive coping behaviors (blaming or threatening others, using angry voice tones, cursing/shouting, acting aggressively). • "We were having a nice conversation, but now you seem angry. Can you tell me what happened?" • "The group is upset with your shouting. They find it hard to concentrate on the discussion." • "Sam is tired of you saying he took your cigarettes. What are your feelings about this?"	Direct responses to the client's defensive behaviors by a trusted nurse help the client identify maladaptive behaviors and their effects on others in the environment and foster a more realistic interpretation of events by the client.
Encourage the client to participate in milieu activities (leisure/occupational/recreational activities, one-to-one/group sessions).	Group participation helps the client decrease anxiety, gain insight into stressors that promote defensive coping behaviors, and acquire more adaptive coping skills.
Help the client select activities that are most rewarding and generally result in success.	Rewarding activities help to increase self-esteem and reduce incidents of defensive coping to meet the client's needs.

Teach the client behavioral strategies: slow deep-breathing exercises, progressive muscle relaxation, simple physical exercises (see Appendix B).

Physical exercises help to divert anxiety-producing energy toward constructive activities and reduce incidents of defensive coping.

Praise the client for using more adaptive methods to meet needs.
- "Your cooperation in group today was appreciated."
- "You expressed yourself clearly and quietly. It was nice that you didn't shout or curse."

Positive feedback when warranted helps to increase the client's self-esteem and ensure continuity of functional behaviors.

Continue to demonstrate concern and caring for the client during times of anxiety, suspiciousness, and mistrust.

Suspicious clients respond well to staff who display concerned, interested attitudes, which can provide the impetus for the client to change or modify dysfunctional behavior.

Refrain from touching the client during times of increased anxiety, paranoia, and impaired reality testing.

Avoiding physical contact prevents the client from misinterpreting motives and possibly reacting with aggression.

Help the client associate maladaptive behaviors with thoughts and feelings that precipitate them (see Appendix B)

This gives the client the opportunity to interrupt the sequence and replace negative behaviors with learned relaxation strategies.

Do not challenge, threaten, or use unnecessary force with a client who is verbally insulting.

The client may react with violence to protect self and self-esteem.

Suggest trying writing or drawing as a means of communication, when the client is capable of cognitive or expressive activities.

Writing or drawing offers a constructive alternative to express feelings and meet needs and can decrease anxiety and minimize defensive coping.

Construct a written behavioral contract with the client, listing acceptable behaviors in clear, concrete terms, if the client is capable of compliance.

Written contracts serve as permanent visual reminders for clients who find it difficult to respond to verbal directives. *Note:* Contracts do not replace ongoing assessment and observations of a client's behavior.

Set limits in a calm, direct, matter-of-fact way when the client begins to demonstrate behaviors that are out of control (accuses, blames, curses, threatens, exhibits hostile/aggressive acts).
- "You may stay in the volleyball game if you do not shove other clients."
- "Threatening others is not acceptable even if you say you're joking. Let's discuss other ways to deal with your feelings."
- "It's OK to leave the group when you feel anxious, but slamming the door shut is disruptive. Let's talk instead."

Setting limits when necessary helps to prevent injury to the client and others and gives the client the opportunity to choose more functional methods to have needs met. The client who is experiencing a loss of control feels comforted knowing staff is in control and will help the client regain composure.

Inform the client that the client's behavior (verbal abuse, persistent anger) is unacceptable, and help the client redirect to other activities.

Redirection helps the client refocus anger toward alternative methods to meet needs and prevents injury to the client and others in the milieu.

For the Client Whose Defensive Coping Is Out of Control and Who Poses a Danger to Self or Others

Initiate seclusion/restraint when warranted, as a least restrictive therapeutic intervention.

Seclusion/restraint is used to help the client gain or regain control when anger, aggression, verbal threats, or physical violence cannot be managed by other therapeutic methods and the client and others need protection.

Continue to support and monitor prescribed medical and psychosocial treatment plan.

Postdischarge support helps the client maintain more functional and adaptive coping methods.

Care Plan

NANDA Diagnosis: Disabled Family Coping

Behavior of a significant person (family member, other primary person) that disables his or her capacities and the client's capacities to address effectively tasks essential to either person's adaptation to the health challenge.

Focus:

For the family and significant persons of a chronically ill client who demonstrates dysfunctional behaviors owing to lack of cognitive, physical, or psychologic resources needed to cope with the effects of mental illness.

RELATED FACTORS (ETIOLOGY)

Extremely ambivalent family relationships
- Members vacillate between withdrawal from and solicitude toward the ill person.

Significant persons unable to express feelings of guilt, anger, frustration, or despair

Ineffective/maladaptive coping strategies used by significant persons

Denial by significant persons of psychosocial/financial impact of illness on client/family/community

Disintegrated client/family role/relationships

Resistance/refusal of significant persons to participate in the client's treatment and care

Physically/developmentally/emotionally impaired significant persons

Defensive/uncooperative significant persons

Knowledge deficit of significant persons regarding illness and management

Family enmeshment, overinvolvement, solicitude, extreme worry regarding client/illness/management of care

DEFINING CHARACTERISTICS

Significant persons are inattentive to the client's basic needs.
- Client exhibits unkempt, unclean appearance on various admissions.
- Client demonstrates progressive weight loss, poor skin turgor, broken skin, and dental caries.
- Client's clothes are dirty, shabby, or sparse.

Significant persons fail to attend to the client's needs for love and companionship.
- Others do not visit during the client's hospitalization
- *Client:* "No one cares about me," "Everyone I know eventually leaves me," "I'm not wanted at home anymore."

Significant persons fail to assist the client in management of the illness.
- Refuse to accompany client on follow-up treatments
- Neglect to help client comply with medication regimen after discharge.

- Are uncooperative with staff regarding client's placement after discharge.

Family members display inappropriate or mixed reactions toward the client's illness and effects on client, family, and community.
- Display little or no emotion when discussing the client's illness and treatment and effects of the illness on all of their lives.
- Express conflicting, emotionally charged content (criticism, disappointment, solicitude, worry, overprotectiveness, overinvolvement).

Significant persons are preoccupied with negative thoughts and feelings regarding the client's illness and management of care.
- Describe feeling overwhelmed with anger, anxiety, fear, guilt, or despair.
- State they are unable to dismiss thoughts of personal inadequacy and hostility toward the client.

Significant persons withdraw from the client during time of need (intolerance, rejection, abandonment, desertion).

Family members demonstrate overprotective behavior or overinvolvement toward the client, which fosters the client's dependency *(enmeshment)*.
- Constantly remind staff of their devotion to the client.
- Phone the unit several times a day.
- Visit day and night and hover around the client.
- Act as the client's protector in the milieu.
- Make demands on staff on the client's behalf.

Significant persons alternate between displays of rejection and overprotection toward the client *(ambivalence)*.

Family members demonstrate distortion of reality regarding the client's illness, such as extreme denial about its existence or severity.
- Carry on usual routines, disregarding the client's needs.
- Act indifferent or apathetic toward serious information given to them about client and illness.

The family makes decisions and performs actions that are detrimental to the client's and family's social or economic well-being.
- Accumulates debts that do not include cost of the client's care, treatment, or placement.

Significant others demonstrate signs of agitation, depression, aggression, or hostility.

The family demonstrates ineffective or neglectful relationships among members, which disintegrate the family support system.

The client develops helplessness, inactivity, and dependence on significant persons and society.

Family members display impaired ability to restructure meaningful lives or to individualize because of their prolonged involvement with the client.

OUTCOME IDENTIFICATION AND EVALUATION

Significant persons verbalize realistic perception of roles/responsibilities regarding the client and the client's illness, care, and treatment.

Express thoughts/feelings about responsibility to client, openly and frequently, in a therapeutic environment.

Demonstrate improved communication, problem-solving, and decision-making skills in relating to other family members and health care personnel regarding the client's illness and treatment.

Exhibit effective coping strategies in dealing with the client's illness and management of care.

PLANNING AND IMPLEMENTATION

Nursing Intervention	Rationale
Assess the family's current level of functioning, and contrast with their level of functioning before the onset of the client's illness.	Assessment determines the degree of the family's dysfunction over time and assists them to develop a realistic plan to support the client according to the family's tolerance and capabilities.
Assess and promote the readiness and willingness of individual family members to participate in the client's management of care.	Aftercare of clients ideally includes family members, as appropriate, if the client is to succeed in meaningful interpersonal functioning.
Examine the extent of expressed family emotions, enmeshment, or disintegration regarding the client, the illness, and management of care.	Clients from families who are overinvolved, enmeshed, or overprotective, or who consistently express criticism, disappointment, hostility, solicitude, extreme worry, or anxiety, are at high risk for relapse.
Encourage family members to join therapeutic family groups, as needed (see Family Therapy, Appendix B).	Groups allow the family to express anger, despair, frustration, guilt, or powerlessness with others who share similar emotions. Realistic expectations and goals regarding the family's role in the client's illness and treatment can be discussed.
Teach family members the facts about the client's illness, emphasizing that it could strike any family. Include the illness course and its chronicity and expected effects on the family/community.	Educating the family helps to dispel myths and decrease the stigma of mental illness (which promotes adaptive coping skills) and encourages the family to rejoin society fortified with accurate information and decreased embarrassment about the client and the illness.
Promote family involvement in the hospital environment. • Family members attend group/family therapy. • Confer with caregivers as often as necessary. • Attend in-service seminars. • Review current literature on the client's illness, its treatment, and related research. • Review Internet sources (if family has access to computer).	Healthy family involvement/participation in the client's hospital setting informs the family of all facets of the client's illness and management, demonstrates that care of the client is a team effort so that the family will not feel isolated and overwhelmed, and offers hope through the client's success in a therapeutic environment. Family involvement can continue after discharge.
Encourage family involvement in behavioral management programs that specifically address the client's problems.	Involvement helps the family acquire strategies that can positively influence the client's life and strengthen the family system.
Inform the family of available community services and personnel to assist when the client's symptoms and behavior are difficult to comprehend or manage. • *Hospital* treatment team includes nurse, physician, social worker, and occupational therapist. • *Aftercare* services include local mental health meetings, day treatment groups, night hospitals, sheltered workshops, rehabilitation services, and private therapists.	Assuring the client/family of the availability of qualified help and support reduces feelings of isolation and powerlessness, encourages use of services to enable clients to remain in the community, relieves the family of its burdens, and strengthens the family system.

## chapter 5

Adjustment Disorders

Adjustment disorders represent a group of diagnostic categories that describe a maladaptive reaction to clearly identifiable stressful events or situations. Stressors may be a *single event* such as the ending of a personal relationship, *several events* such as serious business or marital problems, or *recurrent events* such as those associated with seasonal jobs and business crises or ongoing circumstances such as living in a high-crime neighborhood or working with difficult people. Stressors may affect a single individual, a whole family, a larger group, or an entire community, as in a natural disaster. Some stressors may accompany specific developmental events, such as beginning school, leaving one's home of origin, being married, becoming a parent, or retiring (Box 5-1).

An adjustment disorder is not an exacerbation of a preexisting mental disorder that has its own set of criteria, such as an anxiety disorder or a mood disorder. However, an adjustment disorder can coexist with another Axis I or Axis II diagnosis if the latter does not account for the pattern of symptoms that have occurred in response to the stressor event.

Not only are adjustment disorders associated with an increased risk of suicide attempts and suicide completion but also an adjustment disorder may complicate the course of illness (e.g., decreased compliance with the medical regimen or increased length of hospital stay) in people diagnosed with a medical condition.

In a multiaxial assessment, the nature of the stressor is indicated by listing it on Axis IV (e.g., marital, divorce, work, or academic problem). Box 5-2 contrasts adjustment disorder responses and bereavement responses.

Box 5-1 | **Stressors and Their Relationship to Developmental Stages**

Childhood: Separation from significant others; preschool
Adolescence: Graduation from high school; life choices
Young adulthood: Intimacy; marriage; parenthood; career building
Middle-age adulthood: Financial/emotional care of young/old family members
Older adulthood: Loss of job/spouse; possible major illness

Box 5-2 | **Responses of Adjustment Disorder and Bereavement**

Adjustment disorder: Responses to stress are generally unexpected.
Bereavement (grief): Responses to stress are generally expected, such as death of a loved one.*

*A diagnosis of adjustment disorder may be made if the response in bereavement is in excess of or more prolonged than what is typically expected.

ETIOLOGY

Specific etiologic factors are associated with adjustment disorders (Box 5-3). The etiology of adjustment disorders varies widely. The stressor may be *internal,* such as

Box 5-3   Etiologic Factors Related to Adjustment Disorders*

BIOLOGIC/GENETIC

Physiologic response to crisis and stress, such as acute or chronic illness/injury, that requires a biologic adjustment.

BIOCHEMICAL

Activation of adrenaline and other neurotransmitters, as noted in stress adaptation and crisis models.

PSYCHODYNAMIC

Maladaptive ego defenses or lack of ego strength at critical life stages; inability of the ego to adapt/adjust to crises.

PSYCHOSOCIAL

Psychologic/emotional responses to crisis/stressor events or inability to use existing coping methods or create new ones; may be
    influenced by timing, intensity, or repetition of the stressor event.
A chronic, debilitating illness may require both physical and psychologic adjustments to the ongoing stressors.

DEVELOPMENTAL

Stressors experienced at critical developmental stages of adolescence, adulthood, middle adulthood, and older adulthood.

CULTURAL

Sociocultural adjustment, response to illness, and meaning of illness vary among individuals from different cultures.
An individual's culture may determine whether the reaction to the stressor is expected or exceeds the usual response.

*Although a specific etiology for adjustment disorders has not been established, a combination of factors is implicated. The current
research emphasis is biologic.

development of a medical condition, or *external*, such as loss of a job due to downsizing of employer agency (see Box 5-1).

EPIDEMIOLOGY

Adjustment disorders are common and may occur in any age group, including children; men and women are equally affected. Epidemiologic features vary widely because of the types of populations studied and the assessment methods used. A higher incidence of adjustment disorders, however, seems to occur in individuals from disadvantaged life circumstances than in the general population in that they experience a high rate of stressors, including the results of poverty, unemployment, crime, unwanted pregnancies, malnutrition, single parenthood, drug abuse, and other physical and psychologic abuses.

The percentage of people in outpatient mental health treatment with a diagnosis of adjustment disorder ranges from approximately 10% to 30%.

The onset of symptoms occurs within 3 months of an identified stressor and may occur within days if the event is acute. Duration is usually brief, lasting months, but symptoms may persist if the stressor is prolonged (e.g., threatening neighborhood, persisting marital strife).

ASSESSMENT AND DIAGNOSTIC CRITERIA

The defining characteristic for adjustment disorders is development of emotional or behavioral symptom disturbance in direct response to a psychosocial or environmental stressor. The symptom picture is accompanied by disturbance in social relationships and occupational functioning (school or work) or by marked distress in the individual that exceeds an expected normal response.

Although adjustment disorders do occur alone, they are also associated with preexisting mental disorders, medical conditions, or surgical procedures. Individuals with adjustment disorders often have problems with substance use and abuse; suicide ideation, gestures, threats, attempts and completions; and somatic complaints. Symptoms vary widely depending on the type of disorder.

DSM-IV-TR Criteria

Various categories of adjustment disorder have been identified based on the *Diagnostic and Statistical Manual of Mental Disorders (DSM-IV-TR)* criteria (see box on p. 140; see also Appendix A).

Types of Disorders

The response of the client with an adjustment disorder is considered maladaptive because of noted impairment in

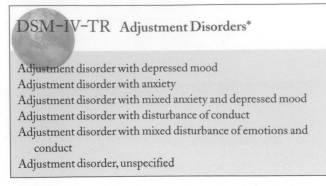

DSM-IV-TR Adjustment Disorders*

Adjustment disorder with depressed mood

Adjustment disorder with anxiety

Adjustment disorder with mixed anxiety and depressed mood

Adjustment disorder with disturbance of conduct

Adjustment disorder with mixed disturbance of emotions and conduct

Adjustment disorder, unspecified

*Adjustment disorders are coded according to the subtype that best characterizes the predominant symptoms.

social, academic, or occupational functioning or because the resultant symptoms or behaviors exceed normal, usual, or expected responses.

Adjustment Disorder with Depressed Mood

The defining characteristics of adjustment disorder with depressed mood are depressed mood, tearfulness, sadness, and feelings of hopelessness/helplessness. More serious responses are melancholia, regression, psychophysiologic decompensation, and depersonalization.

Adjustment Disorder with Anxiety

The defining characteristics of adjustment disorder with anxiety are worry, nervousness, jitteriness, and in children, fears of separation from major attachment figures, resulting in myriad symptoms.

Adjustment Disorder with Mixed Anxiety and Depressed Mood

The defining characteristics of adjustment disorder with mixed anxiety and depressed mood are symptoms of both anxiety and depression, as described in the previous two categories.

Adjustment Disorder with Disturbance of Conduct

The defining characteristics of adjustment disorder with disturbance of conduct is a violation of others' rights or of major age-appropriate societal norms and rules, such as truancy, vandalism, reckless driving, substance abuse, fighting and other inappropriate forms of anger/aggression/impulsivity, and defaulting on legal responsibilities.

Adjustment Disorder with Mixed Disturbance of Emotions and Conduct

The defining characteristics of adjustment disorder with mixed disturbance of emotions and conduct combine emotional symptoms such as depression and anxiety with a disturbance in conduct, as described previously.

Adjustment Disorder, Unspecified

The defining characteristics of adjustment disorder, unspecified, are not classifiable in any of the other sub-types, such as physical complaints, social withdrawal, school or work problems, or other psychosocial stressors.

INTERVENTIONS

Treatment Settings

Clients with adjustment disorders are typically treated on an outpatient basis. Exceptions occur when the stressor or its consequences are greater than the individual's ability to cope and short-term acute care in a treatment facility is necessary. Clients will be admitted to a facility if suicidal. A variety of therapeutic techniques may be employed by an interdisciplinary team, depending on the professional preference, assessment of problem, and desired outcome.

Medications

Medications are used sparingly for clients with adjustment disorders because symptoms of these disorders are expected to resolve after the immediate cause is identified and treated. Also, practitioners prefer to observe the client without the effects of medication because symptoms of adjustment disorder may include symptoms of anxiety and may even progress to include symptoms of a major mental disorder such as depression.

In general, both benzodiazepines and antidepressants mainly of the typical type, are used to treat adjustment disorders, depending on the symptoms (see Pharmacotherapy box on opposite page).

Psychosocial Therapies

Nurse-client relationship

A facilitative therapeutic alliance can be beneficial for the client who experiences an adjustment disorder. Being able to express feelings, thoughts, and behaviors with an empathic and nonjudgmental nurse often brings emotional catharsis, initial organization of thoughts and problem solving, and modification of problematic behaviors that have occurred or worsened as a result of responses to the stressors. With use of therapeutic techniques the nurse can affect or assist client change and provide a necessary affiliation needed by the client during stressful times (see Chapter 1).

Adjunctive therapies

Recreational therapies may be useful for clients diagnosed with adjustment disorder, whether they are in an outpatient or inpatient setting. Leisure activities promote socialization and help clients become more comfortable with others who may have similar problems, even if they do not all share the same diagnosis. Recreational therapies also inspire clients to engage in more self-directed pursuits that may build confidence and increase self-esteem. Exercise can be a constructive anxiety-reducing outlet for some clients; others may prefer relaxation strategies.

Occupational therapy may help clients whose crises are related to role changes or who may have some residual dysfunction as a result of a concomitant physical disability.

PHARMACOTHERAPY **Adjustment Disorders**

ADJUSTMENT DISORDERS WITH ANXIETY

The *benzodiazepines* alprazolam (Xanax) and lorazepam (Ativan) are used to treat anxiety symptoms on a short-term basis only, because of their addictive properties. Doses are administered orally as follows:

- *Alprazolam:* 0.25 to 0.5 mg 3 times daily; not to exceed 4 mg/day.

Dose for older adults: 0.25 mg 2 or 3 times daily.

- *Lorazepam:* 1 to 2 mg 2 to 3 times daily; not to exceed 10 mg/day.

Dose for older adults: half the adult dose daily.

Side effects of benzodiazepine include the following:

- Drowziness, dizziness, confusion
- Headache, anxiety, tremor, stimulation
- Fatigue, depression, insomnia
- Paradoxical agitation (alprazolam)

ADJUSTMENT DISORDERS WITH DEPRESSION

The selective serotonin reuptake inhibitors (SSRIs, atypical antidepressants) fluoxetine (Prozac), paroxetine (Paxil), and sertraline (Zoloft) are nonaddicting substances used to treat depressive symptoms. SSRIs are currently the first-line treatment for clients who have adjustment disorders with depression. Doses are administered orally as follows:

- *Fluoxetine:* 20 mg daily in morning; may be increased to 20 mg twice daily if no improvement is noted in 4 weeks; not to exceed 80 mg/day.
- *Paroxetine:* 20 mg daily in morning; may be increased by 10 mg/day each week if no improvement is noted in 4 weeks; not to exceed 50 mg/day.
- *Sertraline:* 50 mg daily; may be increased to maximum of 200 mg/day. Do not change dose at intervals of less than 1 week; administer in morning and at night.

Side effects from SSRI are less intense and troublesome than those of the typical antidepressants.

Systems affected by one or more SSRIs include the central nervous system (CNS); cardiovascular, genitourinary, gastrointestinal, respiratory, integumentary, and musculoskeletal systems; and eyes/ears/nose/throat. General systemic effects also occur in clients with adjustment disorder who are taking SSRIs.

The client's developmental stage, capabilities, presented problems, and preferences should be considered before adjunctive therapeutic activities are initiated.

Supportive therapies

Clinical nurse specialists, social workers, physicians, and psychologists are prepared and trained to manage the care of clients with adjustment disorders through a therapeutic interdisciplinary team approach. A variety of treatment options are available for outpatients, depending on professional preference, assessment of problems, and desired outcomes. Cognitive therapy, brief strategic therapy, and other types of behavioral interventions may be used effectively in combination with psychodynamic, psychotherapeutic, or interpersonal approaches. Family therapy may be selected when the identified stressor is a crisis within the family system. Group therapy may also be used.

Other therapies

Biofeedback, psychodrama, hypnosis, meditation, visual imagery, and journal writing are other therapeutic modalities that may be helpful for clients with adjustment disorders, depending on individual problems and client/practitioner preference (see Appendix B).

PROGNOSIS AND DISCHARGE CRITERIA

Unless a client is suicidal, out of control, or abusing drugs in addition to having an adjustment disorder, treatment is usually at home or in other outpatient settings. Discharge may mean suspension of outpatient treatment when symptoms have abated. The prognosis for the client with adjustment disorder is usually good based on the symptom duration of six months. Chronic disorders may occur when symptoms persist in response to a chronic stressor (e.g., HIV/AIDS). The following criteria demonstrate the client's readiness for discharge:

- The client verbalizes absence of thoughts of self-harm.
- Verbalizes realistic perceptions of self and capabilities.
- Sets realistic goals and expectations for self and others.
- Identifies psychosocial stressors and potential crises.
- Describes plans and methods to minimize stressors.
- States realistic/positive methods to cope with stressors.
- Identifies signs and symptoms of adjustment disorder.
- Contacts appropriate sources for validation/intervention.
- Utilizes learned techniques to prevent/minimize symptoms.
- Verbalizes knowledge of therapeutic/nontherapeutic effects and potential problems of prescribed medications.
- Makes and keeps follow-up appointments with appropriate staff.
- Expresses feelings openly, directly, and appropriately.
- Engages family/significant others as sources of support.
- Structures life to include appropriate outlets/activities.
- Verbalizes plans for future with absence of suicidal thoughts.

The box on p. 142 provides guidelines for client and family teaching in the management of adjustment disorders.

CLIENT AND FAMILY TEACHING   **Adjustment Disorders**

Nurse Needs to Know

- The client with adjustment disorder has greater difficulty than usual coping with stressors or conflicts.
- Adjustment disorder may coexist with another Axis I or Axis II disorder and may occur in any age group.
- Stressors or conflicts can usually be identified and may be a single (job loss) or recurrent (ongoing relationship problems) event.
- The client may need protection from self-destructive/injurious behavior.
- Hospitalization is necessary when the client is suicidal or a danger to others.
- Adjustment disorder can complicate the course of an existing medical illness.
- Anticipate stress-producing situations and their effects on individual clients and families.
- Recognize emerging signs of an adjustment disorder, and identify appropriate sources to help the client/family cope more effectively.
- Identify client/family strengths and their positive effects on the client's well-being.
- Recognize the importance of medication compliance, if prescribed for anxiety or depression.
- Identify therapeutic/nontherapeutic effects of drugs and the dangers of misuse/abuse.
- Identify the client's use of independent behaviors and ability to cope more adaptively with stress and conflict.
- Reinforce symptom prevention and coping skills with the client/family.
- Provide the client/family with appropriate resources in case of emergency.
- Investigate appropriate community resources for client care after discharge.
- Investigate current Internet and library resources for client/family education.

Teach Client and Family

- Teach the client and family to identify stress-producing situations and events.
- Teach the client/family how to anticipate stress-producing situations and to take steps that may help to avoid/minimize them.
- Teach the family how to protect the client from self-destructive acts and to contact appropriate sources for help immediately.
- Instruct the family to utilize appropriate emergency resources if the client is suicidal or a danger to others and requires hospitalization.
- Teach the client effective coping methods to manage/minimize stressors when possible; include family when feasible.
- Teach the client/family to recognize emerging signs of adjustment disorder and to contact appropriate resources for help as soon as symptoms occur.
- Teach the client/family the importance of medication compliance.
- Inform the client/family about the therapeutic/nontherapeutic effects of medications and the dangers of misuse and abuse.
- Encourage the client to express thoughts and feelings openly and appropriately.
- Reinforce symptom prevention measures with the client/family, and obtain their feedback to validate learning.
- Assess the client continually and at discharge for self-destructive thoughts, future goals and plans, and ability to cope appropriately for age and status.
- Inform the client/family about community groups available after discharge.
- Teach the client/family how to access current Internet and library education.

Care Plans

Adjustment Disorders (All Types)
- Ineffective Coping
- Dysfunctional Grieving

Care Plan

NANDA Diagnosis: Ineffective Coping

Inability to perform a valid appraisal of the stressors; inadequate choices of practiced responses; inability to use available resources.

Focus:

For the client experiencing maladaptive responses to an identifiable stressor event, as demonstrated by impairment in social, academic, or occupational functioning, and behaviors that exceed the normal expected response to the stressor. Symptoms of anxiety, depression, or conduct disturbances may also be present. Stressors can be acute or chronic; psychosocial, physical, or developmental; singular or multiple.

RELATED FACTORS (ETIOLOGY)

Impaired reactions to developmental conflicts (graduation from high school, leaving home for college, marriage, parenthood, retirement)

Maladaptive responses to psychosocial stressors (marital problems, divorce, job dissatisfaction, business failure, moving to a new environment)

Residual effects of physical or psychiatric illness/disability

Depletion of previously existing coping methods and inability to attain new ones

Premorbid life-style of negative coping methods

Developmental lag

Ineffective/absent resources

Dysfunctional family system

Lack of goal-directed behavior/skills

Ineffective problem-solving skills

Knowledge deficit regarding crisis management

Lack of insight regarding own abilities and limitations

Unrealistic expectations of self and others

Low self-esteem

Negative role modeling

Unresolved grief in response to crisis or stressor event

Psychologic or emotional vulnerability

DEFINING CHARACTERISTICS

The client verbalizes inability to cope with stressors/conflicts.
- "I can't make it without my significant other."
- "I'll never find another job that satisfies me."
- "My marital problems are ruining my life."
- "I can't adjust to this new place; it's depressing."

Demonstrates nonacceptance of health-status change.
- Withdraws from social functions.
- Shows loss of appetite/weight unrelated to disability/illness.
- Has saddened affect with intermittent crying spells.
- Demonstrates self-destructive behavior (e.g., smokes, stays up all night).
- Directs anger/blame toward family/friends.
- Demonstrates inability to work or perform activities of daily living.

Demonstrates ineffective capacity to problem-solve or establish goals (cannot make simple choices or decisions).

Exhibits increased dependency on others to complete work and fulfill needs.
- *Child* client depends on parents to complete school assignments and household chores.
- *Adolescent* client overspends allowance and borrows money from family/friends rather than work for it.
- *Adult* client uses fiance/spouse/family members to support the client financially and emotionally.
- *Older adult* client relies on grown children to provide basic needs even though capable of performing own daily tasks.

Demonstrates inability to adjust to maturational changes.
- *Child* client displays regression during toilet-training process.
- *Adolescent* client experiences depression caused by body changes (acne, unfulfilled body image).
- *Adult* client develops depression about weight gain due to pregnancy.
- *Older adult* client experiences depression following "normal" changes of aging.

Continued

Demonstrates inability to meet role expectations.
- *Child* client displays regression at birth of new sibling.
- *Adolescent* client experiences anxiety when attempting intimacy.
- *Adult* client develops depression upon perceiving performance as parent to be inadequate.
- *Older adult* client experiences depression after retirement from valued job/profession.

Manifests alterations in societal/milieu participation.
- Isolates/withdraws from social scene.
- Refuses to engage in community activities.

Fails to follow societal/unit rules of conduct.
- *Child* client demonstrates temper tantrums and other acting-out behaviors upon perceiving needs to be unmet.
- *Adolescent* client steals others' belongings and engages in physical fights with individuals perceived to be "enemies" or opponents.
- *Adult* client commits violent or illegal crimes and misdemeanors with apparent unconcern about consequences of actions.

Expresses self-destructive thoughts/plans/gestures.

Demonstrates noncompliance with therapeutic regimen, including refusal to take prescribed medications.

Verbalizes knowledge deficit regarding stress prevention.

Demonstrates inability to minimize stressors when they occur.

Describes symptoms of grief responses to stressor events and crisis situations.
- Engages in frequent sighing.
- Displays sad, despondent feelings.
- Verbalizes negative, hopeless thoughts.
- Conveys a sense of powerlessness.
- Demonstrates ambivalence and anger.
- Displays low self-esteem.
- Practices yearning and protest.
- Demonstrates inability to plan future goals.

OUTCOME IDENTIFICATION AND EVALUATION

The client verbalizes ability to cope with stressors/conflicts.
- "I can make it now; my friends have given me the support and strength to go on without my husband."
- "I know I have the talent to be successful in another job. I've done it before."
- "Maybe divorce isn't the worst thing in the world. It's better than struggling in an unhappy marriage."
- "I miss my family and friends, but moving to a new place is an exciting opportunity to meet new people."

Demonstrates acceptance of health change status.
- Demonstrates fewer depressive symptoms.
- Laughs and engages with others more often.
- Has better appetite.
- Maintains normal weight.
- Returns to normal sleep patterns.
- Displays healthy expressions of anger.

- Does not blame others for the client's health change.
- Resumes normal activities/interests.
- Discontinues self-destructive behavior.

Demonstrates decreased dependency on others to meet needs.
- *Child* client completes schoolwork/household tasks with minimal supervision.
- *Adolescent* client works for allowance and spends within means.
- *Adult* client supports self and family/significant other adequately.
- *Older adult* client is supportive adjunct to grown children/grandchildren or significant others, as age and circumstances allow.

Demonstrates effective adjustment to maturational changes.
- *Child* client achieves mastery of stages (trust, autonomy, initiative) without significant regression.
- *Adolescent* client achieves puberty and identifies with appropriate role models, with minimal conflicts and stress.
- *Adult* client accepts generative processes (pregnancy, weight gain) with absence of midlife crisis.
- *Older adult* client accepts normal changes of aging with integrity versus despair.

Meets role expectations with minimal stress.
- *Child* client accepts changes (preschool, school, new sibling) with minimal regression.
- *Adolescent* client achieves healthy peer relationships with minimal anxiety and conflict.
- *Adult* client exhibits strong, flexible parenting and other mentor skills and successful job/career performance.
- *Older adult* client accepts retirement as part of life and transfers productivity to alternate worthwhile activities.

Actively participates socially with family, friends, and community groups.

Follows societal/unit rules of conduct.
- *Child* client is directable and adaptive with minimal acting out or oppositional behaviors.
- *Adolescent* client relates well with peers and accepts adult supervision/directives with minimal opposition.
- *Adult* client refrains from hostile, illegal acts toward society or other clients.

Demonstrates absence of self-destructive behaviors.

Complies with therapeutic regimen, including medication.

Verbalizes knowledge/plan to prevent stress.

Minimizes inevitable stressors when they occur.

Demonstrates stress prevention/reduction skills (see Appendix B).
- Engages in physical exercise/activities.
- Writes in a log/journal.
- Practices cognitive therapeutic strategies.
- Uses reframing techniques.
- Demonstrates assertive response behaviors.

Cites knowledge of appropriate community resources for ongoing follow-up care, as necessary (e.g., self-help groups, day treatment program, individual or group therapy).

PLANNING AND IMPLEMENTATION

Nursing Intervention	Rationale
Encourage discussion of feelings and emotions (anger, fear, sadness, guilt, hostility) with the client according to developmental level.	Talking about feelings and emotions helps the client identify actual object of stress/crisis and develop the trust to begin to work through unresolved issues.
Provide physical outlets for healthy release of pent-up anger/anxiety and hostile feelings (punching pillows, running, jogging, simple stretching and breathing exercises, as appropriate).	Physical exercise is a safe and effective method to reduce stress/tension.
Promote independent behaviors, role, and life-style experienced by the client before adjustment disorder symptoms. *Child:* Assign simple age-specific tasks related to school and home with appropriate rewards/tokens for each completed task. *Adolescent:* Construct with the adolescent a written daily log/diary of completed school/household work and amount of money/privilege earned for each task. *Adult:* Encourage adult support groups (cognitive, behavioral, brief strategic, assertive, relational, retirement planning, psychodrama, or process groups, as appropriate). Suggest family therapy for all age groups as it applies to individual situations (see Appendix B).	Increased responsibility for age-appropriate life tasks and roles promotes coping skills, self-esteem, and independent functioning. The client's success or failure depends in part on the client's choices.
Assist the client to adhere to unit or program rules and discuss consequences of noncompliance. Carry out consequences in a matter-of-fact manner if unit or program rules are broken. *Child:* Facilitate "chair time" (quiet time) or reduction in rewards/privileges. Engage in role playing and role modeling as appropriate. *Adolescent:* Deny a special recreational activity (group outing, field trip). Engage in role playing and role modeling. Facilitate behavioral contracts. *Adult:* Deny movement to higher level of privilege in the unit. Engage in individual, group, family, or didactic therapies, appropriate to coping/adjustment problem.	Adjustment problems related to conduct disorders and related diagnosis require clear guidelines and directives by the staff to increase client compliance and coping. Also, other clients are entitled to a safe, nondisruptive, therapeutic milieu, without fear of manipulation. Adults who continue to be noncomplaint with unit rules or do not engage in milieu programs may be recommended for alternative treatment (partial hospitalization, crisis centers, rehabilitation facilities, discharge to own support system).
Help the client recognize aspects of life in which the client has maintained control and order.	Awareness of personal control during critical developmental stages decreases powerlessness and enhances self-esteem. It also provides hope that the client can transfer those abilities to resolve present conflicts/stressors.
Identify with the client the stressor or stressor event that precipitated the maladaptive coping and other symptoms of adjustment disorder, and assist the client through the problem-solving process. Prioritize possible alternative coping methods appropriate to client's age and life circumstances. Discuss positives and negatives of each alternative. Examples: • Suggest that the client construct a double column on a sheet of paper and write positives on one side and negatives on the other side for each alternative coping method. • Choose the best alternative method and apply it to the identified problem, first in a role-play situation, then in actual life.	Identifying stressors or stressor events that result in maladaptive coping and continued negative consequences is the first step in formulating effective alternative solutions and coping methods.

Continued

PLANNING AND IMPLEMENTATION—cont'd

Nursing Intervention	Rationale
• Evaluate the effectiveness of the alternative methods. Did the method minimize the stressor and its effects? • Develop awareness of areas of limitations, and learn effective responses that create more distance between the self and the stressor or stressor event (see assertiveness training, Appendix B). • Continue to consult with nurse or therapist for assistance and modification of plan, as necessary.	
Provide realistic praise for the client's attempts at adaptive coping and finding solutions for adjustment problems, even when they are not always successful.	Positive reinforcement for continued attempts at adaptive coping skills promotes hope and repetition of effective, desirable behaviors.
Encourage client to discuss life-style before health status change, including coping methods used during those times.	Identification of client's strengths, support system, and healthy coping style is useful in facilitating adaptation to current change or loss.
Give client permission to express normal grieving emotions (fear, anger, sadness) related to health status change and actual or perceived loss.	Some people may not be aware that anger, fear, and sadness are normal, healthy responses to critical life crises that need to be expressed, although if symptoms persist, it may indicate a more serious depressive disorder that requires further treatment.
Teach the client/family/significant others about the emotional, psychologic, and physiologic responses to stressors and stressor events, as appropriate. Provide understandable current reading material and Internet resources regarding adjustment disorders and related symptomatology.	Appropriate knowledge empowers the client/family and increases hope, cooperation, and compliance. Information can result in preventive measures that can minimize or eliminate future stress-related problems.
Locate with the client/family the community resources geared to each individual's adjustment crisis, including health status change, marital discord, maturational/developmental crisis, and occupational/academic problem.	Community resources provide a wide variety of professionals, including community health nurses, social workers, psychologists, marriage/family therapists, school/occupational counselors, and clergy, who are available for ongoing help with adjustment problems.

Care Plan
DSM-IV-TR Diagnosis   **Adjustment Disorders (All Types)**

NANDA Diagnosis: Dysfunctional Grieving

Extended, unsuccessful use of intellectual and emotional responses by which individuals/families/communities attempt to work through the process of modifying the self-concept based on the client's perception of loss.

Focus:

For the individual who demonstrates a sustained or prolonged detrimental response approximately several months to a year following a loss of a loved one or valued occupation/object/life-style. Individuals in clinical settings are often at high risk for dysfunctional grieving because they frequently experience unsuccessful emotional/societal reintegration after a loss.

A diagnosis of adjustment disorder may be made if the response in bereavement (grief) is in excess of or more prolonged than what is typically expected; for example, if the individual remains fixed in one stage of the grief process for an extended period or if the normal symptoms of grief become exaggerated.

RELATED FACTORS (ETIOLOGY)

Physiologic/Psychologic

Loss of physiologic/psychologic functioning as a result of physical/mental/emotional disorder/trauma

Situational

Changes in life-style or status
- Unanticipated death of a loved one
- Unwanted or unplanned pregnancy
- Complications of childbirth
- Physically/mentally ill family member
- Divorce
- Loss of career/finances/occupation
- Victim role (rape, robbery, abuse)

Maturational

Losses associated with aging: eyesight, hearing, mobility.
Forced retirement
Death of spouse/old friends
Leaving home to live with grown children
Moving to a retirement home or skilled nursing facility

Other Losses

Multiple or cumulative losses
Feelings of guilt and loss of self-esteem engendered by
    ambivalent or difficult relationships with the deceased
Lack of support systems
History of vulnerability, as noted by response patterns
    associated with crisis/stressor events (loss)

DEFINING CHARACTERISTICS

The client verbalizes expressions of distress (grief
    symptoms) regarding loss, change, or stressor event
    (anger, guilt, sadness, crying, labile mood,
    yearning/protest, sighing) inappropriate to normal
    stages of grieving.
Demonstrates alterations in functioning (loss of
    appetite, libido, sleep, concentration, pursuit of
    tasks). Displays fatigability and anxiety (agitation,
    irritability).
Makes statements about unresolved issues and inability to
    move forward in life, with negative dream patterns,
    reliving of past experience, and idealization of previous
    life-style or the deceased.
Projects excessive, inappropriate anger toward self and
    other family members/friends, rather than focusing
    anger appropriately toward the loss.

Displays continued ambivalence and loss of self-esteem,
    indicating high risk for self-destructive behavior.
- "I should have died instead of her."
- "He was so wonderful. I was the bad one."
- "It was my fault that she died. I don't deserve to live."
Demonstrates unsuccessful adjustment/adaptation to the
    loss: prolonged denial, delayed emotional response,
    preoccupation with loss experienced by others.
Displays social isolation or withdrawal.
Fails to resocialize with current friends, develop new
    relationships/interests, and restructure life following the
    loss.
Demonstrates idealization of the deceased or lost valued
    object, situation, role, status, or occupation, with
    concomitant nonacceptance of current life
    circumstances.

OUTCOME IDENTIFICATION AND EVALUATION

The client acknowledges the loss and expresses
    feelings/emotions associated with the loss experience
    (anger, sadness, guilt) appropriate to the grief
    process
Demonstrates a decreasing response in the intense pain
    associated with the grief process, appropriate to the
    stages of grieving.
Demonstrates increased functional abilities (sleep,
    appetite, sexual activity, concentration, and pursuit of
    tasks).
Attempts to resolve issues associated with the loss in a
    healthy, meaningful way; discusses both positive and
    negative qualities (realistically) about the deceased or
    lost object, status, or occupation.
Moves forward and beyond the grief experience in a timely
    manner: makes future plans, seeks others for
    socialization, experiences healthy dreams, focuses on
    more positive aspects of life.
Resolves ambivalence and self-blame about loss or lost
    valued object or concept, with concomitant increased
    self-esteem.
Seeks support persons and community resources (self-help
    groups, counseling, clergy) as needed.

PLANNING AND IMPLEMENTATION

Nursing Intervention	Rationale
Identify the tasks of mourning that the client must accomplish (acknowledging the loss, experiencing the pain, adjusting to the loss, reinvesting, goal setting).	Such identification helps to establish the client's place on the grief continuum and begins to help with grief work and reintegration of life.
If denial persists and the client continues to deny feelings associated with the loss, assure the client that feelings/emotions are normal, healthy responses to loss and should be expressed in a safe, nurturing environment.	Unexpressed feelings result in pent-up emotions that may be directed inward and may eventually lead to depression or other disorders.

Continued

PLANNING AND IMPLEMENTATION—cont'd

Nursing Intervention	Rationale
If anger is excessive and inappropriately expressed, help the client/family understand that anger is a normal response to loss and powerlessness and needs to be vented, but that it is best to channel anger toward the loss and its actual consequences rather than project it toward self or others.	Such assurance provides structure and control for the client's emotional expressions while still giving permission to vent.
Encourage the client/family to talk about both positive and negative qualities of the deceased or lost object, status, or role.	Realistic appraisal of the loss gives the client a clearer perspective of the situation, minimizes idealization, and promotes acceptance of current life circumstances.
Engage the client in motor activities (brisk walks, jogging, physical exercise, volleyball, exercise bike).	Physical exercise provides a safe, effective method for expending anxious energy, anger, and tension associated with the loss.
Assess the client's levels of functioning: sleep, appetite, dream patterns, sexual activity (if appropriate), socialization.	Increase in levels of functioning indicates successful movement toward health and reintegration and a reduction in the pain of grief and despair.
Evaluate whether the client is goal directed and making future plans or regressing and withdrawing from life.	Goals and plans for the future are indicators of health and reintegration, whereas regression and withdrawal signify that the client is at risk for depression and needs further evaluation and follow-up care.
Continue to engage the client in social activities and meaningful interpersonal interactions.	People experiencing grief and loss need to be involved with others to minimize isolation and withdrawal and to regain trust that others will help bear the pain of grief and that "life goes on."
Identify effective supports in the family and community (self-help groups, individual/group counseling, clergy) for the grieving individual.	Appropriate support can help clients more readily do the grief work that will move them toward health and integrity.

## chapter 6

Personality Disorders

*P*ersonality is that unique and distinctive human quality that defines and determines the essence of a person's character, "what the person is really like." An individual's personality serves to distinguish the person from everyone else in the world yet at the same time reflects qualities shared by all individuals.

Personality traits are specific features or behavioral patterns that make up an individual's overall personality. Personality traits are defined in the *Diagnostic and Statistical Manual of Mental Disorders (DSM-IV-TR)* as "enduring patterns of perceiving, relating to and thinking about the environment and oneself." Traits represent an individual's lifelong style of viewing and interacting with the world. Traits begin to emerge early in life, develop over time, and are manifested within a broad range of experiences and social situations.

Personality disorders develop when those enduring, deeply ingrained traits or patterns become maladaptive and inflexible and cause difficulty for the person in relating to, working with, or loving others. The disorders are stable over time and eventually lead to distress and impairment. Frequently a personality disorder may be annoying to others or troubling to society or the law yet not viewed as a problem by the person with the disorder. Because the behavior has been so long-standing, it often feels "comfortable" *(ego-syntonic)* to the individual. Therefore the person believes that he or she is right and the world is wrong and attempts to manipulate the environment to fit his or her needs.

Another factor that promotes resistance to change or treatment is that these individuals rarely experience the pain and discomfort of *anxiety* as a cue to their maladaptive behavior or its consequences. This lack of anxiety reinforces their perceptions that change is unnecessary. They may seek treatment only when they become depressed because others can no longer tolerate the dysfunctional behaviors and proceed to make it difficult for them to continue to function in the same manner. In other words, societal demands exceed their ability to cope.

Personality disorders become evident in childhood or adolescence, but an actual diagnosis is usually not made until adulthood, when the person is 18 years or older. A formal diagnosis of personality disorder is sometimes assigned to a child or adolescent in cases when the maladaptive traits are stable and persistent over a long time and occur in various situations. Diagnosticians say the diagnosis is warranted because characteristics are *crystallized,* or fixed and unchanging.

ETIOLOGY

In the past it was thought that environment was the primary factor in shaping and influencing the development of personality. Although environmental and psychosocial influences undoubtedly play a part, more recent studies demonstrate that biologic factors are also evident and have been specifically identified in some personality disorders. In addition, psychoanalytic and psychologic theories offer explanations for healthy and deviant personality formation. As with many other disorders, the current consensus is that a combination of biologic, environmental, and psychologic factors is most likely the source of personality dysregulation (Box 6-1).

Box 6-1   Etiology for Personality Disorders

BIOLOGIC FACTORS

Genetic/familial factors
- Higher incidence in first-degree relatives with disorder
- Higher incidence in monozygotic twins

Neurotransmitter dysregulation
- Increased serotonin level in suicidal behaviors
- Increased dopamine level in aggressive/violent behaviors

Disruptive neurointegrative function

PSYCHOSOCIAL/ENVIRONMENTAL STRESSORS

Parenting styles
- Punitive/rigid
- Excessively permissive/overindulgent
- Abusive/neglectful
- Poor parent-child bond

Acquaintance influences

Availability/lack of resources

Poverty, losses

War, oppression

Violence (home, school, gang)

PSYCHOANALYTIC FACTORS

Impaired psychosexual stage development

Psychic structure impairment (id, ego, superego)

OBJECT RELATIONS

Individuation/separation obstruction

Object constancy disruption

SOCIAL LEARNING

Learned responses/behaviors

EPIDEMIOLOGY

In general, definitive epidemiologic statistics are not clearly specified because individuals with personality disorders are not usually formally diagnosed. Incidence is higher among those whose first-degree relatives have personality disorders or related disorders. Antisocial, schizoid, and obsessive-compulsive personality disorders occur more often in men, whereas borderline, dependent, and histrionic personality disorders are more common in women.

Diagnosis of personality disorders has increased since the 1980 edition of the *DSM* was published, in which criteria were revised to be more specific and to produce standardized classification.

An exact figure for the number of personality disorders is not known. Many personality disorders go undiagnosed, and affected individuals frequently are unaware that they have such a diagnosis as they perform routine activities of daily living. Their lives may be disruptive or disrupted, but if not identified through family, friends, bosses, or other influential persons in their lives who insist that they seek help, these individuals often continue living with their disorder.

For example, a woman who has dependent personality disorder and dreads taking responsibility for her life may remain in a submissive, degrading, or abusive relationship in exchange for having someone who will take care of her. She may never be aware of her disorder. A man with antisocial personality disorder may make large sums of money by taking advantage of others who are unaware of his bogus business scheme and investment promises for riches. He charms, manipulates, and lies his way to wealth on the backs of his victims' willingness to believe his Pied Piper magic. Only after taking all their money and disappearing is his diagnosis known and repeatedly discussed. Unless exposed, these diagnoses can exist under cover, or may be known only to psychiatric professionals, for a lifetime.

Interpersonal relationships are disturbed on some level in all personality disorders. People with the diagnosis of personality disorder rarely seek help voluntarily for their condition. They may seek help for anxiety or depressive symptoms that result from functional obstacles or barriers. Clients may not see the relationship disturbance as their fault because of the nature of the disorder (ego-syntonic), but they may seek professional help when faced with the threat of relationship severance from a spouse, friend, or boss. They seek help for their personal loss, not for the sake of the significant other; they lack empathy for others. At this point the person may be diagnosed.

Personality disorders are also discovered in conjunction with comorbid Axis I diagnoses when a person presents for psychiatric intervention for another mental disorder, in any setting.

Diagnosis of a personality disorder is assigned to adults 18 years or older. Exceptions are children or adolescents under 18 who have demonstrated the enduring patterns of maladaptive symptoms for at least 1 year. Their symptoms have remained stable in various situations, pervading all aspects of the youngster's life, and are not the result of a developmental stage or accepted cultural deviation or other Axis I mental disorder. The diagnosis of *antisocial personality disorder* is not made before age 18; however, if those traits do exist, the diagnosis of *conduct disorder* is assigned until the person is 18 years old.

Personality disorders occur in approximately 0.5% to 3% of the general population. Depending on type of disorder, however, this prevalence increases as to high as 20% in the psychiatric clinical population. *Dependent personality disorder* is by far the most prevalent type reported in clinical settings, especially day treatment centers or clinics that treat clients with chronic disorders.

ASSESSMENT AND DIAGNOSTIC CRITERIA

The diagnosis of personality disorder is made when the enduring pattern of maladaptive characteristics for each type of disorder exists over an extended period and is not the result of another mental disorder or a response to a current psychosocial stressor. This type of disorder is fixed. The person is not experiencing a passing state, but rather symptoms that remains stable over time and in many different situations. Other criteria are significant in making the diagnosis (Box 6-2).

Personality disorders are reported on Axis II of the multiaxial DSM system. When the client has more than one personality disorder, these are listed in order of importance. The individual is rarely admitted to an acute care psychiatric facility for a personality disorder. Often it becomes apparent after admission, however, that a comorbid Axis II diagnosis interrelates with the admitting Axis I diagnosis and may influence or even interfere with treatment goals. Consider these examples: Axis I/paranoid schizophrenia with Axis II/paranoid personality disorder or Axis I/major depression with Axis II/dependent personality disorder.

Clients often are admitted to legal facilities for traits and behaviors associated with some Axis II diagnoses. One notable example is the lack of guilt, remorse, or hesistance to perpetrate acts of overt or covert aggression against others. These symptoms are hallmarks of antisocial personality disorders and enable major and minor white-collar covert crimes or overt physical violence toward any victim who suits the perpetrator's current personal or collective needs or long-term plan.

The personality disorders are clustered according to similarities as follows:

Cluster A: Paranoid, schizoid, schizotypal (eccentric, cold)

Cluster B: Antisocial, borderline, histrionic, narcissistic (emotional, erratic, dramatic)

Cluster C: Avoidant, dependent, obsessive-compulsive, passive-aggressive (anxious, fearful)

DSM-IV-TR Criteria

Regardless of the type of personality disorder diagnosis, most clients tend to manifest self-focused and self-serving behaviors. Various categories of personality disorder have been identified according to *DSM-IV-TR* criteria (see box below; see also Appendix A).

Paranoid Personality Disorder

The defining characteristics of paranoid personality disorder are pervasive, long-standing suspicion and distrust of others and expectations of being threatened, harmed, exploited, or degraded. These individuals are secretive, guarded, and devious; they search for hidden meanings in harmless or benign remarks or situations. They are invariably argumentative, hostile, defensive, and stubborn. They are acutely aware of rank and power and are frequently intolerant of superiors and authority figures. Rigid and uncompromising behaviors make it difficult to work with these individuals in groups. A persistent search for the injustice directed at them permeates their lives. Individuals with paranoid personality disorder hold grudges and refuse to forgive others.

Schizoid Personality Disorder

The defining characteristics of schizoid personality disorder are a lifelong, pervasive, voluntary withdrawal from familial and social relationships and restricted emotional expression. These individuals have no close friends or confidants and have little or no desire for intimacy or sexual contact with another person. They prefer solitary activities

---

Box **6-2**   General Diagnostic Criteria for Personality Disorders

1. Enduring pattern of behaving, or personal inner experiences that deviate from one's cultural norm, relating to *two or more* of the following:
   a. Ways of perceiving and interpreting others and the environment
   b. Emotional responses (range, appropriateness, lability, intensity)
   c. Control of impulses
   d. Interpersonal function
2. Pattern of responses is stable over time and situation (inflexible, unchanging).
3. Responses impair functioning (personal, social, occupational).
4. Pattern is long-standing over time (identifiable in childhood or adolescence).
5. Pattern is *NOT* caused by other mental or medical disorders or substances.

DSM-IV-TR Personality Disorders

Paranoid personality disorder
Schizoid personality disorder
Schizotypal personality disorder
Antisocial personality disorder
Borderline personality disorder
Histrionic personality disorder
Narcissistic personality disorder
Avoidant personality disorder
Dependent personality disorder
Obsessive-compulsive personality disorder
Personality disorder not otherwise specified

and seem lonely, isolated, and eccentric. Individuals with schizoid personality disorder appear aloof and cold and seldom, if ever, express strong emotions or respond to others with gestures or smiles.

Schizotypal Personality Disorder

The defining characteristics of schizotypal personality disorder are odd or strange appearance, ideations, and behaviors and an inability to attain or maintain relatedness. These individuals have peculiar beliefs; experience magical thinking, bizarre fantasies, and unusual perceptions; and are extremely uncomfortable in the company of strangers. They tend to be suspicious, often experience ideas of reference, and may believe that they have special powers or insight. Affect is generally bland or silly, and interpersonal interactions are impaired in persons with schizotypal personality disorder.

Antisocial Personality Disorder

The defining characteristics of antisocial personality disorder are an enduring pattern of violation of social norms and an inability to conform that results in impaired life functioning. Antisocial personality disorder is common in first-degree relatives of those with the disorder. The pattern may include a generally irresponsible attitude toward duties, obligations, and the rights of others; lying; cheating; stealing; running away from home; drug abuse; and unusual sexual behavior. Criminal activity and disregard for the rights of others are prevalent. In fact, up to 75% of people in prisons have been diagnosed with antisocial personality disorder.

These individuals may be witty, charming, seductive, and manipulative to have their needs met, but they invariably lack a social conscience or feel remorse about mistreating others. Reckless, demanding, cunning, conning, abusive, and aggressive behaviors are common. Interpersonal skills are generally ineffective, with resultant difficulties in sustaining close, warm, or lasting relationships. These individuals are often incapable of leading self-supporting, independent, rewarding lives and seldom have success in meeting the needs of others. Manipulation and impulsivity are hallmarks.

Many people with antisocial characteristics have manipulated the environment to achieve political or economic power. Most likely, they were exposed to a life-style in which such traits were considered necessary adjuncts to success.

Borderline Personality Disorder

The defining characteristics of borderline personality disorder are a pervasive disturbance in self-image, mood, and affect; impulsivity; and an excessive need state, with resultant unstable, ineffective interpersonal relationships. These individuals appear to be in a perpetual state of crisis. During periods of extreme stress they may experience transient psychotic symptoms that are generally not severe enough to warrant a formal diagnosis of psychosis.

Individuals with borderline personality disorder may demonstrate disturbances in identity, sexual orientation, and value-belief system and may make poor choices in career goals, friends, or romantic partners. They invariably experience chronic feelings of boredom and excessive fears of abandonment, whether real or imagined. They tend to manipulate the environment to satisfy their needs and assuage their fears.

Persons with borderline personality disorder often display sudden, unpredictable outbursts of anger as a result of their labile and unstable mood and affect. Their anger is often intense and uncontrolled and may be demonstrated as general irritability, temper tantrums, verbal abuse, physical assaultiveness, anxiety, or depression.

Because of intense feelings of *ambivalence* (two opposing feelings occurring at the same time), these individuals tend to view others as either "all good" or "all bad" at any given time and are unable to perceive others as being able to integrate these characteristics. Because affected individuals see the world only in terms of "black and white," they can act on only one extreme feeling at a time. This defense process, known as *splitting*, is considered a hallmark of the borderline personality.

Often these individuals tend to overidealize people or groups in a momentary effort to become close. Because of their fear and distrust of attachments, however, they just as quickly devalue them as an expression of rejection. They also tend to project their own feelings of discomfort onto others to protect themselves from any anxiety that may be provoked by such feelings. These manipulative, dysfunctional behaviors distance the individuals from others and perpetuate unstable, unsatisfying relationships.

Impulsive behaviors may lead the individual to activities that are self-damaging, such as excessive shopping sprees, shoplifting, casual sex, binge eating, or substance abuse. In more severe cases, self-mutilation and other suicidal gestures are common, generally because attempts to manipulate others have failed or because of intense anger or feelings of depersonalization, described by the individual as numbness or detachment. Often these persons with borderline personality disorder may feel no pain as a result of self-abusive behavior.

Histrionic Personality Disorder

The defining characteristic of histrionic personality disorder is an excessively dramatic, extroverted or flamboyant, attention-seeking display of emotions. These individuals need to be the center of attention, want immediate gratification, and exhibit poor tolerance for frustration. They constantly seek approval, praise, and reassurance from others and often resort to crying spells, temper tantrums, or accusations when their needs are not met.

Although individuals with histrionic personality disorder may readily form relationships, their ingenuine, superficial, and egocentric charm generally dissipates quickly when others tire of their immature, histrionic behaviors. Once they form a relationship, they either attempt to control their partner or become dependent. Seductive, coy, and flirtatious behaviors are common in persons with histrionic personality disorder. These individuals are impressionable, demonstrate poor judgment, and are easily influenced by others.

Narcissistic Personality Disorder

The defining characteristics of narcissistic personality disorder are a grandiose sense of self-importance and feelings of entitlement. These individuals believe that they are unique and thus deserving of special treatment and consideration. They actively seek praise or approval from others, are hypersensitive to evaluation, and become humiliated or enraged by others' criticism. They may hide their feelings of shame or anger by outwardly appearing indifferent.

These individuals often lack empathy for others and may exploit people to have their own needs met or for self-aggrandizement. Interpersonal relationships are generally disturbed and ineffective because "friendships" and romantic or sexual encounters are formed primarily to serve the individual's own needs.

Avoidant Personality Disorder

The defining characteristics of avoidant personality disorder are excessive shyness and timidity and hypersensitivity to negative evaluation or rejection by others, which usually results in social withdrawal. Close interpersonal relationships are rare with these individuals; before making any commitments, they require a guarantee of constant, unconditional acceptance without the threat of criticism.

The extreme shyness and timidity these individuals experience often leads to avoidance of social situations, which greatly interferes with attaining and maintaining lasting friendships, as well as their choice of occupation. They generally avoid any new situation that may involve potential risk, danger, or difficulty, even though the possibilities are remote.

Unlike persons with schizoid personality disorder, who socially isolate themselves with no desire to engage with others, individuals with avoidant personality disorder may have strong desires for social contact, acceptance, and affection but are unable to reach out and relate to people. As a result, their interpersonal relationships are severely restricted.

Dependent Personality Disorder

The defining characteristics of dependent personality disorder are extreme submissiveness toward others and a pattern of dependence on others to assume responsibility for their lives. These individuals generally lack self-confidence, cannot make decisions for themselves, and require constant reassurance and advice. They avoid leadership roles and find it extremely difficult to initiate or complete a project or task. These people intensely dislike being alone and consistently seek others on whom to depend. They may tolerate unhappy or even abusive relationships to satisfy their strong dependency needs.

Obsessive-Compulsive Personality Disorder

The defining characteristics of obsessive-compulsive personality disorder are exaggerated orderliness, perseverance, stubbornness, indecisiveness, and restricted emotionality. These individuals tend to be rigid, inflexible, and perfectionistic and often fail to complete projects because of their inability to achieve their own high performance and outcome standards. They are invariably preoccupied with correct form, rules, details, and efficiency and usually appear overconscientious when involved in a task. They generally insist that a project be done their way; if not, they prefer to do it themselves.

Individuals with obsessive-compulsive disorder are not generous with material goods, praise, or affection and find it almost impossible to part with even worn-out or worthless possessions. Because of their rigidity, inflexibility, stubbornness, and selfishness, they have difficulty maintaining close friendships.

Personality Disorder Not Otherwise Specified

This category is reserved for personality functions that do not meet criteria for any specific personality disorder; for example, a personality disorder that consists of features of more than one disorder *(mixed personality)*. These combined personality functions can cause significant clinical impairment in one or more important areas of functioning (e.g., social, occupational). Examples include depressive personality disorder and passive-aggressive personality disorder.

▌ INTERVENTIONS

Long-term psychotherapy may be effective in bringing about behavioral changes, but the long-standing, enduring traits or patterns inherent in all personality disorders may be obstacles to treatment. Defining characteristics and behavioral styles that have become ingrained are naturally resistant to change.

Behavioral, cognitive, group, and family therapies and assertiveness training have proven helpful in symptom management and modification.

A person who has a personality disorder (Axis II) generally does not require hospitalization unless suicide threats, gestures, or attempts are present, or the personality disorder occurs with a major Axis I disorder that requires intervention.

Medications

A variety of medication categories are used for personality disorders, when necessary, for symptoms of anxiety, depression, or uncontrolled rage or aggression (see Pharmacotherapy box on p. 154).

Pharmacotherapy is used for the following symptoms of personality disorders:

COGNITIVE-PERCEPTUAL SYMPTOMS

Derealization, depersonalization, illusions, suspiciousness, odd or eccentric thinking, anger, hostility, and psychotic behavior.

INITIAL TREATMENT WITH LOW-DOSE ANTIPSYCHOTIC MEDICATIONS

1. Four- to six-week treatment trial.
2. Prolonged treatment (up to 22 weeks) may result in high rate of noncompliance and side effects.
3. If the client's response is less than optimal, symptoms should be reevaluated to determine etiology and appropriate treatment.
4. May be augmented with selective serotonin reuptake inhibitor (SSRI) antidepressants if affective symptoms are also present.

AFFECTIVE DYSREGULATION

Lability, rejection, sensitivity, inappropriate intense anger, depressive "mood crashes," temper outbursts, anhedonia, constricted affect, and excessive anxiety may be caused by serotonin dysregulation.

INITIAL TREATMENT WITH SSRIs

1. Four- to six-week treatment trial with fluoxetine (Prozac), 20 to 80 mg/day or sertraline (Zoloft), 100 to 600 mg/day
2. Prolonged treatment (up to 1 to 3 years) has been reported to retain improvement.
3. Standards for continuation and maintenance phases of treatment are inadequately defined for personality disorders.

4. May be augmented with a low-dose antipsychotic if the client is experiencing poor behavior control or with a benzodiazepine, such as alprazolam (Xanax), lorazepam (Ativan), or clorazepate (Tranxene), if client is experiencing significant anxiety. Benzodiazepine therapy needs to be closely monitored because of the high risk for abuse.
5. Additional pharmacotherapy may include
   - Tricyclic antidepressants
   - Monoamine oxidase inhibitors (MAOIs)
   - Anticonvulsants such as valproate (Depakote) and carbamazepine (Tegretol)

IMPULSIVE/BEHAVIORAL SYMPTOMS

Clients with personality disorder may demonstrate self-destructive or assaultive acts, somatic behaviors (binge eating, spending, sexual activities, drugs), cognitive impulsivity (rash judgment), suicide, or homicide. The etiology may be low serotonin level in the central nervous system (CNS).

INITIAL TREATMENT WITH SSRI ANTIDEPRESSANTS

1. Effects on the client's impulsivity usually are noted before the effects on the client's depression or affect.
2. May be augmented with a low-dose antipsychotic if the client's response is inadequate.
3. Carbamazepine and valproate are often used in clinical practice based on their efficacy in bipolar disorder.
4. Atypical antipsychotic medications may be effective for treating self-mutilation and other impulsive behaviors arising from psychotic thinking. However, few data are available to support their use.
5. Opiate antagonists, such as naltrexone (Trexan), may be used for the treatment of repetitive, self-injurious behavior. Treatment trials primarily involve clients with mental retardation.

Nurse-Client Relationship

The nurse must accept that the client with personality disorder is unable to change his or her basic personality. The nurse therefore establishes objectives to reflect the following:

- Be prepared for the client's manipulative behaviors toward nurses and other clients, and be ready to set reasonable limits, regardless of the diagnosis. Clients need to have nurses demonstrate strength without being punitive.
- Assist the client to achieve a reduction (versus elimination) of extreme or self-defeating behaviors.
- Assist the client to state and practice healthy strategies for coping with inner experiences of discomfort or omnipotence and impulses to manipulate others to meet own needs.
- Use firm but kind constructive confrontation to effect behavior change.

- Praise the client's efforts to practice learned strategies.
- Keep expectations reasonable; avoid rescue fantasies. Clients with personality disorders will not demonstrate a "cure" on your shift.
- Avoid punitive remarks or imposing limits that punish or exclude the client in the interest of appeasing the nurse's frustration.
- Consistently review cognitive associations with the client to help eliminate self-defeating traits and reinforce behavioral efforts.
- Constant autodiagnosis and review of therapeutic principles are necessary for the nurse/staff to be effective in meeting the client's needs.
- Supervision and interdisciplinary treatment teams are imperative for validation of staff perceptions/interventions.

PROGNOSIS AND DISCHARGE CRITERIA

Because of the long-term, deeply ingrained patterns of maladaptive perceptions, feelings, cognitions, and behaviors that accompany personality disorders, the prognosis for these clients is generally poor and at best is guarded. It is difficult to change a person's lifelong patterns of living. Prognosis is not hopeless, however, and the nurse and staff must think in degrees of "either/or" rather than "all or none." In essence, any healthy changes are praised and rewarded. Discharge criteria are as follows:

- The client controls impulses to manipulate others to meet own needs.
- Demonstrates ability to postpone immediate gratification.
- Verbalizes anger without acting out.
- Utilizes learned strategies to reduce anger.
- Refrains from harming self or others.
- Identifies dependent, interdependent, and independent behaviors.
- Demonstrates independent thinking (decision making).
- Verbalizes realistic goals toward independence.
- Expresses needs and opinions assertively.
- Demonstrates ability to overcome procrastination, negativism, and resistance.
- Identifies events/situations that trigger anxiety and obsessions/compulsions.
- Manages anxiety with multiple stress-reducing techniques.
- Employs cognitive-behavioral techniques to control obsessions/compulsions.
- Initiates and completes projects effectively.
- Recognizes own mistrust and projection.
- Validates perceptions with others.
- Seeks interaction and socialization with others.
- Refrains from idealizing, blaming, and devaluing others.
- Demonstrates respect for the needs and rights of self and others.
- Voices realistic appraisal of own talents and achievements.

The box below provides guidelines in the management of personality disorders.

CLIENT AND FAMILY TEACHING   Personality Disorders

Nurse Needs to Know

- The client with personality disorder often tests the limits of the treatment team.
- The client may need protection from self-mutilation or injury to self or others.
- The client may become suicidal and require suicidal precautions and a safety-ensured milieu.
- Assess and identify the client's functional and dysfunctional behaviors.
- Establish therapeutic trust with the client, but avoid a personal relationship.
- Focus on the client's strengths, assets, and accomplishments when possible.
- Recognize manipulative and splitting behaviors when they occur.
- Set limits on the client's manipulative behavior in a simple, direct manner.
- Challenge the client's splitting behavior in a firm but gentle manner.
- Intervene with strategies to manage the client's anxiety and obsessive-compulsive behaviors.
- Provide mature, assertive role modeling for the client/family.
- Help the client verbalize anger rather than act aggressively or in a passive-aggressive way.
- Learn assertive communication and behaviors and their benefits to the client.

Teach Client and Family

- Explain to the family that the client may challenge them and test their limits.
- Inform the family that the client may self-mutilate or attempt to injure self or others, requiring safety precautions and professional interventions.
- Caution the family that the client may become suicidal and need protection and hospitalization.
- Teach the family to assess the client's functional and dysfunctional behaviors, and encourage them to seek professional help when necessary.
- Advise the family to develop trust with the client but to set appropriate limits when necessary.
- Instruct the family to focus on the client's strengths and accomplishments whenever possible.
- Teach the family to recognize manipulative and splitting behaviors and how to set limits on negative behaviors in a simple, direct way.
- Teach the client/family strategies to manage the client's anxiety and obsessive-compulsive behaviors.
- Teach the client/family how to use assertive communication skills when dealing with each other, such as "I" messages versus "you" statements.
- Instruct the client/family to verbalize their anger rather than use aggressive or passive-aggressive behaviors.
- Tell the client/family to make opportunities for the client to practice social and assertive skills with others.

Continued

CLIENT AND FAMILY TEACHING | **Personality Disorders—cont'd**

- Provide opportunities for the client to practice social and assertive skills in the milieu, including individual and group interactions.
- Encourage the client/family to seek others for interactions and socialization.
- Learn cognitive-behavioral activities that promote a realistic self-appraisal and increase self-esteem.
- Reinforce the client/family's expressions of positive feelings and behaviors.
- Reinforce the client's realistic thoughts, perceptions, and appraisals.
- Assess and identify the client's dependent, interdependent, and independent behaviors.
- Reinforce the client's independent, responsible behaviors.
- Provide opportunities for the client to practice decision-making skills (e.g., facilitate a client meeting, lead a therapeutic activity, monitor a craft group).
- Praise the client for respecting the needs and rights of self and others.
- Praise the client for making attainable goals and for efforts to achieve them.
- Reinforce the importance of taking medications that may be prescribed for anxiety or depression.
- Recognize psychosocial stressors and how to manage and prevent symptoms.
- Investigate community groups and resources to help the client/family after discharge.
- Investigate current educational resources available on the Internet and in the library.

- Encourage the client/family to continue cognitive-behavioral therapy with a designated therapist after discharge.
- Advise the family to reinforce the client's realistic self-perceptions and realistic appraisal of others.
- Encourage the family to reinforce the client's positive feelings and behaviors.
- Teach the client/family that the client needs to have simple, achievable goals.
- Tell the family to reinforce the client's independent behaviors when possible.
- Inform the client/family that the client needs opportunities to practice simple decision making (take medications, make medical appointments).
- Instruct the family to praise the client for respecting own and others' rights.
- Teach the client/family about the importance of medication compliance.
- Teach the client/family to identify psychosocial stressors and how to recognize, manage, and prevent symptoms.
- Inform the client/family about community groups available after discharge.
- Teach the client/family how to access current Internet and library resources.

Care Plans

Personality Disorders (All Types)
- Defensive Coping
- Chronic Low Self-Esteem
- Ineffective Coping

Care Plan

DSM-IV-TR Diagnosis **Personality Disorders (All Types)**

NANDA Diagnosis: Defensive Coping
Repeated projection of falsely positive self-evaluation based on a self-protective pattern that defends against underlying perceived threats to positive regard.

Focus:
For the client whose behavior patterns or personality traits result in lifelong ineffective interpersonal relationships because of the client's denial of problems, weaknesses, failures, and responsibility; projecting blame; hypersensitivity, anger/aggression, lying; and perceived grandiosity or superiority over others.

RELATED FACTORS (ETIOLOGY)

Personal identity disturbance
Self-esteem disturbance
Depletion of effective coping methods
Low impulse control
Role-relationship disturbance
Ineffective problem-solving skills
Lack of insight and judgment
Self-centeredness
Perceived threat to self-system
Life-style of defensive behaviors
Developmental conflicts
Psychosocial stressors
Environmental stressors
Knowledge deficit regarding adaptive coping methods

DEFINING CHARACTERISTICS

Mistrust/Suspicion
The client interprets others' words or actions as demeaning or threatening.
- "What did you mean by that remark? Were you making fun of me?"
- "Why were you and the other clients laughing when I came into the room?"
- "I didn't get chosen as group leader because they're all out to get me."

Views benign remarks or events as if they contained hidden meanings or messages.
- "My check bounced because the bank deliberately held back money from my account."
- "The board and care manager warned me to pay my rent on time. He's just looking for a reason to throw me out."
- "The phone company sent me another notice. They take advantage of my emotional problems."

Avoids confiding in others for fear they may use the information to harm or belittle the client.
- "I'm afraid to tell anyone how I feel. They may turn against me."
- "I don't trust anyone enough to tell them my personal thoughts."
- "How can I ever be sure what I say will not be used against me?"

Demonstrates hypervigilant or extremely cautious behaviors toward persons perceived as threatening or hostile.
- Scans the environment during group meetings and activities.
- Observes other clients from a distance.

Verbalizes suspicion that others are saying rude, vulgar things about the client.
- "I just know they're spreading horrible rumors about me around here."
- "They're probably making up all kinds of ugly, dirty stories about me."

Anger/Aggression
The client reacts impulsively with anger toward people, groups, or situations perceived as threatening or belittling.
- "How dare you spend all that time talking to Ted. You're supposed to be my staff person."
- "I'm very angry at you for ignoring my comments in group today. You gave Joy lots of time to talk."

Continued

- "I hate you for not choosing me to be community leader."

Bears long-term grudges toward others for slights, insults, or injuries.

- "I wasn't invited personally to join the card game, so I want nothing to do with them."
- "I'll never forgive my sister for treating me badly when we were kids."
- "I'll never speak to my mother again. She always criticizes me."

Assaultive/Destructive

The client engages in physical fights with other clients for no apparent reason.

- "I hit Nick because his bragging really irritated me."
- "Joy's attitude really made me mad, so I tore up her diary."
- "If you come anywhere near me, I'll punch in your face."
- "You think you're so smart. But I bet I can beat you up."
- "I messed up Kate's room because she made me mad."

Relates history of child or spouse abuse.

- "Sure, I beat my kids. It'll make them tougher."
- "Every once in a while my husband and I get into a real fistfight."

Blaming/Projecting

The client avoids accepting blame for actions or inaction, even when blame is warranted.

- "Don't blame me for not cleaning the dining room. There were still clients in it at 9 PM."
- "It wasn't my fault that I missed the 7 o'clock activity. Staff should have reminded me."
- "I don't understand why the group is so mad at me all the time. What did I do?"

Blames others for own thoughts, feelings, or behaviors.

- "It was Nick's idea to go AWOL. He wanted us to smoke some pot."
- "You never cared about me. I'm not one of your favorite clients."
- "Everything was perfect today until *you* came in and started to tell everyone what to do."
- "The other clients are just jealous of me. That's why they don't talk to me."
- "You didn't help me get my laundry together. How can I wear clean clothes?"

Passive-Aggressive

The client expresses indirect resistance toward fulfilling responsibilities based on covert aggression.

- "It's too hard for me to be the client leader. I can't wake up everyone in time for community meeting every day."

Reacts resentfully, resistively, and oppositionally to others' demands and requests.

- "Your idea seems OK, Joy, but I don't think we can fit it in at this time."

Procrastinates when asked to complete a task, project, or activity.

- "I'll get going on that project eventually. Just give me some time."
- "I know I keep promising to take my turn at cleaning the craft room. I'll try to get to it today."
- "Next time, I'll be sure to bring the tools we need to complete that project."

Uses subtle sarcastic remarks instead of overt anger.

- "Jay, I thought you might like this sandwich. You're such a good eater." (Jay is overweight).
- "You're such a good nurse; you're always so busy. I hardly ever see you."

Obstructs and thwarts the efforts of others by failing to do own share of duties and responsibilities.

- "I know I signed up to bring the dessert. I just didn't feel good."
- "I just didn't find the time to do that favor you asked me to do."

Avoids obligations by conveniently "forgetting" (forgets important appointments, birthdays, special events, names).

- "I can't understand how I forgot to prepare my half of the speech for today's meeting."
- "Joy, I can't believe I forgot to get your magazine when I was out on pass. I did remember Nick's cigarettes."

Demonstrates intentional inefficiency.

- "No, I just didn't have enough time to call the board and care home."
- "I tried to bake the cake, but I'm not good at it, so I brought some doughnuts."

Withholds information (conveniently "forgets").

- "I'm sorry, Kate. I guess I forgot to tell you about the meeting."
- "I forgot Jay was going home today. I would have told you if I remembered."

Impulsivity

The client engages in impulsive acts without regard for consequences.

- "I don't know why I started doing drugs again; I suddenly got the urge."
- "Bill collectors are always after me; I'm a compulsive spender."
- "I have several unpaid speeding tickets; I can't resist driving fast."
- "I have no regular home address; I like to get up and go."

Lying

The client verbalizes untruths to staff and other clients.

- "I would never 'cheek' my medications; I always take them when I should."
- "I swear that I attended the assertiveness group yesterday; you just didn't see me."
- "Joy said I lied about smoking her cigarettes; I never take anyone else's things."

* "Jeff insisted that he saw me eating his snack, but it wasn't me."

Narcissistic/Antisocial

The client demonstrates self-important, grandiose behaviors.
* Takes command of community meetings and activities.
* Interrupts groups/individuals in authoritarian manner.

Exaggerates achievements and talents.
* "I'm the best client leader in the world."
* "If it wasn't for my organizational skills, nothing would get done around here."
* "I almost became a psychiatrist, so I understand most of the clients' problems."

Verbalizes belief that he or she is entitled to special treatment or privileges.
* "I simply have to play my radio at night or I can't fall asleep."
* "I deserve a pass. I'm a model client."
* "I don't care if there isn't enough space in the meeting room. I'm going in anyway."

Ignores hospital rules and policies as if they do not apply to the client.
* Leaves the unit without telling staff or signing out.
* Smokes in nonsmoking areas.
* Makes phone calls when the client should be attending group activities.

Exploits others to meet own needs.
* Asks other clients to give up contact time with staff to have staff's time for self.
* Feigns friendship with roommate to gain something (more closet space, bed near window).

Cannot express feelings or emotions.

Lacks empathy and understanding for others.
* "I don't feel sorry for Sam just because his wife left him. Other people have gone through the same thing."
* "I can't worry about these other clients. I have better things to do."

Irresponsibility

The client exhibits irresponsible, insensitive behaviors toward others and the environment.
* Fails to clean room, pick up clothes, or remove dirty dishes/ashtrays after use.
* Leaves shower/bathroom messy or dirty after use.
* Eats food/snacks that belong to other clients.

Neglects to fulfill obligations or duties.
* "Why should I have to help clean the craft room? That's what they pay housekeepers for."
* "Oh, well, I missed the relationship meeting. I hope someone else took the minutes."

Fails to recognize consequences of irresponsible actions.
* "I don't see why Joe is so mad at me for 'borrowing' two lousy dollars. I intend to pay him back."

* "So what's the worst thing that could happen if I smoke a little marijuana at the board and care home?"

Maladaptive Denial

The client fails to recognize own weaknesses or limitations.
* "I don't have any problems with the other clients. They all love me."
* "No one can say I don't do my share of work around here, even if I'm not a regular client."

Denies client role and reason for hospitalization.
* "I'm only here for a rest. I had to get away from my crazy family."
* "I can't imagine what the other clients here are going through. I try to help them whenever I can."

Denies consequences of actions.
* "I don't know why everyone is so 'crazy' because I was AWOL."

OUTCOME IDENTIFICATION AND EVALUATION

Mistrust/Suspicion

The client establishes trusting relationships with staff, peers, and significant others.
* Expresses meaningful thoughts and feelings to trusted clients and staff.
* Participates in group meetings and activities.
* Shares personal confidences with a special person.
* Verbalizes trust in clients, family, and staff.

Demonstrates decreased or no suspicious behaviors toward others and the environment.
* Accurately interprets meanings of others' words or behaviors.
* Refrains from searching for "hidden" messages or agenda in others' statements or actions.
* Ceases to believe that others' statements or behaviors refer to the client.
* Ceases to believe that others are making up "lewd" or "vulgar" stories about the client.
* Ceases to interpret others' words or actions as demeaning or threatening to the client.

Demonstrates absence of scanning, guarding, or hypervigilant behaviors.

Anger/Aggression

The client exhibits decreased or no verbal expressions of anger.

Exhibits decreased or no aggressive outbursts or demonstrations.

Refrains from bearing grudges against significant others, clients, or staff.
* "I think it's time I gave my parents another chance."
* "I'm not mad at Kate any longer. She didn't mean to hurt me."
* "I realize the staff was only trying to help me when they put me in seclusion."

Demonstrates assertive rather than aggressive behaviors.

Continued

Assaultive/Destructive

The client ceases to engage in physical fights or altercations with others.
Demonstrates absence of violent or destructive behaviors.
Verbalizes desire to seek help for abusive behaviors.

Blaming/Projecting

The client accepts blame or share of blame when warranted.
- "It wasn't only Nick's idea to leave the unit. I also wanted to go."
- "I know now that it was my angry behavior that drove people away. It wasn't that they didn't care."
- "The meeting was postponed because of my lateness."
- "I'm sorry for accusing staff of being 'bossy' and 'protective.' I've been acting like a child."
- "I admit I did my share to mess up the clients' lounge, and I apologize."

Ceases to blame others for own behaviors.
- "I realize that no one made me smoke the marijuana. I wanted to smoke."
- "It was my problem with alcohol that broke up my marriage, not my wife's nagging."
- "I started the fight with my bad temper. Paul was just defending himself."

Passive-Aggressive

The client directly expresses anger, irritation, and frustration without resorting to indirect or covert responses.
- Ceases to use humor, sarcasm, or messages with "hidden" meanings when expressing anger, irritation, or frustration: "I'm angry that staff is too busy to give me much time today."
- Verbalizes angry feelings overtly: "I'm feeling angry about . . . "; "It made me angry when . . . "; "I was angry because. . . . "

Ceases to use indirect behaviors as covert expressions of aggression to resist fulfilling responsibilities.
- No longer resists others' reasonable ideas, wishes, or responsibilities.
- Ceases to withhold critical or relevant information from staff.

Refrains from procrastinating when asked to complete a task, project, or activity (begins and ends work on time).
Completes full share of work in client community so that others' efforts are not obstructed.
Fulfills client duties and obligations willingly.
- Cleans up after self without being urged.
- Takes turns with other clients at group tasks.

Demonstrates efficiency and reliability.
- Attends groups and activities.
- Arrives on time to groups and activities.
- Participates satisfactorily in groups and activities.

Demonstrates assertive rather than passive-aggressive behaviors (see assertiveness training, Appendix B).

- Uses "I" messages, eye contact, and congruent verbal and facial expressions in communicating with others.

Impulsivity

The client verbalizes decreased need to act impulsively.
Uses learned techniques to control impulsive behaviors: slow deep breathing, counting to 5 before responding to stimulus (see Appendix B).
Demonstrates significant decrease or absence of impulsive acts or behaviors: refrains from speeding, shopping, spending, moving from place to place, taking drugs.

Lying

The client makes truthful statements to staff and clients.
Refrains from using lies or fabrications to meet needs.
Shares information relative to health and safety of self and others; does not withhold information.

Narcissistic/Antisocial

The client demonstrates no or significant reduction in self-important, grandiose behaviors.
- Refrains from interrupting or "taking over" group activities.
- Resists exaggerating or flaunting own talents and achievements.
- Praises others' talents and accomplishments.

Exhibits consideration for others rather than demonstrating self-entitlement.
- "I'll turn off my radio at 9 PM so others won't be disturbed."
- "Since I've already been on a field trip, I'll give up my window seat to another client."

Obeys hospital rules and policies.
- Informs staff when leaving the unit.
- Smokes only in designated smoking areas.
- Makes phone calls at times other than during scheduled activities.

Meets own needs without exploiting others.
Facilitates genuine interpersonal relationships.
Expresses feelings and emotions more readily.
- "I'm feeling sad . . . angry . . . anxious . . . happy." Expresses empathy and understanding for others.
- "I feel sorry for Sam since his wife left him."
- "It was difficult for Kate to be client leader. She was nervous."
- "Nick had a tough day. I know what it's like when visitors don't show up."
- "It's sad that Ken has no place to go when he's discharged."

Irresponsibility

The client demonstrates mature, responsible behaviors toward self and others.

- Maintains neat, clean environment (room, clothing, self).
- Completes fair share of client responsibilities (helps set up for meals and activities, relays messages regarding meeting times and places).

Fulfills client role and obligations.

- Engages in therapeutic treatment regimen.
- Participates in milieu groups and activities.

Verbalizes awareness of consequences of actions.

- "I'm going to pay back the money I borrowed from Nick as soon as possible. I don't want to ruin our relationship."
- "I'll wait for my break to smoke. If I smoke in my bathroom, my roommate and I could get into trouble."

Accepts accountability for own behavior.

- "It was my job to help the group prepare for the party. I just didn't go to enough meetings."
- "I should have been dressed and ready for my appointment with the social worker. Now I'll have to wait to select a board and care facility."

Maladaptive Denial

The client recognizes own limitations and weaknesses.

- "I realize I haven't done my share as a client."
- "I admit that I have problems being accepted by other clients."

Accepts consequences of actions.

- "I don't blame staff for being angry that I left the unit without telling anyone. I deserve to be placed on restrictions."
- "I understand now that the other clients resented me because I didn't act like a client."

Accepts client role and need for treatment.

- "I realize now that I'm here because I need help with my emotional problems."
- "I can understand what the other clients are going through. I'm going through similar experiences."

PLANNING AND IMPLEMENTATION

Nursing Intervention	Rationale
Mistrust/Suspicion	
Identify own level of anxiety, and use strategies to reduce anxiety.	Anxiety is transferable and can foster the client's mistrust and suspicion.
Approach the client face-to-face, *not* from behind.	The client is likely to become startled if he or she cannot immediately see the approaching person. Face-to-face contact decreases suspicion and mistrust.
Use a calm, matter-of-fact manner when interacting with the client. Use low, steady voice tones, *not* high-pitched or urgent tones. Use slow, smooth body movements, *not* sudden or erratic motions.	A calm approach creates a secure, nonthreatening environment and reduces the client's suspiciousness.
Initially, assign the same staff person(s) to work with the client.	This practice helps to establish consistency and trust in staff and environment.
Engage the client in brief one-to-one interactions initially, progressing to longer interactions, informal groups, and finally more structured groups and activities.	This sequence gives the client more opportunities to establish trust and develop interpersonal relationships.
Employ assertive, not aggressive or authoritarian, responses ("I," *not* "you," statements).	Assertive, nonaggressive, appropriate responses and behaviors by an understanding nurse help to provide clear directives, increase the client's trust in staff and the environment, reduce suspicion and hostility, and give the client the opportunity to interpret the meaning of his or her behavior.

Therapeutic Responses

"I noticed that you sat alone during lunch and seemed upset when you looked at Kate and me."

- The nurse meets the client's eyes with a calm, unemotional facial expression, without constantly staring, so as not to seem demanding or threatening (uses eye contact).
- Uses facial expressions consistent with verbal responses.
- Maintains an unemotional facial expression and affect while relating facts and meaning regarding a benign incident or situation.

Continued

PLANNING AND IMPLEMENTATION—cont'd

Nursing Intervention	Rationale
Mistrust/Suspicion—cont'd	

Nontherapeutic Responses

"*You* shouldn't feel threatened just because Kate and I sat together at lunch today"
- The nurse smiles inappropriately with little or no eye contact while giving the client serious directives.
- Acts impatiently or angrily while asking the client to clarify the meaning of the client's behavior.

"You" (versus "I") statements imply that something is "wrong" with the client (see assertiveness training, Appendix B).
Acting impatiently and/or angrily is authoritarian may send a message that the nurse disapproves of the client.

Offer the client clear, simple explanations of environmental events, activities, and the behaviors of other clients, when necessary.
- "That remark was not meant for you, Ted. It was directed to everyone in the group."
- "I noticed you looked uneasy at the community meeting, Joy. The other clients were pleased that you came."
- "Joe, the clients were laughing at a funny story that Sam told them. They weren't laughing at you."

Explaining events in a direct, simple way helps to lessen the client's doubts, fears, and suspiciousness and promotes trust.

Inform the client in a direct, matter-of-fact manner that you do not share the client's interpretation of a statement or event, while still acknowledging feelings.
- "I know you think we planned to change your staff person, Pam, but actually she was assigned to another unit."
- "Mark, I know you believe that Jay and Nick don't want to sit with you, but they need to sit in front of the bus because sitting in the back makes them nauseous."

Offering simple, accurate interpretation of statements or events helps the client foster realistic rather than irrational thoughts and conclusions and brings the client closer to reality.

Assist the client to interpret statements or events more concretely.
- "Jeff, it's very likely that your landlord sends a notice to anyone who is late with the rent."
- "Joy, the phone company has no way of knowing about your mental disorder. They just want a payment."
- "Nick, the clients don't leave dirty ashtrays around just to upset you, although it can be annoying."

Helping the client accurately interpret events or statements discourages concerns that they may contain "hidden" meanings or ulterior motives directed toward the client.

Clarify the meanings and intent of remarks or situations that are misinterpreted by the client.
- "Jeff, the board and care manager told the social worker that you will not be thrown out of the facility as long as the rent is paid."
- "Joe, your check bounced because there wasn't enough money in your account, not because the bank stole your money."
- "When Kate said she was 'sick and tired,' she did not mean that you made her 'sick and tired,' Ted."

Clarifying meanings and intent that are misinterpreted by the client provides factual information that helps to promote the client's trust.

Assure the client that, although other clients and staff discuss the client, they are not spreading vicious, ugly rumors.
- "Nick and Joan do talk about you, Joy, but they have not spoken about you in an unkind way."
- "Sarah did say she had lunch with you, Ann, and she also said she enjoys spending time with you."

Assuring the client that other clients are discussing the client favorably helps to decrease the anxiety that can perpetuate suspicious behaviors. This assurance also helps to increase the client's self-esteem.

Direct the conversation toward reality-based topics when the client becomes bogged down in irrational beliefs or paranoid ideations.

Talking about universally shared topics with the client helps to reestablish logic and decrease suspicious thoughts and perceptions.

- "Sam, a few minutes ago you were talking about movie stars. Let's talk about your favorite movies."
- "Kate, just before the meeting we were discussing music. I'd like to hear about your music collection."

Identify the client's expressions and behaviors during interactions.
- "Joe, I notice that you hesitate when you begin to talk about your problems with me."
- "Sarah, you have a puzzled look on your face. I wonder if you believe what I'm saying."
- "Jeff, I think you might be uneasy about sharing your experiences with the group."

Clarification of the client's suspicious concerns helps to expose areas of mistrust and gives the client an opportunity to challenge and correct the concerns.

Set limits on the duration and frequency of the client's suspicious concerns during one-to-one and group interactions.
- "Kate, I know you have concerns about some things, and staff will listen for about 10 minutes each shift. The rest of the time needs to be spent in scheduled activities."

Setting appropriate limits on the client's suspicious concerns helps to discourage perpetuation of negative behaviors and encourages time spent in therapeutic activities.

Share a benign, nonthreatening personal fact or feeling with the client.

Sharing universal feelings and simple facts helps to establish rapport and trust and encourages the client to confide in the staff.

Therapeutic Responses
- "I'm a student nurse. I like to help others."
- "I sometimes feel sad when others have problems."
- "I also get upset once in a while."

Nontherapeutic Responses
"I know just how you feel. I'd feel the same way in your situation."
"I worry too when I think people are talking about me."
"It's normal not to trust banks or any big businesses."

Nontherapeutic responses indicate that the nurse could not possibly know how the client feels.
Agreeing with the client in this case justifies the client's suspicions.
The client relies on the nurse to present and interpret reality.

Assure the client that anything discussed with staff is confidential information and will be shared only with staff persons who are responsible for the client's treatment and care.
Note: Clients who reveal suicidal thoughts or plans must be advised that such intents will be shared with other appropriate staff and physician to protect the client.

Assurance of confidentiality promotes trust and encourages the client to share thoughts, feelings, and beliefs that are relevant to the client's treatment and care.

Explore situations in which the client often feels suspicious, and discuss alternative problem-solving methods.
- "Jeff, at other times when people were laughing, what did you do to determine whether they were laughing at you? Sometimes asking people directly to explain their behavior can prevent you from thinking the wrong thing."
- "Joe, rather than assume others are saying bad things about you, what about talking to a trusted staff person or client about your concerns first?"
- "Joy, have you thought about approaching the board and care manager with your concerns about being evicted? You may find out if there actually is a problem."

Helping the client solve problems when the client is capable provides the client with more realistic and appropriate methods to deal with situations that provoke suspiciousness.

Continued

PLANNING AND IMPLEMENTATION—cont'd

Nursing Intervention	Rationale

Mistrust/Suspicion—cont'd

Nursing Intervention	Rationale
Discuss with the client the consequences of not validating actual meanings behind situations or events that provoke suspiciousness. • "Jay, by not finding out what actually is happening, you may continue to feel left out." • "Ted, your feeling of isolation may not go away if you don't ask about situations that seem troubling to you."	Discussing the importance of problem-solving the meanings behind situations may prevent the client from misinterpreting situations or events and helps to promote trust in others and the environment.
Assist the client to examine and clarify his or her own thoughts and beliefs. • "Kate, what do you think about the incident that happened in group today?" • "Joy, think more about what happened in the community meeting." • "Ted, what do you actually believe about the clients' responses to you during the activity?"	Clarification helps the client evaluate thoughts and beliefs more accurately and realistically and thus avoid misinterpretation.
Encourage the client to raise healthy doubts about his or her suspiciousness and erroneous beliefs. • "Jay, do you really believe the telephone company disconnected your phone because of your mental illness?" • "Ted, is it actually possible that everyone here is saying bad things about you?" • "Mark, I find it hard to believe that the staff can't be trusted with information that will help you."	Raising doubts helps the client challenge and analyze his or her beliefs more closely and realistically and thus reduces suspiciousness.
Offer the client feedback when, as a result of doubts and suspicions, the client erroneously accuses others of behaviors. • "Kate, when you say Nick has spread vicious rumors about you, he gets upset." • "Joy, Ted said he felt hurt when you accused him of taking your share of the staff's time."	Genuine feedback helps to increase the client's awareness that his or her behaviors can affect others negatively and can result in rejection by others.
Praise the client for efforts made toward correct interpretation of the meanings and intent of others' responses and situations. • "Ted, I was impressed with your clear understanding of the group's response today." • "Pam, the clients appreciated our accurate interpretation of their remarks during the community meeting. I could tell by the way they all listened to you."	Warranted praise helps build the client's self-esteem and trust, encourages continued efforts through positive reinforcement, and decreases paranoid thinking.
Engage the client in activities, crafts, or exercises during unstructured or "free" time.	Activities distract the client from preoccupation with suspicious thoughts and beliefs and fill the time with actions that bring quick rewards and increase self-esteem.

Anger/Aggression, Assaultive/Destructive

Nursing Intervention	Rationale
Approach the client in a calm, nonthreatening manner. Set limits on the client's behavior if it appears that anger may escalate to physical aggression or violence. Suggest to the client that he or she take "time out." • "Kate, that is not acceptable behavior. Some time spent in your room may help you gain control." If time-out does not relieve the client's feelings, offer as-needed (prn) medication. Seclusion/restraint may be the least restrictive intervention.	Using a calm, nonthreatening approach and setting necessary limits help to assuage the client's anger and can prevent violent behavior.

Assure the client that he or she is entitled to angry feelings but may not impose angry outbursts on other clients.
- "Jeff, I realize you're angry, but cursing in group is not acceptable behavior."
- "Pam, I know you're upset that the chocolate pudding is gone, but slamming your tray down in the cafeteria is disruptive and not acceptable."

Establishing guidelines while acknowledging the client's angry feelings helps the client manage behavior that interferes with other clients' rights or disrupts milieu activities.

Give the client feedback regarding impulsive, angry outbursts.
- "Sam, your screaming and yelling during the community meeting upset you and the others."
- "Kate, your roommate asked staff to change her room because your episodes of rage frighten her."
- "Ted, staff are concerned because your anger is interfering with your progress and disrupts others."
- "Tom, the group stops listening to you when you scream and wave your arms; they get anxious."

Clear, direct observations of the client's negative behavior help the client recognize the negative effects of volatile behavior on the client and others.

Teach the client quick, effective stress management strategies (see Appendix B).
- The client walks way from the immediate area to a less stimulating environment.
- Performs slow, deep-breathing techniques.
- Engages in progressive relaxation exercises.
- Uses visual imagery techniques.

Stress management activities assist the client to reduce the physical manifestations of anger and help to promote a calm internal state.

Assist the client to put angry feelings into words during one-to-one interactions.
- "Ted, when you feel angry, talk about your feelings with staff."
- "Kate, you seemed upset at lunch today. You slammed your tray down hard. Let's discuss your feelings."
- "Sarah, you say you're not angry, but you shouted at several people this morning. Let's talk about your feelings during our session today."

Putting angry feelings into words with a trusted staff member helps the client express feelings and emotions in a nonthreatening setting and avoids directing anger toward other clients.

Encourage the client to identify situations or events that generate angry feelings.
- "Ted, I noticed you were calm until the topic of intimacy came up in group. Then you immediately began to shout."
- "Jim, you seemed relaxed until your roommate spoke to someone else. Then you cursed and stomped out of the room."

Identification of anger-inducing situations helps the client connect behaviors to specific stimuli so that the client can begin to take steps to manage or prevent impulsive, angry outbursts in subsequent similar situations.

Discuss with the client possible fears or frustrations that may provoke impulsive, angry outbursts.
- "Jim, when your roommate talks to other people, you lose your temper. Do you feel ignored or left out?"
- "Kate, it seems that whenever other clients talk about their boyfriends, you get angry. Are you feeling lonely or sad?"

Discussing fears and frustrations helps the client recognize that anger can be a response to a real or imagined threat and prepares the client to respond more appropriately in the future.

Assist the client to clarify the intent of situations that the client perceives as threatening.
- "Jim, when your roommate talks to other clients, it doesn't mean he's forgotten you. He speaks to you often."
- "Kate, it's OK to feel sad or lonely when others discuss their boyfriends. But they don't do it to make you sad or mad."

Clarifying potentially threatening situations allows the client to view them more realistically and can prevent angry outbursts.

Continued

PLANNING AND IMPLEMENTATION—cont'd

Nursing Intervention	Rationale
Anger/Aggression, Assaultive/Destructive—cont'd	

Help the client reevaluate the perceived threat involved in the anger-producing situation before reacting explosively.
- "Ted, when a situation begins to anger you, count to five before reacting and think of what is upsetting about the situation."
- "Jay, if discussing intimacy upsets you because you don't have a relationship now, think of ways to work on your relationships with others instead of getting angry."
- "Kate, use your learned strategies when you begin to feel anger. Then rethink the situation."

Reevaluation of a perceived threat helps to extend the time between the anger-inducing stimulus and the client's response and gives the client more opportunity to control anger (see Appendix B for learned strategies).

Use assertive responses when the client resorts to angry outbursts to have needs met.

Assertive therapeutic responses help to set limits and guidelines for the client who has impulsive outbursts. Firm but gentle reminders that staff are available to all clients help defuse client's fears and generally reduce anger, whereas aggressive, authoritarian responses may challenge or irritate the client and provoke anger or fear of abandonment (see assertiveness training, Appendix B).

Therapeutic Responses (Assertive)
- "Jeff, I asked Bob to be the group leader because it was his turn. You were the leader last week."
- "Kate, Joy talked more than you in community meeting today because she had many concerns, as you did yesterday."
- "Sam, I spoke with Ted a lot today because he needed my help. I also help you. Remember our talk yesterday?"

Nontherapeutic Responses (Aggressive)
"Jeff, don't be so selfish. You know it's not your turn to be group leader."
"Kate, you're being unreasonable. Joy talked more because she has more problems than you."
"Sam you're acting childishly. Ted needed me more than you did today."

Engage the client in a physical exercise program for use throughout the day (e.g., stationary bicycle, brisk walks, exercises, Ping-Pong, volleyball), especially before and after stress-producing experiences.

Physical activities help redirect anger-inducing energy toward productive, psychomotor activities.

Assure the client that the client does not need to resort to angry outbursts to have needs met.
- "Nick, it's not necessary to scream at staff. We'll help you when you need us."
- "Joy, you don't need to bang on the door of the nurses' station. We'll open it when we see you."
- "Ted, the group will listen to you better if you speak without cursing."

Assurance that needs will be met helps to decrease the fear and frustration that accompany the client's unmet needs and promotes more socially acceptable behavior.

Discuss with the client how angry outbursts can discourage social relationships and foster threats of loneliness and abandonment.
- "Joy, when you direct your frustrations toward others in an angry way, they won't want to be around you. And the very thing you fear [abandonment] may occur."

This information increases the client's awareness of the consequences of negative behaviors and encourages more functional responses by the client.

Initiate a written contract (if feasible) that sets limits on the client's angry outbursts, with clear strategies to help reduce their frequency.

A contract gives the client access to a tangible reminder of acceptable milieu behaviors and ways to maintain them.

Engage the client in cognitive or behavioral strategies and therapies: role playing, cognitive-behavioral therapy,

Use of learned therapeutic techniques helps the client manage anger effectively, increase self-esteem, and

thought substitution/stopping, assertiveness training, process/focus groups (see Appendix B).

express angry feelings in more socially acceptable ways.

Praise the client for efforts made to manage angry feelings and express self in a socially adaptive manner.
- "It was a positive decision to approach me to discuss your feelings before attending the community meeting."
- "The staff has noticed a significant improvement in your behavior since you began cognitive therapy."
- "You are really making an effort to use exercise and physical activity to manage your anger."

Genuine praise helps to promote continued efforts by the client and increases self-esteem.

Blaming/Projecting

Make short, frequent contacts with the client throughout the day.

Frequent contacts help to establish a trusting nurse-client relationship.

Assess the client for the risk for violence to self or others (e.g., angry out bursts/threats/gestures directed toward self or others; pacing/scanning the environment).

Careful assessment of the client's behavior, especially changes that may indicate violence, helps to protect the client and others from harm or injury.

Refrain from reacting with anger or hostility to the client's accusations. Instead, use a calm, matter-of-fact, but not overly casual approach.

Matter-of-fact responses help to decrease the client's feelings of alienation and discourage blaming and overly projection.

Collaborate with staff to use consistent responses when the client refuses to accept blame or blames and accuses others.

Consistent responses by staff help to clarify unacceptable or maladaptive behaviors with the client.

Use assertive responses to gently challenge the client's false accusations: "I" versus "you" messages, eye contact, congruent facial/verbal expressions.

Assertive responses help to discourage validation of the client's beliefs and accusations without inciting anger or aggression. They tend to increase self-esteem.

Therapeutic Responses (Assertive)
- "I don't think it was Nick's idea to go AWOL, Jay. He never mentioned wanting to leave."
- "I find it hard to believe that the other clients are jealous of you, Joy. I've seen nothing to indicate that."
- "I don't believe it's up to me to do your laundry, Nick. All clients do their own laundry."
- "I care about you and all the clients equally, Kate. I can't always give everyone all the time they want."

Nontherapeutic Responses (Nonassertive)
"You know you deliberately missed the 7 o'clock activity, Sam. *You*'ve done this before."
"You could have cleaned the dining room even if there were clients in it, Ted. *You* just didn't want to do it."
"You and every client here must do their own laundry, Nick. That's the rule, and *you* know it."

Nonassertive or aggressive responses convey an accusatory, harsh tone that may incite defensiveness and anger in the client and diminish the client's trust and self-esteem.

Refrain from responding prematurely in the assessment process to the client's accusatory or "disgruntled" remarks that reflect the client's dissatisfaction.
Client: "I don't know why I have to go to every meeting. This place expects too much."
"This food is terrible. You'd think they would hire a decent cook."

Allowing the client to vent negative feelings in the initial stages of an admission helps the staff to assess the extent of the client's anger and to plan interventions accordingly.

Engage the client in groups that encourage social interactions (e.g., community meetings, relationship groups, outings).

Social gatherings help to increase the client's social skills, build trust among peers, and discourage the client's blaming and projection.

Continued

PLANNING AND IMPLEMENTATION—cont'd

Nursing Intervention	Rationale
Blaming/Projecting—cont'd	

Nursing Intervention	Rationale
Assist the client to identify when blaming or projection is hurtful or threatening to others. • "Ted, the clients are upset because you've been saying they take your belongings." • "Joy, when you say that everything was fine until I came into the room, I feel annoyed." • "Kate, allowing Pam to take the blame for not reminding you about your responsibility in the group project may hurt your friendship."	This information helps the client recognize the negative impact of the client's accusations and blame on others.
Assist the client to analyze his or her belief systems and situations that result in blaming others. • "Jeff, you say you missed the meeting because Sarah didn't remind you. Actually, I told you several times about the meeting." • "Pam, you say it was Joy's idea to leave the unit without permission, but you left as well." • "Ted, you're telling me everything was fine until I came into the room. What do you think happened when I came into the room?"	This type of analysis helps the client develop a more realistic belief system and decreases the incidence of blaming or accusing others.
Engage the client in milieu activities that are productive and rewarding (physical exercise, sports, arts/crafts).	Involvement in rewarding activities helps the client build self-esteem/self-worth and reduces opportunities for blaming.
Assign milieu responsibilities to the client. • Request that the client notify other clients for meetings and groups. • Ask the client to plan activities with staff. *Note:* Assigned tasks should not be punitive or demeaning.	Duties and assignments help to occupy the client's time with activities that increase responsibility and self-worth and promote awareness of positive versus negative behaviors.
Praise the client whenever the client accepts responsibility for actions and refrains from blaming or accusing others. • "Kate, it was good to hear you say you left the dining room messy without blaming anyone else." • "Nick, the group said they appreciated your apology for playing the radio so loud."	Genuine praise increases the client's self-concept/self-esteem and helps to reinforce positive behaviors.
Passive-Aggressive	
Observe the client's nonverbal behavioral clues that may indicate anger. • The client avoids groups/one-to-one interactions. • Procrastinates when asked to complete tasks. • Resists or rejects suggestions/ideas. • Conveys impatience/frustration/boredom. • Uses sarcasm, often disguised as humor.	Assessment of passive-aggressive behaviors is the first step toward helping the client connect behaviors with angry feelings.
Assist the client to identify and label angry feelings underlying passive-aggressive behaviors. • "Joy, what were you actually feeling when you left in the middle of our discussion?" • "Joe, when you told the group you were 'bored' with the discussion, what emotions were you experiencing?" • "Kate, describe what you were feeling when you ignored me today."	Identifying angry feelings helps the client develop an awareness of the physical and emotional sensations of anger and begin to consider management strategies.

Assist the client to recognize the negative effects of passive-aggressive behavior on self and others.
- "Ted, when you use sarcasm with humor, the other clients tend to avoid you."
- "Kate, did you notice the group's irritation when you said you found them 'boring'?"

Help the client identify the source of angry emotions.
- "Joe, you were very sarcastic in group today. I also noticed that your folks didn't visit you this afternoon. Let's talk about that."
- "Kate, you've been avoiding people all day. Are you still upset because you haven't been discharged yet?"

Teach the client strategies to express repressed anger in accordance with the treatment plan.
- The client engages in regular physical exercise or activity (e.g., stationary bike, Ping-Pong).
- Uses punching bag/batakas, with supervision.
- Participates in art/music therapy.
- Expresses angry feelings in a nonthreatening setting; talks, cries, or shouts in presence of trusted staff member.

Encourage the client to express anger directly rather than using sarcasm, avoidance, procrastination, or ignoring others or responsibilities.
- "Jeff, tell staff when you feel angry or irritable so we can help you deal with the cause of your anger, if possible, or help you manage it in a healthy way."
- "Sarah, it's better to express your anger when you begin to feel it rather than let it build up. Talk to staff when you're angry, and we will help you."

Assure the client that expressions of anger will not bring retaliation or chastisement from staff.
- "Jeff, it's OK to express angry feelings. Staff are here to help you cope with them."
- "Kate, expressing anger with staff is therapeutic and not wrong."

Assist the client to identify areas of procrastination and ineffective performance.
- "Donna, you haven't begun your share of the art project. The other clients can't continue without your help."
- "Sally, you didn't collect the names we need to elect a client leader. The group can't vote without a list of names."

Discuss with the client the positive results of initiating projects and performing tasks effectively.
- "Donna, your work on the quilt contributed to your group's prize. Could that be part of the reason that you're feeling so good today?"
- "Steve, you said at the community meeting that you're feeling happier than you have for a long time. Did the compliments you received for leading the group contribute to that feeling?"

Giving feedback to the client for negative behaviors can reduce the frequency of insensitive or hostile remarks.

Helping the client discover the source of angry emotions (when possible and evident) enables the client to deal more directly with the cause and avoid displacing hostile feelings toward others.
Note: Underlying causes of anger may be too deeply hidden or too complex to uncover and may require long-term psychotherapy.

Helping the client express anger though safe stress-reducing activities and behaviors allows the client to demonstrate anger through acceptable channels, which reduces anger and stress and promotes safety.
Note: With repressed behaviors, even if the cause cannot be exposed, the nurse can assist the client to safely manage anger.

This approach enables the client to have needs met from appropriate sources, reduces anxiety, and can prevent aggression resulting from built-up anger.

This assurance helps to lessen or eliminate the client's fear of consequences of demonstrating angry feelings in a safe setting.

Factual feedback helps the client develop an awareness of negative behaviors and their effects on others.

Discussing positive results of the client's behavior helps the client see that the rewards of initiating and completing tasks are greater than covert acts of aggression.

Continued

PLANNING AND IMPLEMENTATION—cont'd

Nursing Intervention	Rationale
Passive-Aggressive—cont'd	
Acknowledge those experiences regarding hospitalization that typically cause anger, irritation, or resentment: being away from a familiar living situation, sharing space with others, talking to strangers about problems.	Acknowledgment of experiences helps to assure the client that anger related to loss of control and feelings of powerlessness is a normal, human emotion and can be expressed openly, in a safe setting.
Share with client similar experiences that provoked anger, resentment, or irritation in yourself. *Note:* Sharing universal feelings (anger, sadness) is acceptable as long as the discussion focuses back to the *client's* needs as soon as possible.	Sharing common human feelings helps to assure the client that certain events or experiences provoke similar responses in most people, and that the client is not alone with these feelings.
Explore with the client situations, topics, or experiences that result in feelings of anger, resentment, or irritation.	Although some deep causes of anger may not be readily known, exploration helps the nurse and client determine more common causes of anger and begin to plan strategies to best help the client in each situation.
Engage the client in groups and activities: behavioral-cognitive therapy, assertiveness therapy, process/focus groups, role playing/sociodrama. *Note:* Sociodrama is not a mainstream therapy, but its elements may be used in role-playing activities.	Participating in therapeutic groups/activities helps the client disclose angry feelings and learn to cope with them and communicate them more effectively (see Appendix B).
Praise the client for efforts made toward direct expression of anger versus use of passive-aggressive behaviors. • "Joy, you expressed your angry feelings appropriately in group today." • "Nick, it was good that you told me how angry you were when I forgot our meeting."	Praise given for efforts made and for positive results helps to increase the client's self-esteem and reinforce more direct expressions of anger.
Impulsivity	
Assess the degree and destructiveness of the client's impulsivity.	Assessment helps to determine the effects of impulsivity on the client and others and can protect the client and others from injury or harm.
Protect the client and others from injury when the client loses control as a result of impulsive behaviors (see seclusion/restraint interventions, Chapter 3).	Staff who use appropriate safety measures for clients with impulsive/threatening behaviors are the best protection against harm or injury to the client and others in the milieu.
Identify with the client, the client's impulsive behaviors, and the resulting problems. • Alcohol or drug abuse • Spending or credit card abuse • Driving too fast with unpaid speeding tickets • Drunk-driving citations • Moving from place to place with no permanent home base • Changing jobs for a variety of reasons • Trouble with the law or legal system	Problem solving with the client about the consequences of the client's impulsivity makes the client aware of associated problems and provides incentive to have needs met in more functional ways.
Identify resources and support systems available for the client: family/friends, employers, conservator, Veterans Administration, insurance, religious affiliates, parole officer. Facilitate collaboration between hospital/health care personnel and other resources/systems to meet the client's needs: social service referral, short-term inpatient milieu therapy, outpatient therapy, county mental health ervices, legal system.	Following up problem-solving with helpful resources to address impulsive behaviors helps the client have needs met in a more functional way.

Assist the client to recognize feelings that precede impulsive acts (anxiety, anger) (see preceding interventions for passive-aggressive client).

Teach the client strategies to increase the time between the stimuli that trigger feelings and the impulsive actions (see Appendix B).
- The client uses slow, deep-breathing exercises.
- Practices relaxation techniques.
- Counts slowly to five when feelings that precede impulsive behaviors emerge.
- Removes self from stimuli (takes "time out") when senses feelings are escalating out of control.
- Occupies free time with meetings, activities, and groups.

Collaborate with the client and interdisciplinary team members to identify the best therapeutic approach to the client's impulsive life-style.

Engage the client in an appropriate therapeutic regimen in the hospital/community that helps the client modify impulsive behaviors.
- Chemical dependency rehabilitation program
- Classes for drunk driving
- Legal counseling
- Family counseling
- Groups that deal with addictive behaviors (e.g., gambling, drinking, prostitution, spending, shoplifting, speeding).

Recognizing feelings that occur immediately before an impulsive act helps the client reduce impulsive incidents.

Increasing the time between the provoking stimulus and the impulsive act interrupts the stimulus-response cycle and helps the client gain control over maladaptive responses.

A multidisciplinary approach provides consistency and thus is an effective way to meet the client's needs.

Both the hospital and the community offer programs that are critical to the client's recovery and ongoing care.

Lying

Assess the degree, frequency, and consequences of the client's use of lies to meet needs.

Gently challenge the client's lies by pointing out the discrepancies in the client's stories.
- "Paul, you say you never 'cheek' your medications, yet you were refused a pass because of that."
- "Sarah, you told your doctor that you attend every group, but you didn't attend the assertiveness training group today."
- "Mark, the snack you were eating had Jeff's name on the label, so Jeff was correct about you eating his snack earlier."

Teach the client to approach staff directly to have needs met rather than resorting to lies or fabrications.
- "Paul, if you have problems with taking your medication, talk to staff or your doctor about it. Not taking the medication will not solve your problem."
- "Sarah, it's better to discuss the reasons you don't attend your assertiveness training group than to tell your doctor you never miss it."
- "Mark, if you want a snack, tell staff or check it on your menu. Don't take another client's food."

Assessment of the client's lying behaviors helps the staff plan interventions that eliminate or minimize the client's lying.

Pointing out discrepancies in the client's stories, when it is therapeutic, helps make the client aware of lies and discourages their repetition.

This information lets the client know that his or her needs will be met without the use of lies.
The client is informed that lying and "stealing" in the milieu are not acceptable behaviors, especially in regard to the other clients and the staff.

Continued

PLANNING AND IMPLEMENTATION—cont'd

Nursing Intervention	Rationale

Lying—cont'd

Nursing Intervention	Rationale
Inform the client about the effect of the client's lies on others. • "Mark, lying about eating Jeff's snack makes it difficult for him to trust you." • "Paul, 'cheeking' your medication is serious. Staff will have to put you on a behavioral contract." • "Sarah, lying about attending the assertiveness training group will not gain trust. It will hurt your treatment and progress."	Clients need to be aware of the negative consequences of lying behaviors to work at reducing lies and other fabricated stories.
Initiate activities that build the client's self-esteem: physical activities (e.g., Ping-Pong, volleyball), arts and crafts, music, games (e.g., Scrabble, chess).	The client's involvement in activities that are fun and satisfying helps to discourage use of lies and fabrications to gain attention and meet needs.
Construct a behavioral contract that clearly describes acceptable behaviors and consequences of lying. *Note:* Behavioral contracts are used in conjunction with other therapeutic methods and may not be the standard treatment for all clients or facilities.	A written contract is one method that staff can use to establish guidelines and help set limits on the client's use of lies.
Assure the client that direct, truthful behaviors are more rewarding than lying. • "Mark, everyone appreciates you asking staff for snacks instead of taking other clients' food." • "Paul, sharing your concerns about medication effects rather than 'cheeking' pills was helpful in changing the dosage." • "Sarah, apologizing for not being truthful about attending the assertiveness group has helped your relationship with staff and other clients."	Clients who are rewarded by staff for positive behaviors, when warranted, begin to realize that it is more beneficial to be open and honest than to lie or hide the truth.
Engage the client in activities: role play/sociodrama, cognitive-behavioral therapy, assertiveness training, process/focus groups (see Appendix B).	Activities involving other clients' reactions and opinions reinforce staff responses to the client's lying behaviors and promote continuity of open, honest interactions.
Praise the client for efforts made toward use of open, honest interactions and reduction or absence of lying. • "Kate, the staff say they have noticed your efforts to be direct and honest." • "Sarah, the staff and clients say they appreciate your truthfulness."	Positive feedback by trusted staff helps to build the client's self-esteem and reinforces repetition of truthful behaviors.
See later care plan for the client with ineffective coping for additional interventions.	

Narcissistic/Antisocial

Nursing Intervention	Rationale
Assess the client's level of narcissism and grandiosity (e.g., how self-focused and self-serving is the client?).	A thorough assessment of the client's behaviors helps to determine how they interfere with the client's role and interactions with other clients and assists in the planning of interventions.
Assure the client that he or she does not need to resort to narcissistic or antisocial behaviors to have needs met. • "Pam, it's not necessary to interrupt groups to make your needs known. It's more effective for you to ask staff for assistance." • "Ted, breaking hospital rules will not get you the kind of attention you need."	Open, direct discussion with the client on how to have needs met helps to decrease the client's concerns about needs not being met and discourages narcissistic/antisocial behaviors.

Assist the client to recognize the negative effects of self-centered behaviors on others.
- "Sam, the rest of the group gets upset when you occupy their time with long, exaggerated stories."
- "Jeff, staff doesn't appreciate it when you walk into their private areas without asking permission."
- "Joe, playing music after 9 PM disturbs the other clients."

Detailing how the client's negative behaviors affect others helps the client develop an awareness of the impact of his or her behavior and begin to modify it.

Encourage the client to challenge his or her narcissistic beliefs.
- "Nick, the other clients find it hard to believe the stories you tell about your accomplishments."
- "Kate, what makes you believe you should have more privileges than the other clients?"
- "Kate, you have done a commendable job as client leader. Other clients have also done well."

Assisting the client to challenge erroneous beliefs in a nonthreatening way helps to present reality and diminish the client's feelings of entitlement and exaggerated self-importance.

Tactfully confront the client with his or her attempts to exploit other clients to meet own needs.
- "Jeff, it seems as if you're only nice to Jeff when you want a favor from him."
- "Sarah, you offered to make your roommate's bed and clean the room just before you asked for $10. She says you ignored her before that."

Tactful confrontation helps to make the client aware of negative behaviors and can reduce their frequency.

Initiate a written contract that sets limits on the client's antisocial behaviors.
Note: Contracts may not always be effective with these clients because contracts provide opportunities for further manipulation. Also, it is difficult for staff to monitor behaviors.

A written contract is useful for some clients as a tangible reminder of acceptable milieu behaviors and methods to achieve them.

Encourage the client to participate in milieu activities: physical games (e.g., Ping-Pong, volleyball, shuffleboard), intellectual games (e.g., Trivial Pursuit, Scrabble), other group activities (e.g., bingo, arts/crafts, group sing-alongs).

Therapeutic activities help to modify narcissistic, self-important behaviors through the cooperative group process.

Engage the client in therapies that will help the client recognize and manage narcissistic, grandiose, and exploitive behaviors: role play/sociodrama, cognitive-behavioral therapy, assertiveness training, group therapy (see Appendix B).

Individual and group-oriented therapies are time-tested treatments that help clients reduce negative behaviors through education and practice.

Demonstrate appropriate, mature behaviors through role modeling.

Appropriate role modeling shows the client acceptable, effective interpersonal interactions.

Use role modeling to express feelings and emotions (joy, sadness, laughter) in a variety of appropriate situations.

It is difficult for persons with narcissistic and antisocial personality traits to confront feelings and express emotions. The nurse can facilitate this through role modeling.

Give positive feedback whenever the client expresses self in relation to others and situations outside the self.
- "Joan, it's good to see you laughing with the other clients. The community meeting was fun today."
- "Barbara, it's OK to cry when you feel sad for other people. It can be healthy to release emotions."

Praising the client for relating to others and reacting to situations in ways that are not self-serving or self-aggrandizing lets the client know that expressing feelings toward and with others is acceptable and beneficial to a person's emotional health.

Inform the client directly when actions are inappropriate or interfere with the rights of others.
- "Paul, it's not acceptable to put your arm around other clients or to touch them, unless it's part of a game or activity."

Giving the client feedback immediately for unacceptable behaviors reminds the client which behaviors are inappropriate and helps set limits for the client to better control negative behaviors.

Continued

PLANNING AND IMPLEMENTATION—cont'd

Nursing Intervention	Rationale

Narcissistic/Antisocial—cont'd

- "Sarah, taking cigarettes, snacks, or anything else that belongs to other clients is not tolerated."

Praise the client for relating to others without use of narcissistic, grandiose, or exploitative behaviors. • "Sally, you really were an equal team member in the volleyball game." • "Jay, staff appreciate that you knock on the door and wait for a response before walking into staff areas." • "Sam, the other clients were happy with your cooperation in group today. You didn't interrupt anyone."	Praising the client in a genuine way for positive behaviors reinforces appropriate behaviors and increases self-esteem.

Irresponsibility

Evaluate the effects of the client's irresponsible behaviors on the client's progress and interactions with others in the milieu.	A thorough evaluation of the client's behaviors and the effects on others helps the staff plan appropriate interventions that promote responsible behaviors.
Inform the client in a calm, direct manner each time the client demonstrates irresponsible, insensitive behaviors. • "Jeff, you need to clean the shower after you use it. That's the responsibility of every client here." • "Mark, the group waited 20 minutes for you to lead the meeting. You didn't tell us you were out on pass."	Reminding the client of negative behaviors increases the client's awareness of his or her actions and promotes positive behaviors.
Point out the consequences of the client's irresponsible actions on other clients. • "Pam, Joe lent you money that you promised to pay back the next day. When you didn't, he was unable to pay his way into the movie." • "Bob, hiding marijuana in your room caused serious problems for your roommate."	Reinforcing the negative impact of the client's behaviors on others and the milieu increases the client's awareness of the harmful consequences of his or her actions and promotes more responsible behaviors.
Construct a verbal or written behavioral contract (if feasible) with the client, listing specific responsibilities and obligations that the client is expected to achieve. • Maintaining neat, clean room and client areas. • Cleaning shower and bathtub after use. • Attending all meetings and activities. • Arriving on time for all meetings and activities. • Informing other clients and staff when unable to keep appointments and commitments. Specify in the contract the behaviors that are restricted. • Borrowing money, clothing, cigarettes, or other valued items from other clients. • Smoking or keeping illegal drugs in or around hospital area. • Having alcoholic beverages in or around hospital area.	A contract of either type promotes positive, responsible behaviors and sets limits on irresponsible actions. A written contract also provides tangible guidelines that are constant reminders of the client's responsibilities and restrictions.

Maladaptive Denial

Assess situations in which the client uses maladaptive denial. Possible causes of denial include fear of mental illness and its outcome, client roles/responsibilities, low self-esteem, limitations/weaknesses, resistance to treatment regimen/poor compliance, guilt/shame.	Assessing the client's dysfunctional use of denial helps the nurse and the treatment team determine areas of conflict that are too anxiety provoking for the client to confront and that prevent progress.

Assist the client to identify threats that precipitate denial.
- "Paul, staff realizes the other clients often ask your advice. You are also a client and need help, too."
- "Steve, it's difficult for you to admit that you have a mental health problem. But it's the first step toward getting better."
- "Mark, you say you're not a 'regular' client, yet you're experiencing what many clients experience."
- "Sam, while it may be true that your family has problems, you're here because it was difficult for you to cope as well."

Helping the client identify obstacles to treatment through simple, direct communication skills encourages the client to confront conflicts that inhibit compliance with treatment, promoting movement toward health.

Explore with the client the consequences of resistance or refusal to admitting the need for treatment.
- "Paul, attending groups and meetings is part of your treatment plan; to ignore that will delay your progress."
- "Mark, saying you're not a 'regular' client doesn't mean you don't need therapy. Your chances for recovery are better with treatment."
- "Kate, leaving the hospital without telling staff shows us that you're not taking your client role seriously. That will make it harder for you to recover."

Exploring with the client the negative consequences of the client's resistance to treatment helps the client abandon maladaptive denial and begin to comply with the medical regimen.

Teach the client anxiety-reducing strategies to manage threats to the self-system (see Appendix B).

Anxiety-reducing strategies help diminish the use of denial and increase compliance with the treatment plan.

Provide opportunities for the client to express thoughts and feelings of fear, low self-esteem, guilt, and shame.
- "Jeff, staff is here to listen to your feelings about your illness and hospitalization."
- "Kate, it will help staff with our treatment approach if you talk about your concerns with us."

Giving the client opportunities to express painful feelings and thoughts helps the client bring fears and conflicts into the open and can reduce the incidence of denial.

Help the client recognize that the unrealistic "optimism" of denial does not reduce the client's illness or symptoms.
- "Nick, your inability to be viewed as a client may reduce anxiety for awhile, but your illness must be treated to reduce painful symptoms and behaviors."
- "Ted, ignoring or negating your problems will not make you feel better. The treatment plan is for that."

It is critical to help the client overcome maladaptive denial until the client ultimately recognizes that denial is not conducive to health and well-being.

Allow the client to use defenses such as denial adaptively when he or she is unable to cope in a more functional way.

Denial may be used adaptively for a brief time to reduce the client's anxiety when it threatens to overwhelm the client and when the anxiety cannot yet be managed in a more functional way.

Identify the client's expressions of fear, guilt, and shame as possible signs of progress, and encourage these expressions.

Encouraging the client to continue to express feelings that provoke denial offers hope for movement toward recovery.

Challenge the client's belief that weaknesses are synonymous with illness by teaching client about mental illness.
- "There are several theories of mental illness, Pam, but a mental disorder is not a character weakness."
- "Jeff, a mental disorder is as real as a physical illness. Both can be treated, and neither is considered a weakness."

Replacing the client's erroneous beliefs about mental illness with factual, scientific information reduces the stigma of mental illness, minimizes denial, and reinforces the client's progress and hope for recovery.

Encourage the client to participate in groups and activities within the milieu.

Participation in therapeutic activities helps to distract the client from the use of denial by reducing anxiety through pleasurable activities.

Engage the client in cognitive and behavioral therapy groups (assertiveness training, role play/sociodrama, process/focus groups) (see Appendix B).

Group activities encourage the client to share feelings with other clients, elicit helpful feedback through the group process, and reduce maladaptive denial.

Continued

PLANNING AND IMPLEMENTATION—cont'd

Nursing Intervention	Rationale
Maladaptive Denial—cont'd	
Praise the client for a reduction in or absence of maladaptive denial and for compliance with treatment regimen. • "Jeff, talking about your illness and problems shows real progress." • "Pam, bringing your concerns out into the open is a big step in coping with them more effectively." • "Kate, admitting that you need help as do the other clients is a sign of your growth." • "Mark, sharing your guilt about your illness in group today is a sign of your increasing strength."	Genuine praise increases the client's self-esteem, promotes continuity of functional coping behaviors, and encourages hope for recovery.

Care Plan
DSM-IV-TR Diagnosis   **Personality Disorders (All Types)**

NANDA Diagnosis: Chronic Low Self-Esteem

Long-standing negative self-evaluation/feelings about self or capabilities.

Focus:

For the client who demonstrates a life-style of overt or covert behavior patterns that reflect a negative self-concept. Behaviors may manifest as dependency or jealousy, among others, and may greatly interfere with the patient's ability to function at an optimal developmental stage.

RELATED FACTORS (ETIOLOGY)

Personal identity disturbance
Disturbance in self-perception/self-concept
Powerlessness
Lack of insight/judgment
Ineffective problem solving
Perceived abandonment/rejection
Developmental conflicts
Psychosocial stressors
Environmental stressors
Role/relationship disturbance
Life-style of dependence/avoidance
Perceived victimization
Knowledge deficit regarding effective social skills

DEFINING CHARACTERISTICS

Dependency

The client demonstrates dependency on others to have needs met.
Appears frequently at nurses' station with nonurgent requests and asks for help with tasks that can easily be done by the client.
• "I need help with my laundry. I can't do it alone."
• "Could you get my cigarettes for me? They're in my room."

Demonstrates inability to make decisions without excessive advice from others and procrastinates.
• "I just can't make up my mind. Please help me decide what I should do."
• "What should I do now? Make my bed? Get dressed? Or take a shower?"
Needs constant reassurance from others.
• "Am I doing this checklist right?"
• "Does this place setting seem OK?"
• "Should I take my medication now?"
Allows others to make important life decisions.
• "You decide what board and care home I need."
• "I wish you would call my husband and tell him I can't see his mother anymore."
Lacks self-confidence or belittles own abilities and assets.
• "I just can't seem to do anything right. You do it so much better."
• "I'm a flop and a failure as a wife and mother."
• "I don't blame my husband for leaving me. I'm not even attractive."
Displays difficulty in initiating projects.
• "How should I get started on my assignment?"
• "It's too hard to begin this project on my own."
Fears abandonment and is uncomfortable when alone.
• "I'll die without my husband to take care of me."
• "I can't imagine leaving my mother's home."
• "Why does everyone always leave me alone?"

Isolated/Withdrawn/Avoidant

The client demonstrates inability to form close, personal relationships with others.
• Rejects intimacy with one significant partner.
• Referred to as a "loner" by significant others.
Avoids social contact in the milieu.
Remains isolated in room for long periods.
Responds minimally when approached.
Exhibits cool, detached behavior toward others.

Easily hurt by criticism.

Fears being embarrassed or humiliated.

- Blushes or cries when others offer praise or criticism.

Exaggerates risks or danger in ordinary situations or events.

- "I'm not going on the field trip. The bus could skid and go over a cliff in the rain."

Arrives late for milieu activities; leaves early.

Abandonment Fears/Attention Seeking

The client demonstrates a need to avoid actual or perceived abandonment.

Makes frequent appearances at the nurses' station.

Makes unreasonable demands for staff's time and attention.

- "I hate to bother you during your lunch hour, but I won't take up much of your time."
- "Why do you only talk to me for a few minutes and then leave?"

Seeks contact person or other staff members with a sense of urgency that is incongruent with the actual need.

- "I really *need* to see you now. I'm out of clothes."

Demands that staff call attending psychiatrist several times throughout the day.

- "I *have* to see my doctor. I know he is in the hospital now."
- "Can you call my doctor at home? There's something I forgot to ask."
- "I saw my doctor leave the unit without talking to me. Could you *please* catch her before she leaves the hospital?"

Questions loyalty of friends and family members.

- "I doubt that my best friend will be waiting for me when I get out of here."
- "I'm scared that my father will give up on me and *never* let me back in the house again."

Telephones significant others for reassurance many times throughout hospitalization.

Hysteria

The client responds in dramatic, urgent, or exaggerated manner toward persons or situations that do not warrant such reactions.

- "I absolutely *must* see my doctor right now."
- "If I don't get my weekend pass, I'll just *die*."
- "You simply *have* to speak to my roommate. I can't tolerate her abuse one more day."

Increases voice tone and uses gestures.

Displays intense emotional expressiveness inappropriate to situation.

Seductiveness

The client exhibits seductive, flirtatious, or teasing behaviors with sexual overtones.

- Gazes suggestively; poses seductively.
- Wears tight, scanty, or revealing clothing.
- Discusses personal or sexual topics.

- Directs seductive behavior toward favored person or toward the milieu in general.
- Makes excuses to see the favored person as often as possible.
- Writes love notes to objects of affection.

Jealousy

The client expresses extreme feelings and thoughts of jealousy regarding suspected infidelity of spouse, sexual partner, staff, or other clients.

- "I can't even trust my wife with my own brother or father."
- "I'm sure my husband is attracted to most of the female clients when he visits me."
- "I realize my boyfriend flirts with all the nurses here. I'll bet he's going out with the whole neighborhood while I'm in here sick."
- "My roommate thinks she's so great and that everyone loves her. I can't stand her."
- "Everyone thinks Tim is so wonderful. He's really a big phony."

Accuses staff of giving more attention to other clients or spending more time with them.

Makes frequent phone calls home to check up on spouse or partner.

Hypersexuality

The client makes frequent sexually suggestive statements, generally in an attempt to increase self-esteem.

- "Why should anyone care if I put my arms around Mary? After all, I'm a man."
- "It's no big deal that the staff caught us in bed together. It's normal."
- "I don't know why I can't even kiss someone I like just because we're in a hospital."
- "Gosh, Kate, that blouse really shows off your figure. It gives me ideas."

Behaves in a sexually provocative manner.

- Winks; thrusts hips or chest in suggestive manner.
- Tells sexually oriented stories and jokes.
- Sits next to individuals in positions that result in physical contact.

Rigid/Perfectionistic

The client is unable to complete tasks because of fear of substandard performance and product.

- "I just can't finish my assignment. I don't have enough time to do it right."
- "It will take me forever to do justice to this project. I'd rather not try it at all."

Is preoccupied with details to such a degree that activities and projects go uncompleted.

- "I don't know if I can finish this project. There are so many details that need my attention."
- "I want to complete my activities, but I have other things on my mind."

Continued

Demonstrates excessive rigidity regarding values, ethics, and morals, which inhibits task performance and completion.
- Preoccupied with verbal or written accounts of ethical or moral issues to the exclusion of assigned tasks or projects.
- Discusses spiritual beliefs during activity times without regard for task assignment.

OUTCOME IDENTIFICATION AND EVALUATION

Dependency

The client verbalizes independent statements.
- "I can take care of my own basic needs."
- "I'm going to shower and do my laundry today."

Demonstrates independent behaviors.
- Approaches nurses' station only when necessary.
- Performs self-care and other tasks without help.

Makes decisions related to illness and treatment.
- Discusses possible change in medication dose with nurses and physician.
- Plans and organizes daily task and activities.

Makes decisions unrelated to illness and treatment.
- Enlists family or friends to take care of personal business (e.g., pay rent/bills, feed pets, water plants) during hospital stay.
- Chooses own place to live after discharge.

Verbalizes self-confidence in abilities and assets.
- "I know I'm a darn good parent."
- "When it comes to my work, I'm very capable."
- "I've always been a good artist."

Demonstrates confidence in abilities and tasks.
- Initiates and completes projects successfully.

Expresses comfort in spending time alone.
- "I actually enjoy having some time to myself."
- "I love my family, but it's good to be alone once in a while."

Makes independent choices regarding life-style.
- "I need to leave my parents' home and be on my own."
- "I'm no longer afraid to live without a partner."

Isolated/Withdrawn/Avoidant

The client seeks social contact with clients and staff.
Spends majority of time in client areas rather than alone in room.
Responds with brightened affect when approached.
Initiates interactions with others.
Participates with others in milieu activities.
Arrives at milieu activities on time; stays for entire session.
Engages in conversations and dialogue with others.
Forms close personal relationship with a significant other.
Accepts constructive criticism without crying or retreating.
Accepts praise without blushing or retreating.
Seeks praise for accomplishments.

Attends outdoor activities and field trips without expressing exaggerated risks or dangers.

Abandonment Fears/Attention Seeking

The client approaches nurses' station only when necessary.
Approaches staff at convenient times rather than during their breaks or lunch hour.
Seeks staff's time and attention for relevant reasons rather than nonurgent requests.
Acknowledges loyalty of family/friends.
- "I know my family cares about me."
- "I'm sure that my friends will always be there for me."
Refrains from frequent telephone calls to family/friends.
Ceases to make frequent requests of staff to contact attending physician.
Makes requests of staff without an exaggerated sense of urgency.
Expresses comfort in spending time alone rather than feeling fearful or anxious.
- "I actually enjoy being alone once in a while."
- "The times I spend by myself are peaceful."
The client with *borderline personality disorder* with intense abandonment fears no longer requires a "transient object" (picture, note, stuffed animal) when left alone.

Hysteria

The client demonstrates absent or decreased dramatic or exaggerated affect when interacting with others.
Uses a low to moderate tone of voice.
Displays appropriate emotional response congruent with the situation.

Seductiveness

The client responds appropriately toward others, with absence of seductive, flirtatious, or teasing behaviors.
- Refrains from using sexually provocative dialogue.
- Assumes appropriate positions rather than seductive or suggestive body language.
- Ceases to demonstrate provocative or suggestive gestures or expressions.
- Resists wearing tight-fitting, revealing clothing inappropriate to the setting.
Stops seeking out favored staff person or physician for personal, "romantic" reasons.
- Reports absence of romantic notions, daydreams, or fantasies directed toward others in the environment.

Jealousy

The client demonstrates fewer or no jealous behaviors.
Decreases number of phone calls to spouse or significant others during hospitalization.
- Refrains from accusing partner of infidelity or flirting with others.
Ceases to accuse staff of giving more time and attention to "all the other clients."

Verbalizes trust toward significant partner.
- "I really do trust my wife."
- "I have faith in my boyfriend. I know he will be loyal to me while I'm in the hospital."

Hypersexuality

The client refrains from making lewd, sexually provocative statements.

Resists touching others in a sexually suggestive manner and rarely needs reminders.

Demonstrates appropriate behaviors, with absence of sexually provocative gestures, poses, or expressions.

Rigid/Perfectionistic

The client completes majority of tasks without fear of substandard performance and product.

Accomplishes assignments without being overly preoccupied with details.

Completes activities and projects without being diverted by rigid moral and ethical preoccupations.

Demonstrates more flexible and less rigid behaviors.
- Makes sufficient time for all scheduled activities and projects and rarely needs reminders.
- Reacts in a more calm, matter-of-fact manner to imperfect, substandard task or project.

PLANNING AND IMPLEMENTATION

Nursing Intervention	Rationale
Dependency	
Assess client's level of dependence in a variety of areas.	Initial assessment helps the nurse plan interventions and measure the client's level of progress against expected outcomes.
Formulate a nursing care plan outlining the client's basic needs and activities of daily living. • Activities the client can perform independently (independent) • Activities with which the client requires help (interdependent) • Activities the client needs the nurse to perform for him or her (dependent).	A comprehensive treatment that addresses the client's dependence, interdependence, and independence helps determine and encourage appropriate independent behavior.
Positively reinforce the client's independent behavior. • "Pam, I see you showered and put on some makeup this morning." • "Ted, you made out your own menus without help for 3 days." • "Jeff, you were on time for all the group activities today." • "Jay, start to do your laundry and I'll be here if you need help."	Reinforcing the client's independent behaviors increases confidence and self-esteem and encourages continuity of appropriate independent behavior.

Establish clear boundaries between nurse and client and client and others.
• Separate nurse's duties from client's responsibilities.
  "Pam, I will set the trays on the tables, and you and the others can arrange the napkins and utensils."
  "Paul, I'll put your clothes in your room, and you can fold them and put them away."
• Distinguish between the client's responsibilities and those of other clients.
  "Ken, it's your turn to clean the clients' dining room. Bob volunteered to empty ashtrays and wash out the coffeepot."
  "Beth, you can be the leader of the clients' group this afternoon. Sarah hasn't been here long enough."
	Establishing clear boundaries helps the client from becoming too enmeshed with others, which may result in a dependency on others to get needs met.

Encourage independent decision making in accordance with client's level of progress. • When the client asks, "What shall I do now?" you can reply with the statement, "What are some of the things you want to do now?"	Encouraging the client to make decisions within level of capability increases the client's self-worth and self-esteem.

Continued

PLANNING AND IMPLEMENTATION—cont'd

Nursing Intervention	Rationale
Dependency—cont'd	

- If the client cannot make up his or her mind about which activity to attend, you can ask, "What do you think would be most helpful to you now?"

Clarify with the client both negative and positive feelings that accompany dependency.
"Ken, how do you feel when you do something for yourself? Do you feel that way when others do things for you?"

Clarifying feelings the client experiences when performing dependent acts helps to show the client that there are more negative aspects connected to dependency and discourages dependent behavior.

Identify with the client the positive results of independent behaviors and accomplishment.
- "Sam, the clients really enjoyed the article you wrote in the clients' newsletter."
- "Kate, the placemat you made for the clients' holiday meal brightened their day."
- "Ken, your planning Sam's farewell party was a nice surprise for everyone, especially Sam."
- "Susan, your starting the sing-along was appreciated. Will you do it again when the group is together?"

Identifying positive results of the client's independent actions and accomplishments reinforces repetition of independent behaviors.

Offer the client choices whenever possible.
- "Mark, are you going to take your shower now or after the community meeting?"
- "Susan, you choose which game to play during activity time."
- "Ted, you can select the clients' prizes at the Bingo game tonight."

Offering choices that are within the client's capability helps to increase independence and encourages the client to participate in his or her own care and treatment.

Encourage the client to make decisions regarding his or her own care and treatment whenever feasible, rather than ask staff's permission.
- If the client asks, "Is it OK if I go to my room to rest?" ask the client, "Do you want to rest?" and if the response is yes, encourage the client to restate: "I *am* going to my room to rest."
- If the client asks, "Can I take my shower now?" ask the client, "Do you want to shower now?" and if the response is yes, have the client restate: "I *prefer* to take my shower now."
- If the client asks, "Is it OK if I attend Dr. Jones's lecture instead of playing bingo?" ask the client what she or he wants to do, then, based on the client's reply, encourage the client to state: "I *want* to attend Dr. Jones's lecture this afternoon."

Encouraging the client to make decisions to meet needs by using assertive language helps to increase the client's independence, judgment, and decision-making abilities regarding care and treatment.

Increase decision-making opportunities as the client progresses in treatment.
- "Ted, when you leave on your pass today, what are the things you'd like to do?"
- "Pam, you'll need to decide between staying in your parents' home and going back to independent living."
- "Susan, after you're discharged, it will be up to you to return for follow-up treatment."

Increasing the client's decision-making opportunities as he or she progresses promotes problem solving and assertive skills and prepares the client for life after discharge.

Respond with approval to the client's efforts toward independent decision making, as long as the decision is not harmful.

Approving the client's decision-making efforts, even if the decision itself is not perfect, helps reinforce continued independent behaviors.

- "Pam, it was good that you made a decision about where to live after you are discharged."
- "Ted, it's good that you arrived at the decision to pay your bills while you were out on pass."

Demonstrate respect for the client's feelings, even when he or she is unable to perform independently.
- "Donna, it's OK to feel bad that independent living didn't work out for you this time."
- "Kate, you're saying you're feeling frustrated, but it's OK to ask for help with difficult tasks."
- "Jane, you're feeling mad at yourself for not having decided where to live when you're discharged. You can begin working on that tomorrow. How can we help?"

Respecting the client's feelings and offering help when decisions do not meet the client's expectations assures the client that he or she is worthwhile and accepted.

Engage the client in physical activities that offer quick rewards.
- Brisk walks
- Exercises
- Stationary bicycle
- Ping-Pong
- Volleyball

Rewarding activities and healthy exercise increase the client's energy level and promote self-esteem.

Help the client set realistic, attainable goals.

Setting realistic, achievable goals helps to avoid or minimize failure, provides hope for behavioral change, and increases the client's feelings of independence and control over life.

Therapeutic Responses
- "Ted, it's good that you're making plans for your discharge; what did you think about the board and care homes you visited?"
- "Sally, I know you want your own apartment; what are your thoughts about independent living for a while?"
- "Pam, your desire to become a psychiatrist makes me think that you would like to do something to help people feel better."

These therapeutic statements are based on the nurse's judgment of the client's capabilities, rather than based on the client's wishes and desires, and more closely reflect achievable goals.

Nontherapeutic Responses
"Ted, if you really want to live by yourself, give it a try."
"Pam, you want to become a psychiatrist, why not talk to a college counselor about the course work?"
"Sally, you can do almost anything if you put your mind to it."

These nontherapeutic statements, however well-meaning, may encourage the client to pursue or attempt goals that may be beyond the client's capabilities. This could result in a sense of failure and diminished self-esteem.

Gradually help the client to decrease secondary gains (assistance from others, avoidance of responsibilities) that accompany dependent behaviors.
- "Paul, since you've been on time for the morning community meeting for 3 days, you don't need to be awakened by staff anymore."
- "Ken, you've made some real progress; staff thinks you're ready for the responsibility of client leader."

Using positive reinforcement to encourage the client's independence and responsibilities discourages continuance of dependent behaviors.

Teach the client to challenge unrealistic beliefs (e.g., failure, unattractiveness, lack of initiative) by pointing out factual information.

Pointing out realistic facts that challenge the client's negative self-perception helps decrease the client's negative self-concept and promotes self-worth.

Therapeutic Responses
- "Susan, you say you haven't succeeded at anything in your life, yet your children visit you and phone you every day."
- "Jeff, you say you never had ambition, yet you've achieved a bachelor's degree in history, which is an accomplishment."

These therapeutic statements challenge the client's unrealistic, negative beliefs by presenting actual facts versus opinions in an effort to replace negative beliefs with realistic, factual information (see Appendix B).

Continued

PLANNING AND IMPLEMENTATION—cont'd

Nursing Intervention	Rationale

Dependency—cont'd

• "Kate, you keep saying you're unattractive, yet I've heard clients and staff compliment your hairstyle and taste in clothes many times."

Nontherapeutic Responses

"Susan, how can you say you're unsuccessful? You have a nice family."

"Jeff, anyone with a college degree has to be successful."

"Kate, you have the prettiest blue eyes; I find that very attractive."

Challenge the client's exaggerated fears of abandonment and perceived consequences with factual information.

These nontherapeutic statements, however complimentary, distract the client from his or her real concerns and do nothing to diminish the client's negative self-perceptions.

This helps the client to develop an awareness of his/her actual capabilities and strengths.

Therapeutic Responses

• "Sarah, you say you 'can't make it' without your husband, yet you left him to enter the hospital for help and you've done well for 3 weeks."

• "Pam, no doubt your mother has helped you; she will continue to be supportive even if you live apart from each other."

• "Ted, you stated that you're hesitant to leave your roommate because you don't want to be alone, even though you fight a lot. Is being alone more stressful than tolerating frequent fighting?"

These therapeutic statements gently and accurately challenge the client's self-defeating beliefs while preserving the client's strengths and self-esteem.

Nontherapeutic Responses

"You know, Sarah, you really shouldn't feel you need a man to make your life complete; you're doing fine without one."

"Pam, everyone has to leave his or her mother behind; it's part of growing up."

"Ted, you can always get another roommate; why put yourself through all that stress?"

These nontherapeutic statements tend to chastise the client rather than challenge the belief system, which may perpetuate the fears rather than decrease them.

Assist the client to evaluate resources that will encourage and promote independence.

• "Sam, the social worker is an appropriate person to help you inquire about places to live."

• "Ted, the pharmacist teaches a class for clients every Tuesday; he may be another source of information about medication effects."

This assists the client in using reliable sources of help when necessary.

Identify with the client and family the strength and assets of the family unit and the client's contribution to the functioning of the family, as appropriate.

Note: Some families need help to maintain strength and integrity, before the client is able to succeed in his or her role within the family unit.

This helps to reinforce the importance and value of the client's role as a family member in accordance with the strength and capability of the family unit.

Discuss with the client and family the family behaviors that are no longer necessary but continue to interfere with the client's need for independence.

• "It may be that Jeff can now make more decisions for himself, since he is taking the new medication that helps him to function more independently."

• "It's understandable for the family to be concerned about Pam wanting to try independent living; her doctor and staff believe she's capable of doing it with your support."

Discussing the client's progress and capabilities with family members (with the client's permission) helps the nurse and treatment team gain insight into family behaviors that may interfere with the client's need for independence. This may pave the way for the nurse to do some family education.

Teach and assist the family to work with the client, doctor, and staff in promoting and encouraging the client's independent behaviors. • "It's to everyone's benefit that we all work together with Jeff so he can reach goals that are achievable." • "Everyone will gain when Pam's goals for independent living are successful; she needs all our support to do it."	Education and support of family members regarding the client's independent needs and goals help foster more autonomous family functioning for all members.
Engage the client in appropriate group, cognitive, and behavioral therapies. • Role play • Cognitive-behavioral therapy • Assertiveness training • Process groups • See Appendix B	Participation in a variety of therapeutic activities and groups tends to increase self-esteem and foster independent functioning and behaviors resulting from support, acceptance, and the universality of group dynamics.
Problem-solve with the client to identify the following: • Problems that realistically require some assistance • Goals that the client can achieve independently • Issues that need to be deferred to other sources • Alternative solutions for each problem • Solutions that consider both positive and negative aspects	Practicing problem-solving skills with the client helps to maximize the client's independent functioning and minimize dependent behaviors.
Praise the client for efforts made toward independent functioning. • "Jeff, your leading the community meeting in Ken's absence showed real initiative." • "Pam, making the final decision to find a roommate rather than move back in your parents' home is a big step for you."	Giving praise for the client's genuine efforts toward independence increases the client's self-esteem and reinforces independent behaviors.

Isolated/Withdrawn/Avoidant

Assess the degree of the client's isolation and level of progress in the self-imposed treatment regimen.	The client may be newly admitted and need time to adjust to the facility and milieu.
Make short, frequent visits to the client's room.	This shows the client that staff is caring and empathetic and understands that long, drawn-out interactions may be overwhelming.
Provide assistance with basic needs and activities of daily living, as needed. • Initially accompany the client to the shower, laundry room, and other new places. • Provide the client with toothbrush, toothpaste, comb, and hairbrush. • Offer literature, magazines, writing paper, and pencils. • Provide the client with a copy of the milieu-structured activities.	Assisting the isolative client with basic needs, as needed, helps the client to maintain self-respect and increases self-esteem.
Provide the client with his or her own clothing and valued personal belongings, as feasible. *Note:* This may not be possible if the client is suicidal or assaultive and clothing or personal effects can be used to inflict harm.	Having the client wear own clothing and use personal belongings, if safe and appropriate, reinforces the client's self-identity, promotes comfort and trust, and minimizes isolative behavior.
Engage in short, simple verbal interactions with the client. • "Here's the new toothbrush I promised you." • "I see you have pictures in your room." • "Is there anything else you need?" • "Did you fill out your menu for the day?"	Brief, nonchallenging interactions with the client throughout the day may begin to draw the client into the therapeutic community and reduce isolative behavior.

Continued

PLANNING AND IMPLEMENTATION—cont'd

Nursing Intervention	Rationale
Isolated/Withdrawn/Avoidant—cont'd	

Nursing Intervention	Rationale
Sit with the client for brief periods, interrupting silence only if it appears uncomfortable for the client (fidgets, paces, has worried or strained facial expression).	This helps the client to feel safe in an interpersonal relationship.
Gradually increase time of one-to-one interactions with the client. • Begin with 5-minute one-to-one interactions; progress in increments of 5 minutes until the client can engage in a 20-minute interaction without demonstrating discomfort or verbalizing the need to withdraw.	Gradually extending the time of interactions with the withdrawn client helps to promote socialization in a nonthreatening way and decreases periods of isolation.
Encourage the client to *gradually* join other clients in the milieu. • Begin in the dining room. Have the client first sit near the door, then graduate to a more populated, central area; progress to an informal or casual group setting; participate in one-to-one games with trusted staff, eventually including one or two trusted clients; progress to noncompetitive group activities (e.g., exercise, drawing, cooking, singing); attend a didactic class (e.g., cognitive-behavioral or assertive therapy); participate in more structured formal or process groups.	Gradually exposing the client to simple-to-complex milieu activities will give the client an appropriate amount of time to adjust to less challenging social situations before becoming involved in more challenging ones. This will increase socialization skills and reduce the client's isolation in a healthy, nonthreatening way (see Appendix B, Desensitization Techniques).
Promote involvement in physical activities (e.g., exercise, walking, Ping-Pong).	Physical activities increase the client's energy level and social accomplishments, which increase self-esteem.
Provide the client with plants or pets, if appropriate. (Most facilities use a pet therapy service).	Contact with nonthreatening living plants or animals will promote the client's expressions of love and nurturing and reduce isolation.
Set limits on naps and the amount of time client spends alone in room.	This will ensure that the client will sleep at night and be awake and rested for daytime milieu activities.
Provide the client with a balanced nutritional regimen.	This will prevent dehydration, constipation, and deterioration of physical health that may exacerbate the client's isolation and delay progress and recovery.
Gradually promote closeness, if appropriate, in accordance with the healthcare team's assessment of the client's tolerance. • Allow the client more space when beginning the interaction, gradually narrow the space between yourself and the client to arm's length, and progress to a comfortable social distance. *Note:* Two feet is a comfortable social distance.	Gradually reducing space between nurse and client during interactions gives the client time to develop trust and tolerance and reduces the client's isolation in a nonthreatening way.
Facilitate nonverbal expression of painful feelings through writing, drawing/painting, typing, playing piano/singing, and physical exercise.	These expressive activities can provide a release of painful feelings when the client cannot verbalize them and may help reduce isolation.
Engage the client in casual conversations at various intervals throughout the day. • Call the client by name; ask how he or she is doing; discuss nonthreatening topics of interest; share a soft drink or cup of tea with the client.	These simple acts of socialization show caring and interest and help promote the client's ease and comfort in social interactions.
Accept the client's refusal to joint staff or group in every activity or interaction without personalizing it.	Accepting the client's refusal on occasion prevents personal feelings from interfering with the therapeutic relationship and gives the client some control over decisions that may increase self-worth.

Role model positive social and interactive skills that can be readily achieved by the client.

Avoid placing the client in social situations or activities where he or she may fail or feel uncomfortable.

When the client is ready, provide the client with opportunities to discuss situations that may influence social withdrawal and isolation.
- "Ted, what makes it difficult for you to join the community?"
- "Tod, what situations cause you to want to leave groups and activities?"
- "Pam, how can staff help you feel more comfortable here in this community setting?"

Point out situations that seem to result in the client's withdrawing from the milieu.
- "Nick, I noticed that when there's too much noise you tend to leave the client areas."
- "Pam, whenever the clients get into a 'heated' discussion, you retreat to your room."
- "Joy, it seems that you find it difficult to attend group activities after a meeting with your doctor."

Problem-solve with the client the available methods to manipulate the environment or modify stress-inducing situations.
- Reduce stimuli (e.g., lower volume settings on radio, stereo, television; reduce lighting).
- Accompany the client to a less stimulating area and assign less stressful activities with fewer people.

Collaborate with physician and staff to schedule intense one-to-one interactions with the client during times that do not interfere with milieu groups and activities.

Demonstrate respect and interest in the client's desire for aloneness and isolated activities (e.g., reading, painting, listening to music or favorite radio or television program, praying), as long as the client participates in the therapeutic regimen.
- "Tod, I think it's good to enjoy such valuable interests and hobbies as long as you also participate in the treatment plan."
- "Kate, it's important to be alone occasionally; you also need to attend community meetings."
- "Kate, reading and painting in your room can be therapeutic; so are group activities and interactions."
- "Joy, your faith is important to you, and staff can help you plan your day so you will have time to pray."

Explore with the client realistic and unrealistic components of the client's perceptions about situations and events that cause him or her to withdraw.
- "Joe, you say you left because Ted seemed to criticize you. I didn't see it that way; let's discuss it with Ted."
- "Joy, your face turned red and you walked away when the group complimented you; it's OK to accept praise for a job well done."

Involve family, friends, and other support systems in the client's social activities.

This will help to illustrate healthy, effective socialization skills for the client's benefit and encouragement.

This will prevent decreasing the client's self-esteem and further withdrawal from others.

Discussing situations that may provoke the client's isolative behavior and social withdrawal will allow the client to accept painful experiences and move on with life.

Pointing out stressful situations that may provoke the client's withdrawn behavior helps prepare the client to begin to manage environmental stressors that promote isolation.

Problem solving with the client to create a less stressful environment may facilitate his or her increased participation in milieu activities and decrease isolation.

Adjusting the schedule to meet client needs may decrease the client's withdrawal from the milieu and promote participation and socialization in groups and activities.

Acknowledging and respecting the client's preferred activities, even if performed in isolation, validates the client's life choices and increases self-worth and self-esteem.

Exploring situations that impact the client in a negative way helps the client to distinguish between rational and irrational thoughts and encourages the client to begin challenging irrational ideas (see Appendix B).

This will help to strengthen the client's social network and decrease alienation and isolation.

Continued

PLANNING AND IMPLEMENTATION—cont'd

Nursing Intervention	Rationale

Isolated/Withdrawn/Avoidant—cont'd

• "Pam, your sister and brother-in-law are coming to visit you this evening; perhaps they can join the family group activity."	
Praise the client for efforts made toward contacting others, attending groups, participating in activities, and decreasing withdrawal and isolation. • "Kate, you attended all group activities this week; your participation contributed to their success." • "Sam, returning to the community meeting after talking to your doctor showed real progress."	Genuine praise for efforts by the client to minimize isolative behavior tends to reinforce continued socialization and increase self-esteem.

Abandonment Fears/Attention Seeking

Assess the frequency and intensity of the client's attempts to seek out staff for unreasonable nonurgent demands or requests.	Assessment of the client's attention-seeking behaviors helps the nurse to plan interventions that minimize abandonment fears and interrupt attention-seeking behaviors.

For the Client with Borderline or Mixed Personality Disorders with Exaggerated Fears and Dread of Abandonment

Leave the client with a symbolic or "transient" object (e.g., a note, card, or picture).	This will help bridge the gap between actual contacts with the client and relieve the intensity of the client's abandonment fears.
Assure the client that everything necessary is being done for his or her treatment and care while acknowledging concerns. • "Paul, we realize you worry about your care; staff meet regularly to discuss your treatment plan and progress."	This assurance by staff will help to relieve the client's fears of being alone, ignored, or abandoned.
Address the client's major concerns in a timely manner whenever possible.	This will help to reduce the client's attention-seeking behaviors.
Assure the client that staff are available to meet needs when necessary.	This assurance helps to reduce the client's fears of abandonment and interrupts attention-seeking behaviors.

Therapeutic Responses

• "Kate, staff are here when you need our assistance; seeking us out for things you can do yourself is not necessary." • "Paul, it's not necessary to approach the nurses' station so often; staff will be available when you need us."	These therapeutic responses by staff help to assure the client of staff availability and may help minimize attention-seeking behaviors.

Nontherapeutic Responses

"Kate, you know better than to bother the staff with unnecessary requests; we're not going to leave you." "Paul, standing in front of the nurses' station all day is very irritating to the staff. We're not going anywhere."	These nontherapeutic statements reflect a parental type of disapproval that may result in exacerbation of the client's abandonment fears and attention-seeking behaviors.
Teach strategies that help the client to cope with the feelings of urgency that accompany perceived abandonment. • Slow, deep-breathing exercises • Relaxation techniques • Count slowly to five before seeking staff • Take a brisk walk • Use visual imagery • See Appendix B	Effective stress-reducing strategies help to channel emotions toward productive activities and exercises, which distract the client from fears of abandonment and other irrational feelings.

Assist the client in a tactful way to replace perceived fears of abandonment with actual situations. • "Kate, you say you're afraid of being left alone; actually, you're seldom alone with the staff so near." • "Paul, it seems you have a real concern about being alone; in reality there's always someone close by." • "Joy, you say you're afraid your friends will leave you, yet they visit you almost every night." • "Joe, you're worried that your dad won't let you live at home when you leave here, yet he phones every day asking when you'll be able to go home."	Pointing out actual facts and situations that contradict the client's irrational perceptions helps focus the client on reality and discourage attention-seeking behaviors.
Help the client structure activities throughout the day.	A well-structured program helps to minimize the client's periods of free time and discourages attention-seeking behaviors.
Plan with the client solitary activities he or she is interested in pursuing. • Writing letters • Riding a stationary bicycle • Keeping a diary	This will help to maximize the client's periods of aloneness and reduce his or her need to seek others to fill each moment of free time.
If warranted, develop a behavioral contract with the client that sets limits on attention-seeking behaviors. • Set up a schedule with the client for times the client may approach the nurses' station. • Have the client bring problems to assigned staff person only. • Limit personal telephone calls to three per day; have client decide on times.* • Construct a list with the client that defines urgent versus nonurgent concerns for requests.	A written contract may be used as a tangible reminder that will help the client gain control over dysfunctional behavioral patterns and develop greater self-sufficiency.
Encourage the client to participate in therapeutic group activities. • Role play, sociodrama • Behavioral therapy • Cognitive-behavioral therapy • Assertiveness training • Process or focus groups • See Appendix B	Group activities help the client maximize strengths and capabilities and learn strategies for coping with abandonment fears by listening to how others cope with similar fears and anxieties.
Gently challenge the client's fears of abandonment. • "Kate, you often say you can't bear to be alone, yet you accomplish a lot during those times." • "Paul, you may think you need to be around people all the time, but you are quite capable on your own." • "Mark, you have concerns about free time, yet you do good things for yourself when you're alone."	This type of gentle challenge helps to show the client his or her actual capabilities and strengths.
With the client's permission, engage family and friends in therapeutic sessions with the client and therapist, or psychiatrist, if appropriate.	This may help to address the client's concerns about loyalty of loved ones and reduce fears of abandonment.
Consult with appropriate sources (e.g., social services, adjunctive therapists, psychiatrist) for collaborative solutions to problems.	Interdisciplinary collaboration may generate ideas that will help to minimize the client's attention-seeking behaviors and fears of abandonment.

Make sure the client agrees with limited phone calls so as not to interfere with "patient rights."

Continued

PLANNING AND IMPLEMENTATION—cont'd

Nursing Intervention	Rationale
For the Client with Borderline or Mixed Personality Disorders with Exaggerated Fears and Dread of Abandonment—cont'd	

Nursing Intervention	Rationale
Use assertive responses tactfully and consistently. • "Kate, I can't talk now; we'll talk in 45 minutes." • "Sam, I'll help you when you need it; you don't need my help to wash your clothes." • "Mark, you spoke with your doctor just a few minutes ago; we'll call her office after the 2 o'clock activity." • "Sarah, we spent a lot of time together this morning; I'll plan to spend time again with you in 2 hours. We can plan about 15 minutes talking at that time." • "Jeff, your frequent use of the telephone is interrupting your treatment; we need to set up a phone schedule."	Assertive responses used by nurses and other staff in a consistent manner help set limits on the client's occasional unreasonable demands for time and attention.
Praise the client for decreased attention-seeking behaviors and ability to cope with free time without making unreasonable demands on staff. • "Kate, staff have noticed your efforts to work out some problems on your own before you seek us out." • "Paul, it shows real progress that you don't need to approach the nurses' station so often." • "Jeff, your decreased use of the telephone is a sign of growth." • "Mark, making less demands on staff's time shows you're able to be alone successfully."	Genuine praise for the client's efforts to reduce attention-seeking behaviors and to cope successfully with free time helps reinforce repetition of positive behaviors and increase self-esteem.

Hysteria	

Nursing Intervention	Rationale
Assess the frequency and intensity of the client's melodramatic or exaggerated responses.	Assessment of the client's hysterical behaviors assists the nurse and other staff members to plan interventions that will help the client subdue his or her dramatic responses.
Assure the client that it is not necessary to resort to dramatic or exaggerated behaviors to get needs met. • "Kate, it's not necessary to respond so dramatically; staff will listen to your concerns." • "Ted, responding in such an exaggerated way isn't necessary; the doctor already agreed to give you a pass." • "Joy, staff will speak to your roommate about your concerns; there's no need to be talking in this manner."	Letting the client know his or her needs will be met without having to resort to hysterical or exaggerated behaviors will relieve his or her anxiety and reduce the incidence of hysterical responses.
Point out to the client the incongruence between the actual situation and the client's response. • "Joy, your roommate left her laundry on your bed for 5 minutes to answer the phone. Screaming that she 'abused' you is an overreaction." • "Ted, your weekend pass was granted 3 days ago; yelling that you'll 'die' if you don't get it is an exaggerated response."	Pointing out the client's unnecessary overreactions to mundane situations may help the client adapt his or her responses to match the intensity of the situation and refrain from overreacting.
Inform the client of the negative impact of his or her hysterical behavior on others. • "Kate, your responding in this manner is troubling to the other clients." • "Ted, it bothers the other clients when you respond so dramatically to simple events." • "Joy, screaming demands at the staff is distracting and won't get your needs met."	Telling the client how his or her hysterical behaviors negatively affect others may encourage the client to reduce overly dramatic responses.

Teach the client therapeutic strategies.
- Slow, deep-breathing techniques
- Relaxation exercises
- Count slowly to five before responding
- Physical exercises and activities
- See Appendix B for deep-breathing and relaxation strategies

Therapeutic strategies help channel the client's emotions toward productive physical activities and exercises, which may interrupt hysterical responses and overreactions.

Use role-play exercises in formal and informal situations.
- Create a hypothetical situation between nurse and client (formal).
- Demonstrate appropriate responses to events that occur in client areas such as dining room or lounge (informal).
- Discuss the client's feelings and perceptions after the role-play exercises.

Role-playing activities, when appropriate, help to teach the client to tone down overreactions and dramatic responses.

Engage the family and client in therapeutic group sessions with an appropriate therapist with the client's permission and physician collaboration.

Therapeutic group sessions can be an effective format for discussing the family's interaction pattern and its influence on the client's hysterical behavior (see Appendix B, Group Therapy).

Encourage the client to approach assigned staff for one-to-one interaction whenever he or she feels overwhelmed by a sense of emotional urgency.

Talking out feelings with a trusted staff person will help the client to minimize use of hysterical behaviors in the milieu.

Instruct the client in therapeutic group participation.
- Role play, sociodrama
- Behavioral therapy
- Cognitive-behavioral therapy
- Assertiveness training
- See Appendix B

Therapeutic groups can be very effective in helping clients to learn strategies to reduce hysterical, dramatic responses through the dynamics of group process and interactions among group members.

Praise the client for efforts made to reduce or eliminate hysterical, melodramatic responses.
- "Jane, your responses lately have been appropriate to the situation and show real maturity."
- "Ted, staff have said that they appreciate your efforts to react to situations without being overly dramatic."
- "Kate, the clients have commented favorably on your attempts to respond in moderation."

Genuine praise for the client's efforts to respond with more moderate tone and affect helps to increase the client's self-esteem and reinforce repetition of positive behaviors.

Seductiveness

Assess the degree and frequency of the client's seductive behaviors.

Assessing the client's seductive behaviors helps the nurse and other staff to plan interventions that interrupt and minimize the client's seductive behavior patterns.

Inform the client that staff will meet needs related to hospitalization but will not accept seductive behaviors.
- "Nick, staff are available to help you with your problems, although your suggestive behaviors will not be tolerated."
- "Pam, staff cares about your well-being, but flirting with other clients or staff is not allowed."
- "Kate, staff request that you ask your assigned staff person for help and stop seeking out male staff."

This will assure the client that his or her needs will be met, yet staff will continue to set limits on seductive or other inappropriate behaviors.

Explain to the client the negative reactions of others toward his or her seductive behaviors.
- "Nick, the other clients want you to stop your sexual advances; it makes them uncomfortable."

This will help make the client aware of the impact of seductive behaviors on others and begin to take steps to eliminate them.

Continued

PLANNING AND IMPLEMENTATION—cont'd

Nursing Intervention	Rationale
Seductiveness—cont'd	

- "Pam, your continuous flirting is annoying to the other clients, and they ask that you stop."
- "Donna, staff and clients are uncomfortable when you wear such tight clothing; we request that you stop."
- "Mark, sending seductive notes to other clients angers them and must stop."

Collaborate with staff to plan treatment strategies for the client's seductive behaviors.	Interdisciplinary collaboration helps to ensure consistency in the client's care and treatment.
Assign a staff person who can be firm about the client's seductive behaviors yet flexible enough to accept the client's vulnerabilities.	Clients with seductive behaviors need a balance of structure and discipline and acceptance and understanding. Rigid disapproval decreases self-esteem and inhibits trust.
Engage the client in therapeutic group sessions with an appropriate therapist in collaboration with the psychiatrist.	Therapeutic groups can be effective in helping the client to discuss his or her seductive behaviors and to problem solve effective management strategies by interacting with other clients.

Praise the client for positive qualities and behaviors.
- "Nick, you were a very effective client leader during the community meeting."
- "Pam, it was thoughtful of you to lend your sweater to Kate when she said she was cold."
- "Kate, your suggestions for the group activity today were very helpful."
- "Mark, sharing your visitor's time with your roommate was very considerate."

Genuine praise for the client's efforts to minimize seductive behaviors, and reach out in a sincere way to other clients helps to increase self-worth and diminish the need for seductive behaviors.

Use role play with the client in one-to-one situations, if appropriate.	Role-play can help to show the inappropriateness of seductive behaviors and teach the client mature, appropriate interpersonal skills.

Discuss the role-play exercises with the client.
Examples (nurse to client):
- "When I responded to your request with suggestive behaviors, how did you feel? Did you feel valued or devalued as a person?"
- "How did you think I reacted when you interacted with me without using a seductive approach? Was I more, or less, receptive to your actual needs?"

Discussing the role-play exercises will help elicit the client's perspective of the different behaviors and their effects on client and nurse.

Engage the client in milieu activities.

Mileu activities help the client use free time productively and refrain from using seductive behaviors to promote self-worth and meet needs.

Engage the client in therapeutic group activities.

Therapeutic group activities help build the client's self-esteem and teach him or her more mature methods of interacting with others through the dynamics of the group process.

Examples:
- Role play, sociodrama
- Behavioral therapy or cognitive therapy
- Assertiveness training or process groups
- See Appendix B.

Construct a behavioral contract, if necessary. Consequences vary according to hospital policy. Examples of contract:	A behavioral contract may help to set limits on the client's seductive behaviors and direct the client toward mature, effective interactions.
- Refrain from using seductive behaviors (e.g., flirting; teasing; suggestive statements, poses, or gestures).	

- Cease wearing tight, revealing clothing; must wear undergarments.
- Stop sending sexually provocative notes or messages to staff or other clients.

Give the client positive feedback whenever he or she refrains from seductive behaviors or ceases to wear revealing clothes.
- "Donna, staff have noticed that your choice of clothing is appropriate and not suggestive."
- "Mark, the clients are pleased that you've stopped sending seductive notes to them."
- "Kate, approaching your staff person for assistance instead of seeking out male staff shows real progress."
- "Nick, refraining from making sexual advances is a sign of growth and maturity."

Feeding back positive client behaviors helps to increase the client's self-esteem and reinforce repetition of positive, mature behaviors.

Jealousy

Assess the degree and risk for injury to the client and others as a result of the client's jealousy.

Assessing the client's jealousy toward others in the milieu helps the nurse and other staff to plan interventions that will protect the client and others from emotional or physical harm.

Protect the client and others from injury when the client loses control as a result of jealous rage (e.g., client may need to be separated from the milieu, or placed in seclusion) (see seclusion and restraint interventions in Chapter 3).

Protecting other clients and staff by removing an aggressive client from the milieu helps prevent injury to the client and others.

Evaluate situations that provoke the client's jealousy and loss of control.

This will help the nurse and other staff members to plan interventions that will assist the client to manage jealous thoughts and behaviors (whether jealousy is justified or out of proportion to the actual situation).

Encourage the client to put jealous thoughts into words.
- "Pam, you seem to become agitated each time your sister visits you. I know she's caring for your kids; let's discuss it."
- "Ted, it may be helpful to talk about your jealous thoughts with staff to clarify some points."

Assist the client to challenge unwarranted or exaggerated jealousy by helping the client separate facts from misperceptions.
- "Paul, you say your wife is out with other men every night while you're in the hospital, yet she visits you every night and works all day."
- "Sarah, you tell us how your husband flirts with the nurses when he visits you; none of the nursing staff has observed that."
- "Nick, you say staff spends more time with other clients. Let's talk about the time we spend with you."

Getting the client to openly express jealous thoughts when he or she is capable helps prevent the client's behaviors from escalating to uncontrolled rage and aggression and provides opportunities for client self-expression and understanding.

Provide activities (e.g., occupational therapy, therapeutic recreation).

Therapeutic activities help the client to vent negative feelings and increase self-worth and control, which in turn may minimize jealousy that may stem from the client's low self-concept and powerlessness.

Suggest physical outlets.
- Stationary bicycle
- Brisk walks
- Ping-Pong, volleyball, shuffleboard

Physical exercise tends to divert anger-producing energy toward productive, rewarding activities.

Discuss with the client and family (if appropriate) the situations and behaviors that provoke anger, jealousy, and rage.

Discussing anger-provoking situations with the client and family helps them to problem-solve and modify those behaviors and situations that promote jealous episodes among family members. The client's jealousy may reflect a family pattern and may require more intense family therapy after discharge.

Continued

PLANNING AND IMPLEMENTATION—cont'd

Nursing Intervention	Rationale
Jealousy—cont'd	

Nursing Intervention	Rationale
Engage the client in the milieu and group therapies. • Community meetings • Behavioral therapy • Cognitive-behavioral therapy • Assertiveness training • Role play • Relationship groups • See Appendix B	Participating in milieu activities and groups encourages the client to ventilate feelings and thoughts and to evaluate input from other clients, nurses, and adjunctive therapists that will increase the client's self-esteem and control and reduce jealousy.
Praise the client for successful management of jealous thoughts. • "Paul, it shows real progress that you haven't made any jealous accusations about your wife for a week." • "Sarah, it was good to hear you tell the group that you no longer feel jealous of the nurses when your husband comes to visit you." • "Jeff, you deserve credit for bringing your feelings of jealousy out into the open; that's the first step toward resolving them."	Genuine praise for the client's efforts to control and minimize jealous thoughts helps to build the client's self-esteem and reinforce positive behaviors.

Nursing Intervention	Rationale
Hypersexuality*	

Nursing Intervention	Rationale
Assess the extent and frequency of the client's hypersexual behavior.	Assessing a client's hypersexuality helps the nurse to plan interventions that interrupt or eliminate hypersexual behaviors.
Inform the client that staff will meet his or her needs but that hypersexual behavior will not be tolerated. • "Sam, staff wants to help you, but placing your arm around clients or touching them in a suggestive manner is not allowed here." • "Nick, we're here to assist you with your problems, but talking to others in a sexually provocative way will not be tolerated." • "Kate, staff wants to help you, but it's against hospital policy to lie in bed with another client or engage in sex; it may get you dismissed from the hospital." • "Pam, staff care about you, but kissing other clients, or anyone else here, is not acceptable."	This type of information assures the client that his or her problems will be addressed while staff will continue to set limits on disruptive, hypersexual behavior.
Construct a behavioral contract to set limits on the client's hypersexual behavior. Consequences vary according to hospital policy. • Refrain from demonstrating inappropriate sexual behaviors (e.g., hugging, kissing, touching in sexually provocative manner, lying in bed with other clients) • Cease using sexually suggestive body language, gestures, or poses. • Stop sexual, lewd dialogue or innuendo.	A written contract can be a tangible reminder that will help the client to control disruptive behavior and also teach the client appropriate, effective methods of interacting.
Engage the client in therapeutic sessions with an appropriate therapist in collaboration with the client's psychiatrist. This will give the client more opportunity to work on problems associated with hypersexual behaviors and learn to replace them with mature, effective interactions.	

Hypersexual behavior is generally more intensely manifested than seductive behaviors and may be noted in clients with mania and antisocial personality disorder. See Sexual and Gender Identity Disorders, Chapter 11, for additional information.

Point out the negative impact of the client's hypersexual behavior on other clients and staff.
- "Nick, when you use sexual language in front of others, they tend to leave the area."
- "Pam, your frequent kissing and hugging attempts are annoying to the other clients and they ask that you stop."
- "Kate, lying in bed with another client was upsetting to everyone and cannot be repeated or you may be dismissed from the hospital."

Pointing out the negative consequences of the client's hypersexuality on others helps show the client the disruptive effects the behavior has on the milieu and encourages the client to reduce or eliminate the behaviors.

Collaborate with staff to ensure consistent management of the client's hypersexual behaviors.

Clients with long-standing inappropriate behaviors require consistent treatment strategies.

Assign a staff person who can be firm about the client's hypersexual behavior, not intimidated by it, and flexible enough to address problem areas without negating the client.

Clients with hypersexual behavior patterns require firm control and direction yet also need acceptance to preserve their feelings of self-worth.

Praise the client for positive qualities and behaviors.
- "Kate, showing the new client around the unit was very considerate."
- "Nick, offering your place at the card game to Joe was generous."
- "Pam, it was nice of you to take notes at the community meeting."

Genuine praise for client efforts to modify negative behaviors and use more mature approaches increases self-esteem and diminishes the need for hypersexual behaviors.

Encourage the client to participate in physical activities.
- Aerobic exercises (unless contraindicated)
- Brisk walks
- Stationary bicycle
- Jump rope
- Volleyball, Ping-Pong

Physical exercise helps direct sexual energy toward productive activities and may reduce the incidence of hypersexual behaviors.

Engage the client in therapeutic group activities.
- Behavioral therapy
- Cognitive-behavioral therapy
- Assertiveness training
- Group therapy
- Role play
- See Appendix B

Participating in therapeutic activities and group process helps build the client's self-esteem and enables the client to learn mature, effective methods of interacting without resorting to hypersexual behaviors.

Give the client positive feedback whenever he or she refrains from using hypersexual behaviors.
- "Nick, staff have noticed that you no longer use sexual terms when you interact with others."
- "Kate, you've made real progress; your behaviors are mature and appropriate."
- "Pam, the other clients say they enjoy being around you since you've stopped trying to kiss them."
- "Sam, refraining from touching and hugging other clients shows growth and maturity."

Positive feedback for the client's use of positive behaviors helps to build self-esteem and reinforce repetition of mature, positive behaviors.

Rigid and Perfectionistic Behaviors

Assess the frequency of the client's inability to complete tasks or projects owing to concerns that the task performance or finished product will be imperfect or substandard.

Assessing the client's perfectionism will help the nurse and staff plan interventions that will help the client complete tasks.

Assess the extent of the client's preoccupation with details that tend to hinder his or her job performance.

This will help the nurse and other staff determine the level of rigidity and perfectionism that inhibit the client's task completion.

Continued

PLANNING AND IMPLEMENTATION—cont'd

Nursing Intervention	Rationale
Rigid and Perfectionistic Behaviors—cont'd	

Nursing Intervention	Rationale
Assess the degree of the client's rigid preoccupation with values, ethics, and morals.	This will help the nurse and other staff determine the possible source of task incompletion or substandard performance.
Assure the client that completion of a task, project, or activity is more valued than the quality of the product or performance. • "Pam, it's more important to finish the volleyball game than to win it; your participation is needed for that." • "Joy, the art therapist is not concerned with artistic ability; your interpretation of the completed drawing is valued."	Letting the client know his or her work is valued for its own sake will help reduce the client's fear of imperfection and encourage task completion.
Assist the client to set limits on rigid preoccupation with values, ethics, and morals. • "Ted, staff agree that it's appropriate to spend 15 minutes each shift on your spiritual beliefs and the remainder of the time on completing assigned projects." • "Kate, it's acceptable to take 10 minutes each shift to discuss your ethical views with your staff person. The rest of the time needs to be spent on therapeutic activities."	Setting limits with the client on rigid, perfectionistic behaviors helps the client to make time for task performance and completion.
Construct a written behavioral contract for task completion, if warranted.	A written contract provides the client with a tangible reminder of the amount of time required for task performance and completion.
Assign the client one task or project at a time to be completed within a specific time frame. • "Pam, your job is to collect each person's contribution to the collage, including your own, by 2 PM next Monday." • "Nick, your assignment is to read the first section in the cognitive therapy book by Friday at 10 AM" • "Joy, you're expected to be up and dressed by 8 AM every morning. Tomorrow we'll discuss other responsibilities." • "Mark, this week you'll be responsible for cleaning and tidying up your room. Next week you can begin to do your laundry."	A client with rigid, perfectionistic qualities generally prefers to complete an assignment to the best of his or her ability before moving on to the next project. Time constraints are necessary to minimize the client's preoccupation with details and promote task completion
Engage the client in group activities in which each person's contribution is required for the task or project to reach completion. • Community jigsaw puzzle • Preparing food for picnic or barbecue • Development of collage or poster • Sing-along session	Being part of a group in which each member is expected to contribute a task for the project to reach completion may encourage the client's successful performance through the dynamics of the group process.
Encourage the client to attend structured groups. • Role play, sociodrama • Behavioral therapy • Cognitive-behavioral therapy • Assertiveness training • Process or focus groups • See Appendix B	Therapeutic groups may assist the client to develop an awareness of rigid, perfectionistic behaviors and may offer strategies that will help the client overcome the constraints they place on task performance and completion.
Engage the client and family in therapeutic sessions with an appropriate family therapist in collaboration with the client's psychiatrist and with the client's permission.	This will help identify rigid and perfectionistic interactions within the family that inhibit the client's ability to complete tasks and to suggest alternate methods for enhancing performance and project completion.

Encourage the client to select activities, tasks, and projects that he or she chooses to perform and complete.

Praise successful completion of assigned tasks, projects, or activities.
- "Pam, you successfully completed your job of collecting the collage contributions from the clients on time."
- "Nick, you were well prepared for group Friday morning after reading your cognitive therapy assignment."
- "Joy, staff noticed you were dressed and ready for the day by 8 AM every day for 1 week."

Refer to Impaired Social Interaction Care Plan in Chapter 2 for additional interventions for clients whose preoccupation with details or rituals are the result of an obsessive-compulsive disorder.

Having choice and control over selected tasks and projects may help the client accept responsibility for completing tasks and projects.

Genuine praise for the client's efforts to complete tasks and for actual project completion helps reinforce repetition of positive behaviors; minimize rigid, perfectionistic qualities; and enhance the client's self-esteem.

Care Plan
DSM-IV-TR Diagnosis **Diagnosis: Personality Disorders (All Types)**

NANDA Diagnosis: Ineffective Coping
Inability to form a valid appraisal of stressors; inadequate choices of practiced responses; inability to use available resources.

Focus:
For the client whose behavior patterns or personality traits result in significant impairment in coping with personal, social, or occupational demands or stressors. The defining characteristics are generally typical of the person's long-term functioning and are not limited to isolated episodes of illness.

RELATED FACTORS (ETIOLOGY)

Depletion of coping methods/resources
Disturbance in self-concept/low self-esteem
Low impulse control
Ineffective or absent support systems
Ineffective problem-solving skills
Lack of insight/judgment
Knowledge deficit regarding societal rules, norms, and
     interactions
Fear of abandonment/isolation
Perceived self-victimization
Self-involvement
Life-style of dependence
Developmental conflicts
Psychosocial stressors

DEFINING CHARACTERISTICS
Splitting

Splitting is a hallmark defense mechanism of individuals
     diagnosed with borderline personality disorder.

Splitting is defined as seeing the world in terms of black or
     white. The individual often views others as either all
     good or all bad, which can change for no obvious
     reason.
The client expresses conflicting alternate responses of
     acceptance and rejection at different times toward
     individuals or groups.
- During a morning session with her psychiatrist, Kate tells
     the physician she "loves" his approach. Later that
     afternoon, Kate vents her rage at her physician's
     "incompetence."
Demonstrates routine use of "splitting" statements.
- "I like you so much better than all the other nurses. You're
     so understanding, and they don't seem to care at all."
- "You're the only staff person here who really notices me.
     No one else will even talk to me."
- "I hate the day staff; the nurses are so bossy and cold.
     The evening people are much nicer and friendlier."
- "I thought you were my friend, but now I see the only one
     I can really count on is my roommate."
- "I'm so mad at my roommate I could scream. She was so
     much nicer when we first met. I guess you're my best
     friend now."
- "Don't you dare tell the staff about my wish to die. I don't
     trust anyone but you."

Idealizes

The client exaggerates others' attributes and capabilities.
- "You're so wonderful. I just adore your personality. You're
     nicer than anyone I've ever known."
- "I love the way you deal with clients. I want to be exactly
     like you someday."
- "I just admire Kate so much. She's more like a nurse than
     a client. She's so helpful to me."

Continued

- "My life was in complete ruin until I found Dr. Smith. He's a god to me."

Devalues

The client demeans and degrades others; typically follows idealization (see "Kate" example under Splitting).

- "I'm afraid to tell anyone here how I feel. They'll all turn against me."
- "I'm sure that whatever I say here will be used against me."
- "You're the worst nurse I ever saw. How did you ever get a job in a psychiatric hospital?"
- "You don't know the first thing about helping people; I feel sorry for all your clients."
- "If you tell anyone about my suicidal thoughts, I'll always think of you as a dirty traitor who can't be trusted."

Manipulation

The client manipulates others and the environment to meet own needs.

- "You're the sweetest nurse in the whole world. I know you'll help me get a weekend pass."
- "If you'll just watch out for the staff while I stay in my girlfriend's room, I'll do your laundry for a week."
- "Couldn't you spare me one of your cigarettes? After all, I defended you when Joy complained about you to the other clients."
- "Since you were sick yesterday and didn't work, do you think we could have more time to talk today?"
- "If I can't be client leader I'll just have to leave this place and go where I'm wanted."

Intense/Unstable Relationships

The client expresses intense, extremely emotional responses toward interpersonal relationships.

- "The relationship between me and my boyfriend is so exciting. We're either hugging or kissing or yelling and screaming at each other."
- "My girlfriend and I can be completely in love one minute, then we're tearing each other apart. It's maddening but never dull."
- "My roommate and I fight constantly, but we really love each other to death."

Boredom

The client verbalizes feelings of boredom frequently.

- "I can't stand this place. There's nothing to do here."
- "There's nothing in this hospital that interests me; the staff, the clients, and the activities are all boring."
- "If I don't find something exciting to do in this place very soon, I'm really going to go crazy."
- "If I have to attend craft group one more time, I'll scream."

Demonstrates bored behaviors (rule out depression).

- Displays frequent sighing or yawning during group activities.

- Demonstrates disinterested facial expressions throughout meetings.
- Leaves room in middle of group function or activity for no apparent reason.

Restricted Affect/Humor

The client demonstrates lack of humor and restricted range of emotions, which the client may view as normal *(ego-syntonic)*.

- "I'm glad I can remain unemotional about my problems."
- "It's just not in me to express my feelings."
- "I see nothing funny about these jokes that all the other clients were laughing about."

Remains aloof and detached during situations that normally warrant strong emotional responses (e.g., joy, sadness).

Displays indifference or disinterest toward the praise or criticism of others (blunted affect, no eye contact).

OUTCOME IDENTIFICATION AND EVALUATION

Splitting

The client expresses consistent responses toward groups and individuals rather than the conflicting "splitting" responses of acceptance and rejection.

- Interacts with others as if they are multifaceted rather than either "all good" or "all bad."
- Demonstrates significant reduction in extreme, alternate responses toward groups or individuals.

Idealizes

The client refrains from idealizing or exaggerating others' attributes or capabilities.

Expresses more realistic view of the qualities of others.

- "I don't always agree with my doctor, but she has always been there to help me."
- "My roommate gives some good advice, but she's also a client with her own problems."
- "You're a caring nurse and I appreciate that, even if I don't always agree with you."

Devalues

The client ceases to devalue, degrade, or demean others.

- "Now that I've had a chance to think about it, I don't believe my roommate is a 'dirty traitor' for telling the staff I was suicidal."

Resists making rude, cruel, or derogatory statements directed toward others.

Responds in a mature manner.

- "I'm very upset with my doctor for not issuing my pass as he promised, but I'll deal with it."
- "I'm angry at you right now for not keeping our appointment. Let's talk about it."
- "After being here a while, I feel that the staff mean well and can be trusted."

Manipulation

The client refrains from use of manipulation to have needs met.
- Makes requests clearly and openly without apparent hidden messages.
- Ceases to use covert bribes or threats when interacting with others.

Demonstrates significant reduction in manipulative behaviors as a way to meet needs.
- Engages in mature, open interpersonal interactions.
- Expresses needs directly without apparent ulterior motives or agenda.

Exhibits appropriate verbal and behavioral expressions.

Intense/Unstable Relationships

The client expresses feelings toward relationships in realistic, moderate terms, with absence of intense, volatile emotions.
- "My boyfriend and I no longer scream at each other one moment and kiss and make up the next."
- "My girlfriend and I have a much more calm and stable relationship now."
- "My husband and I have our ups and downs, but they are not as emotionally charged as they used to be."

Demonstrates calm, consistent emotions when interacting with others.

Boredom

The client verbalizes increased feelings of interest and excitement toward milieu groups and activities.
- "I really get a lot out of the groups and activities."
- "There's always something to do during our free time, like riding the stationary bicycle or listening to a relaxation tape."

Demonstrates increased interest in scheduled groups, activities, and individuals.
- Participates in milieu activities without signs of boredom (e.g., frequent sighing, yawning, sleeping).
- Displays brightened or animated facial expression while engaged in groups and activities.
- Initiates interactions with staff and clients frequently rather than avoiding social contact.

Restricted Affect/Humor

The client demonstrates a wide range of emotional responses, from joy to sadness.

Expresses heightened interest and emotions toward others' praise and criticism (e.g., animated affect, eye contact, increased feeling in voice tone).
- "I'm interested in what others think about me, even though it's hard to take negative comments."
- "Thank you for the compliment. It's important to me."
- "I'm not happy about being criticized. In fact, it's upsetting."

Displays increased humor in appropriately humorous situations.
- "The jokes that Jeff told during lunch were funny."
- "I laughed at Kate's stories with the other clients."

PLANNING AND IMPLEMENTATION

Nursing Intervention	Rationale
Splitting	
Assess the degree and frequency of the client's attempts to divide others through the defense mechanism of splitting.	A thorough assessment helps to determine the extent of the client's dysfunctional behaviors and assists in planning appropriate interventions to counteract the splitting.
Using feedback with the client in a nonaggressive manner helps share observations that challenge the client's perceptions that individuals or groups are either "all good" or "all bad."	Observational challenges help correct the client's distortions and reduce the incidence of splitting.

Therapeutic Responses
- "Donna, you say the evening staff treats you badly, but just last week you said good things about them."
- "Ted, you're angry at me now, but this morning you said our discussion really helped you."
- "Pam, you get really upset with your assigned staff nurse when she's with other clients. At other times, though, you can't wait to talk to her."
- "Kate, you say no one else here cares about you as I do. What has the staff done to show they care?"
- "Kate, you seem angry with your doctor now, yet at other times you say she helps you a lot."
- "Ted, you're asking me not to tell anyone else about your suicidal feelings because you don't trust them. But each

Therapeutic responses point out client behaviors and situations that factually challenge the client's distorted perceptions. This type of consistent feedback by the treatment team can reduce splitting behaviors and prompt the client to use more functional methods to have needs met.

Continued

PLANNING AND IMPLEMENTATION—cont'd

Nursing Intervention	Rationale

Splitting—cont'd

staff member is here to help you, so we all need to be aware of your feelings."

Nontherapeutic Responses

"Donna, how can you say the evening staff treats you badly when they gave you a birthday party last week?"

"Ted, what did I do to make you so angry? You seemed OK during our discussion earlier."

"Kate, you know your doctor means well. She would be hurt if she knew how upset you are."

Nontherapeutic responses defend against the client's accusations and place the nurse and staff in a vulnerable position. Such responses fail to point out behaviors that would challenge the client's splitting attempts.

Develop a contract with the client stating that the client will approach only his or her assigned staff nurse on each shift for requests and questions.

- "Donna, you said Kim told you it was OK to have a cigarette now. That's my role as your staff person, and you'll have to wait 10 minutes when we go to the patio as a group."
- "Mark, asking me to phone your doctor at home to order a pass for you for tomorrow needs to be discussed with Sally, your staff person."

A written contract acts as a tangible reminder of expected behaviors and discourages the client from splitting staff to have needs met.

Assist the client to redirect angry or ambivalent feelings through constructive activities: physical exercise, art/music therapy, relaxation techniques (see Appendix B).

Therapeutic activities help the client release negative energy and reduce stress and frustration in a socially acceptable way.

Assist the client to take responsibility for having needs met.

- "Kate, you say the staff isn't meeting your needs. What do you think we could do that would meet your needs?"
- "Joy, how can you work with the staff to best meet your needs?"

Open-ended questioning by staff places expectations for care on the client and discourages the client from splitting the staff.

For the client ready to confront the source of the problem, assist the client to recognize the benefits of refraining from splitting to have needs met.

- "Donna, understanding that nobody can please everyone all the time will greatly improve your relationships with others."
- "Mark, the knowledge that most people are not either all good or all bad is helpful in your interactions and important to your recovery."

Nonaggressive confrontation by staff encourages mature, functional responses by the client.

Engage the client in progressive, nonthreatening situations in which the client can practice mature, effective responses without splitting. Begin with one-to-one nurse-client interactions; gradually include one or two trusted clients; proceed to an informal group setting (dining room); progress to a more structured group (community meeting); and finally, engage client in a formal group discussion.

Exposing the client gradually to social situations in a simple-to-complex manner helps the client develop mastery of effective responses and gradually reduces splitting behaviors.

Encourage the client to keep a record of times when he or she used mature, effective responses versus ineffective splitting responses.

This exercise helps the client compare and contrast the different effects of the two types of responses on others and promotes continued use of mature, effective responses.

Praise the client for attempts to reduce splitting responses and to use mature, effective communication.

- "Donna, staff and clients have noticed your efforts to communicate in a responsible way."
- "Mark, clients and staff said they appreciate your hard work in changing your method of interaction."

Positive reinforcement promotes repetition of effective responses and increases self-esteem.

Idealizes	
Challenge the client's idealistic views, which are a component of splitting, with realistic responses.	Nonaggressively challenging idealization helps to correct the client's unrealistic, exaggerated perception, substituting a more realistic assessment.

Therapeutic Responses

- "Donna, you say I'm better than all the other nurses, but good nursing care is the goal for all of us."
- "Joy, your doctor isn't a 'god,' but it's clear that you're satisfied with his care."
- "Joy, I know you often go to your roommate for advice, but she's also a client and needs help from the staff as you do."

Therapeutic responses effectively contradict the client's idealization and weaken the attempt to split staff and others.

Nontherapeutic Responses

"Donna, thanks for the compliment, but the other nurses try hard, too."

"Joy, lots of clients think of their doctors as 'gods.'"

"Joy, it's good that you admire your roommate so much, as long as you realize she doesn't know everything."

Nontherapeutic responses encourage the client's idealistic views and fail to correct the distortion or challenge the splitting behaviors.

Engage the client in therapeutic groups, including role play/sociodrama, behavioral-cognitive therapy, assertiveness training, and process/focus groups (see Appendix B).

Therapeutic groups help the client explore splitting behaviors and their effects on self and others through the dynamics of the group process and feedback from other clients and group leaders.

Devalues	
Use firm directives to set limits on the client's attempts to devalue persons or groups, another component of the client's splitting behavior.	Firm limit setting may be necessary to stop the client's verbal attacks toward staff or other clients who need protection from verbal assaults.

Therapeutic Responses

- "Pam, your angry words directed toward others are not appropriate and won't be tolerated."
- "Joy, you cannot remain in group if you curse and accuse people."

These therapeutic responses firmly set limits on the client's inappropriate, angry accusations and challenge the devaluation component of the splitting behavior.

Nontherapeutic Responses

"Bob, what makes you think your doctor is a pompous fool?"

"Mark, how dare you say I'm a bad nurse after all I've done for you?"

These nontherapeutic responses defend against the client's accusatory remarks and place the nurse in a vulnerable position. The responses fail to clarify consequences for the client's unacceptable behavior.

Manipulates	
Assess the extent and frequency of the client's manipulative behaviors.	A comprehensive assessment helps the nurse and treatment team to recognize situations that provoke a client's manipulation and to plan interventions to reduce manipulative behaviors.

Direct attention to the client's manipulative behavior.

Therapeutic Responses

- "Mark, when you give me all those compliments, you usually want something from me."
- "Bob, what makes you think I can give you extra attention today because I was out sick yesterday?"
- "Sam, asking Jeff to 'watch out' for staff while you sneak your girlfriend into your room is taking advantage of Jeff."

Focusing on manipulative behaviors helps the client develop an awareness of his or her manipulation and begin to take steps to reduce such behavior.

Continued

PLANNING AND IMPLEMENTATION—cont'd

Nursing Intervention	Rationale
Manipulates—cont'd	

Explore the consequences of manipulative behavior with the client. • "Mark, when you compliment people because you want something from them, they are not likely to trust what you say." • "Bob, when you say I owe you extra time because I was out sick yesterday, it annoys me." • "Sam, asking Jeff to 'watch out' for staff while you sneak your girlfriend into your room would cause trouble for all of you."	Informing the client about the negative effects of his or her manipulative behaviors on others helps prompt the client to use a more genuine approach to meet needs.
Assist the client to mobilize feelings of anxiety, when appropriate. • "Sam, what feelings do you experience when you realize your behavior can seriously harm your friendship with Jeff?" • "Mark, when people no longer believe your compliments, how does that make you feel?"	Individuals with long-standing use of manipulative behaviors generally fail to experience anxiety. Activating anxiety can help the client to anticipate the threat of consequences of manipulative behaviors and eventually learn to control them.
Refrain from responding to the client's manipulative behaviors, such as self-pity, flattery, sexual innuendo, risqué jokes, and use of vulgar language.	Negative reinforcement of inappropriate behaviors reduces the chances that the client will repeat manipulative approaches to others.
Assist the client to clarify his or her needs when the client uses manipulation. • "Pam, when you say Kate owes you a favor because you defended her in group, what do you really need from Kate?" • "Ted, you use a lot of flattering remarks with your staff persons. What do you actually expect from them?"	Needs clarification helps the staff and the client to determine what needs the client is trying to meet through manipulative methods.
Assure the client that his or her needs will be met without resorting to manipulative behaviors. • "Kate, staff will spend an appropriate amount of time with you when you need it. It's not necessary to threaten to leave the hospital." • "Paul, when you have a request, the best way to get results is to ask your assigned staff person directly, rather than telling everyone you're being ignored."	Assuring the client that needs will be met as part of the therapeutic regimen can reduce the client's use of manipulative behaviors.
Refrain from being judgmental while the client examines his or her manipulative behavior.	A nonjudgmental approach demonstrates staff confidence in the client's attempts to recognize, reduce, and eventually eliminate manipulative behavior.
Engage the client in therapeutic and didactic group activities: milieu therapy, behavioral-cognitive therapy, process/focus groups, assertiveness training (see Appendix B).	Therapeutic groups and activities teach the client more effective, socially appropriate methods of interacting with others.
Set limits on the client's manipulative behaviors when it interferes with the client's progress and the rights and safety of others. • "Jeff, telling vulgar stories to get others to pay attention to you is not appropriate and will not be tolerated." • "Donna, your frequent complaints about staff to the other clients are not helping you or them. From now on, direct all your comments to staff."	Setting limits when necessary helps the client to control dysfunctional behaviors and recognize that there are consequences for breaking rules.

Construct a behavioral contract consistent with the client's capability.

A written contract is a tangible reminder that may help the client to set limits on manipulative behaviors when other methods fail.

Document the client's methods of manipulation and effective nursing strategies.

Effective documentation ensures consistent interventions among staff members and can yield more positive client outcomes.

Demonstrate consistency in limit setting and following through with nursing strategies.

Inconsistency places the nurse in a vulnerable position and encourages manipulative behavior.

Express your willingness to admit your errors to the client.
- "Kate, I did forget that you signed up for the field trip. I'm glad you reminded me."
- "Donna, I'm sorry I'm late for our meeting. I'll do my best to give you the time you need."

Clients who use manipulative methods are quick to recognize others' mistakes and will use them to gain control of a situation or interpersonal relationship. On the other hand, clients tend to respect staff who can admit a genuine mistake.

Assist the client to identify when needs are actually met and situations in which the client is treated with respect and dignity.
- "Sarah, you got to go on the field trip after all without having to use unpleasant words or behaviors."
- "Bob, your staff person spent some extra time with you today, and you requested it politely."

Identifying with the client when needs are met in a dignified way helps the client recognize that needs can be met while he or she engages in appropriate interpersonal interactions.

Relate staff's expectations of the client's behavior in a clear, direct manner.

Clearly discussing staff expectations prevents the client from claiming "misunderstanding" as an excuse to manipulate and role models direct communication.

Teach the client strategies to delay need gratification.
- The client uses relaxation techniques.
- Counts to five slowly.
- Thinks about consequences of behavior.
- Discusses alternative behaviors with staff (see Appendix B).

These simple strategies provide time for the client to problem-solve a method of interaction rather than automatically respond in a manipulative manner to meet his or her needs.

Engage the client in the treatment planning process.
- "Paul, how do you think *we* can help meet your needs?"
- "Sarah, what do you feel is most helpful for you here?"
- "Kate, what can *you* do to meet your needs?"

Including the client in the treatment plan increases motivation, participation, and self-esteem, which will diminish the need for manipulation.

Provide mature role modeling in interactions with the client and others.
- Demonstrate respect and consideration toward others (see Therapeutic Nurse-Client Relationship, Chapter 1.)
- Use assertive behaviors such as "I" messages, eye contact, and consistent verbal/facial expressions (see Appendix B).

Role modeling mature, effective interactions teaches the client socially acceptable behaviors that yield positive results and helps the client use effective behaviors rather than manipulative methods.

Assist the client to perceive manipulative behavior and its results realistically.
- "Joy, when you say things to make people feel sorry for you, they see you as a victim. How do you *really* want to be treated by others?"
- "Jeff, when you tell vulgar jokes, ask yourself if you get the response and respect from others that you really want."

Pointing out the negative effects experienced by the client when he or she uses manipulation helps the client recognize that manipulative behavior is not satisfying and can be self-defeating.

Explore with the client the problems in interpersonal relationships that develop as a result of manipulative behavior.
- "Jeff, the other clients are avoiding you because your vulgar jokes offend them. What can you do to improve your relationship with them?"

Exploring social problems caused by manipulating others helps to reinforce the client's awareness of manipulative behavior, especially if the client has difficulty learning from experience.

Continued

PLANNING AND IMPLEMENTATION—cont'd

Nursing Intervention	Rationale

Manipulates—cont'd

- "Donna, the staff wants to meet your needs. But it's difficult to know if we do when you say we avoid you. How can we improve communication?"

Discuss with the client alternative ways of relating to others that do not include flattery, intimidation, and invoking guilt.

- "Bob, when you want a favor from me, ask me directly. Say, 'I need a favor,' rather than tell me the reasons why you think I owe you a favor. I'd be more likely to agree because the approach is honest and doesn't make me feel guilty."
- "Joy, it's easier to tell the other clients the reasons why you would make a good client leader than to flatter them with compliments and gifts. People resent it when they feel forced to do something and are likely not to vote for you."

Giving actual examples of more effective ways to ask for help and comparing them with the client's usual manipulative method teach the client that clear, direct, assertive methods of interacting yield positive results and improve interpersonal relationships.

Spend time with the client when he or she is not using manipulative methods to be noticed.

The client sees that needs can be met through socially acceptable behaviors.

Engage the client in a group setting that helps individuals who manipulate to confront one another through role play or sociodrama.

Group interactions and feedback foster the client's awareness of the negative effects of manipulation on self and others.

Include family in therapeutic counseling sessions (see Appendix B).

Family therapy teaches family members strategies that disrupt the client's manipulative behaviors and promote cooperation in treatment planning.

Praise the client for behaviors that are free from manipulative methods and that indicate consideration and respect for others.

- "Donna, asking me to spend more time with you without telling me why I should shows real progress in communication."
- "John, staff noticed that you no longer tell vulgar stories to gain attention. It is much more pleasant to spend time with you."
- "Pam, it's a positive sign that you've stopped giving compliments when you want something. We have all noticed your new behavior."

Behaviors that are positively reinforced by staff are likely to be repeated by the client.

Praise the client's continued use of mature behavior and social skills.

- "Jeff, you're dealing with your new role as client leader with more confidence."
- "Sarah, your relationships with other clients show caring and consideration."
- "Donna, your communication with staff is clear and honest and reflects growth."

Genuine praise by staff increases the client's self-esteem and personal growth and reinforces positive behaviors.

Provide situations in which the client takes responsibility for choices and decisions to reduce dependency on others to satisfy needs and to learn to be self-reliant rather than manipulate others to gain support and acceptance.

- "Jeff, as client leader, *you* are responsible for getting the other clients together to choose the activity for tonight."
- "Paul, you have several alternative places to live when you leave here. The final decision is *yours*."
- "Kate, whatever *you* choose to make for the cooking session will be OK with the group."

Providing real opportunities for the client to take responsibility for choosing *not* to use manipulative behaviors indicates to the client that staff is ready to trust the client to make the decision to meet needs in a direct, mature manner, which encourages the client to succeed.

Intense/Unstable Relationships	
Assess the intensity and frequency of the client's emotional expressions.	Assessment helps the nurse plan interventions that will help the client modify intense responses.
Share observations of the client's intense responses through feedback regarding his or her interpersonal relationships.	

Therapeutic Responses

• "Sarah, one minute you tell me how much you love your boyfriend, and the next minute you're ready to kill him." • "Donna, you say you adore your roommate, but you also say you fight with her all the time."	These therapeutic responses illustrate genuine feedback on the client's unstable relationships that helps the client develop an awareness of his or her extreme emotional expression and how inappropriate it appears to others.

Nontherapeutic Responses

"Sarah, how can you say you love someone and then feel as though you want to kill him?" "Donna, it's impossible for you to adore someone that you fight with all the time."	These nontherapeutic responses negate the client's feelings and invoke doubts that the client is capable of love.
Nonaggressively challenge the client's perception that extremes of feelings and emotions are necessary components in a relationship. • "Bob, what makes it necessary for you and your wife to react so intensely when expressing your feelings to each other?" • "Mark, how come you and your girlfriend find it necessary to express such intense emotions in your relationship?" • "Sarah, what do you think your relationship with your boyfriend would be like without the extremes of emotions?"	Challenging the client's erroneous perceptions in a matter-of-fact way helps to show the client that relationships can survive without the drama of intense, extreme responses.
Assist the client to recognize that extreme emotional responses can be more harmful than beneficial to a relationship. • "Sarah, when you and your boyfriend react to each other with such intense emotions, it's likely to put a strain on your relationship." • "Donna, the extreme emotions that you and your roommate express to each other may be stressful to your relationship."	Recognizing extreme responses helps the client understand that dramatic, volatile emotions can foster instability in a relationship and can prompt the client to evaluate the relationship differently.
Teach the client strategies to increase the time span between the stimulus and the client's response. • The client practices slow, deep breathing. • Uses relaxation techniques (see Appendix B). • Counts to five slowly. • Engages in physical exercises and activities.	These strategies give the client time and opportunity to choose an alternative, less volatile response and thus reduce the incidence of sudden intense emotional expressions by the client.
Engage the client and his or her partner in appropriate therapeutic counseling sessions as recommended.	Therapeutic counseling provides opportunities for the client and partner to discuss intense emotional responses, their effects on the relationship, and methods to modify or control them in a safe setting.
Praise the client and his or her partner for attempts to control excessive emotional responses. • "Donna, you and your roommate have modified your extreme responses to each other very well. The improvement in your relationship is evident." • "Bob, it's obvious that you and your wife are really working on reducing your intense emotional responses."	Positive reinforcement increases self-esteem and promotes repetition of appropriate responses.

Continued

PLANNING AND IMPLEMENTATION—cont'd

Nursing Intervention	Rationale
Intense/Unstable Relationships—cont'd	
Act as a role model by responding to colleagues and clients within a socially appropriate emotional range.	Role modeling teaches the client socially appropriate emotional expressions and discourages the use of extreme, intense responses.
Relate to the client the benefits of responding within a socially appropriate emotional range. • "Bob, you say you and your wife have never been happier. The change in your responses to each other has improved your relationship." • "Donna, it's good to see you and your roommate getting along so well. The work you've been doing to modify your emotional reactions has helped your relationship."	Discussing the benefits of acceptable emotional behaviors helps to reinforce the client's socially appropriate emotional responses.
Engage the client in therapeutic and didactic groups such as role play/sociodrama, behavioral-cognitive therapy, assertiveness training, process/focus groups (see Appendix B).	Therapeutic group involvement teaches the client how to modify extreme emotional responses through group dynamics and using feedback from other clients and group leaders.
Boredom	
Assess the degree and frequency of the client's boredom.	Assessment assists the nurse to plan interventions that will interrupt periods of boredom.
Assure the client that occasional feelings of boredom are natural and acceptable. • "Pam, it's OK to be bored once in a while." • "Nick, being in a hospital can occasionally be boring."	Assuring the client that occasionally being bored is a natural reaction for everyone validates the client's feelings.
Engage the client in therapeutic activities: physical exercise, recreational activities (e.g., Ping-Pong, volleyball, shuffleboard), arts/crafts, board games, field trips/outings.	Therapeutic activities offer quick, productive rewards that interrupt excessive moments of boredom and release pent-up emotions underlying "bored" behaviors.
Provide the client with a variety of activities.	Variety promotes interest in the milieu and discourages boredom. The greater the selection of activities, the more likely the client is to participate.
Share observations of the client's demonstration of boredom using appropriate feedback. • "Jeff, you often make the comment that you're 'bored.' Are you aware of that?" • "Joy, you frequently fall asleep during the community meeting." • "Kate, you often leave before the activity is over." • "Pam, I notice you seldom participate in the group functions."	Genuine feedback regarding the client's responses, when warranted, helps the client develop an awareness of the client's frequent use of "bored" behaviors.
Assist the client to recognize the feeling state that accompanies expressions of boredom. • "Jeff, when you say you're 'bored,' what feelings are you experiencing?" • "Joy, just before you fall asleep in group, how do you feel about what's happening?" • "Kate, how do you feel as you leave a group activity before it's over?" • "Pam, what do you feel when you sit quietly while the rest of the group participates?"	Recognizing the actual feeling state that may be at the root of boredom helps the client identify the true source of bored behavior.

For the client with difficulty identifying feelings *(alexithymia)*, help the client name the feeling that accompanies expressions of boredom.

- "Kate, when you leave in the middle of a meeting, are you feeling anxious or fearful?"
- "Joy, do you feel frustrated or angry just before you fall asleep in group?"
- "Pam, could it be that you're not participating in group because you're feeling fearful or anxious?"
- "Jeff, when you say you're 'bored,' might you be feeling angry or frustrated?"

Labeling the actual feeling is the first step toward understanding the emotions underlying "bored" behaviors.
Boredom is often a way to deny other feelings.

For the client who is ready, explore the possible threats that provoke feelings underlying "bored" behaviors.

- "Kate, what is it about the group process that you find threatening or scary?"
- "Jeff, what causes you to feel frustrated?"
- "Joy, you said you felt angry when you fell asleep during the group. Let's discuss what makes you feel angry enough to fall asleep during the activities."
- "Pam, it may help to talk about the anxiety that prevents you from joining the group."

Exploring threatening feelings that may be hidden beneath the client's boredom helps the client begin to acknowledge these feelings.

Engage the client in therapeutic groups, such as role play/sociodrama, cognitive-behavioral therapy, assertiveness training, process/focus groups (see Appendix B).

The dynamics and interactions of group activities help the client further explore the threats that promote "bored" behaviors.

Assist the client to confront threatening feelings or situations that result in the use of bored behaviors.

- "Joy, let's talk about the possible reasons for your anger during the group. The group can help you with this."
- "Kate, you say you leave meetings because you're afraid to share your feelings. The group would accept that."
- "Pam, the anxiety you feel about performing in groups is understandable and can be dealt with."
- "Pam, playing Bingo may not be as exciting as other activities, but being part of the client community is therapeutic."
- "Jeff, there are more entertaining events than walking around the lake, but interacting with one another during the activity is important."

Confronting threatening feelings and situations helps the client challenge his or her perception of the threat, which may reduce the client's view of the threat.

Praise the client for refraining from use of bored behaviors and for expressing actual feelings.

- "Jeff, you haven't mentioned being bored for several days. It's a real sign of progress that you're discussing your feelings."
- "Joy, the staff and clients have noticed that you stay awake during the meetings and talk about your frustrations."
- "Kate, talking about your fears rather than ignoring the group is a step forward in your recovery."
- "Kate, we've noticed that you stay until the end of the meetings. Discussing your anxiety with the group has helped."

Positive reinforcement promotes continuity of effective behaviors and increases the client's confidence and self-esteem.

Continued

PLANNING AND IMPLEMENTATION—cont'd

Nursing Intervention	Rationale

Restricted Affect/Humor

Nursing Intervention	Rationale
Assess the client's range of emotional expressions and ability to display humor. Take into account the effects of mental illness and medications on the client's mood and affect.	Assessment of the client's ability or inability to express emotions assists the nurse to plan interventions that will help the client express pent-up feelings and emotions when capable.
Encourage the client to participate in pleasurable activities, such as games, sports, and field trips.	Participating in rewarding activities exposes the client to others who are responding with a wide range of emotions, which in turn may stimulate the client's responses.
Assure the client that it is acceptable at times to refrain from emotional displays, but at other times it is beneficial to express emotions.	This assurance by the nurse demonstrates acceptance while giving the client reasons to express emotions and permission to do so.
Help the client accurately perceive humorous situations and statements by indicating the humorous aspects. • "Sam, when Ted imitated that comedian during the activity today, it was really funny." • "Donna, did you notice how funny it was when all the clients told a different version of the same story at the recreational activity?" • "Mark, the group and staff really enjoyed the part in the movie where everyone thought the main character was a prince instead of a butler." • "Kate, the joke that Jeff told at dinner tonight was quite humorous."	By accurately perceiving humor, the client can experience the joyful feelings promoted by humor and is encouraged to independently look for the humor in things.
Engage the client in frequent individual discussions that include interjections of humor.	Frequently exposing the client to humor draws the client out of his or her detached or withdrawn state.
Use role playing to demonstrate to the client a wide range of expressions (e.g., joy, sadness, laughter).	Role playing presents to the client an appropriate range of emotions in a nonthreatening environment and encourages use of a broad emotional range.
Assure the client that it is acceptable and beneficial to display emotions that are consistent with feelings, situations, and circumstances. • "Kate, it's OK to express sadness when your roommate is discharged. You're going to miss her, and you need to talk about your feelings." • "Mark, laughter is a healthy expression of positive feelings and can help you feel better."	Assurance by a trusted nurse will help the client to release emotions and to understand the benefits of using emotions.
Engage the client in therapeutic groups (e.g., art/music therapy, cognitive-behavioral therapy, assertiveness training, process/focus groups; see Appendix B).	Participating in group exercises and discussions with other clients helps to bring out a wide range of emotional expressions in a safe setting.
Praise the client for displaying humor and using a wider range of emotional expressions. • "Nick, staff really notice your efforts to participate more in group and share amusing stories." • "Kate, it's nice to see you laughing with others more often." • "Donna, your ability to smile and joke with others shows real progress." • "Mark, showing that you felt sad when your roommate left is a big step toward your goal of expressing yourself more."	Genuine praise, when warranted, helps to increase the client's self-esteem and reinforce continuity of positive behaviors.

## chapter 7

Disorders of Infancy, Childhood, and Adolescence

Mentally healthy children and adolescents are recognized as being free of psychopathologic symptoms and as enjoying a safe, satisfying, quality of life that includes secure attachments and positive functioning at home and school and in the community. Mental health in this age group is marked by achievement of expected developmental milestones in the areas of (1) cognition, (2) emotional stability, (3) socially acceptable coping skills, and (4) appropriate socialization within and outside the family.

Mental and emotional disorders may occur at any age; some are identifiable even in infancy (e.g., reactive attachment disorder and developmental disorders). The defining characteristics for several disorders—schizophrenia, mood disorders, psychoactive substance use disorders, anxiety disorders, somatoform disorders, adjustment disorders, and sexual disorders—with a few intrinsic exceptions, are generally the same for children and adolescents as for adults. Diagnosis of personality disorder is usually reserved for people over age 18 but may be assigned earlier if maladaptive characteristics of the disorder have been stable, inflexible, and crystallized.

Children and adolescents have the inevitable task of progression through developmental stages that result in physical, mental, emotional, and sexual changes. Cultural, subcultural, social, and interpersonal influences play an important part in successful coping, adaptation, and integration of these factors by all individuals on the journey to adulthood.

Ideally, the following developmental tasks are achieved during maturation:

- Evolution of identity (self, gender; in relation to family/society)
- Individuation and independence from parental control
- Clarification and prioritizing of values, beliefs, and interests
- Establishment of meaningful relationships with individuals of same and opposite sex
- Achievement of intimacy
- Understanding and appropriate expression of emotion
- Development of meaningful purpose in life
- Building of competence and honing of skills
- Determination of career goals
- Practice of life-styles

Childhood and adolescence are more dynamic than any other human developmental period and are characterized by continual change, transition, and reorganization. "Normal" includes a wide range of thoughts, emotions, and behaviors for these developmental stages. The nurse must always consider "normal" within the context of the child's family, culture, and society rather than focus on the individual alone. Mental disorders that develop in infants, children, and adolescents deviate from the normal range, however, and are outside the anticipated parameters that define these rapidly transitional times in their lives.

ETIOLOGY

Precise etiology of childhood and adolescent disorders is largely undetermined, but it is widely accepted that mental disorders result from a convergence of biologic, psychologic, social, and environmental influences (Box 7-1). Recent studies show correlations and interactions among risk factors, such as the combination of environmental/social risk factors and physical risk factors of the

Box 7-1 Etiology of Mental Disorders of Infancy, Childhood, and Adolescence

BIOLOGIC FACTORS

Genetic predisposition
In utero environment (toxic agents, injuries, viral infections, drugs)
Low birth weight
Neurotransmitter deficits
Structural central nervous system defects
Early childhood diseases

PSYCHOSOCIAL FACTORS

Interrupted or inadequate maternal-infant bonding
Difficult temperament of child
Poor parent-child "fit"
Poverty
Deprivation or neglect
Abuse (emotional, physical, sexual)
Mental disorder of parent(s)
Parental/familial discord
Divorce
Exposure to traumatic events
Exposure to toxins, viruses, or other noxious substances
Difficulty with peer relationships
Parental criminality

child (low birth weight, neurologic damage at birth, learning impairment, autonomic underarousal, fearlessness/stimulation-seeking behavior, insensitivity to physical pain/punishment).

▌EPIDEMIOLOGY

A significant number of children and adolescents have mental disorders. The Methodology for the Epidemiology of Mental Disorders in Children and Adolescents (MECA) study revealed that 21% of those ages 9 to 17 years had a diagnosable mental or addictive disorder associated with at least *minimum* impairment; 11% had *significant* impairment, and 5% had *extreme* functional impairment (Shaffer et al, 1998).

Disorders may improve or worsen depending on several factors, including the fluidity of development itself. Environmental factors often play a major role in the improvement or worsening of disorders in any age group. In this age group, for example, an affected child may improve as parental, sibling, school, and peer relationships improve or positively change. On the other hand, disorders may develop or worsen if an adolescent finds little or no relief from real or perceived traumatic stressors.

Table 7-1   Prevalence of Mental Disorders in Children and Adolescents Ages 9 to 17 Years

Category	Percentage
Anxiety disorders	13.0
Mood disorders	6.2
Disruptive disorders	10.3
Substance use disorders	2.0
Any disorder	20.9

Environment is not the sole source of more severe disorders, and the child is not cured if only the psychosocial environment changes. In some cases the environment is healthy, but disorders still occur or continue. For example, mental disorders with identified genetic components, including autism, bipolar disorder, schizophrenia, and attention-deficit/hyperactivity disorder (ADHD), may erupt in seemingly normal environments (National Institute of Mental Health, 1998).

Prevalence

The prevalence of certain mental disorders is remarkable in children and adolescents (Table 7-1). Anxiety disorders occur more often than any other mental disorder in this age group. ADHD is the most common behavioral disorder of childhood. Development at all levels is interrupted when mental disorders occur in a young person's life, as evidenced by developmental delays, prolonged developmental periods, and other deviance from standard norms of performance.

Suicides

Statistics for suicidal activity in the younger population remain fairly constant, and the numbers continue to be difficult to accept. According to the Centers for Disease Control and prevention (1999), during the last decade the following numbers of children and adolescents committed suicide according to age groups:

- 1.6:100,000 population for ages 10 to 14 years
- 9.5:100,000 population for ages 15 to 19 years
  — Four times more boys than girls commit suicide in this group
  — Twice as many girls attempt suicide in this group
- 13.6:100,000 population for ages 20 to 24 years

These numbers have changed across time. Since the 1960s the number of male suicides in the 15- to 19-year-old group has tripled, whereas the female numbers have remained constant. The rate for white adolescent males reached a peak in the late 1980s (18:100,000 in 1986) and declined somewhat by the end of the 1990s. Hispanic high school students are more likely than other students to attempt suicide. African-American male suicides increased from 1986 (7.1:100,000) to 1997 (11:100,000). Male American-Indian adolescents and young adults in

> **Box 7-2** **Epidemiologic Factors in Disorders of Infancy, Childhood, and Adolescence**
>
> From 10% to 12% of all children have mental or emotional disorders severe enough to be disabling as adults.
> Only 5% to 7% receive adequate mental health intervention.
> Disorders of boys outnumber those of girls 2:1 before adolescence; girls equal or outnumber boys during and after adolescence.
> Emotional disturbances increase in children ages 9 to 12 years and 13 to 16 years.
> Prolonged stressors increase incidence prevalence.
> - Parental marital discord/divorce
> - Overcrowded living conditions
> - Low socioeconomic status
> - Parental psychiatric condition or trouble with the law
> - Family breakup, separation; foster home placement of child or adolescent
> - Child abuse (physical, emotional, sexual)

> **Box 7-3** **Etiology of Mental Retardation***
>
> **BIOLOGIC FACTORS (25%)**
> Chromosomal (e.g., Down syndrome)
>   Metabolic (e.g., phenylketonuria)
>   Prenatal factors (e.g., rubella, cytomegalovirus, toxoplasmosis)
>   AIDS, syphilis, other viruses/infections
>   Enzyme deficiencies
>   Accidents (e.g., head trauma, near-drowning)
>
> **PSYCHOSOCIAL FACTORS**
> Lower socioeconomic groups
>   Social deprivation
>   Inadequate medical care
>   Lack of intellectual/language stimulation
>   Living with parent who has psychiatric disorder
>
> *Cases with no known cause are usually mild.

American-Indian health service areas had the highest rate in the United States 62:100,000 (Wallace et al, 1996).

Box 7-2 lists additional epidemiologic information for this age group. The statistics show that even among the younger U.S. population, mental disorders take a substantial toll on quality of life and on life itself.

ASSESSMENT AND DIAGNOSTIC CRITERIA

Many mental disorders that affect adults also occur in children and adolescents, including anxiety disorders, mood disorders, substance use disorders, and schizophrenia. With a few exceptions, symptoms of these disorders are the same in young people as they are in adults.

DSM-IV-TR Criteria

Various categories of mental disorders have been identified for infants, children, and adolescents according to *Diagnostic and Statistical Manual of Mental Disorders (DSM-IV-TR)* criteria see box on p. 208; see also Appendix A.

MENTAL RETARDATION

Mental retardation refers to a deficiency in intellectual function coupled with an impairment of adaptive function. *Intellectual function* is measured by standardized intelligence tests that yield an intelligence quotient (IQ); individuals scoring below 70 are considered to be mentally retarded (Table 7-2). IQ is believed to be a relatively stable factor that generally is unaffected by remediation.

Adaptive function is the individual's ability to perform effectively consistent with expectations for age and culture in the following areas: communication, daily living skills, social skills, social responsibility, and independence.

Etiology

The specific etiology of mental retardation may be directly attributable to one or more factors (Box 7-3). A combination of factors (biologic, psychosocial, environmental) appears to be influential in many cases.

Epidemiology

Approximately 1% of the U.S. population are mentally retarded, and the disorder is about 1.5 times more common in boys than in girls. The diagnosis is made before 18 years of age; the highest incidence occurs during school years, with a peak between ages 10 and 15. The percentages of the retarded population can be categorized as follows: mild, 85%; moderate, 10%; severe 3% to 4%; and profound, 1% to 2%.

Mild Mental Retardation

Approximately 85% of the retarded population belong in the mild category and often are not noticed as "different" from the general population of schoolchildren until well into the school years. They usually can learn vocational and social skills sufficient to support themselves and achieve academically to about the sixth-grade level.

Moderate Mental Retardation

The 10% of retarded individuals in the moderate group can learn to take care of themselves with supervison. They may be able to perform at jobs in sheltered environments or in the regular job market under strong guidance. They usually

DSM-IV-TR Mental Disorders of Infancy, Childhood, and Adolescence

Mental Retardation*
- Mild mental retardation
- Moderate mental retardation
- Severe mental retardation
- Profound mental retardation
- Mental retardation, severity unspecified

Learning Disorders
- Reading disorder
- Mathematics disorder
- Disorder of written expression
- Learning disorder NOS

Motor Skills Disorder
- Developmental coordination disorder

Communication Disorders
- Expressive language disorder
- Mixed receptive expressive language disorder
- Phonologic disorder
- Stuttering
- Communication disorder NOS

Pervasive Developmental Disorders
- Autistic disorder
- Rett's disorder
- Childhood disintegrative disorder
- Asperger's disorder
- Pervasive developmental disorder NOS

Attention Deficit and Disruptive Behavior Disorders
- Attention-deficit/hyperactivity disorder
- Conduct disorder
- Oppositional defiant disorder

Feeding and Eating Disorders of Infancy or Early Childhood
- Pica
- Rumination disorder
- Feeding disorder of infancy or early childhood

Tic Disorders
- Tourette's disorder

Elimination Disorders
- Encopresis
- Enuresis

Other Disorders of Infancy, Childhood, or Adolescence
- Separation anxiety disorder
- Selective mutism
- Reactive attachment disorder of infancy or early childhood
- Inhibited type
- Disinhibited type
- Stereotypic movement disorder

NOS, Not otherwise specified.
*These diagnoses are coded on Axis II.

Table 7-2	Categories of Severity for Mental Retardation
Category	Intelligence Quotient
Mild	50-55 to about 70
Moderate	35-40 to about 50-55
Severe	20-25 to about 35-40
Profound	Below 20-25

are educable to about a second-grade level and live in group homes or with family.

Severe Mental Retardation

The 3% to 4% of retarded individuals in the severe group are recognizable early in life because they fail to develop adequate motor skills or speech for communication. They may eventually learn to talk, tend to basic hygiene, and perform simple tasks with close supervision.

Profound Mental Retardation

Approximately 1% to 2% of the retarded population are included in the profound category. They have very limited sensorimotor function, may have other physical handicaps, and require constant care and supervision. With supervision, they may learn to perform simple tasks.

LEARNING DISORDERS

A diagnosis of learning disorder is noted when an individual is unable to achieve designated scores on standardized tests of reading, math, or writing proficiency for specified ages, level of education, and IQ. In addition, the lack of these skills hinders progress in school and interferes with activities that require the skills. Disturbances in sensory, perceptual, or cognitive processing may underlie the learning disorder and are often found in conjunction with other medical conditions, such as fetal alcohol syndrome, birthing traumas, or neurologic disorders. The individual with deficient learning skills frequently has low self-esteem and self-concept, negative self-worth, and inept social skills.

Reading Disorder

The defining characteristic of reading disorder, commonly referred to as **dyslexia**, is the inability to achieve specific scores on standardized tests that measure reading comprehension, speed, and accuracy. In addition, the skill deficiency interferes with school progression and daily living activities in which the skills are required. When reading aloud, the child may omit, substitute, or distort content, and the process is usually slow. Reading disorder is usually associated with math and writing disorders.

Mathematics Disorder

Mathematics disorder is noted when an individual is unable to achieve specific scores on standardized tests that measure mathematics competence. The deficiency interferes with progress in school and daily activities in which the skills are important. Competence in mathematics includes several skills, such as recognizing and naming math symbols and signs, changing written problems with math symbols, understanding math concepts and terms, learning tables, and following sequences. Math disorder is often associated with writing and reading disorders.

Disorder of Written Expression

The defining characteristics of disorder of written expression are the inability to achieve standardized test scores and the resulting interference with school progress and daily activities that require writing skills. The disorder is manifested by difficulty organizing content into paragraphs; multiple errors in grammar, spelling, and punctuation; and poor handwriting. Written expression disorder is usually associated with reading and mathematics disorders.

MOTOR SKILLS DISORDER

The primary motor skills disorder in children involves impaired developmental coordination.

Developmental Coordination Disorder

The defining characteristic of developmental coordination disorder is impaired motor coordination. The diagnosis, however, is made *only* in the absence of an underlying medical condition and *only* if the impairment significantly interferes with progress in school or with daily activities. The impaired developmental coordination is age specific, for example, crawling and walking in infants, climbing and buttoning in toddlers, and throwing or catching a ball and printing words in school-age children.

COMMUNICATION DISORDERS

Expressive and Receptive Language Disorders

Expressive language disorder is noted when expressive language development is impaired. Manifestations of the disorder are poverty of speech, short sentences, omission of parts of sentences, limited variety of speech, and use of unusual wording.

Receptive language disorder is coupled with expressive language disorder, as noted by results on standardized assessment tests. Symptoms are the same as for expressive language disorder. The *DSM-IV-TR* diagnosis for these children is *mixed receptive-expressive language disorder*.

Phonologic Disorder

Phonologic disorder is evidenced by nonuse or misuse of sounds of speech for an expected age, as evidenced by sound omissions, sound substitutions, or sound distortions. Examples include omitting the last consonant ("truh" instead of "truck"), use of the letter *b* instead of *p* ("bretty"), and use of "ax" for the word "ask." The individual's cultural background with its specific sound differences must always be assessed in this regard to avoid misdiagnosis.

Stuttering

The defining characteristic of stuttering is impaired flow and pattern of speech, resulting in discontinuous sentences. Manifestations are varied and may include repeated words or sounds ("can-can-can-can-I . . ."), prolonged sounds ("the sssssssssun is warm"), pauses in speech, and other impairments.

PERVASIVE DEVELOPMENTAL DISORDERS

The term **pervasive** is used to describe the category of disorders in which several areas of development—social interaction, verbal and nonverbal communication, behavior, and activity—are severely affected. Pervasive developmental disorders result in severely impaired social function.

Autistic Disorder

Autistic disorder, known in the past as infantile autism, Kanner's syndrome, childhood schizophrenia, and symbiotic psychosis, usually manifests before age 3 years, with a lifelong course. Changes can occur in some individuals, however, including improvement of social and language skills at about 5 to 6 years, improvement or decline in cognitive/social skills at puberty, and escalation of negative behaviors (e.g., aggression, opposition) at puberty.

Individuals with autistic disorder rarely are able to become totally independent because of their impaired IQ, language skills, and social skills. Therefore most affected individuals require a lifelong structured environment and close supervision. Four to five children per 10,000 births are affected by autistic disorder.

Etiology

Biologic and prenatal, perinatal, and postnatal situations and conditions (e.g., anoxia at birth, encephalitis, chromosomal anomaly, phenylketonuria, maternal rubella) may cause brain dysfunction.

Autistic disorder is a severe form of pervasive developmental disorder. Symptoms include the following:

1. *Impaired social interaction* (two of the following must be present for diagnosis):

a. The client is unaware of feelings or needs of others; treats other people as objects.

b. At distressful moments, fails entirely to seek solace from others or seeks comfort in unusual ways.
  • Rather than wanting hugs, may walk in circles or stereotypically repeat a phrase.

c. Does not imitate significant others' actions (waving good-bye), or imitates out of context of situation.

d. Demonstrates impaired social play or total lack of it.
  • Plays alone or engages others only as objects.

e. Demonstrates severely impaired ability to form peer relationships.
  • Shows no interest in others or lacks awareness or understanding necessary to interact socially.

2. *Impaired verbal and nonverbal communication* (one of the following must be present for diagnosis):

a. The client demonstrates total lack of any mode of communication.

b. Engages in abnormal nonverbal communication: inappropriate and out-of-context posturing, facial expression, gazing, gesturing.
  • Fails to smile at or move toward parents or significant others when greeted.
  • Does not cuddle when held; may stiffen instead.

c. Fails to engage in imaginative play.

d. Demonstrates abnormal speech *process:* uses monotone; singsong quality; unusual pitch, rhythm, rate.

e. Demonstrates abnormal speech *content/form:* repetition of speech of other persons, television, or radio *(echolalia);* irrelevant or idiosyncratic use of words, ("want to run the dasher" meaning "I want to take a bath").

f. Displays inability to begin or successfully maintain conversations with others.

3. *Unusual or bizarre activities and interests* (one of the following must be present for diagnosis):

a. The client demonstrates ritualized, stereotyped behaviors: head banging, rocking, body spinning, hand/arm flapping.

b. Displays intense preoccupation with specific objects.
  • Flicks light switches on and off persistently.
  • Watches toy spin for hours without playing with it.
  • Rubs or spins one part of a toy instead of using as intended.
  • Carries one object constantly (jar lid, particular piece of clothing).

c. Demonstrates need for sameness in environment and routine.
  • Becomes upset when furniture is moved from usual spot.
  • Must take same route every time when traveling to grandparent's house.

d. Lacks variety of interests or is preoccupied with one interest.
  • Looks through one book only, repeatedly.

Up to half of autistic children are also mentally retarded at a moderate, severe, or profound level. Interestingly, some children with autistic disorder possess unusual or extraordinary abilities or "islands of genius." For example, a severely retarded person who is unable to make correct change in a store may be able to calculate an extraordinary range of numbers but is unable to understand their significance. An individual may be able to play a musical instrument without ever taking lessons or being able to read music.

Rett's Disorder

Defining characteristics of Rett's disorder (Rett syndrome) are a period of normal functioning prenatally, perinatally, and up to age 5 months, followed by development of multiple deficits. The child has decelerated head growth, loss of acquired hand skills and substitution of stereotyped handwriting or hand-washing movements, changes in social interaction (loss of interest in interpersonal engagement at first, may engage later in course of disorder), and severe problems that develop in coordination and language development, both receptive and expressive.

Childhood Disintegrative Disorder

Childhood disintegrative disorder is marked by a period of normal development for up to 2 years, followed by severe loss of skills before age 10. Loss of skills includes two of the following five areas: language (receptive and expressive), socialization, control of bowel or bladder, play, and motor skills. This disorder has been known in the past as disintegrative psychosis, dementia infantilis, and Heller's syndrome.

Asperger's Disorder

Defining characteristics of Asperger's disorder (Asperger's syndrome) are marked and prolonged impairment in socialization and the development of stereotyped, repetitive behaviors. The individual fails to use social regulators such as smiling directly at others or looking into a person's eyes when talking. There is a lack of sharing with others, and age-appropriate relationships do not develop. Behaviors and interests are frequently stereotyped, rigid, and repetitive (e.g., incessant hand tapping, preoccupation with daily air flights into the city) and of little or no interest to others. Social interaction is severely impaired.

ATTENTION DEFICIT AND DISRUPTIVE BEHAVIOR DISORDERS

Attention-Deficit/Hyperactivity Disorder

Children with ADHD are often referred to as being hyperactive. They have developmentally inappropriate problems in maintaining attention and are impulsive and hyperactive. These difficulties may manifest as inability to stay with a task to completion, listen to the teacher, and finish chores at home. Children with ADHD comment out of turn or cannot wait for a turn, do not follow directions, interrupt others continually, have difficulty staying in a seat, and are constantly "on the go."

Subtypes

Some individuals with ADHD demonstrate symptoms of both inattention and hyperactivity-impulsivity. Others have one pattern more than another, as follows:
- Combined type
- Predominantly inattentive type
- Predominantly hyperactive-impulsive type

Conduct Disorder (Solitary Aggressive Type)

Conduct disorder is characterized by persistent patterns of serious misconduct at home, at school, and in the community. Manifestations of conduct disorder include violation of the basic rights of others and basic rules, laws, or norms (verbal and physical aggression toward other people, animals, and property); stealing, rape, assault; lying; cheating; truancy from school; use of drugs and alcohol; callous disregard for others' feelings; blaming others for own transgressions; and lack of appropriate empathy, remorse, or guilt. If maladaptive behavior persists into adulthood, conduct disorder is changed to a diagnosis of *antisocial personality disorder*.

Oppositional Defiant Disorder

A pattern of defiance, hostility, and negativity characterizes oppositional defiant disorder. Behaviors may include loss of temper; arguments with adults; defiance and refusal to adhere to adult rules; displays of anger, resentment, or vindictiveness; swearing and use of obscenities; and deliberately annoying others.

▌ FEEDING AND EATING DISORDERS OF INFANCY OR EARLY CHILDHOOD

Defining characteristics of feeding and eating disorders are disturbances in feeding and eating during the early years of a child's life. Chapter 10 discusses anorexia nervosa and bulimia nervosa.

Pica

The defining characteristic of pica is the persistent eating of substances that have no nutritive value. This behavior is inappropriate for the specific developmental level or cultural practice. Poverty, developmental delay, neglect, and inadequate parental supervision increase the risk of pica. Specific ingested substances vary with age (Table 7-3). This disorder tends to increase when associated with mental retardation.

Rumination Disorder

Defining characteristics of rumination disorder are repeated regurgitation and rechewing of food that has been swallowed by an infant or child who had normal functioning before the occurrence of this behavior. The child brings food back up into the mouth without retching and either rechews and reswallows or expels the food. Malnutrition may occur with weight loss or failure to gain weight. Children with rumination disorder have a 25% mortality rate.

Feeding Disorder of Infancy or Early Childhood

The defining characteristic of feeding disorder of infancy or early childhood is a persistent failure to eat adequately, with resultant failure to gain weight, or loss of weight, before age 6 years.

▌ TIC DISORDERS

A **tic** is a stereotyped vocalization or motor movement that occurs rapidly and suddenly in a nonrhythmic manner (Table 7-4; see box on p. 214).

Tourette's Disorder

Defining characteristics of Tourette's disorder (Tourette's syndrome) are multiple motor and vocal tics that present several times a day at irregular intervals. Frequently, individuals with Tourette's disorder experience obsessions and compulsions, hyperactivity, self-consciousness, and depression in addition to the tic disorder.

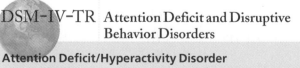

DSM-IV-TR Attention Deficit and Disruptive Behavior Disorders

Attention Deficit/Hyperactivity Disorder
- Combined type
- Predominantly inattentive type
- Predominantly hyperactive-impulsive type

Conduct Disorder
- Childhood-onset type
- Adolescent-onset type
- Oppositional defiant disorder
- Disruptive behavior disorder not otherwise specified

Table 7-3	Age-Significant Substances for Pica	
Age Group	**Substances**
Infants, young children	Paint, plaster, string, hair, cloth
Older children	Sand, insects, animal droppings, pebbles, leaves
Adults	Clay, soil

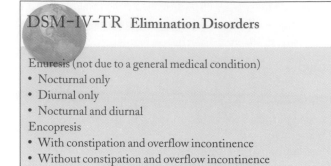

DSM-IV-TR Tic Disorders

Tourette's disorder
Chronic motor or vocal tic disorder
Transient tic disorder
• Single episode
• Recurrent tic disorder not otherwise specified

DSM-IV-TR Elimination Disorders

Enuresis (not due to a general medical condition)
• Nocturnal only
• Diurnal only
• Nocturnal and diurnal
Encopresis
• With constipation and overflow incontinence
• Without constipation and overflow incontinence

Table 7-4	**Tic Manifestations**
Motor Tics	**Vocal Tics**
Simple	
Coughing	Throat clearing
Neck jerking	Grunting
Eye blinking	Sniffing
Shoulder shrugging	Snorting
Facial grimaces	Barking
Complex	
Grooming behaviors	Repeating words out of context
Jumping	Obscene words, swearing *(coprolalia)*
Stamping	Repeating own words *(palilalia)*
Facial gestures	Repeating others' words *(echolalia)*
Smelling an object	Imitation of others' behaviors *(echokinesia)*

ELIMINATION DISORDERS

Enuresis

The defining characteristic of enuresis is repeated urination voluntarily or involuntarily during the day or night into bed or clothing, past the age of expected continence (5 to 6 years). Physical causes must be ruled out before this diagnosis is made.

Primary enuresis refers to the disturbance when it is not preceded by a year of urinary continence. **Secondary enuresis** refers to the disturbance when at least 1 year of continence precedes the disorder.

Nocturnal enuresis, the most common type, occurs during rapid eye movement (REM) sleep, usually in the first third of total sleep, at night. *Diurnal enuresis* occurs during the day and is more common in females. The diurnal type may result from reluctance to use public toilets.

Encopresis

The defining characteristic of encopresis is repeated defecation voluntarily or involuntarily into clothes or areas other than appropriate toilet facilities. Physical causes must be ruled out before the diagnosis is made (see box above).

OTHER DISORDERS OF INFANCY, CHILDHOOD, OR ADOLESCENCE (See box on p. 215)

Separation Anxiety Disorder

When separated from the major figure of attachment (primary caregiver), the child may experience severe to panic levels of anxiety. Symptoms of separation anxiety disorder are unrealistic and persistent and include worry that the parent will not return or will have an accident while away, refusal to go to school, refusal to go to sleep when parent is not near, clinging behaviors, nightmares about separating from parent, physical symptoms (nausea, vomiting, headache, stomachache), or pleading not to be separated.

Selective Mutism

The defining characteristic of selective mutism is failure to speak when speaking is expected, even though the person speaks in other situations. For example, a child may not speak to playmates during school but talks at home. Before a diagnosis is made, the behavior must persist past the beginning of a new class (1 month) and must interfere with educational and social functioning.

Reactive Attachment Disorder of Infancy or Early Childhood

Reactive attachment disorder is characterized by age-appropriate but greatly disturbed social relationships, manifesting as either of two types, as follows:
• **Inhibited type.** Failure to respond to or initiate interactions with others: apathy; lack of spontaneity, visual tracking, curiosity, or playfulness.
• **Disinhibited type.** Indiscriminate socializing: overfamiliarity with strangers, displays of affection toward them, or requests for attention from strangers.

In addition, evidence exists for one of the following regarding negligent or punitive care of the child: (1) disregard of child's needs for affection, comfort, and stimulation *(emotional needs);* (2) disregard of child's needs for food, clothing, and shelter *(physical needs);* (3) disregard of protection from abuse or danger; or

DSM-IV-TR Other Disorders of Infancy, Childhood, or Adolescence

Separation anxiety disorder
• Early onset
Selective mutism
Reactive attachment disorder of infancy or early childhood
• Inhibited type
• Disinhibited type
Stereotypic movement disorder
• With self-injurious behavior
Disorder of infancy, childhood, or adolescence not otherwise specified

(4) frequent changes in primary caregivers, leading to unstable attachments.

Etiology

Reactive attachment disorder is caused by pathogenic care of the infant by the primary caregiver. Lack of bonding or poor parent-infant fit may result from problems that exist with one or both members of the dyad, such as poor parenting skills, low socioeconomic status, deprivation, and presence of mental retardation or a physical anomaly in the child.

Stereotypic Movement Disorder

Diagnosis of stereotypic movement disorder is made when an individual persistently and repetitively performs a nonfunctional motor behavior in a driven way. Examples of behavior include biting self, playing with fingers, head banging, waving hands, rocking, and picking at skin or body orifices. The disorder often occurs in conjunction with mental retardation or in individuals who are institutionalized and receive little stimulation.

▌INTERVENTIONS

When determining treatment related to mental health versus mental disorder in this age group, several factors must be considered. A report of the child's history and past experiences is a valuable tool for gaining correct perspective on present conditions. Knowledge of both normal growth and development and psychopathology are necessary before the nurse can understand the many factors that encompass the development, presence, absence, or continuance of mental disorders. Because of the inherent fluidity of development in this young age group, another consideration is the individual child's capacity and ability to adapt to his or her own internal and external changes and discontinuities when they arise. Also, prevention on all levels plays an important role in treating this population.

Prevention Programs

Prevention programs regarding mental disorders in the younger population have proven statistically successful. For example, Project Head Start for preschool-age children is one of many programs that have demonstrated the importance of (1) *early risk reduction,* (2) *prevention of onset,* and (3) *early intervention* with children and their parents as important factors for ensuring mental health for U.S. children. Through provision of appropriately stimulating and supportive environments, children can make significant advances in knowledge, logic, and reasoning—areas previously thought to be predetermined. Several other national primary prevention programs support this data and the subsequent reduction in mental disorders.

Primary prevention in the form of parenting classes has proven valuable. Parents who learn the patterns of normal growth and development usually have reasonable expectations for their children and their performance. Treatment outlook is generally more favorable if parents have knowledge of healthy parenting skills when their child develops a mental disorder that alters the child's thoughts, feelings, and behaviors and the family's dynamics.

Medications

Medications are used to manage a variety of behaviors resulting from mental disorders of childhood and adolescence, primarily when other therapies do not adequately manage disruptive behaviors that may threaten to harm the child or others. Because these types of medications often need frequent adjustment, parents need to work closely with the physician and pharmacist to provide the child with the optimal medication regimen. The commonly prescribed medications discussed in the box on p. 216 have helped children, parents, teachers, and nurses manage disruptive behavior patterns.

Therapies

Treatment for childhood mental disorders that also occur in adults follows the same general principles, primarily interpersonal therapeutic interventions and psychopharmacology. Medications are frequently used in children with mental disorders, with appropriate dosage modifications for individual age and size.

Interventions for severe and persistent mental disorders, such as severe mental retardation and pervasive developmental disorders, require intensive, specialized care and education of the child and family. Treatment focuses on promotion of the child's language and social development and mastery, with reduction or elimination of behaviors that interfere with learning and functioning in the world.

Nurse-client therapeutic relationship

Nurse-client relationship therapy is ideally suited for this age group (see Chapter 1). The nurse must consider the child's chronologic and developmental stages, cognitive

PHARMACOTHERAPY   Disorders of Infancy, Childhood, and Adolescence*

METHYLPHENIDATE (RITALIN)

Oral methylphenidate is the drug of choice for most hyperkinetic children and has been used to treat attention-deficit/hyperactivity disorder (ADHD) for more than 30 years. Methylphenidate is a mild central nervous system (CNS) stimulant with an unknown mechanism of action. The dose for children 6 years and older is 5 mg before breakfast and lunch, increased by 5 to 10 mg at weekly intervals up to 0.3 to 0.5 mg/kg body weight. The maximum daily dose should not exceed 60 mg.

Therapeutic effects of methylphenidate include increased attention and decreased impulsiveness and hyperactivity in children with ADHD. Side effects include the following:

- Hyperactivity, insomnia, restlessness, talkativeness
- Dizziness, headache, chills, stimulation
- Dysphoria, irritability, aggressiveness
- Impaired normal growth in children (talk with physician)
- Allergic or unusual reactions (call emergency services if serious)

EXTENDED-RELEASE TABLETS

Extended-release methylphenidate (Concerta) is taken whole once daily in the morning. Additional side effects include the following:

- Stomach pain, sleeplessness, decreased appetite
- Nausea, vomiting, nervousness, tics, increased blood pressure
- Psychosis (abnormal thinking or hallucinations)

Concerta is contraindicated in children with anxiety, tension, agitation, glaucoma or eye problems, tics, or Tourette's syndrome.

Focalin (dexmethyl phenidate HCl) is a CNS stimulant and chemically refined form of Ritalin; administered twice a day for the treatment of ADHD. Efficacy of this drug was established in two controlled trials of young clients ages 6 to 17. The recommended conversion doses are:

Ritalin	Focalin
5 mg	2.5 mg
10 mg	5 mg
20 mg	10 mg

Daily doses should be administered 4-hours apart.

Ritalin long-acting (LA) (methylphenidate HCl) is an extended-release capsule that is a long-acting, once daily CNS stimulant for the treatment of ADHD. Ritalin LA has a bimodal release profile with a treatment effect designed to last throughout the school day. The efficacy of Ritalin LA was established in a pivotal controlled trial of young clients ages 6 to 12 years. Available in 20, 30, 40 mg extended-release capsules; the capsule may be opened and its beads sprinkled on warm applesauce, which is helpful for children who have difficulty swallowing an entire capsule.

CLONIDINE (CATAPRES)

Oral clonidine (Catapres) is an adult antihypertensive agent and norepinephrine antagonist prescribed for ADHD. American Psychiatric Association (APA) guidelines for use in childhood disorders have not been established, and clonidine may not be recommended for children under age 12 years. The dose for children with ADHD is 0.2 to 0.6 mg/day, generally given at night. Clonidine should not be stopped abruptly but rather tapered over 3 to 4 days.

Therapeutic effects include the following:

- In ADHD, helps the child relax and sleep during bedtime transition.
- In Tourette's syndrome, improves tic disorders.
- In autism, improves social behaviors, sensory responses, inattention, repetitive behaviors, and affective reactions.

Side effects of clonidine include the following:

- Dry mouth, drowsiness, gastrointestinal symptoms
- Orthostatic hypertention (generally in adults)
- Allergic or unusual reactions (call emergency services if serious)

GUANFACINE (TENEX)

A centrally acting antihypertensive, guanfacine (Tenex) may be prescribed with clonidine to reduce hyperactivity in ADHD or to reduce tics. The dose is clonidine, 3 to 6 µg/kg/day, and guanfacine, 0.75 to 3.0 mg, at bedtime. APA guidelines for use in childhood disorders have not been established, and guanfacine may not be prescribed for children under 12 years of age.

Discuss medication effects with physician or pharmacist before taking guanfacine with other prescribed drugs or over-the-counter substances. Contact physician for any unexpected side effects. Call emergency services for any allergic, adverse, or unusual reactions.

ORAL DEXTROAMPHETAMINE (ADDERALL)

Dextroamphetamine/amphetamine (Dexedrine) or amphetamine (Adderall) is used to treat ADHD and narcolepsy (a sleep disorder) in children ages 3 to 16 years. For ADHD the dose in children 3 to 5 years is 2.5 mg daily and in those 6 years and older 5 mg once or twice daily. Doses may be increased for optimal results but *rarely exceed* 40 mg/day. Lowest effective dose is given and doses are individually adjusted. Long-term effects of amphetamines in children have not been established.

Discuss medication effects of amphetamines with physician or pharmacist. Contact physician for foods to avoid and any unexpected side effects. Call emergency services for any allergic, adverse, or unusual reactions.

NALTREXONE (TREXAN)

A nonaddictive opiate antagonist, naltrexone (Trexan) has significantly improved the management of self-injurious behaviors in children, such as the head banging often seen in autistic disorders.

---

*When children and adolescents demonstrate symptoms of disorders that occur in adults, they will receive the same medications that are given to adults, with careful attention to dosage changes.

level, capacity for change, ability to engage in a therapeutic alliance, and skills that the child has developed in all areas. Modifications in the nurse-client relationship are made as a result of this assessment. The care plans in this chapter support the therapeutic alliance at various levels of intervention and offer other techniques for interacting with younger clients.

Cognitive-behavioral therapy

The nurse assesses and considers the child's capacity for awareness of problematic areas and ability and willingness to participate in an interdisciplinary treatment program. Cognitive-behavioral therapies are currently popular for all age groups, including this population.

In *cognitive therapy* for children and adolescents the client may be assisted in the following steps: (1) recognize troublesome feelings such as anxiety, (2) identify and clarify thoughts associated with the feelings, (3) challenge irrational thoughts, (4) develop a plan to cope with the thoughts, (5) and evaluate the success of coping strategies. Cognitive and problem-solving approaches can often be modified for most ages, but the treatment team will consider the child's capacity and ability to do this work.

Behavioral therapy is often useful in the treatment of children and includes such techniques as contingency management, systematic desensitization, and behavioral contracts. In all instances, priority interventions focus on safety of the child and the environment to prevent and manage violence directed toward self or others. *Contingency management* uses behavioral principles of shaping, positive reinforcement, and extinction to alter behavior by manipulating its consequences. It is most successful when conducted in specialized settings with highly trained staff because consistency and other elements are crucial. Homes and most acute care facilities are usually not prepared to carry through with the rules and have too many distractions. Most settings that treat children incorporate behavior modification methods, but on a level that is less demanding than formal contingency management. Often a points and levels system or token economy is employed so that a child can earn privileges.

Systematic desensitization is used for children and adults to assist them to unlearn fears and phobias by presenting a feared stimulus with a nonfeared stimulus. For example, a client taught to do relaxation techniques whenever a feared stimulus appears (e.g., spiders, heights) frequently learns to control the fear response by reciprocal inhibition.

Behavioral contracts can be adapted for any age group and often are successful adjuncts to other therapies for most mental disorders (Box 7-4) on p. 218. Behavioral contracts are concrete methods for predictability and are easily modified for younger children and for older adolescents, who frequently think of themselves as being more sophisticated. When followed carefully, contracts are successful because they shift the external locus of control (parent, therapist, teacher) to the child's own internal locus of control. The child decides to continue elements of the contract to reap the rewards and avoid the adverse results that were previously negotiated, decided, and agreed on by both the child and the parent/teacher or therapist.

Family therapy

Family therapy is a standard component in the treatment of children with mental disorders. Because the entire family system is involved in the child's disorder, all members require support, empathy, education, and assistance with newly learned skills and techniques that will help them manage the dysfunction. Maintenance of a stable, predictable, healthy environment is necessary in the midst of the chaos that may often accompany a child's mental disorder.

Members are taught to identify early symptoms of the disorder and are encouraged to seek early treatment. Bonding and parenting issues and education are addressed. Parents are encouraged to focus on healthy and growth aspects of other children in the family, in addition to their own union, and not only on the child with the disorder. The family is assisted in expansion of their social support network, including extended family, outside agencies, religious affiliates, school facilities, and support/self-help groups.

When it is impossible for families to manage the multiple symptoms and behavioral disruption that accompany a child's mental disorders, the family must be assisted in placing their child in a facility outside the home. Placement may be temporary or permanent. Often, mixed emotions, relief, and guilt surround such a decision; therefore continued contact with the family to help them maintain their separate and collective healthy function is important.

PROGNOSIS AND DISCHARGE CRITERIA

Prognosis for childhood mental disorders that also occur in adults is essentially the same. Most children and adolescents with mental disorders have a better prognosis if treated early. Severe or persistent disorders (pervasive developmental disorders) carry a less favorable prognosis, but these disorders also can be mild, moderate, or severe, which also affects outcome.

Discharge criteria are individualized according to the client's age, developmental stage, symptom picture, stage of recovery on discharge, and level of care provided in the home/facility. Discharge criteria are used as general guidelines to assist in formulating a plan as follows:
- The client engages in self-care within range of capabilities.
- Demonstrates capacity for emotional control.
- Attends to tasks, schoolwork, and performance without undue anger or frustration.
- Exhibits healthy self-concept and self-esteem.
- Demonstrates functional eating habits and behaviors appropriate for age and stature.
- Uses cognitive, communication, and language skills to make self understood and have needs met.

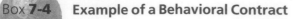

Box 7-4   Example of a Behavioral Contract

Contracts can be very effective tools for compliance with desired behaviors if they are (1) *realistic,* (2) *age appropriate* (younger children require simple, single-level expectations), (3) *consistently maintained* (parent cannot veer from contract by telling child he or she can play first, then fulfill expected behaviors after play), and (4) *valued* by all parties involved.

BEHAVIORAL CONTRACT PRINCIPLES
1. Criteria of the contract are determined through negotiation by all parties.
2. Contract is most effective if written.
3. *Short-range,* attainable goals are defined.
4. Behaviors are rehearsed before final commitment to contract.

PROCEDURE
1. Write clear, concise but detailed description of the client's desired behavior.
2. Set the time and frequency of expected behaviors.
3. Specify positive reinforcements contingent on fulfilling #1 and #2.
4. Specify adverse consequences contingent on nonfulfillment of #1 and #2.
5. Add a bonus clause that includes additional positive reinforcements if client exceeds initial minimal demands.
6. Specify means by which responses are observed, measured, and recorded, (a chart on refrigerator) and specify the procedure for informing the client about achievement.
7. Deliver reinforcement soon after the response (do not prolong giving earned reward).

SCENARIO
Daniel, 10 years old, litters his room and every room in the house with his clothing and belongings. He drops what he does not want to use at that moment on the floor or furniture. He then spends inordinate amounts of time asking where his belongings are. His parents are exasperated, so they begin a contract *with* Daniel, which implies that Daniel and his parents are involved in the behavior change rather than Daniel alone.

Daniel and his parents sit down at a quiet time to quietly discuss the problematic behavior. Daniel usually plays an interactive television game every afternoon after school and almost any time he wants on weekends. Mom, Dad, and Daniel decide together through negotiation and agree how much Daniel is able to do to keep the house and his room clean. As a reward, Daniel will have access to his TV game if he complies. Mom writes the contract, and all agree to 1 week of "rehearsal" before they sign it.

SAMPLE CONTRACT
1. and 2. (See Procedure above.)
   Daniel will:
   a. Dress or undress *only* when in his room, and no other room in the house.
   b. Use one game or toy at a time, putting all other games and toys that he is not using in specific, labeled, designated place in his room (at all times).
   c. Put all clean clothes on hangers or in drawers in his room (by bedtime 18 PM).
   d. Put all dirty clothes in the bathroom hamper (before school/by 7:30 AM and before bedtime/8 PM)
   e. Place backpack next to desk and books on top of desk in his room (immediately after school by 3 PM).
   f. Look over entire house for any of his belongings, picking up any items he may find (before bedtime/8 PM every evening)
3. If #1 and #2 are fulfilled, Daniel may play with TV game each day from 4 to 5 PM on school days and any 2 hours he chooses on weekends and holidays (log of hours posted on refrigerator for Daniel to complete with one parent).
4. If #1 and #2 are unmet, Daniel loses TV game privilege (on that day if unmet in AM *or* next day if unmet at bedtime).
5. *Bonus:* If Daniel meets the contract each day for total of 5 days, he can choose one place from a prepared list for the family outing on Saturday or Sunday.
6. Mom will mark with an X and sign initials on refrigerator poster (every AM); Dad will mark and sign (every PM). If one parent is away, the other will sign off. Contract and performance will be reviewed/discussed by family at dinner each evening. There will be no delayed reinforcements (TV or no TV) at any time or on any day.

Signed (Daniel) _____   Date _____
        (Mom) _____
        (Dad) _____

- Demonstrates interactive skills appropriate for level of development.
- Verbalizes satisfaction with gender identity and sexual preference.
- Interacts meaningfully with staff, peers, and family within capability.
- Seeks attention and assistance appropriately from significant persons, and refrains from undue or unnecessary interactions with strangers.
- Adheres to treatment regimen, including medication as needed.

- Plays appropriately with peers.
- Engages in educational and vocational programs within capabilities.
- Utilizes adaptive coping techniques and stress-reducing strategies.
- Responds satisfactorily to others' attentions and requests.
- Utilizes community resources to enhance quality of life.
- Engages in ongoing individual and family therapy.

The box below provides guidelines for client and family teaching in the management of mental disorders of childhood and adolescence.

CLIENT AND FAMILY TEACHING   **Disorders of Childhood and Adolescence**

Nurse Needs to Know

- Children with mental disorders have developmental and behavioral limitations that may test the patience of parents and caregivers.
- Parents and family members need instruction and guidance about the child's specific disorder, symptoms, treatment, and management.
- Some disorders may result in violent behaviors that may place the child and others in physical danger, requiring immediate emergency interventions.
- Suicide is one of the leading causes of death in adolescents and is becoming more prevalent in younger children.
- Recognizing the signs of depression in children and adolescents may help prevent suicide.
- Because the successful suicide of a peer can precipitate copycat attempts in adolescents, knowledge of the client's history and school experience is critical.
- Learn the age-specific developmental tasks and limitations and apply age-appropriate behavior modification interventions according to facility policy.
- Be sensitive to the child's cultural, spiritual, and ethnic background and how this affects the parents' response and approach to the child's disorder.
- Learn strategies that promote a safe environment, personal safety, and healthy boundaries between the nurse and the client and between nurse and family.
- Because of cultural or educational barriers, some parents require extra time or special instruction to learn about their child's disorder.
- Some parents may be at risk for harming their children and need to be taught nonviolent responses and strategies and how to seek help.
- Provide mature, assertive role modeling for the child/adolescent and parents.
- Provide opportunities for the child/adolescent to practice appropriate social and academic skills through group and classroom activities.

Teach Client and Family

- Educate the parents about age-appropriate developmental tasks, and explain how their child's disorder may disrupt these important milestones.
- Teach the client/parents about the specific disorder, symptoms, behaviors, treatment, and management strategies.
- Explain to the parents/family that children and adolescents with these disorders may test their limits and require patience and understanding.
- Teach the parents/family that some of these disorders may result in aggressive or violent behavior and require emergency intervention.
- Educate the parents/family about the prevalence of suicide among children and adolescents, including copying behaviors of peers who completed suicide.
- Instruct the parents/family about signs and symptoms of depression and suicidal ideation, and provide emergency resources and telephone numbers.
- Emphasize to the parents the importance of reinforcing the child/adolescent's strengths, capabilities, and positive qualities.
- Teach the parents age-appropriate behavior modification strategies.
- Teach the parents/family that medication plays an important role in managing disruptive behaviors and promoting more adaptive functioning.
- Educate the parents about the difficult transitional periods, such as early morning and bedtime, and explain how medication adjustment may help.
- Educate the parents/family about the therapeutic and nontherapeutic effects of medication and when to notify the child's physician.
- Instruct the parents to work closely with the physician, pharmacist, and nurse to provide an effective medication regimen for the child.
- Instruct the parents to educate the client's siblings about the disorder, according to their level of understanding, because they are important to the client's progress.

- Reinforce the strengths, capabilities, and positive qualities of the child and family.
- Help the child/adolescent express anger through appropriate verbal and physical activities rather than using violence or aggression.
- Identify stressors that may promote disruptive or aggressive behaviors, and attempt to avoid or modify them.
- Praise the child/adolescent for efforts made to change or modify disruptive or aggressive behavior patterns and for respecting others' needs.
- Medication compliance is often critical to the child's adaptive behavior, and nurses need to know about therapeutic and nontherapeutic effects of drugs.
- Work closely with the child's physician, pharmacist, and parents to provide the child with an effective medication regimen.
- Take time to understand the parents' point of view, and remain objective rather than taking sides with the child or the parents.
- Know about the availability of alcohol and street drugs and their adverse affects on the health and behavior of the child/adolescent.
- Enforce the facility seclusion/restraint policy if the child/adolescent needs help to control self-destructive or aggressive behaviors.
- Call appropriate emergency resources if the child/adolescent threatens staff or others with weapons or other destructive means.
- Reinforce age-appropriate behaviors and adaptive coping strategies used or attempted by the child or adolescent.
- Reinforce treatment and medication compliance efforts made by parents.
- Investigate community groups and resources to help the client and family after discharge.
- Investigate current educational resources available on the Internet and in the library.

- Instruct the parents to contact appropriate resources if they feel frustrated, out of control, or at risk for harming their child/adolescent.
- Instruct the parents to contact emergency resources if their child/adolescent threatens them or others with a weapon or other destructive means.
- Teach the parents/family that the best approach may be to remove themselves temporarily from a frustrating situation, then count to 10, call a friend, take a soothing bath, or perform a physical activity.
- Teach the parents how to assess for symptoms of alcohol or street drug use, if parents or staff suspect the child/adolescent is using these substances.
- Instruct the parents/family how to maintain safety in the home, personal safety, client safety, and personal boundaries.
- Educate the family in identifying stressors that may provoke the client's disruptive or aggressive behaviors, and teach strategies to avoid or modify them.
- Teach the parents how to use assertive communication skills and mature role modeling when interacting with their child/adolescent.
- Give more time and special instructions to parents with cultural, ethnic, or developmental challenges when educating them about their child's disorder.
- Emphasize to the parents the importance of showing love for their child/adolescent while still setting appropriate limits for disruptive behaviors.
- Reinforce with the parents that compliance with the treatment plan and medication regimen is critical to the client's behavior modification.
- Emphasize to the parents/family the importance of encouraging and reinforcing the client's adaptive functioning and age-appropriate behaviors.
- Praise the client/parents/family for efforts made toward positive interactions.
- Inform the parents about the availability of local support groups for children and adolescents with mental disorders.
- Educate the parents about current educational and supportive resources on the Internet and in the library, and include the client as appropriate.

Care Plans

Attention Deficit and Disruptive Behavior Disorders
- Risk for Self-Directed Violence and Risk for Other-Directed Violence

Mental Retardation or Pervasive Developent Disorders
- Delayed Growth and Development

Care Plan
Attention Deficit and Disruptive Behavior Disorders

NANDA Diagnosis: Risk for Self-Directed Violence and Risk for Other-Directed Violence

At risk for behaviors in which an individual demonstrates that he or she can be physically, emotionally, or sexually harmful to self or others.

Focus:
For the child or adolescent who demonstrates a persistent pattern of behaviors, with conduct and oppositional disorders that violate the rights of others, including potentially physically aggressive or violent acts directed toward self, persons, or property.

RISK FACTORS

Overt, aggressive acts directed toward others and the environment
- The client throws food tray and other objects in presence of others.
- Shouts or curses loudly in classroom or group activity.
- Threatens to harm staff members, peers, and family members.

Self-destructive behavior (active)
- Suicidal thoughts/gestures/plans

History of destructive or violent behaviors self-directed or directed at others

Frequent use of curse words or obscene language without obvious provocation

Pattern of resistance, defiance, or opposition toward authority figures, rules, and regulations
- Running away from home with foster home/institutional placement
- Sexual promiscuity or acting-out behaviors

Pattern of cruel, hostile, or destructive behaviors
- Cruelty to animals
- Starting fires

Inability to attend to tasks or activities, with concomitant hyperactivity (rule out mania)

- The client is easily distracted during schoolwork and in group activities.
- Wanders restlessly around classroom or unit and is intrusive to others

Frequent loss of temper (low impulse control)

Low frustration tolerance
- Is quick to anger during task performance
- Gives up in anger before task is completed

Impaired social or school functioning
- Lies, steals, cheats
- Truant; disruptive in classroom

History of alcohol, drug, or tobacco use

History of alcohol-dependent father or absent father or father figure

History of rejection or abuse by parents or parental figures

History of harsh or inconsistent discipline or management of care by parents or parental figures

Frequent shifting of parental figures (foster parents, stepparents, relatives)

Frequent shifting of residences (homes, institutions)

Low self-esteem

Powerlessness

OUTCOME IDENTIFICATION AND EVALUATION

The client verbalizes awareness of factors and situations that precipitate violent behaviors.

Relates understanding of negative effects of aggressive or violent behaviors.

Avoids situations that precipitate aggressive or violent behaviors.

Expresses anger in appropriate ways: physical activities and exercise, sports/hobbies, talking to staff members or peers.

Uses defense mechanisms adaptively to rechannel or reduce angry feelings: displacement, compensation, sublimation, identification.

Uses assertive rather than aggressive communication with adults and peers ("I" *not* "You" statements).

Continued

Participates in stress-reducing strategies to redirect and reduce angry feelings: deep-breathing exercises, relaxation techniques, thought stopping/substitution exercises, visual imagery, positive affirmations via cognitive therapy/assertiveness training (see Appendix B).
Demonstrates absence of hostile, aggressive threats and gestures directed toward environment.

Demonstrates absence of suicidal ideation, gestures, plans.
Identifies and utilizes resources and support systems effectively: trusted significant adults, staff members, social worker, teacher(s), counselor/therapist.
Initiates own behavioral contract to manage anger and avoid aggressive, violent behavior (in the hospital and at home).

PLANNING AND IMPLEMENTATION

Nursing Intervention	Rationale
Assess cues and warning signals: behavioral changes, escalating anger/anxiety, hyperactivity, recently disrupted family, chronic dysfunctional family life.	The child's/adolescent's impulsive or violent reactions to stressful situations may be preceded by behavioral cues or changes. The nurse's keen assessment skills can prevent harm or injury to the client and others.

Demonstrate acceptance of painful feelings that generally underlie the child's/adolescent's behavior, while not condoning the specific behavior.

Anger and aggression often signify a cry for help or a defense against a reality that the child/adolescent finds intolerable. The therapeutic response indicates that acceptance of feelings validates self-worth, even though disruptive or inappropriate behavior is not acceptable.

The nontherapeutic response suggests that the client, his feelings, and his behaviors are all equally undesirable and unacceptable. This could diminish his self-esteem because it does not separate the behavior from the client and his feelings. It may ultimately create a barrier to further communication between the nurse and the client.

Therapeutic Responses
- "Billy, yelling and swearing in the cafeteria is not acceptable behavior. Finish your lunch without using this behavior, and we'll talk about your feelings then."
If the child/adolescent cannot stop using inappropriate behaviors: "Billy, since you are still yelling and cursing, you'll have to leave the cafeteria and finish your meal later. We'll talk about your feelings then."

Nontherapeutic Response
"Billy, you know better than to yell and curse like that. We cannot tolerate it, and you'll have to stop if you want to be accepted in this unit."

Investigate the client's past suicide attempts and violent acts directed toward others to determine the potential seriousness of present behaviors (threats, gestures, plans). Note severity of threatening behaviors (on a scale of 1 to 10, with 1 being least severe and 10 being most severe) and availability of means.

Knowledge of previous patterns of violence helps the nurse assess the client's tolerance for stress so that action can be taken to prevent subsequent destructive acts.

Initiate a "show of concern" with the child or adolescent who cannot control anger and when risk of violence is imminent.
- Gather several trusted staff around the client without putting hands on, unless necessary.

"Show of concern" is a therapeutic intervention used to help the young client manage volatile feelings and behaviors and prevent harm or injury to self and others. It indicates to the client that staff is nearby to help the client maintain control when the client is unable to control self.

Initiate suicide precautions and seclusion/restraint protocol if the client's aggressive behavior escalates to 8 to 10 in severity and the client cannot be managed safely through other methods. (See Risk for Suicide, Chapter 3.)

Suicide precautions and seclusion/restraint may be necessary to prevent the client and others from harm or injury.

Maintain a therapeutic environment with external controls, such as suicide precautions or behavioral contract with clear, specific rules and consequences, if the client can comply.

These interventions may assist the client to maintain control until he or she is able to use internal controls to modify or reduce inappropriate, aggressive, or destructive behaviors.

Approach the adolescent with respect; avoid a judgmental/authoritarian attitude.

Adolescents are attempting to meet the developmental task of identification and avoid feelings of role confusion. They need approval and acceptance from adults as much as they need direction and limit setting.

Avoid use of teenage jargon when interacting with adolescents, for example, "cool," "hot," or "bad."

Adults who try to be "hip" and use teen terminology generally create distance and distrust between themselves and adolescents, who need adult role models they can count on when they are out of control.

Clarify teenage expressions or jargon that are unclear, rather than acting as if you understand everything that is said.

Adolescents respect honesty, especially when they come from troubled or dysfunctional families where honesty is rare or nonexistent. Honesty builds trust when used tactfully and appropriately.

Avoid "why" questions with children and adolescents.

"Why" questions suggest that the client is wrong to think, feel or behave a certain way, which invalidates the individual.

With the adolescent, "why" questions tend to evoke defensiveness or intellectualization rather than awareness and exploration.

Therapeutic Responses

- "Sarah, what happened just before you threw your tray on the floor?"
- "Jimmy, how come you reacted so strongly in group today?"

Nontherapeutic Responses

"Sarah, *why* did you throw your tray?"
"Jimmy, *why* were you so angry in group today?"

Use open-ended instead of closed-ended questions.

With the young child, "why" questions tend to evoke the response "because," with a concomitant "bad feeling."

Open-ended questions allow the child/adolescent to explain feelings, thoughts, or actions rather than be restricted to "yes" or "no" responses.
Open-ended questions are nonjudgmental and allow clients to be the expert about themselves.

Therapeutic Responses

- "Mark, what are your thoughts about the contract?"
- "Susan, how do you feel when the group focuses on you?"

Nontherapeutic Responses

"Mark, do you think your contract is fair?"
"Susan, does it upset you to be the focus of attention?"

Observe and listen for nonverbal cues that may be symptoms of increasing anxiety, anger, or agitation.
- The client looks down or away from the interviewer.
- Takes long, frequent pauses.
- Stutters; has flushed face; wrings hands.
- Looks bored, frustrated, or troubled.

Keen observations and listening skills can alert the nurse-interviewer to impending aggressive or violent behavior so that preventive interventions can be taken early and serious harm or injury avoided.

Teach the child or adolescent simple stress management strategies: deep-breathing exercises, relaxation techniques, thought-stopping exercises, visual imagery, positive affirmations/other cognitive strategies (see Appendix B).

Therapeutic strategies may help the young client to redirect the energy generated by anger and anxiety toward healthy functional anxiety-reducing activities and exercises.

Engage the client in physical activities: Ping-Pong, volleyball, stationary bicycle, brisk walks, running.

Physical activities help the young client use and channel energy toward healthy, productive activities that increase self-fulfillment and reduce uncontrollable anger and anxiety.

Engage the client (with his or her input) in more satisfying, alternative outlets to redirect angry feelings: physical activities such as pillows or batakas to pound; soft balls to throw at inanimate objects; use of "quiet/alone time," or remain with staff member to talk it out.
Note: Staff members can help the client express feelings and begin to recognize the value of appropriately handling anger.

Satisfying alternative outlets that help the client cope with anger or stress reduce the need to direct angry feelings toward the environment in the form of aggressive or violent behaviors. Physical outlets help relieve pent-up tension, frustration, and anxiety. The child or adolescent may initially view quiet time as punitive but may eventually consider it a helpful way to gain control over angry, volatile feelings, as he or she takes more and more responsibility for initiating own "quiet/alone times."

PLANNING AND IMPLEMENTATION—cont'd

Nursing Intervention	Rationale
Provide individual or group counseling that includes the presence of significant others approved by the child or adolescent: parent(s), best friend, sibling(s), group of same gender or with same problem, or mixed group of teens. (See Group Therapy, Appendix B.)	Individual sessions provide opportunities for the client to vent personal problems and conflicts with a trusted nurse. Group work offers opportunities for increased insight and understanding of self and others and for group support. Discussion and practice sessions can be continued at the group's own pace. Angry feelings can be expressed and explored in a controlled setting with professional group facilitators.
Make a contract for confidentiality with the adolescent; state that information shared with staff will not be discussed with parents, foster parents, or others unless teen gives permission to do so. Explain that the only exception would be if the adolescent threatens or plans to harm self or others, in which case protective actions would be taken, including talking with significant others after making the same contract with them.	Assurance of confidentiality between the client and the staff builds trust and self-worth in adolescents who have found few role models to trust. A contract for confidentiality also opens up channels of communication that can be used to further explore and manage angry feelings. *Note:* The adolescent must be capable of complying with the contract.
Engage the client in role-playing situations in individual and group sessions (see Child/Adolescent Counseling). *Note:* Facilitators must be trained in role play and sociodrama theory and strategies.	Role playing provides opportunities for the client to reverse roles with trusted staff and group members, who portray significant others with whom the client can ventilate pent-up emotions.
Help children and adolescents clarify values through exploration of self-awareness (values clarification exercises). When values and beliefs are incongruent with behaviors, the individual experiences conflict, confusion, and ambivalence.	Values clarification exercises help children and teens develop a value system by questioning, learning, and *Note:* trying out alternative value systems. Building a strong, positive value-belief system can influence behaviors and reduce the incidence of aggressive or violent episodes.
Help adolescents compare and contrast their own values and beliefs with others, noting similarities and differences, by devising exercises in which the youngster can state "I strongly agree" or "I strongly disagree." Inform the adolescent that occasional emotional outbursts are normal reactions to accumulated feelings of anxiety, confusion, and ambivalence.	These exercises help the adolescent develop a greater awareness of own values, express own values, problem-solve alternative values, and select from alternative values with consideration of the consequences. They also help to increase awareness of feelings, thoughts, and ideas regarding adolescent issues (relationships with peers, parents, foster families; body image; sexuality).

Therapeutic Responses

- "This is upsetting for you. It would be for most people your age."
- "It's OK to feel angry. What else about that makes you mad?"

Therapeutic responses help assure the client that all adolescents experience unpredictable emotional highs and lows related to hormonal activity, adjustment to puberty, and pending adulthood. The adolescent sees that he or she is like any other adolescent and thus does not need to experience overwhelming guilt, embarrassment or shame each time he or she cannot control angry outbursts.

Nontherapeutic Responses

"Try not to get so angry about these things."
"Don't feel so upset about this; it's not necessary."
Role-model assertive communication skills.

Nontherapeutic responses infer that the adolescent's feelings or reactions are wrong or exaggerated, which could result in shame, embarrassment, or guilt and inhibit further communication.

Assertive Responses

- Use "I" statements (I feel, I want, I don't want, I like, I don't like, I am willing to).
- "I'm angry at your behavior."
- "I'm upset with the way your room is messed up."

Assertive responses teach the adolescent to express his or her needs and negotiate workable compromises instead of responding with aggressive communication to have needs met.

Nonassertive Responses

Use "You" statements.
"You make me so mad."
"You're sloppy. Your room is a mess." (See Appendix B.)

Teach the adolescent to use coping mechanisms appropriately.

- *Displacement* of anger/aggression through physical exercises, activities (e.g., punching bag, batakas, clay therapy).
- *Compensation* for perceived deficiencies by excelling in schoolwork, arts, crafts, sports, music.
- *Sublimation* of aggressive feelings through hobbies, sports, recreation (e.g., video games, boxing, baseball).
- *Identification* with trusted adults and peers who role-model mature, assertive behaviors.

Nonassertive responses tend to diminish self-esteem and evoke aggressive or defensive responses in the individuals to whom they are addressed.

Healthy use of coping mechanisms helps the young client cope more effectively with stress, anger, anxiety, and frustration and to manage uncontrolled outbursts and aggression.

Child/Adolescent Counseling

Engage the client in ongoing counseling with a supportive child/adolescent therapist, in collaboration with the psychiatrist, to help the young client adapt to changes and disruptions in his or her life, such as transition from family home to foster family home, from one foster family to another, or from a home to an institution.

Help the child and adolescent respond and cope with unstable or shifting environments through role-playing situations.
1. Role-play exercise *without* use of learned concepts.
Nurse [role-playing parent figure]: "Jimmy, your room is still a mess [loud, angry voice]. You promised to clean it before you went to school today."
Jimmy [client playing himself]: "You're always yelling at me [loud, angry voice]. Why can't you let me do what I want with my own room?"
2. Role-play exercise *with* use of learned concepts.
Nurse [role-playing parent figure]: "Jimmy, your room is still a mess [loud, angry voice]. You promised to clean it before you went to school today."
Jimmy [client playing himself]: "Mom, I realize I didn't clean my room when I said I would [calm, low to moderate voice]. I'll get to it right away."
Note: Role playing can be used in a variety of situations with young clients, some of which include providing opportunities for risk taking and problem solving as the child makes the transition into adolescence and the adolescent moves into adulthood. Separation from family, gaining independence, forming peer groups, developing intimate relationships, and expressing unique values and interests, while adhering to social norms when necessary, are all critical skills for a successful, satisfying life. For the young client with a conduct disorder whose significant adult role models and home life are not always stable, role playing can be a helpful adjunct to the client's overall therapy.

Practice assertive behaviors with adolescents in individual and group settings, using situations that occur in everyday life, progressing from simple, nonthreatening situations to more difficult, threatening situations.

Children and adolescents with ongoing conduct disorders and behavioral problems are often shifted from one place of residence to another and need help to learn how to respond and adapt to different environments, some of which may be dysfunctional.

Role playing helps the client practice responses and behaviors in simulated real-life family situations. Role playing can be used to help young clients explore different responses and behaviors, choose those behaviors that yield more positive results, and begin to problem-solve as they incorporate learned concepts of values clarification and assertive responses in the role-playing exercises.
The first role-playing situation illustrates the client's lack of assertive communication in response to his mother's angry statement. Instead, Jimmy matches his mother's emotion with an equally angry response, which only perpetuates the volatile situation.
The second role-playing situation illustrates the client's use of assertive communication in response to his mother's angry remark, which reflects the young person's growing awareness that words have the power to change a negative situation into a positive one. As the child/adolescent gains more satisfying results through assertive communication, the client will incorporate those skills into his or her own value system and continue to use them in subsequent relationships with peers and other adults.

This type of simulated role playing helps prepare the adolescent for similar real-life events with the individuals in his or her life and avoids explosive emotional encounters with significant others.

Continued

PLANNING AND IMPLEMENTATION—cont'd

Nursing Intervention	Rationale
Child/Adolescent Counseling—cont'd	
Give the adolescent honest feedback regarding the effectiveness or ineffectiveness of learned assertive responses used during role-play practice sessions.	Genuine feedback helps to support and strengthen the client's successful responses and discourages unsuccessful communication.
Behavior Modification Systems	
Construct a behavior modification system. In a *token system,* for example, the child/adolescent earns tokens that can be exchanged for personal items or benefits, contingent on the client's behaviors.	Behavior modification systems reinforce positive behaviors by offering personal rewards as incentives. Some systems include loss of tokens for negative behaviors, such as lying, stealing, aggression, and violence.
Design a level system in which young clients gain access to more privileges, consistent with improved behaviors.	The level system is a behavior modification system that offers higher client status along with more privileges, contingent on the client's behavior. Some level systems include demotion to lower levels for negative behaviors or regression to earlier level behaviors.
Construct a written behavioral contract (when appropriate) that clearly states which behaviors are acceptable and which behaviors are unacceptable. Describe specific consequences expected for each unacceptable behavior while adhering to reward systems for acceptable behaviors. Include a time frame in which consequences begin and end.	Children and teens need to test limits as part of learning about themselves and acceptable behaviors in different situations. Firm, fair limit setting tends to promote trust and to prevent acting-out, disorganized, or violent behaviors. Although certain behaviors may be negotiable, stipulating those that are and are not acceptable teaches young people to learn how to set their own limits, a necessary adult skill.
Family Education and Therapy	
Engage families and foster families in ongoing family therapy sessions with and without the identified client (see Appendix B).	Family members need to be aware of the effect each of their roles has on the client's dysfunctional behavior and on the dysfunctional behavior of the family as a unit. The child/adolescent's behavior is a reflection of the entire family's dysfunction, and generally the entire family system needs therapy.
Praise the child/adolescent and the family/foster family for engaging in more functional, socially appropriate interactions that produce positive relationships and reduced or absent aggressive or violent episodes.	Positive feedback reinforces repetition of functional, appropriate behaviors and increases self-esteem for the individual client and the family unit.

Care Plan

DSM-IV-TR Diagnosis **Mental Retardation or Pervasive Developmental Disorders**

NANDA Diagnosis: Delayed Growth and Development
Deviations from age-group norms.

Focus:
For the child or adolescent with a developmental disorder who demonstrates a predominant disturbance in the acquisition of cognitive, language, motor, or social skills, such as a general delay (mental retardation) or a failure to progress in a specific area (speech, motor skills) or in multiple areas in which there are qualitative distortions (pervasive disorder, e.g., autism)

RELATED FACTORS (ETIOLOGY)
Cognitive/mental/emotional deficits
Biologic/psychologic/sociologic factors

DEFINING CHARACTERISTICS
Demonstrates significantly below-average intellectual functioning (IQ of 70 and below, or clinical judgment in infants)

Mild Mental Retardation: Childhood

The client demonstrates social and communication skills that may be indistinguishable from children of the same age (0 to 5 years).
Participates appropriately in children's games activities.
Interacts socially with children of average intelligence.

Mild Mental Retardation: Adolescence

Demonstrates social and communication skills slightly below abilities of peer group.
Exhibits deficits in academic abilities (in contrast to peers) that are noticeable in classroom situations requiring problem solving beyond the client's capacity.

Mild Mental Retardation: Young Adulthood

Demonstrates social and vocational skills adequate for minimum self-support.
Demonstrates ability to care for self: grooms, cooks, cleans own home.
Establishes intimate relationship consistent with social abilities.
Performs at skilled job commensurate with educational/social skills.
Demonstrates ability to live independently with minimal support, but requires guidance and assistance during times of unusual social, emotional, or economic stress.
Note: The client may live in an independent living complex supervised by managers who are trained to assist developmentally challenged tenants in crisis or emergency situations.

Moderate Mental Retardation: Childhood

The client demonstrates ability to talk or learn to communicate during preschool years with greater effort than children of same age.

Moderate Mental Retardation: Adolescence

Demonstrates ability to care for self with moderate supervision and guidance.
Displays difficulty adhering to social conventions, which disrupts peer relationships.
Exhibits pronounced intellectual impairment (unlikely to progress beyond second-grade level).

Moderate Mental Retardation: Young Adulthood

Demonstrates ability to improve skills with individualized social, occupational, or vocational training.
Performs unskilled or semiskilled work under close supervision (sheltered workshop, competitive job market).
Requires extra supervision and guidance during times of stress or crisis.
Needs the structure and supervision of a group home.

Severe Mental Retardation: Childhood

The client displays poor motor development during preschool period (uncoordinated, slow, hesitant).
Acquires little or no communicative speech during preschool period.
Exhibits ability to learn to speak and perform simple hygiene skills during school-age years.

Severe Mental Retardation: Adolescence

Demonstrates only limited ability to learn the alphabet and master simple counting.
Displays ability to learn sight-reading of some "survival" words (men, women, stop).

Severe Mental Retardation: Adulthood

Demonstrates ability to perform simple tasks under close supervision: housework, short simple errands, unskilled job, simple games activities.
Demonstrates ability to live in group home or with family under close supervision.

Profound Mental Retardation: Childhood

The client displays minimal capacity for sensorimotor functioning. Requires highly structured environment with constant aid and supervision to perform self-care.
Note: Some clients may not achieve this goal.
Performs simple tasks under close, individualized supervision by a caregiver.

Profound Mental Retardation: Adolescence

Demonstrates some improvement in motor development, self-care, and communication skills with continued training.

Profound Mental Retardation: Adulthood

Resides in group home, intermediate care facility, or with family.
Performs simple tasks under close supervision in day programs or sheltered workshops.
Note: Some clients may not achieve this goal.

Pervasive Developmental Disorders (Autistic Disorder)

Impaired Social Interactions
The client demonstrates marked lack of awareness of the existence or feelings of others.
Treats others as if they were pieces of furniture or other inanimate objects.
Fails to notice the distress of other individuals.
Lacks awareness of the need for others' privacy.
Displays absent comfort-seeking behaviors when ill, hurt, tired, or distressed.
Seeks comfort in a bizarre, stereotypic manner.
Says "Go, go, go," or other phrase/term whenever hurt.
Exhibits impaired or absent modeling of others' social behaviors.

Continued

- Fails to wave good-bye.
- Does not imitate parents' domestic activities (dusting, sweeping).
- Copies others' actions in robotic, out-of-context manner.

Demonstrates absent or abnormal social play.

- Does not actively engage in simple games.
- Manifests solitary play activities.
- Responds to other children in play only as "mechanical aids."

Displays impaired ability to engage in peer friendships.

Lacks awareness of conventions of social interactions.

- Reads or recites phone book to uninterested peers.

Impaired Verbal/Nonverbal Communication and Imagination Activity

The client demonstrates absent mode of communication.

- Displays lack of verbal babbling, facial expression, gestures, mime, or spoken language.

Displays abnormal nonverbal communication.

- Uses eye contact, facial expression, body posture, or gestures to initiate or modulate social interactions.
- Fails to anticipate being held.
- Stiffens when held.
- Does not look at the person or smile when making a social approach.
- Fails to greet parents or visitors.
- Has a fixed stare in social situations.

Manifests absence of imaginative activity.

- Displays lack of play acting of adult roles, fantasy characters, animals.
- Shows no interest in imaginative stories or events.

Demonstrates marked abnormalities of speech, including pitch, volume, rate, rhythm, stress, and tone (e.g., monotonous tone, "question like" melody or high pitch)

Displays marked abnormalities in the form or content of speech, including stereotypic and repetitive use of speech.

- Demonstrates immediate echolalia (repeats the words of others).
- Repeats television commercials in mechanical manner.
- Uses "you" when "I" is meant (e.g., states "you" want a drink while actually meaning "I" want a drink).
- Uses idiosyncratic words or phrases (e.g., states "go fast riding" to mean "I want to ride in the car").
- Makes frequent irrelevant statements (e.g., starts talking about baseball during a conversation about music).

Demonstrates marked impairment in the ability to initiate or sustain a conversation with others despite adequate speech.

- Indulges in lengthy monologues on one topic regardless of others' interjections.

Greatly Restricted Repertoire of Activities and Interests

The client displays stereotypic body movements: hand flickering, hand twisting, hand flapping, head banging, spinning, complicated bizarre whole-body movements.

Manifests persistent preoccupation with objects or parts of objects.

- Sniffs or smells objects.
- Repeatedly feels texture of materials.
- Spins wheels of toy cars and trucks.
- Shows attachment to unusual objects (e.g., insists on carrying around article of clothing or piece of string).

Displays marked distress over trivial environmental changes (e.g., when a vase/lamp is moved from its usual place or position to another).

- Cries, screams, or stamps feet.
- Repeats words that generally indicate trouble or distress.

Demonstrates unreasonable insistence on complying with routines in precise detail.

- Insists on viewing a particular television show regardless of priorities or circumstances.

Exhibits greatly restricted range of interests and a preoccupation with one narrow or specific interest.

- Plays with toothpicks and places them in rows.
- Gathers facts about astrology.
- Discusses characters on favorite television show.

Note: It is beyond the scope of this care plan to include every possible specific developmental disorder. Please refer to theory section for further information.

OUTCOME IDENTIFICATION AND EVALUATION

The client demonstrates self-care in daily activities within level of cognitive, emotional, and behavioral capabilities.

Displays control of angry, impulsive emotions.

Demonstrates absence of aggressive acting-out behaviors.

Uses communication and language skills to express self clearly and have needs met.

Verbalizes a variety of feelings in appropriate manner.

Exhibits meaningful interactions with staff, peers, and parents consistent with developmental level.

Demonstrates ability to perform satisfactory age-appropriate tasks with minimal assistance.

Displays significant control of stereotypic, ritualistic behaviors (hand flapping, whirling).

Participates appropriately in milieu, group, and individual activities and in classroom setting.

Seeks attention appropriately from known persons, and refrains from unnecessary interactions with unknown individuals (autistic children often cannot distinguish between strangers and significant others).

Complies with treatment regimen, including medication as needed.

Demonstrates increase in self-concept and self-esteem: brightened mood/affect, increased play/laughter, active participation in activities/groups, absence of apathy/dysphoria/acting-out behaviors.

Note: Include family in outcome criteria as relevant.

PLANNING AND IMPLEMENTATION

Nursing Intervention	Rationale
Mental Retardation	

Assess the following in collaboration with other health care team members: the individual's intellectual function via such tools as the Stanford-Binet Intelligence Scale (IQ) and other assessment tools; gross and fine motor skills; behavior, cognition, mood, affect, language, play, self-care skills (e.g., hygiene, toileting, grooming); social communication and interactive capabilities; level of independence; ability to work; ability to solve own problems; adaptation to environment; development of relationships with family, peers, teachers, nurse, therapist, and intimacy with significant person.	Initial assessment of the individual's capabilities and levels of function by nursing and the treatment team helps to focus on strengths rather than weaknesses and serves as a guide for more accurate, meaningful interventions.
Contrast the client's present developmental task with standard age-related tasks as indicated in Erikson's psychosocial stages of man, Piaget's stages of cognition, or Sullivan's interpersonal stages (see developmental theories in texts and other sources).	Review of stages of growth and development by expert theorists such as Erikson and others helps the nurse and treatment team identify the client's growth and developmental strengths and weaknesses and plan interventions relevant to problem areas.
Approach the client in a calm, nonjudgmental manner rather than with an intense, hurried approach.	A calm demeanor by the nurse helps to reduce anxiety, promote trust, and elicit calm responses from the client. Anxiety is transferable.
Communicate and interact with the client in an age-appropriate manner, being careful not to infantilize the client and not to use an authoritarian approach.	Communicating according to the client's age and level of development helps maintain the client's dignity and promote self-esteem. Infantilizing the client or using an authoritarian approach increases dependence and may cause resentment.
Accompany the client and family on a tour of the mental health facility.	A tour of the facility by nursing staff helps to promote familiarity and comfort, reduce anxiety, and orient the client to the environment.
Introduce the client to staff members and other clients slowly (no more than three persons per day).	A slow introduction phase helps to decrease fear and confusion and build trust at a pace consistent with the client's tolerance.
Instruct the client and family slowly in relevant unit rules regarding activities of daily living, safety factors, and behavior toward peers (no more than three rules per day).	This instruction helps to facilitate the client's/family's understanding at a pace consistent with their tolerance and ability.
Supervise the child/adolescent closely for at least 2 days. *Note:* Hospitalization or institutionalization can cause the client to regress; therefore more time may be needed to determine the client's capabilities.	Close supervision in the early stages of hospitalization helps the nurse and treatment team assess the client's strengths and capabilities and specific areas that require assistance.
Allow the child/adolescent to be as independent as possible, offering assistance when necessary.	Independence encourages the client to maximize his or her developmental potential. Infantilizing the client could foster regression.
Schedule group activities in a progressive manner and increase as tolerated. • Engage the client in one group activity per day during the first week. • Ensure that at least one group activity consists of peers in the same age group as the client. • Allow group activities to last no longer than 20 minutes for the first week.	Scheduling activities in a routine manner helps the client gradually become acquainted with peers and learn to interact with them at a tolerable pace.

Continued

PLANNING AND IMPLEMENTATION—cont'd

Nursing Intervention	Rationale
Mental Retardation—cont'd	
Engage the client in more structured groups initially (occupational therapy), and progress to more informal activities (recreational therapy).	Individuals with developmental disabilities learn more quickly from a structured, individualized activity that can help prepare them for less structured groups.
Establish a routine; schedule meals, naps, medications, and treatments at the same time each day to maintain consistency and structure.	Children and adults with developmental disabilities perform better when they know what to expect.
Inform the client of each daily activity immediately before the activity, rather than recite the entire daily schedule only once in the morning.	This approach helps to facilitate attendance, establish a routine, and allay anxiety and confusion. Persons with developmental disabilities need extra reinforcement and reminding.
Construct activities and groups that will meet the needs of the participants and that consist of tasks and strategies that are realistic for clients' intellectual and social levels of function.	Activities should be modified and planned so that they allow the individual to succeed and thus enhance self-esteem, rather than exceed the level of the client's capabilities. Success is the best reinforcement for repetition of positive behaviors.
Engage the client in activities and exercises: arts and crafts, Bingo, volleyball (regular or "sit down"), Ping-Pong, simple stretching exercises, walking, running.	Activities and exercises enhance fine and gross motor skills and promote the client's social interactions with peers and staff.
Schedule small group outings with the activity therapist: a trip to the grocery store or fast-food restaurant, a movie, the zoo, a picnic at the beach, a hike in the park.	Outings and activities facilitate "normal" recreation and social activities and promote verbal and motor skills.
Help each client maximize his or her individual developmental potential by offering as many "normal" experiences as possible (supervise as necessary). • Allow the client to make minor purchases in a grocery store or fast-food restaurant. • Assign unit tasks (e.g., setting the table, decorating the unit). • Engage the client to help set up for activities and clean up afterward. • Assign a different client each day or week to help in the classroom.	Offering normal experiences to maximize the client's developmental potential enhances the client's age-related tasks and builds self-esteem.
Provide assistance as needed with personal hygiene, toileting, grooming, and other self-care needs, making certain that nothing is done for the client that he or she can do alone.	This approach helps to promote the client's comfort, dignity, independence, and self-esteem and protect the client from the ridicule of peers.
Engage the client in "normal" experiences: eat meals in the dining room with other clients, attend all activities.	Normal experiences promote the client's healthy adjustment to the environment, mental and physical growth, independence, and self-esteem.
Provide the client with personal space so that he or she will have room for personal belongings that can remain visible and accessible to the client: alphabet board, books, chalkboard; blocks with numbers and letters; clothing, shoes; hairbrush, comb, toothbrush.	Belongings that are constantly put away and hidden from view may be forgotten by the client and therefore not used, which could inhibit the client's progress.
Help the child/adolescent take care of personal belongings and personal, physical environment.	Helping young clients with personal responsibility promotes independence and increases self-esteem.

Develop with the child/adolescent and parents a teaching plan in daily living skills based on regular periodic assessments.
- Do not overwhelm the child/adolescent with too many tasks at once; assist with each skill individually until client masters it, then move on to the next skill.
- Repeat skills as often as necessary.
- Praise frequently for efforts and accomplishments.
- Be realistic in expectations and assist the family to be realistic as well.

Growth and development are continuous and can be enhanced if both the client and family agree on basic strategies. Continued assessment is critical because the client's physical and emotional state fluctuate and may influence the level of self-care functioning.

Provide opportunities for parents to ventilate feelings of frustration without the threat of shame or guilt.

Unresolved feelings could promote hostility and resentment and interfere with the parent-child/adolescent relationship.

Pain Assessment

Educate parents in signs and symptoms of physical illness, for example, signs of pain or distress.
- Sudden change in behavior
- Restlessness
- Facial grimacing
- Diaphoresis
- Change in body temperature, heart rate, skin color
- Loss of appetite, loss of weight
- Change in bowel, bladder function
- Altered sleep patterns
- Vomiting, spitting up blood
- Frequent or sudden crying, moaning
- Holding affected body part (stomach, side, limb)
- Favoring affected body part (not using a hand or limping to avoid use of a leg)
- Bending over in apparent pain or distress
- Seizure activity (may be mistaken for hyperactivity)
- Consult with physician as necessary

Physical illness can be masked by the client's developmental disability or inability to communicate pain or distress. Parents need to be especially alert to signs and symptoms and means of identifying them.
Use of a pain rating scale with faces depicting levels of pain on a scale of 1 to 10 may assist in identifying the client's level of pain.

Construct a daily behavior rating scale, such as Connor's Behavior Rating Scale, with the parents, teacher, and other multidisciplinary team members.
If Connor's scale is not available, devise a Likert scale with responses such as "never," "some of the time," "most of the time," or "always," which offers a valid rating of the client's observable behaviors.

A behavior rating scale is one tool that helps to determine the client's impulse control, attention span, and activity level and assists staff in planning interventions.

Reinforce the client's appropriate behaviors and decrease or defuse unacceptable behaviors (temper tantrums, other acting-out responses) by constructing a behavior modification program consistent with the client's age, intellectual and social capabilities, and ability to comply with the program rules.(See the following interventions for examples of behavior modification.)

Children and adolescents with mental retardation need special guidance and direction to help manage impulsive, angry outbursts that interfere with their own growth and progress and with others' rights and physical space. Reinforcement of appropriate behaviors promotes repetition of positive responses.

Manage lewd or provocative language with a verbal warning initially.
- "Tommy, that language is not permitted."

Limit setting is necessary for management of inappropriate milieu behavior.

Express a second verbal warning if lewd or provocative behavior continues.
- "Susan, if you do not stop talking like that, you will have to go to your room for 15 minutes."

Consequences should be added to the warning as an additional incentive to stop negative behaviors.

Continued

PLANNING AND IMPLEMENTATION—cont'd

Nursing Intervention	Rationale
Mental Retardation—cont'd	

Nursing Intervention	Rationale
Initiate a 15-minute quiet/alone time if provocative behavior persists. (Quiet time should be part of the client's overall treatment program and used only when all else fails. It should not be used as a punitive, random measure.)	This time alone helps to reinforce verbal warnings with a behavior modification technique. Two verbal warnings should be followed by a quiet time because the client's inability to stop inappropriate behaviors illustrates the need for external control by staff.
Help the parents design a behavioral program similar to the one used in the facility and in the child's classroom. *Note:* Behavioral programs are most effective when combined with other therapies, psychosocial interventions, and medications, such as Ritalin.	This program helps to provide consistency and structure for the client, which reinforces appropriate behavior.
Administer prescribed medications as needed. (See section on medications for drugs used to treat hyperactivity.)	Prescribed medications are administered to help manage the child's uncontrolled, hyperactive behaviors so that the child can attend to daily activities and social and academic functions.
Review the therapeutic and nontherapeutic effects of medications with the child's teacher, parents, clinical psychologist, and social worker.	Knowledge promotes awareness of the role of medication as an adjunct to other therapeutic modalities and thus decreases anxiety.
Reward and praise the client for genuine efforts to comply with unit rules and regulations. For example, give verbal praise, points, stickers, or tokens that can be applied toward special privileges or activities. • "Billy, you picked up all your toys today. You will get 5 points for a treat." • "John, you get 10 points for not talking when others were talking. You can use them for a special activity." • "Kate, you didn't throw anything this afternoon. You will get five tokens to use in the gift shop." Place a sticker on the child's clothing whenever he or she is actively involved in self-care or other activity of daily living.	Genuine reward and praise for efforts to comply with unit rules help to reinforce positive behaviors. Children with developmental disabilities need frequent praise and rewards for their efforts, which serve as a method of behavior modification.
Instruct parents, guardians, and teachers to praise or reward the child/adolescent for paying attention to instruction and progressively increasing his or her attention span consistent with the client's level of developmental ability.	This instruction helps ensure consistency with the behavior modification programs used in the hospital or child/adolescent program.
Talk to the child/adolescent about the relationship between his or her behaviors and the incidents that preceded them. • "Sam, you were upset because. . . ." • "Sue, when that incident occurred, you became upset." • "Joe, this situation happened just before you got upset." • "Kate, just after that incident, you became upset."	This communication helps increase the client's understanding of incidents that may provoke overresponsive behaviors so that the client can choose a more acceptable response or behavior.
Help the client label his or her feelings. • "Kate, you were angry or mad because. . . ." • "Mark, you were feeling bad or sad and. . . ." *Note:* Children with autism find it difficult or even impossible to identify feelings and emotions.	Naming feelings is the first step toward increasing awareness of feelings and connecting them with the behaviors that follow. Naming feelings also enhances language development and allows the client to put angry or troubled feelings into words instead of destructive actions.
Permit the client to express feelings of anger and frustration (see Appendix B for relaxation techniques).	This helps the nurse and treatment team develop an awareness of the source of the client's feelings so that they can help direct the client's energy toward

Collaborate with special education teachers to provide opportunities to explain bodily changes, sexual functions, and issues of intimacy to the preadolescent/adolescent client, with specific, concrete examples and simple illustrations as needed.
Note: Parental or guardian permission and collaboration with the client's psychiatrist are recommended.

constructive activities and assist the client to cope with anger-provoking situations that cannot be changed through relaxation and other techniques.

Individuals with mental retardation often have neither the cognitive ability nor the coping skills to deal with adolescent issues, bodily changes, sexuality, and intimacy. Therefore they may become frightened and confused when normal changes occur (breast growth, menstruation, sexual arousal, penile erection, orgasm). Feelings and emotions such as sexual attraction and love may cause ambivalence and concern in parents and other caregivers, which could result in fear and guilt within the client, who may sense that he or she is "feeling bad things," "thinking bad thoughts," or "doing something wrong." Special sexuality education classes are needed to help these individuals develop a positive self-concept and sexual identity and a greater understanding of their bodies and emotions without fear, guilt, embarrassment, or shame.

Assess the child or adolescent for symptoms of depression, which may be masked by developmental problems such as apathy, dysphoria (anguish), acting out, isolation, or a sudden change in usual behavior patterns with no obvious cause.
Note: Suicide in children and adolescents is generally an impulsive act, often preceded by acting out or apathy (see Chapter 3).

Suicide assessment is critical to prevent self-destructive behaviors.

Explore plans for the possibility of group or independent living with the client, social worker, parents, guardian, and primary therapist after assessing the client's readiness for discharge.

It is important for the staff to facilitate aftercare discharge planning appropriate for the client's needs and consistent with family and community resources.

Encourage the client and parents or guardian to discuss with the social worker all information regarding appropriate facilities for the client.

Exploring available aftercare facilities and community resources appropriate for the client helps to identify alternative residential facilities from which to choose.

Explore cultural considerations with the client, parents, and social worker when selecting a permanent residence for the client.

This helps to assure the client and parents that cultural issues and preferences will be strongly considered in the decision-making process.

Consult with the client, teacher, social worker, and occupational therapist to provide the client with a vocation in the community through a program that prepares individuals with developmental disabilities for jobs consistent with their skills and capabilities.

Providing the client with a job commensurate with capability and potential helps to maximize the individual's vocational skills and ability to participate as a productive, independent citizen and to build a positive self-concept and self-worth.

Autistic Disorder

Use a team approach (parents, counselors, special education teachers, nurses, other significant individuals) to assess the needs of the child with autistic disorder.
- Special education teachers construct a weekly check sheet of the child's behavior and progress in the classroom.
- Parents use learned strategies consistent with team approach to promote structure in the home and elicit the child's cooperation.
- Counselors work with the child and family to promote positive interpersonal interactions.

An interdisciplinary approach to assessment, with the nurse as the team leader, helps to collect the necessary baseline information regarding the child's physical, emotional, and social functions and assists the team in achieving specific, consistent goals and client outcomes (see Chapter 1 for more information on data collection and the nursing process).

Continued

PLANNING AND IMPLEMENTATION—cont'd

Nursing Intervention	Rationale
Autistic Disorder—cont'd	

• Nurses use the nursing process to collect baseline data such as possible organic disorders (seizures) that could be masked by behavioral problems and coordinate all the multidisciplinary findings within an ongoing treatment plan.

Engage team members, teachers, and parents in frequent meetings.
Note: Evaluation of children with long-term developmental disabilities also includes frequent informal assessments and meetings.

Frequent meetings with all concerned people in the child's life are necessary to evaluate the child's progress and outcome attainment and to modify approaches and interventions as needed.

Help the autistic child develop a relationship with a significant person in the facility.
Note: Such a significant person can serve as a liaison between the client and others in the environment and can help minimize the client's isolation.

Developing a special or any relationship with at least one team member helps the autistic child to increase socialization skills and build trust. Autistic children often isolate themselves socially and cannot easily discriminate between parents and strangers. However, they can become attached in an unemotional way to a person who, with patience and consistent interactions, can enhance their social and developmental skills.

Structure scheduled daily activities to resemble the usual routine followed by the child at home or in a residential treatment center.
• Medications: administer at same time, in same manner as usual.
• Meals: serve favorite, usual foods and drinks.
• Naps: plan at usual time; allow client familiar blanket/pillow.
• Play objects: allow favorite toys/objects from home or residential treatment center.
• Routines: continue usual routines (TV shows).

Autistic children are especially resistant to change; therefore structured programs that are similar to usual, consistent routines tend to allay fear and anxiety.

Teach the autistic child one task at a time: washing hands, putting belongings away, buttoning shirt, zipping up zippers.

This approach helps to maximize the child's success and minimize failure and frustration.

Schedule one-to-one times with a primary staff member, such as 2 hours per shift at the same time each day.

Consistent staff and meeting times help develop a trusting relationship and maximize the client's language and communication skills.

Provide a quiet environment and decrease unnecessary sound, noise, and talking.

A quiet environment is soothing to the child and helps to protect him or her from injury and distress. Autistic children may overrespond to sound and behave erratically if there is too much noise, may cover ears in distress to escape sound, or may run from noisy area, injuring self in the process.

Place furniture as close to walls as possible, leaving as much open space in client area as feasible.

Autistic children experience disturbances in motion, such as whirling, lunging, darting, rocking, hand flapping, and head banging, and have a greater chance for injury in a crowded or cluttered area.

Provide the autistic child who has average to above-average intelligence with opportunities and experiences that enhance developmental growth and special interests, such as music, arts, and crafts.

Approximately one quarter to one third of autistic children have average to above-average intelligence but lack the social skills necessary for activities that will promote their special qualities. Significant patience is necessary for caregivers to enhance opportunities for peak development.

Avoid unnecessary or sudden touch when interacting with a child with autism.

The autistic child may be unable to accurately interpret or process sensory input such as touch and may overrespond, as if in pain or panic.

Ignore the autistic child's temper tantrums only if they are *not* harmful or life-threatening.

Ignoring tantrums decreases their frequency. Injurious or life-threatening behaviors should be stopped while the tantrum itself is ignored. Even though it is negative, focusing attention on the behavior will reinforce it.

For the child who impulsively hits or strikes out, hold the child's hands down and firmly state, "No hitting [child's name]."
If the child persists, use quiet time for approximately 2 minutes as a behavior modification strategy.
Note: Quiet time should take place in a quiet, nonstimulating area.

Allowing the child to spend some quiet or alone time, with staff supervision, helps the child to control impulsive behaviors and teaches the consequences of inappropriate actions in a nonthreatening way.

For the child who is easily distracted and has difficulty attending, hold the child's head gently between your own hands so that he or she faces you and looks directly into your eyes.
Establish eye contact and speak to the child slowly, simply, and clearly.
Note: This strategy is useful for all youngsters with attention deficits or who are easily distracted.

This basic strategy is often effective in helping to make the child aware of who is engaging him or her in the interaction and that the interaction is meaningful and requires attention.

Assess the environment and circumstances in which temper tantrums or overresponses occur.
- Sudden change or break occurs in daily routine or activities.
- The child is touched inadvertently by another person.
- The child is startled or troubled by noise or overstimulation.
- A favorite object (e.g., piece of string, cloth, article of clothing) is lost or misplaced.
- A routine television program is cancelled or interrupted.
- The child's ritual is disturbed with no alternative activity to replace it.

Assessing environmental and situational events that trigger temper tantrums or overreactive responses by the child helps the nurse and treatment team plan preventive strategies and interventions.

Speak to the child in short, concise sentences.

This helps to enhance the child's understanding and to hold his or her attention.

For the child with psychomotor rituals, call the child by name when stereotypic body movements occur, such as hand flapping, spinning, or lunging.

This approach helps to distract the client from the activity by gaining his or her attention.

Redirect the child to a constructive activity.

Redirection helps the child displace energy in a beneficial, productive way rather than through exhausting ritualistic behaviors.

Praise the child immediately for positive behaviors, such as attending to verbal instructions by teacher, nurse, parents, or therapist; interacting with peers versus parallel play activities; and engaging in constructive activities.

Immediate praise for positive behaviors reinforces appropriate behaviors. Children with autistic disorder especially need instant, frequent reinforcement for work well done.

Positive Feedback
- Give verbal approval: "Jimmy, you're doing a good job picking up your toys."
- Place a "praise sticker" on the child's shirt during an activity in which the child's behavior is appropriate or demonstrates improvement.
- Allow the child to continue with a favorite activity or game for 15 minutes longer because of appropriate behavior.

Continued

PLANNING AND IMPLEMENTATION—cont'd

Nursing Intervention	Rationale
Autistic Disorder—cont'd	
Provide toys, games, educational supplies, teaching aids, and vocational tools.	Educational aids and learning tools help promote the client's interest and enthusiasm for learning while increasing his or her knowledge base, social behaviors, motor skills, and cognitive abilities.
Explore with the client, social worker, and parents appropriate aftercare facilities if the child cannot reside with parents. *Note:* Refer to the first part of the intervention section in this care plan for additional interventions relevant to the child with autistic disorder.	A thorough exploration of aftercare facilities helps provide a permanent residence that will best meet the client's needs and maximize his or her strengths and capabilities.

## chapter 8

Delirium, Dementia, and Amnestic and Other Cognitive Disorders

Over the next decade the mental disorders in the categories of delirium, dementia, and amnestic and other cognitive disorders will result in extraordinary losses in terms of human despair, interrupted relationships, functional disturbances, and economic costs that will affect individuals, businesses, and governments. The most notable monetary loss will be attributed to cost of treatment for involved individuals and their families and to the loss of productivity associated with "the graying of America." Increasing numbers of aging people will develop these disorders. Productivity is also lost by caregivers, who often must interrupt or completely stop their occupations to care for the client. Cognitive disruption will occur especially in individuals diagnosed with dementia, a disorder that primarily targets the population with the greatest projected growth over the next several decades—the elderly.

Great hope was injected into these gloomy predictions in the form of an antimyloid vaccine (AN-1792) that promised to halt progression of Alzheimer's-type dementia. Research began with trials on mice that were genetically engineered to develop the neuritic amyloid plaques of dementia of the Alzheimer's type. The animal vaccine trials were successful, and studies were done in the United States and Great Britain on humans. The disappointing outcome was that participants developed brain inflammation and the trials were stopped. It is inevitable that research will continue to proliferate in an effort to find treatments and cure for these disorders.

COMMON CHARACTERISTICS

Dementia, delirium, and amnestic and other cognitive disorders are biologic illnesses with two defining characteristics in common. The first characteristic is a clinically significant *decrease in cognitive function* that is a marked change from the person's previous level of function. *Cognition* refers to multiple, interrelated mental processes that include memory, reasoning, judgment, orientation, problem solving, abstraction, and acquisition and use of knowledge and language. Without these processes working together in a synchronous way, dysfunction is inevitable.

The second characteristic common to delirium, dementia, and amnestic categories is that each disorder is caused by a general medical condition or by use of a substance (or a combination). Specific medical conditions may be diagnosed or undiagnosed at the time of symptom eruption, and may or may not be identified during the course of the disorder.

Substances may be in the following forms, with examples:

1. **Toxins:** industrial chemicals used in manufacturing that are inhaled or absorbed through skin; ingested gardening or cleaning products in the home that cause inadvertent poisoning of a very young child.
2. **Medications:** elderly person seeing more than one physician and using multiple incompatible prescription medications; intentional overdose of a prescribed narcotic in a suicide attempt by a person with chronic depression, disease, or pain.
3. **Drugs of abuse:** young people experimenting with and mixing illegal designer drugs at a rave party; heroin abuser who unintentionally overdoses on substances that are more potent than expected; housewife who drinks excessive amounts of alcohol every day.

Box 8-1 Etiology of Delirium, Dementia, and Amnestic and Other Cognitive Disorders

DELIRIUM

Central nervous system: head trauma, epilepsy, brain tumor
Vascular: stroke, hypertensive encephalopathy
Degenerative: Pick's disease, infections
Metabolic: renal/hepatic disease, fluid/electrolyte imbalance, hypoxia
Cardiopulmonary: congestive heart failure, shock, arrhythmias
Systemic: septicemia, urinary tract infection, pneumonia, neoplasms
Sensory deprivation: postoperative state, visual/hearing impairment
Substance induced: intoxication or withdrawal
Medications
- Anticholinergics: traditional antidepressants, antiparkinsonian agents, neuroleptics
- Antihistamines: over-the-counter remedies for cold, flu, sleep
- Antiarrhythmics: quinidine
- Sedative-hypnotics: benzodiazepines
- Narcotic analgesics
- Histamine-2 receptor blockers: cimetidine
- Anticonvulsants
- Beta-blockers
- Antihypertensives
- Corticosteroids
- Antibiotics
Toxins

DEMENTIA

Genetic factors: chromosomal mutations
Acetylcholine loss
Alzheimer's disease: neuritic plaques, neurofibrillary tangles
Vascular impairment: multiinfarct disorder
Human immunodeficiency virus (HIV)
Head trauma
Parkinson's disease
Huntington's disease (chorea)
Pick's disease
Creutzfeldt-Jakob disease
Substance induced, persisting: drug abuse, medications, toxins

AMNESTIC AND OTHER COGNITIVE DISORDERS

Primary systemic: hypoxia
Cerebrovascular disease
Closed head trauma
Brain surgery
Herpes simplex encephalopathy
Seizures
Substance induced: chronic alcoholism

ETIOLOGY

As noted, delirium, dementia, and amnestic and other cognitive disorders have an organic etiology, and the cause is always either a medical condition or a substance, or toxin, or a combination of these (Box 8-1).

EPIDEMIOLOGY

Delirium

The onset for delirium is usually rapid, and the course fluctuates. One of the most preventable, reversible, undiagnosed, underdiagnosed, and untreated mental conditions, delirium is often mistaken for other disorders, such as depression or dementia (Table 8-1). Delirium may be superimposed on other disorders, making it even more difficult to identify, and then may be missed. Although difficult to identify because of its fluctuating nature, delirium is one of the more treatable mental conditions when recognized. When unrecognized, clients can suffer irreversible brain damage or die.

Early recognition of delirium by nurses and other medical professionals is key in the prevention and treatment of delirium. Risk factors for delirium include the following:
- Elderly clients
- Recent major surgery
- Preexisting cognitive dysfunction
- Multiple drug therapy, especially polypharmacy of high-dose psychotropic drugs
- High doses of hypnotics

Delirium is a prevalent disorder. Study results vary because of the different populations studied who develop delirium, including *children* who swallow poisons or have high fevers, *adolescents* or *adults* who abuse drugs, and *elderly persons* who are hospitalized for surgeries or who have dementia. Depending on the study, estimates for elderly clients who are hospitalized for acute physical illnesses and then develop delirium range from 14% to 80%. Clients who have delirium while hospitalized have longer hospital stays than those without delirium, experience greater decline in function, and have higher rates of nursing home admissions. Hospital mortality rates for clients who have delirium are high. The belief that delirium is rapid, transient, and temporary is a myth. Approximately two thirds of elderly clients who experience delirium while hospitalized demonstrate the symptoms after discharge. More than half these clients live alone and are expected to carry out postdischarge medical and nursing orders in addition to their daily activities while in this compromised state. In addition, the cost of caring for clients who are delirious is increased because of the need for more demanding and continuous intervention from staff or other caregivers.

Table 8-1	**Comparison of Delirium, Dementia, and Depression**		
	Delirium	**Dementia**	**Depression**
Onset	Sudden, rapid	Insidious, gradual	Episode usually develops over days to weeks
Course	Fluctuates over hours to days	Progression over 8 to 10 years	Variable; 4 months or longer if untreated
Cognition	Acutely disrupted; may change rapidly	Chronic, progressive deterioration	Generally intact; slowed, distorted
Behavior	Mixed agitation and lethargy	Psychomotor restlessness, wandering, apathy	Psychomotor retardation or agitation
Sleep/wake cycle	Disturbed; sleep deprivation caused by symptom fluctuation	Widely variable; may mistake night for day (differential variation)	Variably disturbed; insomnia, hypersomnia, early-morning awakening
Defining characteristics	Fluctuating levels of consciousness and cognition; impaired short-term memory	Memory impairment (short-term/long-term global memory loss)	Depressed mood, anhedonia
Diagnosis	Difficult to diagnose; often missed or misdiagnosed	Delayed due to gradual progression of symptoms	Readily recognizable by professional
Treatment	Acute Identify/treat cause Alleviate symptoms	*Early stages:* medications to prolong onset *Late stages:* complete client support; caregiver education/ support	Suicide prevention Antidepressants Cognitive-behavioral therapy Client support Family education
Prognosis	Maybe reversible if recognized	Irreversible (Alzheimer's type): steady, slow decline to death	Complete remission occurs in majority of clients Depression may recur

Dementia

Dementia of the *Alzheimer's type* is the most prevalent dementia. The onset and course for this disorder is slow, insidious, progressive, and terminal. It usually takes 8 to 10 years from onset of symptoms to death, but some individuals live for 15 years or more with this stealthy, relentless thief of life.

The trend of lengthening life span will continue throughout the twenty-first century. By 2010, approximately 300 million people will live in the United States, 15% of whom will be over age 65. Alzheimer's-type dementia, one of the diseases most dreaded by elderly persons, their families, and the government, will strike 8% to 15% of those over age 65. That number doubles every 5 years after age 65. Costs of caring for clients with dementia are currently estimated at $80 to $100 billion annually, and costs will continue to increase.

The recent Surgeon General's Report on Mental Health states that education, measured by number of years of schooling, is a reliable predictor of late-life cognitive functioning. Highest percentages of Alzheimer's-type dementia occur in those with the least number of years of education. Conversely, those with higher education who remain cognitively active and engaged in their environment and interests have less incidence or have symptoms later in life.

Amnestic and Other Cognitive Disorders

Onset and course for amnestic and other cognitive disorders vary widely depending on the primary cause. For example, traumatic brain injury, sudden stroke, or neurotoxic poisoning from any source may erupt into an *acute amnestic syndrome.* On the other hand, chronic alcoholism, other prolonged drug abuse, malnutrition, or continuous exposure to toxic chemicals over an extended period usually results in a more insidious onset. Amnestic disorder may be *temporary,* as in a brain injury from which the individual may fully recover, or *permanent,* as in individuals who chronically abuse alcohol and fail to eat a nutritional diet.

ASSESSMENT AND DIAGNOSTIC CRITERIA

A shared symptom in delirium, dementia, and amnestic disorders is **memory impairment.** As noted, making a definitive diagnosis within this category of disorders may be difficult, and a thorough assessment helps to distinguish the cause of delirium (Box 8-2). The disorders differ in regard to additional symptoms that accompany memory disturbance, defining characteristics, and in some cases etiology.

Delirium

The defining characteristics of delirium are disturbances of consciousness and cognition. Delirium occurs over a short period, usually hours or days, and levels of consciousness fluctuate without following a set pattern, as evidenced by increased or decreased awareness of the environment. Ability to focus, sustain focus, or voluntarily shift attention is greatly impaired; therefore the client may be easily

> ### Box 8-2   Delirium Assessment
>
> **Physiologic assessment** based on the following workup:
> - Vital signs/electrocardiogram (ECG)/oxygen saturation
> - Pain (as fifth vital sign)
> - Medication/alcohol/substance use history (see Chapter 9)
> - Neurologic examination
> - Mental status examination
> - Step-by-step physical examination by organ system
> - Electroencephalogram (EEG)
>
> **Vital signs/ECG** offer a baseline of the client's physical status (e.g., blood pressure, cardiac problems).
>
> **Medication/alcohol/substances** can contribute to the client's delirium and confusion.
>
> **Neurologic examination** can rule out a stroke or transient ischemic attack (TIA). Examination of the cranial nerves and extraocular (eye) movements can reveal neurologic impairment. Older adults with cataracts are at risk for delirium, which is why patching one eye at a time prevents "black patch" delirium.
>
> **Mental status examination** can rule out depression and other treatable mental disorders. Persons with delirium or acute confusion are often distracted during this examination, whereas persons with dementia struggle to come up with answers that they often nearly miss.
>
> **Step-by-step physical examination by organ system** searches for metabolic disturbances: cardiovascular and pulmonary (arterial blood gases, chest radiograph, oxygen saturation/hypoxia), renal (electrolyte imbalance, uremia, dehydration), endocrine (thyroid panel, diabetes, glucose, calcium), and liver (hepatic function tests). A search for infection (sepsis, occult abscess, meningitis, urinary tract infection, pneumonia) is critical.
>
> **EEG** may be normal in dementia but is often abnormal in delirium (shows diffuse slowing); therefore it is a very sensitive test for identifying delirium, although not necessarily pinpointing a cause. EEG abnormalities may show different patterns (low amplitude, fast activity) in alcohol withdrawal and sedative-hypnotic withdrawal. EEG abnormalities may continue after the clinical symptoms of the brain syndrome are gone.
>
> NOTE: Finding the underlying cause of delirium or confusion is important for treatment to be effective. Although there are many causes, the assessment process is consistent.

distracted by any stimulus or may be unable to refocus attention away from a task or thought if asked. The client may become comatose.

In regard to the common symptom of impaired **memory,** recent memory is affected in delirium. For example, when asked to remember a specific item, the client may be unable to recall it after only a few minutes. The client may repeat within minutes what he just told the nurse. The client may ask, "When will the doctor be here?" after the physician has just left.

Disorientation usually occurs in regard to time. For example, the client may arise in the middle of the night and start to dress for breakfast. The client may tell the nurse he is going to sleep for the night when it is noon.

Language and speech disturbances vary widely, as evidenced by impaired ability to articulate *(dysarthria),* to name objects *(dysnomia),* or to write *(dysgraphia).* The client may ramble or may be completely unable to communicate through speech, writing, or signs *(aphasia).* Aphasia may be sensory (receptive) or motor (expressive).

Sensory-perceptual disturbances are common in delirium and may manifest as *illusions* (e.g., thinks slippers are rodents), *hallucinations* (e.g., hears voice of dead mother, sees people who are not actually there walk into the room), or *misinterpretations* (e.g., thinks loud noise in hallway was automobile accident). Delusional thinking may develop around the sensory disturbances as the individual attempts to make sense of the changing symptoms.

Associated **behavioral disturbances** frequently follow cognitive disturbances and range from psychomotor *hyperactivity* (e.g., restlessness, pacing, screaming, cursing) to psychomotor *hypoactivity* (e.g., lethargy, inability to move from bed or chair, moaning).

Emotional disturbances usually occur in delirium. Labile moods with rapid, unpredictable changes from one mood state to another, often without provocation, are common. Shifts among anxiety, depression, irritability, elation, agitation, and fear may occur in no set pattern.

Sleep pattern disturbances frequently occur in delirium. The sleep/wake cycle may be completely reversed, with the client unable to fall asleep at night, lying awake and agitated, then sleeping all day long. In the phenomenon called *sundown syndrome,* the client is relatively alert and has marginally intact cognition, then suddenly becomes confused, agitated, and restless as night approaches. Symptoms may be triggered by changes in light and other environmental stimuli coupled with fatigue at the end of the day and compromised age-related senses (decreased vision/hearing). Sundown syndrome occurs frequently in clients who have dementia.

Dementia

The defining characteristics of dementia are multiple cognitive deficits, especially memory impairment, and one or more of the following: aphasia, apraxia, agnosia, and impaired executive function.

As with delirium, symptoms for dementia are directly related to either a medical condition or ongoing effects of a substance, or a combination of the two. All symptoms represent a decline from previous function and interfere with social function (e.g., family, friends, organizations) and occupational function (e.g., job, homemaker).

The symptoms of dementia are progressive and develop slowly through four stages (Box 8-3). As a result, clients frequently cover up the symptoms as they deny the inevitable and attempt continued functioning. Close family members are usually aware of changes long before casual acquaintances, who may argue that the client "seems normal."

As in delirium and amnestic disorders, the hallmark symptom for dementia that must be present to make the diagnosis is **impaired memory,** which is described as (1) inability to learn new material or (2) inability to recall previously learned material. Clients with dementia usually have both deficits. At first, long-term memory often is retained as clients begin to forget immediate events, situations, and everyday routines. In early stages they forget appointments, where they put the car keys, or where the car is parked after shopping. This progresses to inability to remember their birthday or how to return home from a local familiar place, which causes fright and anxiety. Progressively, the client fails to identify relatives or own name, eventually experiences global memory loss, and is unable to recall either remote or recent events or situations.

Mild cognitive impairment (MCI) describes early neurocognitive dysfunction in which the person can still compensate for deficits in memory, executive function, (making plans, balancing checkbook), attention, language, and perceptual motor ability (integration of information with motor activity). Several studies are in progress for MCI because 15% to 20% of these clients develop dementia of the Alzheimer's type (Surgeon General's Report on Mental Health, 1999).

Speech and language deteriorate noticeably throughout the course of dementia, and *aphasia* develops. An extensive vocabulary acquired over a lifetime diminishes as the disorder progresses. When describing events, the client cannot think of appropriate words and begins to call many items "that thing" or may use extraneous words while searching for the right ones. Poverty of speech occurs, and sometimes unusual patterns of speech occur. For example,

the client may repeat words of the person talking to them *(echolalia).* Eventually all speech may disappear and the client becomes mute.

Another symptom that occurs in dementia is *apraxia,* referring to the inability to use objects correctly or perform intentional motor function and purposive movements, even though comprehension and sensorimotor systems are intact. The client may name objects correctly (fork, shoes, comb) but may be unable to use them as intended.

The loss of ability to recognize, comprehend, and identify objects is known as *agnosia.* The client's vision and sensorimotor systems may be intact, but the client may be unable to name specific indicated objects (e.g., light, table, flowers). As the disorder progresses, the client is unable to recognize own spouse or even own image in a mirror.

Disturbance of executive function refers to the inability to carry out higher level thinking such as planning, organizing, initiating functions, performing tasks in a new way, or sequencing objects or tasks. Clients also have difficulty thinking abstractly. For example, clients find they are unable to take care of finances, organize a trip, or comprehend and participate in discussions unless the topics are concrete.

Sensory-perceptual alterations frequently occur in the later stages of dementia. Psychotic symptoms may manifest as hallucinations, delusions, or illusions.

All symptoms of dementia represent a decline from the client's usual or normal functioning and culminate in an inability to participate in life that eventually leads to death. In addition to cognitive impairments, multiple physical symptoms arise as part of the progressive decline (see Box 8-3).

Amnestic and Other Cognitive Disorders

The defining characteristic of amnestic disorder is **impaired memory** directly related to effects of a general medical condition or to ongoing effects of one or more substances (drugs of abuse, medications, toxins), or a combination of the two. The ability to learn and recall new information is always impaired in amnestic and other cognitive disorders. Depending on the areas of the brain affected, clients are unable to recall verbal or visual information that was communicated a few minutes before. Recent memory is impaired. Remote memory is frequently intact; the client is able to remember stories from the distant past, but may be unable to tell the nurse how he got to the health care facility, who brought him, or the name of the agency. The client may *confabulate* (create information to fill in memory gaps) in early stages of amnestic disorder.

Disorientation to person and place is common in amnestic and other cognitive disorders; disorientation to self is usually associated with dementia. Because of lack of insight in amnestic disorder, the client with severe memory impairment may become argumentative when confronted, even though situational facts and events confirm the memory deficit.

Box 8-3   Stages of Dementia

STAGE 1

The client demonstrates minor short-term memory problems.

Displays subtle mental and physical decline.

Covers up errors.

Has difficulty focusing attention.

Starts to lose interest in environment, events, and situations.

Demonstrates deterioration of social courtesies.

Becomes uncertain in actions.

Probes for right words.

Shows difficulty making decisions.

STAGE 2

The client demonstrates obvious memory deficits.

Hesitates with verbal initiation or responses.

Is disoriented to time.

Complains of neglect.

Forgets appointments, routines, and events.

Accuses other clients of stealing.

Hides possessions, then forgets location.

STAGE 3

The client demonstrates severe memory loss.

Is disoriented to time, place, person.

Displays motor deterioration.

Wanders, then cannot find way back.

Licks lips, and uses chewing motions.

Becomes hyperoral.

Demonstrates immodest behavior.

Has unsteady gait; shows physical imcompetence.

Displays poor communication; repeats words.

Cannot read or write.

Does not recognize self in mirror.

Needs help with all daily activities.

Has catastrophic reactions.

STAGE 4 (TERMINAL STAGE)

The client demonstrates global memory loss.

Displays ataxic movements.

Demonstrates psychotic behavior.

Displays extreme psychomotor retardation.

Recognizes no one.

Needs complete assistance.

Cannot eat; tube-fed.

Becomes susceptible to infection.

Loses weight.

Is incontinent.

INTERVENTIONS

For effective intervention with delirium, dementia, and amnestic and other cognitive disorders, it is imperative to determine the correct diagnosis, which is often missed. Also with this category of disorders, where one diagnosis may be superimposed on another, the examiner must conduct a careful complete history, physical examination, and mental status assessment (including diagnostic laboratory tests) to determine the correct treatment focus. Due to the nature of the symptoms in these disorders, it is usually necessary to interview the family or others who are close to the client to validate that information is correct.

In addition to targeting specific causes, if found, the nurse focuses on (1) symptom alleviation; (2) prevention of mental and physical complications; (3) maintenance of fluid, electrolyte, and nutritional balance; and (4) therapeutic interpersonal support of the client and family.

Treatment Settings

Acute care

When symptoms are acute, hospitalization is required. For example, with acute symptom onset of delirium due to an accident, stroke, neurotoxin, or other systemic medical cause, the client is usually admitted for immediate intervention and close monitoring. This intervention may occur in an emergency room or other acute care center and may require emergency medications, intravenous therapy, or even surgery. With subacute symptoms, clients may be monitored at home or in a long-term care facility, if a responsible person can stay with the client and a nurse or physician is available to assess change.

Home

When symptoms are slow and insidious, as in dementia of the Alzheimer's type, it is sometimes beneficial to keep the client in familiar surroundings for as long as possible. This approach may prolong the inevitable decline if the home environment is benevolent and relatively free from anxiety-provoking situations. If care for a client takes place in a home with children and grandchildren, the normal chaos associated with a busy daily life can be overwhelming for all parties and may exacerbate the client's symptoms. Spouses or families may have difficulty understanding or administering multiple prescription medications to the elderly client, which often leads to additional problems and symptoms associated with polypharmacy.

Day treatment and long-term care

In middle stages of dementia it is recommended to engage the client in a day treatment program outside the home if available. The purpose is to keep the client in the community as long as possible, providing cognitive stimulation, socialization, and physical exercise. An effective program also provides needed respite for the caregivers, who otherwise would have 24-hour, uninterrupted responsibility for the client.

In later stages, continuing care in the home can become too exhausting for the family because of increasing needs to manage unpredictable client responses and behaviors. Family members must also deal with their own grief, emotional responses, and demands on time and energy. Treatment related to the client's physical needs and medication administration often exceed the family's capabilities.

Eventually most families are forced to admit clients with dementia and other chronic cognitive disorders to a special needs facility (e.g., nursing home) for continuous professional monitoring. Generally, although some out-standing long-term facilities exist, the more common problem today is finding quality care for loved ones in this setting. The reasons are largely attributed to a shortage of well-trained health care personnel to meet the challenges of caring for this growing population.

Medications

A variety of medication types are employed to treat these complex disorders. In general, the medications used depend on the symptoms, as well as the underlying cause or causes. Effective results of medication often rely on early detection, in which case the disease process may be slowed. A common rule of thumb for older adults is to begin drug therapy with low doses and proceed slowly with additional medications. Polypharmacy (use of multiple medications) and drug-to-drug interactions can cause confusion or agitation and result in falls or increased risk of falls (see pharmacotherapy box below).

PHARMACOTHERAPY | **Delirium, Dementia (Alzheimer's Type), and Head Trauma**

DELIRIUM

To treat delirium effectively, it is important to find the cause, which may involve medications, specifically those with anticholinergic effects. Many prescription and over-the-counter drugs have significant anticholinergic properties (see Box 8-1). Primary treatment for anticholinergic-induced delirium is **physostigmine** (Antilirium), 1 to 2 mg intravenously, intramuscularly, or subcutaneously, and repeated in 15 to 30 minutes and again in 60 minutes if needed. Total dose should not exceed 8 mg. Treatment may need to be repeated over the next 48 to 72 hours, since some anticholinergic medications have a longer half-life than physostigmine.

For severely agitated clients who have delirium, the antipsychotic **haloperidol** (Haldol) may be used. Clients with delirium are very sensitive to the antiparkinsonian side effects of neuroleptics; therefore the dose should be low and an oral dose instead of injection is recommended as soon as possible.

Additional medications are prescribed and other nursing interventions will be implemented if symptoms appear that require treatment. For example, neuroleptics for psychotic symptoms and anxiolytics, such as lorazepam (Ativan) for anxiety, are often prescribed during episodes of delirium.

DEMENTIA (ALZHEIMER'S TYPE)

Effective pharmacologic treatment for dementia requires early detection. Clinical efficacy of acetylcholinesterase inhibitors in the treatment of dementia of the Alzheimer's type has been demonstrated, particularly when used in the early stages. Progression of the disease may be slowed.

Nonsteroidal antiinflammatory drugs (NSAIDs), including the COX-2 inhibitors, may delay the decline of Alzheimer's-type dementia. Antioxidants such as vitamin E (400 IU daily) may also be effective. For women, estrogen replacement therapy may be initiated.

Newer cholinesterase inhibitors are available for treatment and have replaced tacrine (Cognex) because of an easier dosing schedule (once or twice daily), better gastrointestinal tolerance, and greater safety with less risk of liver damage. These reversible cholinesterases include donepezil (Aricept), rivastigmine (Exelon), and galantamine (Reminyl).

Study trials are being done in an effort to prevent or slow the onset of Alzheimer's-type dementia, such as the Alzheimer's Disease Cooperative Study Trial begun in 1999 that utilizes donepezil and vitamin E (Surgeon General's Report, 1999).

In the middle or later stages of dementia of the Alzheimer's type when clients exhibit disruptive symptoms such as psychosis or extreme anxiety, other medications may be prescribed. Clients may receive antipsychotics, antianxiety medications, and antidepressants in an attempt to alleviate symptoms.

HEAD TRAUMA

For head trauma and resulting delirium/agitation or seizure activity, anxiolytics are used for sedation and include lorazepam (Ativan), diazepam (Valium), and midazolam (Versed). Opioids (narcotics) such as morphine sulfate are used for pain relief and analgesia. Corticosteroids are used to treat brain edema resulting from a tumor or a head injury.

Other Treatments

Support of physiologic function for this population is an ongoing and primary objective for nurses. Because of the symptoms, clients are often unable to communicate their needs effectively. Nurses must be vigilant and observant for physical problems with these clients. For example, the nurse may misinterpret and falsely report physical pain as lethargy, inactivity, depression, agitation, or behavioral acting out when the client does not fully comprehend the problem. Good skills for assessment and alternative communication are essential to meet client needs, which are often unspoken but usually communicated in some way. Box 8-4 presents a general set of strategies for working with these clients.

Therapies

Other therapies that are effective with clients who have cognitive disorders include adjunctive therapies, such as recreational and occupational activities, that provide cognitive, sensory, and physical stimulation.

- The client takes planned outdoor walks with frequent stops to rest and observe pleasant and stimulating objects in nature.
- Uses paints, crayons, and chalk on paper for simple expression of feelings.
- Engages in music therapy.
- Throws ball around circle.
- Pets live animals.
- Manipulates clay or other tactile, moldable substances.
- Solves simple puzzles.
- Cognitive or insight-oriented therapies are usually not effective with this group of clients.

▌PROGNOSIS AND DISCHARGE CRITERIA

Prognosis for delirium depends on cause and early identification to prevent further complications and more serious impairment. For example, results of delirium caused by anoxia from an overdose of street drugs may be reversible if the person is treated immediately, but permanent brain damage may result if the disorder is not identified soon enough.

Prognosis for dementia is unfavorable due to progressive symptoms that manifest in a steady decline of mental function and culminate in eventual physical demise. Prognosis can be more favorable, however, when alert nurses, families, and physicians recognize complications

such as delirium that are superimposed on dementia, and therefore ensuring intervention and treatment.

Discharge criteria include retraining and reeducation programs when symptoms are reversible. When symptoms are irreversible, avoidance of insightful exploration is recommended to prevent anxiety, depression, irritability, and catastrophic reactions. Attention to all physical and medical aspects of care is imperative in the treatment of clients with cognitive disorders. Education for family members of impaired individuals, in addition to support therapy, support groups, and respite for caregivers, are essential elements in total care (see box on opposite page).

Box 8-4   **Treatment Strategies for Clients with Delirium, Dementia, or Amnestic Disorders**

Provide

- Safe, consistent environment
- Freedom from physical/emotional pain
- Calm, relaxing, nonchallenging atmosphere
- Calm, stable personnel
- Trained, observant, compassionate staff
- Skilled, adaptive communicators
- Frequent, appropriate, gentle touch
- Tactful humor
- Frequent contact by staff/family
- Visits by own pets
- Socialization opportunities
- Routine schedule/structure
- Client's personal objects
- Orienting objects (calendars, clocks)
- Program for cognitive stimulation/reminiscence
- Client/family teaching
- Adaptive equipment
- Nutrition/hydration
- Adequate snacks
- Restful sleep/naptimes
- Grooming/hygiene
- Supportive, nonrestrictive medication
- Visual/hearing/sensory aids
- Daily exercise
- Frequent ambulation
- Access to outdoors

| CLIENT AND FAMILY TEACHING | **Delirium, Dementia, and Amnestic and Other Cognitive Disorders** |

Nurse Needs To Know

- Some disorders in this category are reversible, and some are irreversible.
- All disorders in this category significantly impair the client's memory.
- Short-term memory loss is a primary symptom in the early stages of dementia of the Alzheimer's type. Memory loss gradually becomes global.
- Clients with delirium may experience confusion, agitation, or changes in the sensorium, which may be multicausal.
- Certain medications, especially in combination, can increase symptoms of confusion and agitation.
- Clients with these cognitive disorders are at high risk for falls or injuries because of decreased sensorium, memory loss, and age-related factors.
- Safety of the client's hospital and home environment is a primary concern.
- Clients may be unable to communicate pain; the nurse needs to assess the client for pain using alternative measures and close monitoring.
- Sundown syndrome (confusion and agitation resulting from fatigue and changes in stimulation) may be problematic for the client, nurse, and caregivers.
- A structured hospital and home environment with minimal changes in usual stimulation is critical because routine helps to reduce fatigue, confusion, and agitation.
- The learning needs of home caregivers and discharge facility staff need to be evaluated, especially about medications.
- Clients with dementia of the Alzheimer's type may occasionally confabulate (attempt to fill in memory gaps with unrelated information), which is not considered lying.
- Clients who confabulate may need gentle redirection to another topic or activity because confronting them with reality may result in confusion or agitation.
- Intake of nutritional supplements, herbs, and over-the-counter drugs may interfere with the client's prescribed medications.
- Clients may resist outside help and place undue demands on home caregivers.
- Stressors that can provoke client anxiety or confusion should be identified and modified or avoided as much as possible.
- Potential elder abuse may be a result of caregiver role strain, and clients and caregivers need to be evaluated if abuse is suspected.
- Home caregivers need breaks from daily client care to avoid frustration and potential abuse.
- Collaborate with social worker to investigate community resources for client and respite resources for family before the client's discharge.

Teach Client and Family

- Teach the family about the client's disorder, and explain the prognosis so that expectations remain realistic.
- Offer hope to the family, and avoid false reassurance when possible.
- Teach the family and home caregivers techniques to reduce the client's risk for falls or injury (protective devices, appropriate lighting, consistency of care, maintaining safe, uncluttered environment).
- Instruct the family on how to observe and assess for nonverbal signs of pain (e.g., moaning, groaning, restlessness, cold clammy skin, vital sign changes, holding body part, doubling over in pain) and to intervene accordingly.
- Teach the family about sundown syndrome, and provide strategies to reduce fatigue, confusion, and agitation (e.g., provide consistent care, maintain a structured environment, avoid changes in stimulation).
- Instruct the family/caregiver to look for sensorium changes and to contact emergency resources if the client's condition worsens.
- Teach the family/caregiver about the sequence of memory loss in the client with dementia of the Alzheimer's type so that they will not be alarmed or frightened.
- Teach the family/caregiver strategies that promote the client's existing memory (e.g., reminiscence activities, environmental cues, familiar songs/pictures, pets).
- Instruct the family/home caregiver about the client's medications (therapeutic effects, dose, time, frequency, adverse reactions).
- Explain to the family/home caregiver the importance of consistent medication administration.
- Instruct the family not to give holistic or herbal remedies with the client's prescribed medications without consulting with physician because the combination may cause adverse effects.
- Suggest that the client remain in the care of one physician to provide consistent care and medication regimen and to avoid adverse drug reactions (polypharmacy, drug-to-drug interactions).
- Teach the family/home caregiver about confabulation (attempts to fill in memory gaps with unrelated information), and stress that it is not lying.
- Instruct the family/caregiver to direct the client to another topic or activity when the client is confabulating because forcing reality may confuse or agitate the client.
- Teach the family/caregiver to identify stressors in the client's environment that may provoke anxiety or confusion, and offer realistic solutions.
- Explain to the family that there are benefits to outside help as long as caregivers are skilled, reliable, and trustworthy and bond with the client.

Continued

| CLIENT AND FAMILY TEACHING | **Delirium, Dementia, and Amnestic and Other Cognitive Disorders—cont'd** |

- Investigate current resources available on the Internet and in the library.

- Teach the client/caregiver to identify stressors that can lead to client or elder abuse (e.g., anger, frustration, fatigue).
- Offer strategies to prevent client or elder abuse (e.g., take breaks, attend support groups, use day treatment facilities, use respite care, talk to therapist).
- Instruct family how to access community resources for the client (e.g., day care centers, case management, grief/spiritual groups, placement facilities).
- Teach the family how to access current educational Internet and library sources.

Care Plans

- Acute Confusion
- Disturbed Thought Processes
- Impaired Social Interaction

Care Plan
Delirium, Dementia, and Amnestic and Other Cognitive Disorders

NANDA Diagnosis: Acute Confusion

The abrupt onset of a cluster of global, transient changes and disturbances in attention, cognition, psychomotor activity, level of consciousness, and sleep/wake cycle.

Focus:

For the client across the age continuum who experiences acute global transient changes manifested by fluctuations in consciousness; sensory-perceptual alterations; and disturbances in alertness, attentiveness, judgment, cognition, psychomotor activity, and sleep/wake cycle, associated with delirium, dementia, and other related amnestic or cognitive disorders.

RELATED FACTORS (ETIOLOGY)

Neurobiologic Factors

Generally over 60 years of age
Delirium
Dementia
Brain and neurotransmitter changes*

Medications/Chemical Agents

- Sedative-hypnotics
- Psychotropics
- Pain medication (opioids/nonopioids)
- Polypharmacy (more than one medication given at same time)
- Drug-to-drug interactions (effects due to drugs interacting with other drugs in the body)
- Adverse drug reactions (serious or toxic responses to drugs)
- Environmental toxins
- Over-the-counter drugs*
- Street drugs*
- Alcohol*

Physiologic Impairment

- Dehydration (with or without electrolyte disturbances)
- Hypoxia
- Infection (upper respiratory tract, urinary tract)
- Systemic failure (kidney, liver)
- Circulatory problems
- Nutritional/metabolic disturbances
- Vision/hearing changes

DEFINING CHARACTERISTICS

Fear/Anxiety/Apprehension

Abandonment (real or perceived)
Physical/mental/cognitive decline
Life changes (moving from own home to nursing home/hospital or relative's home)
Loss of control over environment

Grief/Loss Issues

Death/loss of spouse/significant person
Actual or perceived loss
Actual loss of functioning/productivity
Actual environmental/life changes

Neurobiologic Factors

The client demonstrates sundown syndrome (confusion/agitation/disorientation due to client responses to changes in lighting and stimulation), generally occurring when the sun goes down.
Demonstrates diurnal disturbances: mistakes night for day (gets up in middle of night, attempts to dress self/cook breakfast).
Displays labile mood (moods change from happy to sad or sad to angry for no obvious reason).

For discussion of disturbed thoughts and memory loss related to brain and neurotransmitter changes, see care plan on disturbed thought processes in this chapter. For discussion of alcohol, street drugs, and other nonprescription substances, see Chapter 9 and related care plans in this text.

Continued

Demonstrates attention span deficit/distractibility (difficulty focusing on a conversation or task).

Has illusions: misinterprets actual stimuli (mistakes shadow or moving curtain for dead spouse; perceives bath or shower as rainstorm).

Has hallucinations: sees objects/persons that are not present.

Chants, pounds on walls/furniture; scratches/picks at own skin repetitively.

Demonstrates impaired judgment/insight: unable to recognize or anticipate threats to physical safety.

Demonstrates impaired memory for recall: unable to recall situations and events (conversation with spouse, dinner with family, visit from grandchild, planned appointment).

Displays impaired memory for recognition: unable to recognize familiar people and places (asks wife of 50 years, "When is my wife coming to see me?"; becomes lost in own home, neighborhood, hospital, treatment center).

Has catastrophic/panic reaction (strikes out suddenly, without warning; screams and yells without being obviously provoked).

Demonstrates loss of impulse control (cries/sobs/moans without obvious external stimuli).

Exhibits regressive behaviors without obvious external stimuli (startled or frightened facial expression; huddles fearfully; withdraws from touch).

Manifests paranoid behaviors: accuses others of abuse (harming client during routine treatment), neglect (not feeding client or caring for client's basic needs), and stealing (actual or imagined possessions).

Medications/Chemical Agents

The client demonstrates increased symptoms of delirium as a result of medication regimen, polypharmacy, drug-to-drug interactions, adverse drug reactions, withdrawal/intoxication from prescribed medications, street drugs or alcohol, or other chemicals/substances.

Physiologic Impairment

The client demonstrates hypotension (may be associated with medications; deficient fluid volume). Demonstrates hypoxia/decreased oxygen saturation (may be associated with respiratory infection, deficient fluid volume, stroke, or seizure activity).

Manifests deficient fluid volume, dehydration (with or without electrolyte disturbances), inadequate urine output (with or without urinary tract infection), impaired circulation (changes in vital signs, sensory-perceptual/cognitive deficits), dry skin with bruises (poor tone/turgor), and pitting edema.

Demonstrates urinary tract infection.

Exhibits respiratory tract infection with productive cough and thick sputum.

Manifests reduced sensory/spatial function (hearing, vision, smell, touch, taste, space).

Exhibits nutrition less than body requirements with or without weight loss.

Psychomotor Disturbances (Associated with Neurobiologic Factors)

The client displays impaired coordination/ataxic gait (unsteady on feet, prone to falls).

Paces the halls with agitation/anxiety/restlessness.

Wanders aimlessly without apparent destination.

Demonstrates seizure activity or possible recent stroke (paralysis, garbled speech).

Falls or is at risk for falling according to reliable fall-risk assessment scale.

Is physically unable to perform activities of daily living (ADLs).

Manifests impaired swallowing ability.

Fear/Anxiety/Apprehension

The client cries out when left alone and when visitors/family members leave (may result from feelings of abandonment, both real or imagined).

Demonstrates frustration and anger when unable to perform simple tasks; shouts, pounds on furniture or wall.

Exhibits fear and agitation when moved from familiar environment (may result from feeling lost or insecure); shouts, strikes out in apparent terror.

Manifests fear and resistance when staff attempts to deliver care and treatment; shouts, strikes out.

- Perceives staff as a feared real or imagined person.
- Misinterprets touch as an assault.
- Misinterprets shower or bath for rainstorm or drowning in ocean.

Grief/Loss Issues

Note: Clients experiencing grief and loss may also be depressed and at risk for suicide when they have the energy and motivation to act on their feelings. Therefore staff need to practice suicide precautions in accordance with hospital guidelines and facilitate a psychiatric consultation for appropriate medication and treatment.

The client mourns loss of memory and cognitive functions.

- Attempts to cover up deficits until no longer possible as illness progresses.
- Talks of not wanting to burden family.

Mourns real or imagined loss of spouse or significant others; may talk of wanting to die or to join deceased spouse.

- "I don't want to be here without him."

Mourns loss of productive and generative functioning.

- Stops engaging in interactions or activities.
- Stops socializing with others.

Mourns changes in environment and life status.

- Stops eating.
- Displays poor hygiene or grooming.
- "My life is not worth living anymore."

OUTCOME IDENTIFICATION AND EVALUATION

Neurobiologic Factors

The client remains free from physical harm or injury.

Demonstrates safe, nonthreatening behavior toward others.

Manifests satisfactory orientation to the immediate environment.

Distinguishes actual from perceived stimuli; sees and hears with clarity.

Accurately interprets objects, people, and events in the environment.

Refrains from repetitive chanting/pounding/scratching and picking at skin.

Distinguishes day from night.

Tolerates procedural touch by caregivers.

Demonstrates reduction in crying and recoiling behaviors.

Smiles appropriately with reduction in mood swings.

Demonstrates ability to focus on brief directives by caregivers.

Demonstrates ability to recall familiar faces of family and caregivers.

Exhibits reduction in paranoid behaviors with family and caregivers.

Medications/Chemical Agents

The client demonstrates decreased symptoms of delirium as a result of changes in medication regimen.

- Lower doses of medication and reduction/elimination of polypharmacy.
- Medication administration follows recommended dose for age and condition.

Physiologic Impairment

The client maintains adequate blood pressure range.

Manifests fluid volume repletion and electrolyte balance.

Demonstrates adequate urine output with absent urinary tract infection.

Demonstrates satisfactory oxygen saturation (O_2/SAT) for age and condition.

Exhibits absent infection or medication/controlled infectious process (respiratory tract clear of rales or rhonchi; absent or decreased productive cough).

Exhibits satisfactory nutritional status and weight (eats appropriate amount of food for age, condition, and metabolism).

Manifests satisfactory skin tone and turgor with absent or diminished bruising, decubiti, or edema.

Exhibits satisfactory swallowing ability (with appropriate dietary/liquid supplements).

Psychomotor Disturbances

The client sits calmly for 10 to 15 minutes at a time.

Remains in brief activities for up to 15 minutes.

Demonstrates reduction in pacing, agitation, and wandering.

Exhibits reduction/cessation of seizure activity (with appropriate medication).

Demonstrates reduction in falls and fall risk (with assistance and assistive devices and careful observation, especially following meds).

Performs minimal ADLs with assistance.

Fear/Anxiety/Apprehension

The client demonstrates an overall reduction in fear/anxiety/apprehension.

- Remains calmer with changes in stimuli.
- Shouts and cries less often.
- Sits for up to 15 minutes.

Demonstrates minimal agitation when alone or when visitors/family members leave.

- Turns attention to others in the milieu.
- Engages in a group or activity.

Manifests reduction in frustration when attempting to perform ADLs or simple tasks.

- Does not shout or pound on furniture as often when unable to perform ADLs/tasks.

Demonstrates less resistance and less anxiety/apprehension during care and treatment.

- Accepts care and treatment from caregivers without yelling or striking out.

Grief/Loss Issues

The client demonstrates reduction in mourning related to actual or perceived losses (affect brighter, appetite/ hygiene/grooming better).

Accepts help with minimal frustration because of limitations in physical functioning.

- Is less resistive to staff assistance.
- Occasionally thanks staff for their help.

Accepts environmental and life changes with the help of family and caregivers.

- Socializes with peers.
- Discusses loss with others.
- Makes future plans.

Note: Caregivers and staff need to remain realistic about outcome achievements as a result of the limited capacity of clients with confusion resulting from delirium, dementia, and amnestic disorders. Outcomes are most often effectively attained through assistance, patience, and helpful guidance and cues by staff and family/caregivers.

PLANNING AND IMPLEMENTATION

Nursing Intervention	Rationale
Safety: Environment	
Secure the client's environment. • Lock appropriate doors and windows, including areas surrounding patio and facility. • Remove harmful objects from the client's environment. Provide safety equipment: nonskid carpets/rugs, low beds, chairs with special features, monitors attached to the client's clothing that detect movement and alert staff. Assist the client in bathroom and when moving from bed to chair or bed to commode, using available transfer equipment and sufficient staff to move client whenever possible (*Note:* utilize hospital "lift team" if available). Help the client use the safety bars and other necessary equipment in bathroom or shower. Ensure that water temperature is regulated in the client's bath and shower area. Provide sufficient lighting from the client's bed to the bathroom or commode area. Display large-print signs and pictures on significant areas: door of client's room, bathroom door, closet door, fire doors, door to outside secured environment. Monitor and document the client's fall-risk assessment daily or according to unit policy.	These actions provide for a safe environment and prevent falls and injury, given the client's neurobiologic changes. Use of pictures and printed signs to signify an area is helpful to clients of all languages and cultures.
Safety: Wandering	
Allow the client to wander in a safe, secure, designated environment. Ensure that the client always wears identification bracelet, and keep the client's photograph on file. Alert staff in other departments or surrounding areas of the client's wandering, and give them a description of the client. Help the client find way around the secured inside and outside environment, and point out clearly printed signs and pictures. Place familiar objects, belongings, and valuables in the client's environment. Provide other activities as alternatives to wandering, limiting activities to 30 minutes. Remove "triggers" from the client's view, which are reminders of wandering activity (e.g., hat, coat, purse/wallet, car keys). Reassure the client in a calm, low-key voice tone about where the client is, why he or she is there, and that family and friends know where to find the client. Use monitoring device to track the client if possible. Increase level of observation for the client whose wandering is difficult to manage.	A reasonable amount of wandering may help reduce the client's anxiety and frustration, provide physical exercise, improve cardiovascular system, and improve self-esteem. Alternatives to wandering that is out of control help to direct the client's restless energy to more structured activities. Monitoring and tracking promote client safety. Check the client's medications because wandering may be related to akathisia, a motor restlessness induced by neuroleptic medication.
Safety: Anger/Aggression/Anxiety	
Maintain consistent daily routine, and avoid surprises or unnecessary changes. Observe and anticipate behaviors that are precursors to violence toward the client and others: threats, yelling, screaming,	A consistent routine, keen observations, and anticipating cues or precursors to violence may prevent harm or injury to the client and others in the milieu.

striking out, escalating anxiety/frustration, angry or labile mood, troubled or angry affect, sudden change in mood/affect, fatigue.

Attempt to defuse/deescalate a crisis situation in the early stages, as soon as the client shows behavioral cues of escalating anxiety or frustration (e.g., labile mood, angry affect, cursing, verbal threats).

- Alert other staff of situation so that they may assist as needed.
- Approach the client with a calm, confident affect and demeanor.
- Avoid reasoning or asking questions that the client may have trouble answering.
- Accompany or assist the client to a less stimulating environment using a gentle touch.
- Reduce unit stimuli (e.g., dim the lights, decrease volume on TV or radio).
- Engage the client in a comforting and supportive low-key conversation.
- Distract the client with a more pleasant, beneficial activity.
- Offer food, beverage, or a favorite snack to the client.
- Administer prescribed medications as least restrictive intervention.

Early deescalation may prevent the need for physical interventions, which will preserve the client's dignity and prevent harm or injury to the client and others. Medication should be used as part of treatment plan only as necessary.

Sleep-Wake Alterations/Sundown Syndrome/Nighttime Restlessness

Provide adequate lighting, nightlights, and a well-lit path to the bathroom in the evening.

Take the client to the bathroom, or ensure use of bedpan or urinal before bedtime.

Restrict caffeine and alcohol intake, and avoid stimulants or diuretics in the evening.

Reduce environmental activity at the end of the day and during change of shift.

Avoid overstimulating interactions and program activities, especially in the evening.

Encourage a brief midday nap, but discourage excessive napping during the day.

Establish a routine bedtime schedule, and "stick to it."

Provide healthy exercise for the client: brisk walk outdoors once a day.

Provide familiar, valued things for the client: stuffed animal, soothing music, favorite food treat, especially during times of anticipated stress.

Place orienting and stimulating objects in the client's room: calendar with large print, big clock, soft nightlight in the evening.

Assign the client a room near the nurses' station if sundown syndrome persists.

Offer the client a backrub, using a favorite body lotion.

Provide medication as prescribed, appropriate for the client's age and condition.

Routine schedules, healthy exercise, and methods of orientation provide structure that may help clients distinguish day from night. The effects of sundown syndrome can be reduced with orienting objects and soft lighting in the client's room. Stuffed animals and soft music bring comfort and reduce agitation.

A soothing backrub can relax the client and reduce/prevent agitation.

Medication may be beneficial as part of the client's treatment plan when necessary.

Sensory-Perceptual Alterations/Deprivation (Hallucinations/Illusions/Chanting/Pounding)

Provide sensory stimulation (e.g., touch, smell, taste, hearing, vision).

Helping the client use all the senses reduces the need for self-stimulation (e.g., chanting, pounding, scratching/picking, illusions, hallucinations). With the loss of

Continued

PLANNING AND IMPLEMENTATION—cont'd

Nursing Intervention	Rationale

Sensory-Perceptual Alterations/Deprivation (Hallucinations/Illusions/Chanting/Pounding)—cont'd

Watch the client around hot foods, hot water, and electrical appliances.

Touch

Touch the client on the hand or forearm in a comforting way (use judgment).

Have the client feel materials with different textures.

Assign brief, simple tasks (e.g., folding towels), but do not tire or demean the client.

Encourage staff to give hand massages or backrubs (be aware of culture).

Smell/Taste

Use scratch and sniff cards with familiar smells (e.g., popcorn, flowers).

Make sure the client's dentures are clean and in place.

Involve the client in a cooking or baking activity (determine favorite foods).

Increase intensity of food flavors with natural herbs (do not use hot spices).

Hearing

Check the client's ears for wax buildup regularly, and have it properly removed.

Determine the client's primary language (an interpreter may be needed).

Approach the client from the front; reduce background noise; speak slowly in low pitch.

Use brief, five-word questions/statements for clients with stroke or aphasia. ("I will help you turn").

Play musical instruments, and have the client play drums or bells.

Play soothing music in the client's environment (radio or audiotapes).

Vision

Encourage the client to wear reading glasses or bifocals as needed.

Administer eye drops as prescribed (clients often forget to do this).

Place bright colors around the client's environment.

Use high-intensity lighting with low-glare bulbs, nightlights, and natural light.

other senses, touch keeps clients involved, and close observation prevents burns, accidents/injury, and skin infections. Older clients have a narrow visual range and need more light and less glare. They cannot hear high-pitched sounds well and are sensitive to loud noises. Use of the client's own language and slow, brief sentences stimulates hearing/understanding for clients with special needs.

Illusions/Hallucinations

Do not contradict the client who experiences an illusion. Instead, simply explain reality, and find some practical solutions to the problem.

Therapeutic Responses

- "The shadow comes from the curtain. I will turn on the light so you can see better."
- "The noise you hear is from the leaky faucet. Let's turn on some soft music."

Therapeutic responses promote reality while offering solutions that help enhance the client's senses and may reduce fear, anxiety, and confusion.

Nontherapeutic Responses

"How could a stranger get in your room? That's just a shadow of the curtain."

"Dead spirits wouldn't make noises like that. It's just an old leaky faucet."

Nontherapeutic responses attempt to present reality but tend to "put down" the client and offer no solutions and may increase fear, anxiety, and confusion.

Do not contradict or challenge a client who is hallucinating. Instead, simply explain reality, and calmly try to distract the client with other activities.

Therapeutic responses present a nonthreatening reality to the client and offer distractions that provide positive sensory stimulation.

Therapeutic Responses
- "I don't see anyone else in this room. Let's take a walk in the patio area."
- "I don't hear any voices except yours and mine. Let's watch TV for a while."

Nontherapeutic Responses
"No, there are no strangers in this room. It's just your imagination."

"If there were other voices I would hear them, too, wouldn't I?"

Nontherapeutic responses attempt to present reality but also challenge the client's view of reality, which could increase confusion and self-doubt.

Give prescribed medications when needed, and document client's therapeutic and nontherapeutic responses (see Medications section and Weblinks).

Clients with sensory-perceptual alterations often respond favorably to medications and generally require drugs before other types of therapy are introduced.

Teach the family/caregiver about sensory-perceptual alterations, and help them learn how to use practical, therapeutic strategies (listed previously). Inform them about the importance of medication compliance and therapeutic and nontherapeutic effects of medications.

Knowledge about the disorder, the strategies to manage client responses, and the importance of medication compliance increase family/caregiver coping skills, decrease client confusion, and reduce frustration for all parties.

Medications/Chemical Agents

Assess the client for common side effects of psychoactive medication.
- Excessive sedation, sleepiness, confusion, agitation, stupor
- Orthostatic hypotension (sudden drop in blood pressure when a client is moved from a lying-to-sitting position or sitting-to-standing position)
- Drug-induced Parkinson's disease (tremors, muscle rigidity, masked facies)
- Anticholinergic effects (dry mouth, blurred vision, urinary retention, constipation, confusion, poor memory, difficulty learning new things)
- Tardive dyskinesia (abnormal tremors of mouth/limbs)
- Akathisia (motor restlessness that may aggravate wandering behaviors)
- Paradoxical agitation, confusion, incontinence, instability (unexpected effects of drug caused by benzodiazepines in older adults)

Find the right dose for each patient that will induce a calming effect without causing excessive sedation, sleepiness, or stupor. Extreme sedation causes confusion and agitation, defeating the desired effect of the drug. An overly sedated client cannot eat well, resulting in nutritional/metabolic deficiencies and physical decline. Side effects such as memory impairment and difficulty learning are also symptoms of dementia; therefore taking a drug that worsens these symptoms is counterproductive. Drugs that cause movement disorders, ataxia, and motor restlessness can put clients at risk for falls and subsequent injury. Medications to counteract these symptoms must be used with care because they also produce serious anticholinergic effects. Benzodiazepines should also be used with care because they can cause paradoxical reactions and may also be addictive. They have been known to exacerbate fall risk and falls in older adults, especially in combination with other drugs.

Observe a client carefully for any unusual behavior and symptoms that may occur when a new drug is prescribed. Contact the physician immediately if these occur.

The new drug may interfere and interact with other medications the client is taking, causing a polypharmacy effect or drug-to-drug interaction that can have many harmful consequences. The physician may need to try several other drugs before finding one that has a beneficial effect with minimal side effects. It is best to use psychoactive drugs sparingly, in low doses, and for a brief time.

Use the hospital or local pharmacist and the physician as an educational resource for current drug information.

Nurses need to be well informed in such areas as adverse side effects, drug-to-drug interactions, polypharmacy, and age-specific dose-appropriate information (see Medications section and Weblinks).

Use nondrug measures when possible, such as problem solving, increasing the client's self-awareness, modifying and simplifying the client's environment, and calming communication techniques.

These therapeutic skills help develop the client's trust and may prevent catastrophic reactions and other crisis events.

Continued

PLANNING AND IMPLEMENTATION—cont'd

Nursing Intervention	Rationale
Attention Span Deficit/Distractibility	
Use brief, frequent eye contact and a quiet, soothing voice tone when interacting with the client who has trouble listening and attending. Gently touch the client's arm or face.	A soothing voice tone, brief eye contact, and gentle touch tend to be calming and reassuring and enhance the client's attention span and listening skills.
Be aware of the client's cultural and spiritual differences when using touch and eye contact. • The client withdraws from the nurse's touch or states, "Don't touch me." • Says, "Stop staring at me," or "What are you looking at?"	Some clients have cultures or religions that hold different viewpoints regarding touch and eye contact and thus may resent or misinterpret their use.
In the previous situations, consider using less touch and eye contact and more repetition, changes in vocal pitch, and other nonverbal communication techniques. • Touch should be gentle and reassuring; consider culture and spirituality. • Eye contact use should be brief, intermittent, and convey no emotional extremes. • Facial expressions should convey kindness and empathy versus anger or surprise. • Posture should be straight and convey confidence versus slumped and relaxed. • Voice should be calm/matter-of-fact with some pitch changes to gain attention. • Gestures should be smooth and used to assist verbal communication; too many hand movements can confuse the client.	These simple methods help to gain the client's attention without being perceived as offensive or threatening.
Paranoia/Suspiciousness	
Do not whisper to someone else in front of the suspicious client, and do not talk about the client as if he or she was not there. Help look for a missing item if the client says, "Someone took it," but search the client's usual hiding places first. Eliminate potential hiding places by removing clutter and locking unused areas. Keep an extra set of items that are often lost; check the wastebasket before emptying. Do not respond defensively when accused by the client; avoid arguing or giving a long explanation or excuse; be calm and understanding.	The paranoid or suspicious client is generally feeling or fearing loss of control over the illness and the environment. A calm, reassuring response assures the client that his or her needs are being met and may reduce suspicious behaviors.
Pain Assessment/Medications	
Assess the client for pain, and if the client admits to having pain, medicate according to the physician's order; reassess each time vital signs are taken or according to policy. Use other indicators to assess pain if patient is unable to identify pain: restlessness, groans, vital sign changes, skin temperature changes, family/significant other reports. A visual pain scale with drawings of facial expressions that correlate with numbers on a scale of 1 to 10 may also be used in several languages to help clients of diverse cultures; clients select the most accurate level of pain: 1 to 3 mild, 4 to 6 moderate, and 7 to 10 severe in most pain scales.	Pain is considered the *fifth vital sign*, and all clients are entitled to effective pain relief as part of patient rights according to the Board of Registered Nursing and Joint Commission Pain Standards for 2001. Clients with delirium and dementia may be unable to identify pain, and other indicators need to be used. Pain, tension, or stress may also cause clients to wander; thus relief is important.

Observe the client for therapeutic effects of pain medication.

- *Mild pain:* Nonopioid (nonnarcotic): aspirin, acetaminophen, nonsteroidal antiinflammatory drug, (NSAIDs) (Arthrotec, ketorolac). Adjuvant may also be used: antidepressant, anticonvulsant, corticosteroid, stimulant.
- *Mild to moderate pain:* Weak opioid/narcotic: codeine, combination products containing hydrocodone (Vicodin) or oxycodone (Percodan). Adjuvant may also be used.
- *Moderate to severe pain:* Strong opioid/narcotic: morphine, hydromorphone, levorphanol, oxycodone, methadone, fentanyl transdermal (patch). Adjuvant may also be used.

Observe client for adverse effects of narcotic analgesics.

- *Respiratory depression* (associated with acute opiate overdoses)
  Rx: Reverse with narcotic antagonist (naloxone) but can also cause withdrawal.
  Prevent: Titrate the dose in patients with compromised respiratory function.
- *Constipation* (all opiates are constipating)
  Rx/Prevent: Increase fluid intake; bran/fluid in diet; stool softeners; stimulant laxatives, and finally bulk laxatives if previous treatments are ineffective.
- *Sedation* (decreases in intensity after 3 to 5 days of continuous drug use)
  Rx: Avoid driving until capable (rarely applies to clients with these disorders).
- *Nausea/vomiting* (worse in ambulating clients because of inner ear disturbance)
  Rx: Hydroxyzine may be helpful; prochlorperazine is better for clients in bed.
- *Itching/allergy* (histamine release causes itching; thus not a true allergy)
  Rx: Treat itching by switching the client to a different chemical class of narcotic.

Keen assessment/prevention/treatment of adverse effects may prevent serious complications and death (refer to physician, pharmacist, and computer Weblinks for more extensive information about pain and pain medication).

Client Resistant to Care

Do a self-assessment and reduce your own tension before approaching the client.

Respect the client's privacy when bathing, toileting, and doing procedures.

Use a calm, matter-of-fact approach; be patient; give simple step-by-step instructions.

Offer the client some simple choices, such as selecting food, clothing, and bath time.

Let the client participate in own care, such as holding a washcloth during bathing.

Use favorite soaps, bath oils, and lotions and play soft music during care/treatment.

Share stories with the client, and encourage the client to talk about a topic of interest.

These strategies give the client some control over own care and make the time spent with the client special and meaningful. Clients who feel as if they matter are less likely to resist care.

Fear/Anxiety/Apprehension

Check the client for any physical problems, such as pain, constipation, or fatigue.

Check for underlying anxiety disorder, depression, or panic disorder.

Physical problems such as pain or constipation should be corrected as soon as possible to increase comfort and reduce apprehension. If the client becomes fatigued, the client will have trouble sleeping and will experience sleep pattern

Continued

PLANNING AND IMPLEMENTATION—cont'd

Nursing Intervention	Rationale

Fear/Anxiety/Apprehension—cont'd

Nursing Intervention	Rationale
Give care during quiet times, not when client is likely to be anxious or fearful, and give care at the same time each day. *Note:* Not all clients do well in the morning. Ensure consistency of care and staff as much as possible; prepare the client for treatments. Alert visitors about the client's mood beforehand, and discourage long visiting hours. Try not to move the client to different rooms; do not leave the client alone in a dayroom. Distract the client from restless, repetitive behaviors, such as swinging crossed leg, pacing, pounding on tray, picking/scratching skin, sobbing, or chanting.	disturbance. Anxiety, panic, and depressive disorders may be at the root of the client's behaviors and can often be treated through a psychiatric consult. Routine care, familiar staff, and keeping the client in the same room reduce fears of abandonment. Preparing the client for care and treatment decreases fear and apprehension. Telling visitors what to expect gives them a chance to prepare themselves and better cope with the client.

Grief/Loss Issues

Nursing Intervention	Rationale
Conduct a suicide assessment if the client appears depressed (see Box 3-7). Assess the client for suicidal ideation: refuses to eat/bathe/groom; voices desire to die; has suicide plans and means. Obtain a psychiatric consult for the client whether the loss is real or perceived. Place the client on suicide precautions as necessary according to hospital policy. Listen closely to the client's expressions of grief and suicidality. Spend time with the client, and arrange for visitors to come more often. Consult with the hospital chaplain or the client's own religious or spiritual advisor. Keep the client busy with activities and groups as much as possible. Avoid losing any of the client's valued possessions or belongings. Initiate pet therapy. Provide for a safe, secure discharge or aftercare.	Grief can often lead to depression, which can be treated with medications and therapy. Clients with energy and motivation may attempt suicide indirectly through refusing food (they may receive nourishment through a feeding tube). Spending time with the client reduces feelings of loss and abandonment that are a part of grief. Spiritual or religious guidance offers hope to a grieving person. Keeping the client busy with peers and activities may distract from grief for a time. Grief groups may help depending on the client's level of awareness. Valued possessions and pets are comforting during times of grief and loss. Continuity of care is critical for the grieving client to ensure safety and support.

Care Plan

DSM-IV-TR Diagnosis **Delirium, Dementia, and Amnestic and Other Cognitive Disorders**

NANDA Diagnosis: Disturbed Thought Processes

Disruptions in cognitive operations and activities.

Focus:

For the client with delirium, dementia (e.g., Alzheimer's type), and amnestic and other cognitive disorders who manifests significant disturbances in processing and expressing thoughts in a meaningful way as a result of neurobiologic changes in areas of the brain that control memory and cognition. Consequently, all areas of cognitive and perceptual operations and activities are affected as the client struggles to retain logic and meaning.

RELATED FACTORS (ETIOLOGY)

Inability to process and synthesize information secondary to neurobiologic changes in the brain (e.g., medical conditions, toxins, medications, and drugs of abuse)

Recent memory loss that progresses to remote memory loss and eventually extends to global memory loss

Disorientation, decreased concentration, confusional state

Loss of judgment, insight, comprehension, and problem-solving abilities

Impaired abstract thinking

Interruptions in logical stream of thought

Sleep-wake pattern alterations

Difficulty in focusing attention (distractibility)
Cognitive-perceptual alterations (delusions, paranoia)
Sensory-perceptual alterations (hallucinations, illusions)
Life-style of dependence
Depressed state (pseudodementia)
Anxiety/apprehension
Fear

DEFINING CHARACTERISTICS

Early Stages

The client demonstrates impairment in abstract thinking and reasoning.
- Is unable to find similarities and differences between related words or objects (bus/train, sun/moon, bird/butterfly, dog/goldfish, window/door, pencil/typewriter).
- Has difficulty in defining words and concepts.
- Assigns concrete meanings to familiar proverbs (interprets "people who live in glass houses shouldn't throw stones" or "a rolling stone gathers no moss" literally).

Manifests impaired judgment and decision-making skills in typical social situations.
- Cannot figure out what to do if a mailman delivered a letter that was not addressed to the client; what to do with a stamped, addressed envelope; what action to take if lost wallet; how to get help in middle of night; what to do if in a theater and a fire broke out.
- Fails to make realistic or reasonable plans for self or others; cannot meet social or family obligations; is unable to put business affairs in order.

Experiences difficulty in calculating simple problems, indicating inability to concentrate and focus on thoughts.
- $4 \times 3, 4 \times 6, 42 \times 6, 162 \times 20$.
- Cannot count backward from 100 in increments of 7.
Note: This commonly used test may be influenced by the person's education level.

Exhibits deficiencies in general knowledge, in accordance with educational, sociocultural, and life experiences.
- Does not know president of the United States or other well-known world leaders.
- Cannot name state capitals or names of oceans.
- Cannot state current issues or news events.
Note: Information should be based on generally known phenomena.

Demonstrates inability to learn or comprehend new knowledge, which indicates deficits in perception, retention, association, and recent memory function.
- Cannot retrieve new content 5 to 10 minutes after it is given.
- Cannot repeat a sentence, such as the Babcock sentence, 5 to 10 minutes after it is given ("one thing a nation must have in order to become rich and great is a large and secure stack of wood").

- Cannot verbalize four unrelated words after 5 to 10 minutes (e.g., boy, window, dog, love).
Note: Persons with dementia have difficulty in recent memory acquisition or learning. This may be a key to early detection of dementia.

Exhibits significant recent memory impairment, as indicated by inability to verbalize remembrances after several minutes to an hour.
- "How long have you been here?"
- "What happened just before you came here?"
- "What time did you get out of bed today?"
- "What did you eat for breakfast today?"

Is able to recall early life events or events from childhood: place of birth, name of school, vocation or profession, place of work.
Note: The accuracy of past memory may not be readily assessed because early life events cannot be refuted by the examiner.

Demonstrates lack of insight or ability to perceive self realistically and to understand self. Cannot respond to the following questions:
- "Why did you decide to come to this facility at this time?"
- "Have you noticed any change in yourself or in your outlook on life?"
- "Have you noticed any change in your feelings?"

Exhibits impairment in semantic or knowledge memory.
- Is unable to develop a scenario on request. Cannot synthesize and think about events (e.g., unable to describe actions from dinner until bedtime).
Note: Semantic memory is used in language, abstraction, and logic and is generally impaired in clients with dementia of the Alzheimer's type.

Advanced Stages

The client demonstrates intermittent confusion, disorientation, and poor conceptual boundaries in strange surroundings, as expressed by inappropriate verbal statements.
Note: Acute or chronic confusion is more common in delirium than in dementia. *Nighttime confusion* may indicate sedative intoxication or age-related sleeping changes. *Daytime confusion* may indicate a bilateral cerebrovascular accident or lingering hypnotic effects.

Uses confabulation (attempts to fill in the memory gaps with fabricated or made-up responses) when unable to remember or recall events.
Note: Confabulation is *not* lying. Often, the person with an amnestic disorder in which memory is lost for a time or for certain life events may still be aware of the environment and may use confabulation in an attempt to "cover up" the deficit versus trying to deceive someone.

Demonstrates *aphasia* (loss of language ability); cannot express thoughts through speech, writing, or via symbols; initially has difficulty searching for words and eventually becomes mute as disease progresses.

Note: The most common cerebral pathologic condition associated with aphasia is vascular disease.

Manifests *agnosia* (inability to recognize once-familiar objects because of impaired ability to interpret sensory stimuli): initially the client has trouble recognizing everyday objects; in later stages the client does not recognize loved ones, self, or own body parts.

Note: Aphasia encompasses agnosia and apraxia.

Exhibits *apraxia* (loss of purposeful movement).

Note: Ideational apraxia means loss of ability to formulate the ideational concepts needed to carry out a skilled motor act; the person cannot conceive or maintain the idea. Comprehension is normal in apraxia. Ideational apraxia accompanies diffuse cerebral disorders such as arteriosclerosis.

- Forgets how to use a once-familiar utensil (e.g., eggbeater, potato peeler).
- Cannot recall how to operate a stationary bicycle, although motor function remains intact.

Motor apraxia is decline of kinesthetic motor patterns necessary to perform a skilled motor act, usually related to a precentral gyrus lesion.

The term *ideomotor apraxia* is applied to a person who has lost the skills for a given complex act but may retain conditioned habits and perform them repetitiously (perseveration); may be associated with disease of the supramarginal gyrus.

Demonstrates *circumstantiality* (digression and extraneous thinking with cumbersome, convoluted detail), as volunteered by the person but unnecessary to answer the examiner's questions.

Note: Circumstantiality results from excessive associations of an idea that reaches the consciousness and interrupts the stream of logical thinking.

Displays *stereotypy* (persistently repeats words or phrases) caused by interrupted stream of thought.

Manifests *perseveration* (multiple repetitions of words, phrases, or movements despite efforts to make a new response) related to interrupted stream of thought.

Uses *circumlocutory phrases* (roundabout, non–goal-directed speech patterns); words or phrases seem to avoid meaning or conclusion; may be caused by interrupted stream of thought.

Demonstrates *delusions* (thought content disturbance, a fixed belief not changed by logic).

- *Ideas of reference.* Object of environmental attention: being watched, spied on, or singled out.
- *Alien control.* Passivity: being guided by external forces.
- *Nihilistic.* Denies reality and existence: "I have no head, no stomach," "I cannot die," "I will live forever."
- *Self-deprecation.* Feelings of unworthiness, sinfulness, ugliness, or emitting obnoxious odors, generally noted in severe depression.

- *Grandeur.* Elated states: great wealth, strength, or power, sexual potency, identification with a famous person or God.
- *Somatic.* Organic preoccupations: having cancer, obstructed bowel, leprosy, or some horrible disease. In severe depression with psychotic features, somatic delusions take on bizarre qualities: a "rotting gut," "heart made of stone," or "brain as a bag of worms." Somatic delusions are to be distinguished from a preoccupation with normal, visceral, or peripheral sensations.

Experiences obsessions and compulsions (thought or impulse disturbance): preoccupation with persistent idea, thought, or impulse that cannot be eliminated by logic, generally followed by an uncontrollable urge to perform an act to relieve anxiety; usually performed in ritualistic fashion according to certain rules held by the individual.

Experiences hallucinations, illusions, depersonalization (sensory-perceptual alterations).

- *Hallucinations* are false perceptions that affect all the senses: sound, sight, touch, taste, smell, and somatic.
- *Depersonalization* is an alteration in the perception or experience of the self in which the usual sense of one's reality is temporarily lost or changed; feeling as if one is detached from body or mind.

Demonstrates emotional lability (may result from delusion, hallucination, illusion, depersonalization, fear, anxiety, confusion, disorientation, memory loss).

- After being relatively calm and passive, suddenly becomes angry and aggressive without apparent provocation.

Manifests depression, which may perpetuate altered thought processes or may result from the client's frustration related to progressive dementia.

OUTCOME IDENTIFICATION AND EVALUATION

The client demonstrates intellect and judgment to the best of ability based on extent of organic pathology and residual cognitive functions.

Reminisces about past life experiences by using long-term memory functions.

Responds coherently to simple, concrete statements.

Demonstrates absence of overt anxiety, fear, and confusion.

Follows repeated, concrete directions.

Maintains residual sensory-perceptual functions.

Participates in basic ADL decisions: selects favorite foods, chooses clothing.

Demonstrates orientation to person, place, and time.

PLANNING AND IMPLEMENTATION

Nursing Intervention	Rationale
Approach the client gently with an open, friendly, relaxed manner.	Clients with cognitive disorders such as dementia of the Alzheimer's type often "mirror" the affect of those around them. A tense, hurried approach would reflect on the client, who may become anxious and resistant. A gentle, calm approach is comforting and nonthreatening.
Identify yourself and look directly into the client's eyes, making sure you have his or her attention. • "Mr. Jones, I'm your nurse, Kathy."	Clients with cognitive and memory impairments need to have their nurse's identity constantly reestablished. If the nurse does not have the client's attention, the client could misinterpret the nurse's words and actions and become confused and frightened.
Speak to the client in a clear, low-pitched voice.	High-pitched tones create anxiety and tension in clients with Alzheimer's-type dementia and other cognitive disorders.
Eliminate competing and distracting background stimuli (e.g., radio, television, extraneous talk) when speaking to the client.	Too much stimulation results in sensory overload and confuses the client.
Ask only one question (or make only one statement) at a time, using short, simple sentences (try not to use more than five or six words at a time). • "Are you cold?" • "Are you hungry?" • "Do you need to urinate?" • "Here is your pill." • "Here is your robe." • "That door goes to the bathroom."	Asking only one question at a time decreases the client's confusion, promotes concentration, and increases attention span.
Repeat the question if the client does not respond or seem to understand your meaning. Use exactly the same words.	Repetition reinforces comprehension. Changing the words further confuses the client.
Therapeutic Response • "Do you hurt?" (pause) "Do you hurt?" **Nontherapeutic Response** "Do you hurt?" (pause) "Are you in pain?"	
Use "yes" or "no" questions whenever possible, and avoid those that require choices or decision making.	Clients with cognitive impairment cannot make complex decisions and feel frustrated when confronted with such a task. (In the early stages of the disease, clients may be able to make simple choices.)
Therapeutic Response • "Would you like to go for a walk?" If the client says, "No," then ask, "Would you like to listen to music?" **Nontherapeutic Response** "Would you like to go for a walk or listen to music?"	
Rephrase the question after a few minutes if the client still does not seem to understand the words. Be patient.	Repeating and rephrasing provides another opportunity to enhance understanding, although the client will need time to process new information.
Break down a task into individual steps, and ask the client to do them one at a time. • "Here are your eyeglasses." (pause) • "Take them out of the case." (pause) • "Put on the eyeglasses." (pause)	Clients with cognitive and memory impairment cannot attend to more than one task at a time. Breaking down a task into individual small steps reduces frustration and promotes self-esteem.
Accompany verbal communication with appropriate nonverbal cues or signals (as long as client has your attention).	Using multiple methods of communication (auditory and visual) enhances the client's understanding of the nurse's meaning and promotes a successful outcome.

Continued

PLANNING AND IMPLEMENTATION—cont'd

Nursing Intervention	Rationale
• "Here is the toilet/urinal" (while leading the client to toilet or placing urinal). • "This is your sweater" (while holding sweater so the client can put it on).	
Use gentle touch when appropriate. • Hold the client's hand. • Place a soothing, supportive arm on the client's shoulder.	Touch communicates the physical expression of caring and empathy. Touch is usually interpreted as therapeutic by most clients but may be misinterpreted by clients who are suspicious, paranoid, or delusional (use judgment).
Use strategies to promote rapid eye movement (REM) or dream sleep. • Allow the client to walk around in a secure area during the day until tired. • Eliminate or reduce naps during the day. • Engage the client in an active daily schedule.	REM sleep promotes rest and avoids confusion, disorientation, and irritability, which may occur as a result of sleep deprivation or disruptions in the client's usual sleep-wake cycle.
Offer the person a little beer or wine at bedtime (when ordered). Offer low-dose sedative or hypnotic medication (with short half-life) if all else fails. If restraints are used, remove them when the client falls asleep.	Alcoholic beverages if ordered can help to relax the client and induce sleep. Low-dose sedating medications may serve the same purpose. Restraints are used only if all other strategies fail and should be removed as soon as the client gains control and/or during sheep.
Increase environmental stimulation if the client appears restless, fatigued, or confused or attempts to wander during the night (sundown syndrome). • Place the client in a room next to the nurses' station. • Maintain soft lighting in the room. • Provide soft music (radio).	Increasing environmental stimulation promotes sensory stimulation that is missing during the quiet bedtime hours. Clients who are suddenly deprived of their routine daily activities require some stimulation at night to prevent restlessness and promote sleep.
Observe the client closely for behavioral cues that indicate pain or discomfort: change in posture (bending over), facial grimacing, increased restlessness, sudden change in behavior.	Pain is considered the fifth vital sign and is assessed according to the client's report of pain and other observations, if the client is unable to verbalize pain (see care plan for Acute Confusion).
Arrange the unit with a reality orientation board that includes easy-to-read clock, calendar (with date, day, time, season, weather), menu, name of facility, and city/state.	Structured, well-placed objects enhance the client's optimal memory function, orientation, and thought processes.
Arrange pictures of familiar objects, utensils, foods, pets, or flowers in key areas on the unit, with appropriate identifying labels.	Accessible, familiar objects stimulate the client's memory function and cognition.
Place familiar and cherished objects in the client's room (e.g., family photographs, pet pictures, quilt, statues).	Personal, valued belongings promote comfort and trust and enhance memory function.
Use concrete language rather than abstractions or slang verbalizations when interacting with patients.	Clients with dementia of the Alzheimer's type and other cognitive disorders have lost the ability to comprehend abstract or slang remarks and are often confused and frustrated by their use.

Therapeutic Responses
• "Are you feeling OK?"
• "It's time to sleep."

Nontherapeutic Responses
"How is it going?"
"It's time to hit the hay."

Maintain routine and structure within the unit rather than submit the client to daily changes in schedule.	The client with Alzheimer's-type dementia and other cognitive disorders has difficulty coping with changes in routine because of short-term memory deficits and emotional lability. A consistent, structured routine supports

Use pictures to communicate with clients who demonstrate aphasia, as well as other cognitive and memory deficits.

memory function and orientation and reduces confusion and frustration.

Visual images enhance the client's understanding of the meaning of the message.

Redirect the client with a simple task or activity whenever he or she mumbles incoherently, rambles in a confused manner, perseverates on the same topic, or engages in stereotypic behaviors.
- Folding towels, pillowcases (familiar tasks are more likely to bring success).
- Stirring cookie, cake mix (familiar smells may have a calming effect).
- Simple exercises (may be done sitting down).
- Sit-down volleyball (use light beach ball).

Engaging in simple tasks reduces confusion, obsessions, and compulsions and provides a direction for the individual's disorganized thought processes and behaviors (refocus and rechannel anxiety-producing energy). Repeating a task such as wiping the kitchen counter or folding linen for 20 minutes or more may be comforting. If the activity seems to be upsetting, gently redirect the client toward another activity.

Initiate a pet or plant therapy session with small, nonthreatening, gentle animals and fresh, green plants.

Plants and animals promote a calming effect; promote comfort, love, and affection; enhance the senses; and support memory function.

Engage the client in frequent reminiscence sessions by reviewing past experiences (e.g., look through family photo album together and identify familiar loved ones).

Reminiscence exercises utilize functional remote memory and promote feelings of enjoyment and belonging or, conversely, feelings of sadness or anger (client may need to vent extremes of feelings in a safe setting.)

Reassure and comfort the client who seems lost and confused being in a new or strange place. Inform the client where he or she is, why, and for how long.

Reassurance decreases fear and anxiety related to feelings of abandonment or confusion and promotes orientation in a simple way.

Therapeutic Responses
- "Mrs. Walker, you are at the day care center for activities today. Your son will come to take you home at 4 o'clock; that's 2 hours from now."
- "Mrs. Long, this is Mrs. Davis's room. I'll walk you to your room now; it's right down the hall."
- "Mr. Campbell, that door leads to the stairs. Are you looking for the bathroom? I'll take you there." (Be sure to pause between each statement.)

Nontherapeutic Responses
"Mrs. Walker, you know you come here 3 days a week. Don't worry; your son will pick you up in a while."

This response assumes that the client will remember that she comes regularly to the day care center.
Also, some terminology may be interpreted concretely ("Your son will pick you up"), which may confuse the client.

"Mrs. Long, you're not supposed to be in the other clients' rooms. Let's go back to your room and read your name on the door again."

This response scolds the client and thus infantilizes her, then assumes that if she reads the name on the door, she will remember her own room thereafter.

"Mr. Campbell, be careful, that door is the fire exit. What are you looking for, the bathroom again?"

This response assumes that the client knows what a fire exit is and that he can respond to an open-ended question ("What are you looking for?"), when it has been shown that the client is usually searching for the bathroom door and simply needs reminding.

Use colors creatively.
- Suggest that the facility paint a different color on the door of each client's room, with clients wearing buttons of the same colors as their doors; include color-coded linen and bedspreads.
- Initiate the painting of colored stripes on the floor to serve as codes to different areas in the facility.

Different colors stimulate the client's visual sense, promote identification and direction, and enhance recent memory function.
A chart with the various colors and the areas each color represents could be placed on the wall of the main room for continual viewing by the clients.

Continued

PLANNING AND IMPLEMENTATION—cont'd

Nursing Intervention	Rationale
Celebrate special events or occasions (e.g., holidays, anniversaries, birthdays) with the client and family. • Have a birthday party with cake and decorations. • Invite clients and staff who are close to the client. • Sing familiar holiday tunes ("Happy Birthday").	Celebration of special events enhances memory function with familiar traditions and demonstrates warmth and caring.
Refrain from arguing with a suspicious client about the truthfulness of a complaint. Instead, listen to the client's feelings and deal with the suspicious behaviors. • Respond with empathy and reassurance to feelings of loss and confusion. • If the suspicion focuses on "theft," help the client recover the lost item (if feasible). • Distract the client from the focus of suspiciousness by directing him or her toward other tasks or activities.	Suspicious clients cannot control this type of behavior; instead, they require empathy, understanding, and therapeutic strategies to reduce agitation and aggression. Persistence may lead to agitation and aggression.
Refrain from confronting or arguing with a suspicious or paranoid client about any misconceptions the client may have. Instead, present a nonthreatening reality in a calm and gentle manner; redirecting also helps if the client persists.	Pursuing the client's paranoid ideation may promote agitation or aggression because the client is unable to respond verbally to logic and reason. Agreeing with confabulation or made-up stories can result in confusing the client even more. Gently correct the client rather than convince the client that he or she is wrong. This approach decreases anxiety and prevents any embarrassment the client may feel if he or she happens to be aware of his or her progressive decline in mental functions. Distraction and redirection may prevent agitation and aggression, especially if the client is persistent.

Therapeutic Response
• *Client to nurse:* "I remember you; you're Hilda who lives next door to me in New Jersey."
• *Nurse to client:* "Mrs. Smith, good morning; I'm Karen, a nurse here at Sunnyvale Home in California; you live here now. Let's join the others in the music group.

Nontherapeutic Responses

"Now, Mrs. Smith, I told you 5 minutes ago; this isn't New Jersey, it's California, and I'm Karen. I don't know anyone named Hilda."	This nontherapeutic approach attempts to convince the person that she is wrong by strongly negating the confabulation, which may increase anxiety and shame and decrease self-esteem. It may also be a futile effort because of the client's short-term memory impairment, which may result in frustration for the client and staff.
"Mrs. Smith, if you want this to be New Jersey, that's fine with me. How am I like Hilda?"	This nontherapeutic approach agrees with the client, which could further distance her from reality. Asking to be compared with "Hilda" requires the client to process information in a way that may exceed her capabilities and be frustrating and confusing.
Refrain from agreeing or disagreeing with the validity of the client's delusion. Instead, respond to the feelings that the client demonstrates (which are real).	Denying or confirming a fixed belief only increases the client's confusion and anxiety because a delusion can be both real and frightening to the client.

Therapeutic Response
• *Client to nurse:* "Everyone here wants to kill me. They want to see me dead."
• *Nurse to client:* "Mr. Brown, you seem frightened; you won't be harmed here. This is a hospital, and these people are nurses."

This response addresses the client's feeling and presents reality in a gentle, nonthreatening manner which will promote the client's trust, comfort, and reality.

Nontherapeutic Responses

"Mr. Brown, don't get excited; no one wants to harm you. We all like you."	This response challenges the client's delusion by defending the staff and avoiding the client's underlying feelings (fear of being harmed).
"Mr. Brown, what makes you think we want to hurt you? This is a hospital; we're your friends."	This response implies that the person has no right to his belief unless he can come up with a reason. Because the

client may not be capable of such reasoning, he may become more confused.

Therapeutic Response

- *Client to nurse:* "Who are you, and what are you doing in my house? You must be a spy."
- *Nurse to client:* "Mr. Jones, I'm Gloria, your nurse. This is your room. It's 5 o'clock, and dinner is being served in the dining room."

In this approach the nurse presents reality by identifying self, the client's room, the time, and the event (dinner) without challenging the delusion, all of which reduce the client's anxiety and paranoia and promote reality and comfort.

Nontherapeutic Response

"Mr. Jones, I live in this house, too. Remember me, my name is Gloria? Let's have dinner together."

In this approach the nurse validates the delusion by stating that she too lives in "this house." She fails to identify her role as a nurse or to orient the client to time or place, which may further confuse and disorient the client.

Avoid argument or confrontation with the client experiencing a hallucination. Instead, listen to the feeling it invokes within the client, and respond in a calm, noncommittal manner, without agreeing or disagreeing with the sensory misperception.

Listening to the client's feelings decreases anxiety, reduces confusion, and presents a nonthreatening reality.

Therapeutic Responses

- "Mrs. Smith, I don't hear the voices you hear, but it must be upsetting (or frightening) to you."
- "Mr. Jones, those people on TV are talking about news events that are going on in the world today."

Nontherapeutic Responses

"Mrs. Smith, there are no voices here; stop worrying about it."

"Mr. Jones, those people on TV are talking to everyone, not just you."

This response argues with the client's perception without presenting a nonthreatening reality and fails to acknowledge feelings, which could increase anxiety and confusion. This response corroborates the client's perception by suggesting that the TV newspeople are "talking to everyone," which could also increase anxiety and confusion. Simple explanations of the client's sensory misperception promote reality orientation and reduce anxiety.

Avoid contradicting or challenging the client experiencing an illusion (misinterpretation of sensory stimuli). Instead, offer a simple explanation of what the individual experiences.

Therapeutic Responses

- "That noise is from the pipes under the sink."
- "The curtains are being moved by the wind."
- "That shadow is from the lamp."

Nontherapeutic Responses

"No, there is not a strange man in the room."
"No one is trying to climb in the window."
"That shadow is not an evil spirit; there are no such things."

Challenging a client's misperceptions is demeaning to the client and may increase fear and anxiety.

Educate the family and significant others about the effects of Alzheimer's disease and other types of organic brain disease on the client's short-term memory function and cognitive processes, as well as the struggle to recall past events.

Awareness of the client's capabilities and limitations helps families acquire more realistic expectations and reduces their frustration.

Teach the family and significant others effective strategies to enhance the client's memory function and decrease confusion.
- Provide reminiscence sessions.
- Maintain structure and routine.
- Convey patience and understanding.

Knowledge facilitates communication, acceptance, and effective interpersonal relationships between clients and families.

Care Plan

DSM-IV-TR Diagnosis   **Delirium, Dementia, and Amnestic and Other Cognitive Disorders**

NANDA Diagnosis: Impaired Social Interaction
Insufficient or excessive quantity or ineffective quality of social exchange.

Focus:
For the client with delirium, dementia, amnestic disorders, and other cognitive disorders that reflect deterioration of mental functions because of the brain's response to disease or damage, resulting in impairment in social skills and inability to relate to others in a healthy, functional manner.

RELATED FACTORS (ETIOLOGY)

Altered thought processes
Confused or disoriented state
Impaired intellect and memory
Sensory-perceptual alterations
Decreased sensorium
Loss of body functions
Self-care deficit
Fear/anxiety/apprehension, depression
Panic or rage reactions
Self-concept disturbance/powerlessness
Compromised physical ability
Social isolation, apathy
Impaired verbal communication
Emotional lability

DEFINING CHARACTERISTICS

The client demonstrates discomfort in social situations with peers, family, and others.
• Is restless and agitated during family meals or gatherings; unable to sit through meals; responds angrily to routine requests such as "pass the salt" or to benign social chitchat.
Exhibits use of unsuccessful social interactions with peers, family, and others.
• Uses *confabulation* (conscious attempts to fill in memory gaps with wrong facts or information, *not* considered intentional lies).
The family reports change of style or pattern of interaction.
The client demonstrates apathy and withdrawal from social interactions and activities.
• Ceases to attend usual social functions (e.g., bridge club, golf)
• Spends more time in room away from family.
Displays lack of spontaneity in interpersonal relations.
• Hesitates when responding to others, even when topic is familiar to the client.
Demonstrates emotional lability (may result from delusion, hallucination, fear, confusion, anxiety, frustration).

• Displays sudden outburst of anger with no obvious provocation when approached by family member, nurse, or another client.
• Begins to shout in the middle of an activity (e.g., exercise class, cooking group).
• Expresses fear when the nurse or a family member attempts to help the client into shower or bathtub (may be experiencing an illusion; shower could be misinterpreted as rain).
Exhibits decreased interest and care in ADLs (e.g., basic hygiene, grooming, household chores, business matters).
• Forgets to bathe, use deodorant.
• Fails to dress completely or appropriately (e.g., looks disheveled).
• Wears same soiled clothing repeatedly.
• Ceases to do laundry, prepare meals, shop for food, feed family pets.
• Stops paying bills, answering mail, attending meetings.
Demonstrates diminished regard for social courtesies.
• Responds to others with rude or vulgar remarks.
• Forgets to thank others or excuse self when appropriate.
• Behaves in stubborn or cantankerous manner in presence of others.
Wanders aimlessly around facility or home without direction or sense of purpose (e.g., may end up in another client's room or bed).
Loses sense of direction in once-familiar surroundings (e.g., may be unable to find way home, inciting neighbors or police to search for the client).
Demonstrates extremely impaired judgment in social behaviors.
• Handles own fecal material instead of flushing it in toilet.
• Smears feces on walls or furniture.
• Disposes of excrement in inappropriate places (under bed, in closet) with no memory of it.
Displays perseveration in the form of compulsive, stereotypic behaviors.
• Rubbing hands together until skin is raw.
• Licks lips, chews lips or inside of mouth repeatedly.
• Explores inedible objects with mouth *(hyperorality)*.
• Taps fingers repeatedly on tabletop or feet on floor when seated (irritates others).
• Folds and unfolds sheets, towels, blankets continuously (may be used as therapy as long as it does not irritate or exhaust the client).
Demonstrates increased agitation when confronted with new or different situations or unfamiliar people.
Exhibits increased restlessness and confusion at bedtime, especially when alone in dark room *(sundown syndrome)*.
Loses ability to read, write, connect lines, or draw figures with any depth or detail *(agraphia)*.

Loses ability to carry out purposeful kinesthetic movement
    (motor apraxia).
Examples:
- Can no longer figure out how to operate once-familiar
  tools (e.g., eggbeater, hammer)
- Cannot recall how to use simple utensils (e.g., cutting
  with knife, fork).
Displays apathy or indifference toward food (e.g., stops
    eating).

Exhibits relaxed posture and facial expression.
Sits through meals and activities for longer periods without
    agitation or restlessness.
Displays decreased emotional lability (e.g., angry outbursts,
    panic, rage reactions) when interacting with others.
Responds favorably to reminiscence activities with staff,
    peers, and family.
Interacts successfully when engaged in tasks and activities
    that are within range of interest and abilities.

OUTCOME IDENTIFICATION AND EVALUATION

The client demonstrates increased comfort during social
    interactions consistent with capabilities.

PLANNING AND IMPLEMENTATION

Nursing Intervention	Rationale
Determine all factors that may contribute to the client's decreased sensorium and would lead to cognitive dysfunction and physical/emotional agitation. • Hypoxia • Electrolyte imbalance (sodium, potassium depletion) • Renal, hepatic, cardiac, respiratory disorders • Pain • Malnutrition, vitamin deficiency • Drug therapy effects (polypharmacy, adverse drug reactions)	Dementia of the Alzheimer's type is often not the only source of the client's impaired thought processes and interactions.
Initiate treatments necessary to correct the client's dysfunctions as much as possible. Provide adequate fluid, electrolytes, nutrition, and vitamins. Administer oxygen as ordered and assess medication effects and restructure medication schedule as necessary.	Early diagnosis and treatment for all possible problems improve the client's sensorium, cognitive abilities, and overall health and increase subsequent social interactions.
Introduce yourself to the client and use eye contact with a calm, reassuring manner and gentle touch while addressing the client by name.	Clients with Alzheimer's-type dementia and other cognitive disorders are very sensitive to others' moods and emotions and can become easily frightened or agitated by an indifferent or negative approach. Conversely, identifying oneself, eye contact, and a calm, gentle approach have a soothing effect on the client and help him or her to focus on subsequent interpersonal interactions. *Note:* Refrain from touching a client who is suspicious or paranoid.
Use simple, concrete terms and a clear, modulated voice tone to explain procedures to the client.	These techniques enhance comprehension because clients with sensory and cognitive deficits have difficulty understanding abstract terms or vague, unclear generalities. Also, soft, low voice tones may be inaudible if the client has a hearing problem.
Reduce extraneous environmental stimuli (loud noise from radio/TV, unnecessary talk/motion), or accompany the client to a quieter area.	These clients are very sensitive to the emotional environment, and reducing distracting stimuli eliminates sensory overload, decreases confusion, prevents agitation, and promotes relaxation.
Ensure that clients who need dentures, hearing aids, or eyeglasses wear them whenever needed.	Such assistive devices enhance the client's senses and reduce frustration and confusion. Clients who have trouble hearing, seeing, or speaking may misinterpret the environment or be misinterpreted by others, which could further impede social interactions.

Continued

PLANNING AND IMPLEMENTATION—cont'd

Nursing Intervention	Rationale
Refrain from challenging or arguing with the client who reacts catastrophically to a situation (rage, aggression). Instead, remain calm, and remove the client from whatever may be upsetting.	Clients with dementia of the Alzheimer's type or other cognitive disorders are sensitive to the behaviors of others and are likely to calm down when distracted by a reassuring nurse. When verbal skills are lost, the client's feelings are generally appropriate, but exaggerated, so that the behavior is socially inappropriate. Distraction is therefore more effective than arguing or reasoning.
Refrain from confronting or arguing with the suspicious, paranoid, or delusional client about the truthfulness of the client's complaint.	The client often cannot respond to reason, and challenging the client may result in anger or aggression.
Refrain from forcing the client to comply with situations that seem to frighten, confuse, or antagonize the client. Instead, wait until the client is more calm and composed.	The client may be experiencing a hallucination or illusion, and the use of force may provoke a panic attack, rage reaction, or aggression and result in harm or injury. Often, the client will calm down after some sleep, rest, or distraction.
Use strategies and responses that reduce or avoid anger, agitation, and aggression. • Demonstrate empathy and reassurance for the feelings of loss and confusion. • If the suspicion focuses on "theft," help the client recover the lost item for as long as appropriate (if feasible). • Distract the client from the focus of suspiciousness with other tasks or activities, rather than pursue the focus of suspicion.	Angry, confused, or suspicious clients need a calm, empathetic approach regardless of the issue. Strategies that reflect empathy and reassurance often reduce negative feelings and protect the client and others from harm or injury. Distraction and redirection also promote a calm emotional state.
Offer prescribed low-dose medication if the client's agitation cannot be managed by other means. (See Boxes 8-4 and 8-5 for *extrapyramidal side effects* and *neuroleptic malignant syndrome*).	Appropriate use of medication as a least restrictive intervention helps reduce the client's agitation and prevent escalation of behaviors that may be harmful. Observe for troubling/untoward effects from medication.
Gently restrain the client if he or she cannot be distracted and behavior escalates to an unmanageable level (release the client from restraints as soon as possible). Follow regulatory standards for restraint use.	Restraint should always be used as a least restrictive intervention to protect the client and others from harm or injury.
Adhere to routine care (ADLs) whether the client is cared for by family or nursing home staff.	A regular ADL routine decreases confusion and agitation and avoids regressive behaviors (e.g., acting out, incontinence, smearing feces).
Redirect the client with a simple task or activity whenever the client perseverates or engages in stereotypic behaviors: rubs hands together; taps fingers on tabletop or feet on floor; folds or unfolds sheets, pillowcases, towels.	Redirection helps to focus anxiety-producing energy toward constructive ends. Folding towels may be comforting for about 20 minutes. If the activity seems upsetting, redirect the client toward another activity or interaction.
Engage the client in short, routine social interactions throughout the day, using a calm, gentle approach, familiar simple topics, and concrete language.	Engaging in simple interactions avoids sensory overload, enhances memory function, and supports clear thought processes and positive social interactions.
Demonstrate patience when the client hesitates before initiating conversation or responding to others' requests; attempt to anticipate the client's needs.	Urging the client to speed up remarks or requests only frustrates and confuses the client. Meeting the client's needs prevents adverse effects.
Use humor when feasible, but not at the client's expense.	Humor is a universal language and an experience that enhances communication and social interactions (use judgment).

Ignore crude or vulgar remarks or actions made by the client while assessing the intent behind the client's words or activity. The client who acts or speaks in a sexually explicit manner may be attempting to get in touch with that part of self that was once sensual and productive. The nurse can engage the client in another rewarding, enjoyable activity such as music, exercise, or preparing a meal.

Clients with Alzheimer's disease and other cognitive disorders occasionally lose their capacity to control socially inappropriate behaviors or expressions. When the family and staff satisfy other important needs, clients may exhibit more positive behaviors as they begin to feel accepted and productive.

Assess the client's ability to perform once-familiar motor acts, such as operating tools, utensils, or instruments (e.g., stationary bicycle, eggbeater, using knife and fork together to cut), and offer assistance when necessary.

Clients eventually lose the ability to carry out purposeful, kinesthetic movements (motor apraxia) and need help.

Assist the client with basic care and personal hygiene needs, such as bathing, dressing, grooming, and applying cosmetics.

A neat, clean appearance promotes comfort, builds self-esteem, and protects the client from rejection or ridicule during social interactions with other clients.

Allow the client to do as much as possible for self, as long as the effort does not become frustrating or confusing.

Encouraging a client's independence as long as possible builds self-esteem and promotes positive interpersonal relationships.

Serve the client simple, easy-to-eat meals and drinks.

Serving simple, convenient meals and beverages decreases the amount of time the client is required to sit in one place and minimizes restlessness and agitation.

Engage the client in interactive therapies: music therapy, stretching exercises, cooking, sit-down volleyball.

Therapies increase the client's involvement and interpersonal interactions with staff and other clients during the day and minimize the client's apathy and withdrawal from social situations and activities.

Arrange schedule so that the client stays awake (avoids naps) during the day.

Sleeping during the day may disrupt or prevent nighttime sleep and result in restlessness and agitation during the night and fatigue and exhaustion during the day.

Assess the effectiveness of medications and any adverse effects (if client is taking them to control agitation).

Drug dosage may need to be reduced or the drug schedule changed if it makes the client sleepy during the day. Some medications may paradoxically increase agitation and confusion and interfere with the client's social interactions.

Schedule tests and treatments for the morning and afternoon.

This will allow the client to wind down in the late afternoon and evening, which helps to avoid excess stimulation before bedtime.

Reorient the client in a calm, soothing manner if the client awakens during the night.

This approach avoids precipitating extreme agitation and possibly aggressive behaviors.

Family Teaching

Inform family members not to be alarmed when the client experiences confusion, anxiety, or rage. Instead, calm the client by decreasing stimulation that may be distressing, or accompany the client to a less stimulating area and stay until the client is calm and composed.

Clients with Alzheimer's-type dementia and other cognitive disorders occasionally experience emotional lability, which may result from neurologic changes in areas of the brain that control mood and affect, as well as from the client's overwhelming frustration and powerlessness. Reducing distracting stimuli helps to calm and focus the client, which may decrease anxiety and prevent behavior from escalating to panic or aggressive states. Remaining with the client when he or she is anxious or confused provides security and safety.

Continued

PLANNING AND IMPLEMENTATION—cont'd

Nursing Intervention	Rationale
Teach family members that the client can no longer fully engage in the social conversation that generally accompanies mealtimes and other similar social situations.	Providing the family with knowledge about the effects of the disease on the client's social capabilities gives realism to their expectations so that they will not make unrealistic demands that may frustrate the client unnecessarily.
Teach the family that the client may use confabulation in social situations to hide memory deficits, not as an attempt to lie, and that arguing or disagreeing will only antagonize the client.	Increased knowledge about the behavioral effects of dementia of the Alzheimer's type fosters more positive interpersonal relationships between the client and significant others.
Inform the family that the client reacts best to reminiscences about the past rather than to "here and now" conversations.	The recent memory stores are impaired early in the disease process, whereas clients can still recall many past events. Reminiscing good or bad times is a positive experience because it brings the client in touch with familiar feelings and engages the client in more meaningful social interactions.
Instruct families to place an identification band around the wrist of the client with Alzheimer's-type dementia that includes the client's name, address, and other critical information.	Clients with serious cognitive and memory deficits may wander away from home and become lost and even die from exposure or dehydration. Proper identification will alert those who may find these clients so that they can be returned home to their families.
Encourage families to enroll clients who live at home in an Alzheimer's day treatment center if possible.	Being part of a group on a regular basis under the guidance of trained professionals stimulates the client's existing memory and enhances the client's daily social interactions. It also gives the family a respite from the challenging care of their loved one.
Arrange for the family to attend an Alzheimer's family support group, if possible, on a regular basis.	Families with loved ones who have dementia of the Alzheimer's type or other cognitive disorders can be helped and comforted by families experiencing the same challenges. Families can also learn effective methods to interact with clients, which will reduce their frustration and enhance the quality of life for clients and families alike.

## chapter 9

Substance-Related Disorders

Since the beginning of recorded time, humans have used mind-altering and mood-altering drugs to change their experience of being in the world. Probably by mistake it was discovered that fermented fruits, vegetables, and grains yielded alcohols and that ingested plants or their extracts could be used to produce various physical, cognitive, perceptual, and emotional states considered desirable. Today, humans continue to use substances for these effects, and substance abuse is a major problem in many areas of the world.

Substances related to mental disorders can be in the form of **drugs of abuse, medications,** or **toxins** (Box 9-1). People may unintentionally be exposed to substances that cause disorders. For example, a person may work with toxic chemicals or mix prescribed and over-the-counter medications and develop substance-related disorders.

Substances are also often used with intent. The trend to use and abuse drugs continues, sometimes with remarkably negative outcomes and complications that affect not only the individual, but also the family, friends, employers, and

---

Box 9-1   Categories of Substances Related to Mental Disorders

DRUGS OF ABUSE	MEDICATIONS	TOXINS
Alcohol	Anesthetics	Heavy metals (lead)
Amphetamines	Analgesics	Rat poisins
Other sympathomimetics	Anticholinergics	Pesticides
Caffeine	Anticonvulsants	Nerve gases
Cannabis	Antihistamines	Antifreeze
Nicotine	Antihypertensives	Carbon monoxide
Cocaine	Cardiovascular agents	Carbon dioxide
Hallucinogens	Antiparkinsonian agents	Fuel
Inhalants	Antimicrobials	Paint
Opioids	Antidepressants	
Phencycladine (PCP)	NSAIDs	
Sedatives/hypnotics/anxiolytics	Over-the-counter medications	

NSAIDs, Nonsteroidal antiinflammatory drugs.

society in general. Examples are evident in every area of life: physical illnesses and diseases (HIV/AIDS, cirrhosis of the liver, fetal alcohol syndrome), mental disorders (substance-induced persisting psychosis), social impairment (substance-related divorce, substance-induced persisting dementia, or alienation by family), legal problems (drug-related injury to others, DUI sentences), and occupational, problems (terminated from job, expelled from school). For some individuals the intentional use of substances may be controlled and considered relatively harmless. Many others, however, experience a loss of control over use of substances, which often results in disruptive disorders, the focus of this chapter.

ETIOLOGY

Despite the physical, emotional, cognitive, social, relational, occupational, spiritual, and legal problems that may occur as a result of substance abuse and dependence, many individuals continue to use and abuse drugs. Theories to describe this compelling phenomenon are plentiful, but none is solely accepted. As with many other categories of psychiatric disorders, it is widely accepted that a combination of biologic, psychologic, psychosocial, and environmental factors converge to perpetuate substance-related disorders.

Although studies of genetics and drug abuse have been widely funded and publicized, specific genetic markers for these disorders are not yet identified. Family studies, twin studies, and adoptee studies strongly suggest a familial predisposition and pattern of drug use. Box 9-2 lists several factors that may be involved in the origination and perpetuation of substance disorders.

EPIDEMIOLOGY

Cannabis (marijuana), often referred to as the "gateway drug" because it is frequently the first or one of the first drugs that young people try, is one of the most commonly abused drugs in America, followed by abuse of prescription drugs.

Although alcohol abuse and dependence remain a major problem in the United States because alcohol is readily available, legal, and relatively inexpensive, alcohol use has decreased slightly over the past 2 decades. Several factors influenced this trend, but the most salient reasons appear to be the swift and sure legal consequences for driving while intoxicated, a growing public intolerance for drunkenness, and the focus on increased health and fitness, which is incongruent with heavy alcohol consumption.

All age groups may be affected by drug abuse. The prevalence of alcohol and drug abuse is higher among men than women, although women abuse prescription drugs more often. Men ages 30 to 45 have the highest abuse rates. Heavy alcohol use across a lifetime is reported by approximately 25% of U.S. adults, and 15% report heavy abuse of other drugs. The fastest growing population of drug abusers is the elderly.

Box 9-2   Etiology of Substance-Related Disorders

BIOLOGIC
Genetic predisposition
Neurobiologic origins
- Low levels of MAOIs
- Dehydrogenase deficit
- Dopamine excess/cravings
Comorbid physical/mental diagnoses
Self-care need/interest deficit

PSYCHOLOGIC/BEHAVIORAL
Depressed mood
Unmet dependency needs
Impulsive style
Inability to tolerate failure
Inability to contend with life stress
Unmet needs for power/attention
Hyperactivity or conduct disorder
Low self-concept/self-esteem
Codependence

SOCIAL
Peer influence/pressure
Detrimental environment
- Deteriorating neighborhood
- Alienating issues
- Illegal behaviors
- Drug trafficking
Dysfunctional family system

MAOIs, Monoamine oxidase inhibitors.

The National Institute on Drug Abuse reported in 1998 that although overall alcohol consumption has decreased, risk for alcohol abuse and dependence is increased among Hispanics and African-Americans. As a result, minorities are at risk for associated social, legal, and health-related problems. Native Americans and Alaskan natives have major problems with alcohol. More than one third of the deaths of native Americans are attributed to alcoholism and associated physical disorders, such as cirrhosis of the liver.

Raves

A growing trend among young people is an increase of drug sales and drug consumption during parties called "raves." Frequently, uninformed parents condone their childrens' participation at these parties because the venue usually includes dancing and is often advertised as being alcohol-free. Naïve parents often think their children will be safe. The need for approval in this developmental stage is strong, and as a result, many youngsters who ordinarily would not try drugs bow to peer pressure when they are encouraged and/or challenged.

The drugs that are abundantly available at these gatherings are dangerous, and the number of fatalities rises each year. Danger exists not only in the chemical compounds but in the inconsistency of the product's content. Users most often do not know the source, strength, or safety of the drugs but use them anyway. The drugs are also referred to as "club drugs," "designer drugs," or as the media calls them "date-rape drugs" because some of them cause amnesia along with other varied symptoms and render their users helpless, easy targets for sexual abuse.

These illicit drugs are considered illegal in some states and include the following:

- *Ecstasy* (MDMA, "E") a synthetic stimulant is one of the most popular club drugs. It was considered safe and used widely by drug users in the 1970s. It is cheap to make and is usually imported from Europe, mainly the Netherlands, where it is legal. Dealers can get $15-$30 per pill here in the United States, so one understands the difficulty stopping sales.
- *GHB* (gamma hydroxybutyrate, "liquid ecstasy") was legally used in this country as a muscle building compound but is no longer legally available. Its intoxicating effects are similar to alcohol, and it is often touted as the "date-rape drug" because it is a clear liquid that can easily be and often is added to the drinks of unsuspecting victims.
- *Ketamine* ("K," "Special K") is an animal tranquilizer used by veterinarians that causes hallucinations in humans. It is often used with Ecstasy and other drugs. The combining of club drugs is called "cocktailing" or "rolling." Mixing drugs may potentiate the effects and increase the dangers.
- *Nitrous oxide* (NO) is a gas that is legally used by dentists and other medical professionals for anesthesia. Partygoers use the drug by filling balloons with the gas and rebreathing it (inhaling and exhaling into the balloon) until their brain oxygen is depleted, causing altered sensations and consciousness and often unconsciousness.

More state governing bodies become aware of this problem each year and act to curtail it, but many argue that laws will not stop the drug use in this population.

Comorbidity

One or more substance-related disorders frequently occur in association with other Axis I mental disorders in the *Diagnostic and Statistical Manual of Mental Disorders (DSM-IV-TR)*. The comorbidity is referred to as a *dual diagnosis*. Other Axis I disorders often coexisting with substance disorders are anxiety disorders; mood disorders, including major depression, bipolar disorder, and dysthymia; attention-deficit/hyperactivity disorder, conduct disorder; and some personality disorders (antisocial, dependent). Clients with thought disorders are also using

and abusing alcohol and illicit drugs more frequently. Clients may be admitted with the diagnosis of schizophrenia coupled with a *DSM-IV-TR* Axis I diagnosis of substance abuse or substance dependence (Table 9-1).

ASSESSMENT AND DIAGNOSTIC CRITERIA

Substance Dependence

The defining characteristic of substance dependence is continued use of substance(s) despite substance-related problems, as evidenced by physiologic, cognitive, and behavioral symptoms. The individual uses the substance(s) in a repeated pattern that can result in **tolerance, withdrawal,** and drug-taking **behaviors that become compulsive.** The person develops strong physical, psychologic, and behavioral drives to use the substance repeatedly. The presence of **three** or more of the following characteristics constitutes dependence:

1. **Tolerance** is the need for greater amounts of the substance to produce the desired effects (e.g., intoxication) or decreased effects when the same amount of substance is used over time.
2. **Withdrawal** refers to the physiologic, cognitive, and behavioral symptoms (a substance-specific syndrome) that occur when heavy use of substance(s) over a long period is stopped, and blood/tissue levels of the substance decline. In addition, the person usually takes the same or similar substance to relieve the symptoms of withdrawal.
3. **Compulsive substance use pattern** is characterized by the following:
   a. The substance is used for longer than intended, or larger amounts are needed.
   b. The person continually wants to stop or decrease use, and the individual tries but fails.
   c. More and more time is devoted to obtaining, using, or recovering from the drug.
   d. Substance use takes the place of previous activities (recreation, work, family/friends).
   e. Use of substances continues despite, physical (cirrhosis, ulcers), legal (DUI, jail), and social/occupational problem (divorce, loss of job).

Substance Abuse

The defining characteristic of substance abuse is at least a 12-month pattern of maladaptive, continuous, or recurrent substance use that results in **one** or more of the following:

1. Failure to complete obligations in home (neglect family), work (take excess absences), or school (fail to complete assignments/get expelled)
2. Continued use of substances despite danger (driving while intoxicated)
3. Legal problems occur as a result of substance intake (DUI; arrest for threatening neighbor while intoxicated)

Continued

Table 9-1 Diagnoses Associated with Class of Substances

	Dependence	Abuse	Intoxication	Withdrawal	Intoxication Delirium	Withdrawal Delirium	Dementia	Amnestic	Psychotic Disorder	Mood Disorders	Anxiety Disorders	Sexual Dysfunctions	Sleep Disorders
Alcohol	X	X	X	X	I	W	P	P	I/W	I/W	I/W	I	I/W
Amphetamines	X	X	X	X	I				I	I/W	I	I	I/W
Caffeine			X								I		I
Cannabis	X	X	X		I				I		I		
Cocaine	X	X	X	X	I				I	I/W	I/W	I	I/W
Hallucinogens	X	X	X		I				I*	I	I		
Inhalants	X	X	X		I		P		I	I	I		
Nicotine	X			X									
Opioids	X	X	X	X	I				I	I		I	I/W
Phencyclidine	X	X	X		I				I	I	I		
Sedatives Hypnotics Anxiolytics	X	X	X	X	I	W	P	P	I/W	I/W	W	I	I/W
Polysubstance	X												
Other	X	X	X	X	I	W	P	P	I/W	I/W	I/W	I	I/W

From American Psychiatric Association: *Diagnostic and statistical manual of mental disorders*, ed 4, text revision. Washington, DC, 2000, APA.

*Also hallucinogen persisting perception disorder (flashbacks).

NOTE: X, I, W, I/W, or P indicates that the category is recognized in *DSM-IV-TR*. In addition, *I* indicates that the specifier With Onset During Intoxication may be noted for the category (except for Intoxication Delirium); *W* indicates that the specifier With Onset During Withdrawal may be noted for the category (except for Withdrawal Delirium); and *I/W* indicates that either With Onset During Intoxication or With Onset During Withdrawal may be noted for the category. *P* indicates that the disorder is Persisting.

4. Recurrent social or interpersonal problems (friends stop inviting person, arguments with spouse about drug use).

Substance Intoxication

Substance intoxication is a reversible substance-specific syndrome that occurs following intake of or exposure to a substance. Maladaptive symptoms result from drug effects on the central nervous system; mood changes (lability, euphoria, depression), cognitive impairment (insight, judgment, reasoning), and behavior changes (aggression, belligerence, submission).

▌ THE SUBSTANCES OF ABUSE

Alcohol

Alcohol is an orally ingested central nervous system (CNS) depressant that affects every system in the body (see care plan for Risk for Injury in this chapter).

Physical, psychologic, and interpersonal dysfunction is a by-product of alcohol dependence. Alcoholism is a chronic disease and is the number-one drug problem in the United States that involves a legal substance.

The three major *patterns of pathologic alcohol use* are as follows:
1. Need for and consumption of large amounts daily
2. Regular and heavy weekend drinking
3. Long intervals of sobriety with intermittent heavy drinking binges that last weeks or months

Reports indicate an intergenerational familial pattern for alcoholism; members of an alcoholic family have a higher inborn tolerance for alcohol. Use and abuse of alcohol are often accompanied by use or abuse of additional psychoactive substances *(polysubstance abuse)*. Nicotine dependence is a common accompaniment; other substances frequently used are cocaine, heroin, amphetamines, cannabis, sedatives, hypnotics, and anxiolytics.

Depression is often a concomitant disorder with alcohol dependence; however, the depression may be secondary to alcohol use, or individuals may drink to "fix" the dysphoria that is already present. Alcoholism and abuse of other substances are often complications in persons with bipolar disorder.

Amphetamines

Amphetamine is a CNS stimulant that is typically taken orally or inhaled but may also be injected. Use often begins because of the drug's appetite-suppressing effects or the feelings of euphoria the drug produces. Binges may be followed by a period when the individual is exhausted, depressed, irritable, anergic, and withdrawn ("crash"). Paranoia, sexual dysfunction, memory, and attention disturbances are also common with amphetamine dependence. Tolerance to this drug may occur rapidly, resulting in an inability to experience euphoria and an increase of adverse symptoms.

Caffeine

Caffeine consumption in the United States is a common daily occurrence, as a majority of people begin the day with one or more cups of coffee or tea. Many individuals continue throughout the day, evening, and night to drink caffeine-laden beverages that include sodas and cocoa (Table 9-2). Other frequently used products that contain caffeine are chocolate, over-the-counter cold remedies, stimulants, analgesics, and weight loss medications.

Symptoms of caffeine intoxication include restlessness, anxiety, insomnia, psychomotor excitement, periods of inexhaustibility, speeded thoughts and speech, increased bowel and bladder activity, tachycardia or cardiac dysrhythmia, muscle twitching, and flushed face. To date, caffeine abuse and dependence have not been clearly defined in *DSM-IV-TR*. However, a caffeine withdrawal syndrome has been described that includes headache and may include fatigue, drowsiness, anxiety, depression, nausea, and vomiting.

Cannabis

The most common drugs in this group are marijuana, hashish, and purified THC (tetrahydrocannabinol), which are usually smoked but may be ingested orally. Cannabis may produce euphoria, calmness, drowsiness, and *oneiroid* states (dreamlike states while awake) *or* anxiety, paranoia, and, in very high doses or with long-term use, hallucinations.

Dependence on cannabis can be insidious because (1) many users are able to continue to function socially and occupationally and (2) the physical disorders that may accompany other drugs (cocaine, alcohol, heroin) are relatively lacking. Major problems related to long-term marijuana use are (1) extreme amotivation that renders the individual unable or unwilling to attend to tasks that require persistence, (2) anxiety states, and (3) physical symptoms such as chronic respiratory diseases, impaired immune responses, and hormonal dysfunction.

Cocaine

Cocaine, legally classified as a narcotic, produces extreme euphoria, so psychologic dependence may occur after the first use. Cocaine can be inhaled, injected, or smoked ("crack" or "freebase"), and in some cultures it is chewed as

Table 9-2	Approximate Caffeine Amounts in Common Drinks and Drugs		
Drink/Drug		**Serving**	**Caffeine**
Coffee		1 cup	100-150 mg
Tea		1 cup	50-75 mg
Cola		1 cup	30-50 mg
Over-the-counter substances and caffeine prescriptions		1 cup	$\frac{1}{3}$-$\frac{1}{2}$ strength of coffee
Migraine prescriptions		1 tablet	100 mg

coca leaves. The clinical effects of cocaine are similar to the effects of amphetamines, and in addition to euphoria the individual may experience increased task performance, both mental and physical, and increased self-esteem. Intoxication occurs rapidly and is followed by a "crash" caused by dramatic depletion of serotonin. Withdrawal brings symptoms of dysphoria, fatigue, irritability, and anxiety; resultant depression is often accompanied by suicidal ideation.

"Crack" or "rock" cocaine has been labeled the most addictive drug known and is even more insidious, addictive, and toxic than cocaine. Cardiac dysrhythmias caused by cocaine use in all forms may lead to death. The number of babies born to mothers who use crack is significant, and they are likely to be born prematurely and have low birth weight and numerous neurologic problems. They are also subject to abuse and neglect, a problem that is currently considered to be of major proportions.

Long term use of cocaine may produce the following:

Inhaled: Stuffy, runny nose; ulcerated or perforated septum

Smoked: Damaged lungs; increased susceptibility to infection

Injected: human immunodeficiency virus (HIV) or other blood-related diseases; infections; embolism

Hallucinogens

Naturally occurring hallucinogens *(psychedelics)* are found in some species of mushrooms (psilocybin), in cactus (peyote), and in synthetic form (LSD lysergic acid diethylamide). Currently, young people are using MDMA (Ecstasy). Animal research has shown that MDMA can damage neurons that contain serotonin.

Hallucinogens are ingested orally and produce physical symptoms of tremors, heart palpitations, tachycardia, blurred vision, and diaphoresis. Psychologic symptoms include euphoria or dysphoria, (extreme perceptual disturbances). The person may experience separation of self from the environment *(depersonalization)* or heightened sensual stimulation. Colors become brilliant; sounds, smells, and tastes are intense; and *synesthesia* (seeing sounds, hearing visions) may occur. Other symptoms include fear of going crazy, labile mood, experiencing two feelings at the same time, or an excessive sense of attachment toward or detachment from others.

Flashbacks and "bad trips" are often associated with the use of psychedelics. *Flashbacks* are a reexperiencing of the drug-induced state that occurs in the absence of recent ingestion of the drug—a reliving of the event. Bad trips refer to a frightening panic reaction to hallucinogen intake. Psychoactive substances may trigger latent psychotic disorders.

Inhalants

Inhalants are volatile substances such as hydrocarbons, esters, ketones, and glycols that are found in paints, glue, gasoline, cleaners, spray can propellants, and typewriter correction fluids, among other substances. When breathed in through the mouth or nose, these substances act on the CNS, producing dizziness, ataxia, excitement, and euphoria that may lead to aggressiveness and impulsivity. Permanent kidney, liver, and brain damage can result, or death may occur because of depressed respiratory centers.

Nicotine

Nicotine is used most frequently by smoking cigarettes, but nicotine may also be taken by smoking pipes or cigars, chewing tobacco, and inhaling snuff. Cigarette smoking is the most difficult of these habits to break, and in 1989 the U.S. Surgeon General declared nicotine to be one of the most addictive drugs in the world. The difficulty in stopping nicotine use hinges on several factors, including the reinforcers of repeating the process so many times per day (one pack per day = approximately 7300 cigarettes per year multiplied by numbers of puffs per cigarette), the availability of cigarettes and the omnipresence of smokers, and the adverse symptoms that occur on withdrawal from cigarettes. Withdrawal symptoms include anxiety, irritability, nicotine craving, restlessness, increased appetite, and weight gain.

The number of smokers has decreased in the general public but has increased among women, adolescents, and African-Americans. Cigarette smoking has been associated with several diseases, including cancer, cardiovascular disease, and emphysema.

Opiates

Opiates are powerful pain relievers. *Opium,* the basic substance in this group, occurs naturally in the opium poppy. Several psychoactive substances are derived from opium, including morphine, heroin, and codeine. Many synthetic opiates are used in the United States, including propoxyphene (Darvon), meperidine (Demerol), and methadone (used in treatment programs to assist in withdrawal from natural opioids, especially heroin).

Opioids may be ingested, smoked, or nasally inhaled. Clinical effects include drowsiness, analgesia, decreased consciousness, mood changes, euphoria, and pleasurable feelings. Heroin, used medically in other countries because of its excellent analgesic properties, is illegal in the United States. Opiates are respiratory depressants and can lead to death through their direct effect on the respiratory centers of the brain. Deaths due to heroin continue at an alarming rate in the United States because of increased use and unknown purity (potency) of the illegal drugs.

Heroin is the most commonly abused opiate; it is estimated that there are more than 600,000 heroin addicts in the United States alone. In countries where opiates originate (mainly the Middle and Far East), the incidence per capita is much higher. Once established, opiate dependence dominates the individual's entire life and is very difficult to stop.

Phencyclidine

Phencyclidine (PCP) and similarly acting arylcyclohexylamines such as ketamine or TCP can be taken orally, taken intravenously, smoked, or inhaled. PCP and ketamine were originally used as general anesthetics but are now used only by veterinarians because of the severe symptoms that clients may experience when emerging from anesthesia.

Users of these drugs find the effects unpredictable, but many experience feelings of euphoria, warmth, floating sensations, and vivid fantasy in the form of hallucinations and oblivion. Users may also experience depersonalization, estrangement, and isolation. Psychosis can occur and may be more prevalent than currently recognized because of the unreliability of commonly used drug detection tests. Intoxication can lead to convulsions, coma, and death. Several deaths occur each year because of increased use of ketamine with other drugs during rave parties and other recreational settings.

Sedatives, Hypnotics, and Anxiolytics

A pattern of use relating to each substance in this category and leading to dependence usually begins through either (1) a prescription given by a physician that eventually fosters prominent drug-seeking behaviors in which the client may subsequently seek several physicians to obtain an adequate supply of the substance or (2) illegal sources obtained for the purposes of "getting high" with peers or for use with other illicit drugs to enhance, potentiate, or counteract effects. All sedatives, hypnotics, and anxiolytics are cross-tolerant with each other and with alcohol.

Benzodiazepines are among the most widely prescribed and abused legal drugs in the United States. Tolerance for remarkably high doses can occur, and, as is true for most other substances in this category, these drugs are capable of producing physical and psychologic dependence. Withdrawal from these substances by addicted individuals can cause death.

POLYSUBSTANCE DEPENDENCE

Frequently, individuals who use psychoactive substances take several kinds either simultaneously or sequentially. For example, abusers of cocaine may also use alcohol or anxiolytics to contend with anxiety, or marijuana and opiate users may counteract the effects of those drugs by taking amphetamines, anxiolytics, or sympathomimetics.

Repeated use of at least three psychoactive substances (not including caffeine or nicotine) for 12 months or more, without the predominant use of one substance, fulfills the criteria for polysubstance dependence when dependence criteria are met.

INTERVENTIONS

Treatment Settings

Multiple levels of intervention are considered when treating clients who abuse or who are dependent on substances. Clients may voluntarily appear for treatment because of their personal needs and decisions for life changes. A client may arrive for treatment as a result of family or employer ultimatums. Clients may also be admitted involuntarily to an acute care facility due to results of drug-taking behavior; the client may be dangerous to self, aggressive or dangerous toward others, or unable to meet basic living needs because of drug abuse. Whether the arrival is voluntary or involuntary, a thorough assessment of the client is imperative.

Treatment is started based on client assessment and history of drug use, including how long the client has been using before admission and the type and amount of drug. The nurse in an acute care setting is prepared to intervene with the client's physical needs and problems in addition to one or more psychiatric disorders. Clients who have been using large doses of drugs over an extended period usually have neglected their physical health and nutrition.

Levels of Treatment

Three levels of intervention are usual for a person who has been using drugs heavily before admission. The *first level* of treatment focuses on acute care for detoxification and withdrawal. Biologic interventions include medications to prevent seizures, alleviate withdrawal symptoms (Box 9-3), and manage other psychiatric and medical symptoms. Replenishing fluids for adequate hydration, attention to nutrition that includes vitamin B supplements, and rest are provided.

 Box 9-3   **Stages of Withdrawal from Alcohol**

Stage 1 (8 hours or more after abstinence from alcohol): Mild tremors, nausea, anxiety, rapid heart rate, increased blood pressure, diaphoresis

Stage 2 Gross tremors, anxiety, hyperactivity, insomnia, anorexia, generalized weakness, disorientation, illusions, nightmares, hallucinations (mostly visual)

Stage 3 (12 to 48 hours after abstinence): All symptoms described in stages 1 and 2 plus severe hallucinations and grand mal seizures; stages 2 and 3 are known as delirium tremens.

Stage 4 (3 to 5 days after abstinence): Initial and continuing delirium tremens manifested by confusion, severe psychomotor activity, agitation, sleeplessness, hallucinations, and uncontrolled and unexplained tachycardia

Box 9-4   Twelve Steps of Alcoholics Anonymous

1. We admitted we were powerless over alcohol—that our lives had become unmanageable.
2. Came to believe that a Power greater than ourselves could restore us to sanity.
3. Made a decision to turn our will and our lives over to the care of God, as we understood Him.
4. Made a searching and fearless moral inventory of ourselves.
5. Admitted to God, to ourselves, and to another human being the exact nature of our wrongs.
6. Were entirely ready to have God remove all these defects of character.
7. Humbly asked Him to remove our shortcomings.
8. Made a list of all persons we had harmed, and became willing to make amends to them all.
9. Made direct amends to such people wherever possible, except when to do so would injure them or others.
10. Continued to take personal inventory and when we were wrong promptly admitted it.
11. Sought through prayer and meditation to improve our conscious contact with God, as we understood Him, praying only for knowledge of His will for us and the power to carry that out.
12. Having had a spiritual awakening as the result of these steps, we tried to carry this message to alcoholics, and to practice these principles in all our affairs.

Box 9-5   Levels of Consciousness in Substance-Related Emergencies

Full consciousness: Alert, responsive; oriented to person, time, place; intact recent memory; verbalizes spontaneously, coherently; articulates clearly

Impaired consciousness: Drowsy, lethargic, loss of recent memory, slowed thought processes with appropriate responses

Confusion/delirium: Transient periods of disorientation, restlessness; dazed, uncooperative, easily agitated, irritable, fearful, noisy; responsive to verbal stimuli and light tactile stimuli

Stupor: Responds only to repeated verbal stimuli and continuous, painful tactile stimuli

Coma: Response to intense stimuli either reflexive or absent

The nurse interacts with the client using principles for substance disorders and comorbid psychiatric diagnoses. Clients who abuse drugs may suffer from withdrawal effects soon after admission, so nurses need good physical nursing skills, clear boundaries, and kind but firm limit-setting skills to contend with the client's unique personality, physical/psychologic craving for the substance, and drug-seeking behavior.

The *second level* of treatment focuses on chronic health problems, both physical and psychologic, that result from overuse or long-term use of drugs. This treatment includes necessary medical support, psychoeducation groups that assist the client toward insight, self-help groups such as Alcoholics Anonymous (AA) (Box 9-4), individual therapy, support therapy, and family therapy.

The *third level* focuses on assisting the client to rebuild a life without drugs. The nurse helps the client develop plans for substituting healthy behaviors for drug-taking activities; replacing drug-using acquaintances with those who support sober living; building relationships; expanding the social support network; ensuring housing; securing finances; setting appointments and keeping a calendar; resolving to stay associated with a healthy therapeutic environment; and continuing to take responsibility for conducting own life without drugs.

Hospitalization

Overdoses of psychoactive substances can result in medical emergencies or death if intervention is not available. When available, intervention is usually focused on dysfunction or failure of the cardiorespiratory system. The person may be hospitalized after emergency treatment if indicated by the drug user's physical or psychologic dysfunction (Box 9-5).

Physical conditions other than an overdose that warrant medical attention include drug toxicity, withdrawal syndrome, infections, and physical debilities such as dehydration, malnutrition, and allergic reactions. Psychologic impairment for which clients may be hospitalized can manifest in one or more psychiatric syndromes (aggressive behaviors that cause danger to self or others, or behaviors causing grave disability of the client). Examples include suicidal or homicidal threats, gestures, and attempts and the inability of the client to meet personal needs because of compromised mental state.

Medications

Clients admitted to treatment facilities may receive medications to alleviate acute symptoms of withdrawal from psychoactive substances. After discharge, Antabuse (disulfiram) is a deterrent drug that causes a violent toxic reaction when alcohol is also ingested. It works by inhibiting the enzyme that prevents accumulation of acetaldehyde in the blood. Clients become nauseated, hypotensive, flushed, hot, dizzy, and numb and experience malaise.

Therapies
Individual therapy

Problems often seen in substance abuse and dependence include denial, low self-concept and self-esteem, anger,

PHARMACOTHERAPY **Substance-Related Disorders**

DRUG SCREENING

Drug screening is useful when a client (with paranoia or schizophrenia) cannot present a reliable drug history. Blood levels are useful in determining the client's degree of tolerance. With multiple drug use the presence of multiple drug levels will help to determine the order of detoxification.

ALCOHOL WITHDRAWAL

Treatment for alcohol withdrawal includes benzodiazepines such as chlordiazepoxide (Librium) and oxazepam (Serax). Other treatments include clonidine (Catapres), an alpha₂-blocker, carbamazepine (Tegretol), and valproate (Depakote). Antipsychotics may be useful in major withdrawals.

General management includes multivitamins and thiamine (vitamin B₁) and folic acid. Injectable thiamine is usually given by large-volume intravenous (IV) solution, or a single-dose intramuscular (IM) injection, followed by daily oral vitamin B₁ tablet. This regimen is used to prevent *Wernicke's encephalopathy*, a condition associated with alcoholism, and *thiamine deficiency*, characterized by confusion, disorientation, and amnesia.

UNCOMPLICATED WITHDRAWAL SCHEDULE

All hospitalized patients should be monitored for vital signs. Minor signs of withdrawal include the following:
- Elevated systolic blood pressure (>160 mm Hg)
- Elevated diastolic blood pressure (>90 mm Hg)
- Pulse >90
- Temperature >100.4° F
- Nausea, vomiting, diaphoresis or tremor

A typical withdrawal regimen with chlordiazepoxide, if the client is able to take oral medications, consists of the following:
- Day 1: 50 mg every 4 hours
- Day 2: 50 mg every 6 hours
- Day 3: 25 mg every 4 hours
- Day 4: 25 mg every 6 hours
- Day 5: none

Chlordiazepoxide as needed (prn) is generally not recommended, and the client should not be awakened if a scheduled dose is due. Dosage should be adjusted upward if withdrawal symptoms occur, or the dose should be decreased if the client is overly sedated. Oxazepam or diazepam (Valium) can be used as an alternative to chlordiazepoxide. Barbiturates are not typically used because of the potentiation of CNS effects.

COMPLICATED WITHDRAWAL

If the patient is NPO or vomiting, IM or IV diazepam (10 to 15 mg) or lorazepam (Ativan) (2 to 4 mg) may be used as an equivalent dose to 50 mg of chlordiazepoxide. Resume oral chlordiazepoxide as soon as possible. Delirium tremens may occur. Rule out medical illness such as pneumonia and meningitis.

Diazepam (10 mg IV) may be given initially, followed by 5 mg IV until the client is stable.

Alternatives to diazepam include lorazepam (2 to 4 mg).

Benzodiazepines should be tapered over a period of up to 5 days.

Prophylactic anticonvulsants such as phenytoin (Dilantin) may be used to prevent seizures if the client has a history of seizures. In general, anticonvulsants are not necessary.

Naltrexone (ReVia) (initial dose 25 mg first day, then 50 mg daily thereafter) may be useful to reduce craving.

Disulfiram (Antabuse) (250 mg) may be used as a deterrent for drinking when the client is motivated and reliable.

OPIATE WITHDRAWAL

Treatment for opiate withdrawal consists of the following:
- Opiate substitution (e.g., methadone, buprenorphine)
- Clonidine (Both patches or tablets can be used. The patch is placed for up to 7 days.)
- Combination of naltrexone and clonidine

ANXIOLYTIC/HYPNOTIC WITHDRAWAL

A typical low-dose benzodiazepine withdrawal schedule is as follows:
1. If the client is using long-acting benzodiazepines such as Librium, the current drug should be used and is tapered 20% per week. The tapering schedule is slowed toward the end if necessary.
2. If the client is using short-acting benzodiazepines such as Serax, a long-acting benzodiazepine should be considered, and the tapering schedule described above is used.
3. Alprazolam (Xanax) is tapered slowly, and a dose reduction should not exceed 0.5 mg every 3 days.

High-dose withdrawal involves the following; tolerance testing is used before a withdrawal procedure is initiated:
1. Diazepam is commonly used with tolerance testing, and if the tolerance test is positive, the client can be started with diazepam at 40% of the test dose, gradually tapering by 10% every week. Daily dosages should be divided.
2. If the client is using long-acting benzodiazepines, begin with 40% of the current dose, and taper 10% every week.
3. Dosages should be adjusted upward if withdrawal symptoms occur and should be reduced if the client is intoxicated.

ACUTE WITHDRAWAL SYMPTOMS

The following regimens are designed to manage the acute medical withdrawal symptoms of opiates such as heroin and morphine. Methadone is a synthetic opioid similar to morphine but tolerated orally.

Methadone and levomethadyl (hydrochloride) acetate (LAMM) maintenance are appropriate for clients with a long history (over 1 year) of opiate abuse.

Naltrexone (ReVia), a nonaddictive substance, is an alternative pharmacologic treatment, and its effectiveness is limited by noncompliance and low treatment retention.

Naloxone (Narcan), a narcotic antagonist and synthetic cogener of oxymorphone, is indicated for the following:
- Complete or partial reversal of narcotic depression, including respiratory depression induced by opioids, as well as natural and synthetic narcotics
- Diagnosis of suspected or acute opioid overdose

There is no clinical experience with naloxone overdose in humans (Du Pont Merck Pharmaceuticals, 1990).

Methadone Dosing Schedule for Opiate-Dependent Clients

Grade	Signs and Symptoms	Initial Methadone Dose* (mg)
1	Lacrimation, rhinorrhea, diaphoresis, yawning, restlessness, insomnia	5
2	Dilated pupils, piloerection, muscle twitching, myalgia, arthralgia, abdominal pain	10
3	Tachycardia, hypertension, tachypnea, fever, anorexia, nausea, extreme restlessness	15
4	Diarrhea, vomiting, dehydration, hyperglycemia, hypotension	20

*Initial methadone dose is determined by the presenting signs and symptoms. initial dose of methadone is then repeated in 12 hours. Supplementary doses of methadone (5 to 10 mg) are provided if withdrawal signs are either not suppressed or reappear during the first 24 hours. Once the initial 24-hour dose is established, the dose is tapered at a rate of 20% per day or every other day for a short-acting and long-acting opiate, respectively. Methadone is given on a q12h or q8h dosage schedule (every 8-12 hours), with vital signs taken before each dose. It is unusual for a client to require more than 40 mg during the initial 24 hours of withdrawal. If the client is initially unable to tolerate oral medications, IM methadone (10 mg) should be given as soon as possible, followed with the initial oral dose of methadone, as calculated from the presenting grade of withdrawal.
NOTE: Hospitals and treatment centers that are not specifically licensed for detoxifiction of opiate dependence with methadone must limit the use of methadone for detoxiciation to 72 hours (Code of Federal Regulations, 1983).

manipulation, and dependency needs. Interventions for these problems are located in care plans throughout the text. *Denial* is a major issue with drug abusers, and the client must admit and face the drug problem before recovery is possible. Another priority includes support of the client in his or her journey to wellness. This support is best provided within a trusting relationship.

The nurse provides a mature, nonjudgmental role model and firm, kind limit setting for manipulative behaviors. Realistic encouragement and support are also given as the client learns new ways to tolerate life's inevitable anxieties without drugs and to expand his or her social support network to include healthy, sober significant others.

Group Therapy

Substance dependence group meeting are an integral part of treatment and provide the individual with support, education, necessary confrontation, coping strategies, and a social network.

Self-help groups

The 12-step program of AA is the model for other self-help groups that provide support for the client as he or she attains and maintains abstinence (see Box 9-4). Al-Anon is a group that provides education and support for spouses or significant others, and Alateen provides support for children of the recovering substance abuser.

Confrontation interventions

Constructive confrontation is often necessary to affect behavioral change. On that premise the family, boss, friends (all significantly involved individuals) meet with the client in this intervention. Each member, openly and honestly states how the client's drug use has impacted his or her life, for example:

Child: "Dad you missed all my games in school because you were drunk". "You really hurt me when you didn't make it to my graduation"

Wife: "We haven't had a romantic or intimate evening in 3 years because you are always intoxicated." "You think you're a good lover but never think of me any more".

Boss: "Your performance has deteriorated to the point that I'm going to have to let you go."

Then each person tells the client what must change (treatment plan) or suffer consequences.

Behavior modification

Modification of behavior is a necessary step to recovery from substance dependence, and learning new strategies and techniques provides a method for mastering the environment. Behavior therapy can supply the individual with skills through relaxation training, thought and behavior substitution for self-control, and assertiveness training, to name a few. (see Appendix B).

Behavioral aversion programs in the form of electric shocks or medications that produce vomiting upon drug intake have lost popularity.

Halfway houses

Transitional living arrangements provide recovering drug abusers interim homes and programs between detoxification and the eventual permanent home. They allow a slow adjustment to the community and ease the client's return home, which may have been a source of difficulty before becoming sober. Family therapy seems to be an essential component of successful recovery.

Employee assistance programs

Many employers have established employee assistance programs (EAPs) to help employees recover from drug or alcohol dependence while retaining their positions; some make participation mandatory if the individual desires continued employment. Statistics for loss of dollars from lost productivity related to substance dependence have risen dramatically in the past decade, and EAPs have proven profitable alternatives to firing trained and skilled personnel.

Family therapy

Family therapy is a critical component in the ongoing recovery of the person who uses alcohol or drugs, as members attempt to eliminate enabling and codependent behaviors that perpetuate the problem. Therapy is directed toward helping the family gain awareness of the negative effects of enabling and codependent behaviors and developing strategies based on confrontational approaches. (Refer to care plan for Disabled Family Coping. Support and encouragement of the client/family unit is emphasized.

PROGNOSIS AND DISCHARGE CRITERIA

Prognosis for substance-related disorders is guarded and depends on many factors, including length of time drugs were abused, type of drugs abused, familial history, unique biology, current stressors, past experience and success at managing own life responsibly, desire (and commitment) to be sober, degree of self-honesty, motivation for life change, support network, access to therapeutic contacts, and involvement with self-help groups.

Some clients with drug problems complete treatment the first time and remain sober. Some clients have to repeat treatment several times *(recidivism)*. Some clients do not succeed. Nurses remain hopeful and appropriately supportive but realistic when treating clients. Avoidance of enabling is crucial, in conjunction with encouragement and healthy support.

Discharge criteria are as follows:
- The client maintains abstinence.
- Admits to lifelong dependence on psychoactive substances.
- Expresses knowledge of continual process of recovery ("one day at a time").
- Verbalizes realistic goals.
- Maintains attendance in support group (AA, NA).
- Expresses increased self-esteem.
- Verbalizes decreased guilt, loneliness, shame, despair, and anger.
- Demonstrates methods and strategies for managing anxiety, frustration, and anger.
- Lists tangible substitutes to replace drug-seeking, drug-taking behaviors (hobbies, school, employment, volunteer work, social functions).
- States feeling in control of own life.
- Expresses hope for future.
- Attends self-help group (client and family).
- Abandons people and situations that influence and contribute to drug-taking behaviors.
- States consequences of psychoactive substances on biopsychosocial/cultural/spiritual well-being.
- States names and phone numbers of resources to contact when unable to cope or feeling a need to revert to substance-taking behaviors.
- Investigates substance abuse assistance programs such as EAPs.
- Continues with AA if warranted.
- Supports family and/or significant others to attend Al-Anon and Alateen.

The box below provides guidelines for client and family teaching in the management of substance-related disorders.

CLIENT AND FAMILY TEACHING **Substance-Related Disorders**

Nurse Needs To Know
- At least one half of all families in the United States have problems with psychoactive substances, including alcohol and nicotine.
- Psychoactive substances may alter mood, consciousness, mind, or behavior.
- A client may be dependent on more than one substance at the same time.
- Abuse of substances or dependence on substances results in major physical, psychologic, emotional, and social complications.
- Depression may be present before or after the substance abuse problem and needs to be treated as well. Other concomitant diagnoses should be explored.
- Suicidal ideation may occur in persons who abuse alcohol and other substances; therefore suicide assessment is critical.

Teach Client and Family
- Teach the client/family about the physical, psychologic, and social complications of drug and alcohol use.
- Inform the client/family that psychoactive substances may alter a person's mood, perception, consciousness, or behavior.
- Explain to the family that the client may use lies, denial, or manipulation to continue drug or alcohol use and to avoid treatment.
- Caution the client/family about possible onset of depression and the dangers of suicidal ideation.
- Teach the family how to assess for suicidal ideation, and instruct them to contact appropriate sources to help the client, as needed.
- Teach the client/family that drug overdose can result in a medical emergency and even death; give the family emergency resources for help.

Continued

CLIENT AND FAMILY TEACHING   **Substance-Related Disorders—cont'd**

- Overdoses of psychoactive substances can result in medical emergencies or even death if help is not available.
- Physical complications may occur either from the direct effect of the drug or from neglect of nutrition, hygiene, or health maintenance problem.
- Alcohol is the third leading health problem and affects all ages, cultures, and socioeconomic classes.
- Withdrawal from alcohol can be a medical emergency that may require specific medications, such as diazepam and vitamin B, to prevent seizures.
- Antabuse (disulfiram) is a deterrent drug that causes a violent reaction when alcohol is also ingested. Only a reliable client should take Antabuse.
- Marijuana is the most widely used illegal drug; it is known as the "gateway drug" because its use may lead to other drugs, such as cocaine or crack.
- Crack or rock cocaine is the most widely used addicting drug, and heroin is the most widely used opiate.
- Hepatitis B and AIDS occur in large numbers of the heroin-injecting public.
- HIV-related diseases such as AIDS are life-threatening complications that may develop in drug-dependent persons who share needles.
- Problems seen in clients with substance abuse and dependence are denial, low self-esteem, anger, lying, manipulation, and dependency.
- Denial is a major issue, and the client must admit and face the drug problem before recovery is possible.
- The nurse needs to develop a supporting, trusting relationship with the client while also providing firm limit setting and realistic encouragement.
- Pharmacologic treatment for client with substance abuse includes medication for acute symptoms and withdrawal phases of psychoactive substances.
- Psychosocial interventions include individual therapy, group therapy, family therapy, and behavior modification.
- Alcoholics Anonymous (AA) is the model self-help program that provides education and support for the person addicted to alcohol.
- Narcotics Anonymous (NA) is a well-known self-help program for persons dependent on opioids.
- There are several other reliable programs for families of dependent persons, such as Al-Anon or Alateen.
- Halfway houses provide transitional living for persons recovering from drug dependence and abuse. Crisis centers are available for emergency situations.
- Employee assistance programs (EAPs) are established in many U.S. companies to help employees recover from drug or alcohol dependence.
- Recognize the psychosocial stressors that may exacerbate the client's drug-taking behaviors, and learn how to manage and prevent them.

- Inform the client/family that substance abuse can lead to poor hygiene and grooming and a life-threatening decline in nutrition and health.
- Caution the client/family about the dangers of alcohol withdrawal and the need for emergency care to prevent complications and possible death.
- Teach the client/family about the deterrent drug disulfiram (Antabuse) and the need to avoid alcohol during use of Antabuse.
- Instruct the client/family about the effects of substances, such as cocaine, crack, heroin, hallucinogens, amphetamines, marijuana, and alcohol.
- Teach the client/family about the dangers of hepatitis B, HIV, and AIDS and their prevalence in the heroin-injecting community.
- Caution the client that sharing dirty or used needles can result in a life-threatening disease such as AIDS.
- Inform the client/family about the dangers of street drugs; explain that their effects cannot always be successfully treated with typical antidotes.
- Instruct the family that a client who abuses substances generally suffers from dependency issues and low self-esteem.
- Teach the family to establish trust with the client and to use firm limit setting, when necessary, to help the client confront drug abuse issues.
- Provide the client with a full range of treatment during hospitalization, such as medication, individual therapy, group therapy, 12-step program (AA), and behavior modification to strengthen the recovery process.
- Describe the benefits of programs (AA, NA, Al-Anon, Alateen), to the client/family, in collaboration with the client's physician and therapist.
- Discuss the possibility of halfway houses for the client in need of alternative or transitional living arrangements. Collaborate with the client's therapist.
- Inform the client of the benefits of employee assistance programs, if appropriate.
- Teach the client/family how to recognize psychosocial stressors that may exacerbate substance abuse problem and how to avoid or prevent them.
- Emphasize to the family the importance of encouraging and reinforcing the client's continued abstinence and efforts made to live a drug-free life.
- Emphasize to the client the importance of changing lifestyle, friendships, and habits that promote drug use to remain clean and sober.
- Teach the client/family to keep drugs and alcohol out of the home while the client is still in recovery to minimize temptation.

- Learn how to reinforce the benefits of abstinence, treatment, and recovery.
- Recognize that the client has to change his or her life-style and friends if the client is to remain clean and sober.
- Provide the client with emergency phone numbers and resources to call when the client feels the urge to break abstinence, until a sponsor is available.
- Investigate local community support groups and other resources, such as AA, that can help the client remain clean and sober after discharge.
- Investigate current available educational resources on the Internet and in the library.
- Recognize that recovery from an addictive substance is a lifelong challenge.

- Instruct the client/family to use emergency phone numbers, sponsor (if one is assigned), and other support sources whenever the client feels the urge to break abstinence.
- Teach the client/family about the availability of local self-help programs (NA, Al-Anon, Nar-Anon), to strengthen the client's recovery and support the family's assistance.
- Educate the client/family about current educational and supportive resources on the Internet and in the library.

Care Plans

- Ineffective Denial
- Disabled Family Coping
- Risk for Injury
- Risk for Self-Directed Violence
- Risk for Other-Directed Violence

Care Plan

DSM-IV-TR Diagnosis | **Substance-Related Disorders**

NANDA Diagnosis: Ineffective Denial

Conscious or unconscious attempts to disavow the knowledge or meaning of an event to reduce anxiety/fear, but leading to the detriment of health.

Focus:

For the client who fails to participate in own health care or treatment program to improve health status or prevent illness, injury, or self-destruction because of prevailing denial of substance abuse or dependency and its deleterious physiologic and psychologic effects on self and emotional effects on family, work, and community.

RELATED FACTORS (ETIOLOGY)

Negative self-concept, low self-esteem, sense of failure or inadequacy
Loss of self-confidence
Guilt, shame, loneliness, boredom, despair
Anxiety, depression, anger, frustration
Ineffective individual coping
Life-style of denial, projection, rationalization
Powerlessness
Hopelessness
Knowledge deficit regarding negative effects of substance abuse or dependency
Culturally permissive attitudes toward alcohol and drug use
Religious sanctions regarding alcohol and drug use
Ineffective problem solving, impaired judgment
Omnipotence (perceives self as indestructible)
Adolescent crisis, peer pressure, feelings of not belonging or being accepted
Adulthood crisis, job stress or loss, spouse or children pressures
Senior citizen crisis, loss of job, spouse, finances, functions; retirement

DEFINING CHARACTERISTICS

The client denies that psychoactive substances such as alcohol or drugs are problematic or destructive to client or significant others.

- "I don't have to give up alcohol/drugs. It's not a problem for me or my family."
- "I know alcohol/drugs can be harmful to some people, but I can stop anytime I want to."
- "I don't have a problem. I only drink on weekends."
- "AIDS is something I don't have to worry about. I'm not the type to contract that kind of disease."

Delays seeking or refuses to accept treatment for substance-related problems to the detriment of own health.

- "I don't need any professional help. I'm feeling fine."
- "I'll get help when and if my drinking/drug use gets out of hand."

Cannot admit negative impact of alcohol/drug problem on activities of daily living.

- "I'm a good parent. I love my family, and they know it."
- "I never miss a day's work. My boss and coworkers have no complaints about me."

Fails to perceive fear of consequences (death or chronic illness) as a result of alcohol/drug use.

- "I've never been sick a day in my life, and I plan to keep it that way."
- "I'm healthy now and I don't worry about getting ill or dying."
- "Longevity runs in my family. I'll live a long, healthy life."
- "Alcohol/drugs will never interfere with my health."
- "I've never had any symptoms related to alcohol/drugs."

Resorts to self-medication for headaches, gastrointestinal problems, sleep disorders, or tremors related to alcohol/drug use.

- "When I occasionally feel bad because alcohol/drugs affect me the wrong way, I get what I need at the drugstore."

Continued

- "I know exactly what to take to relieve my hangovers; I don't need a doctor."
- "I can take care of myself; I have some old family remedies."

Denies potential or actual financial crisis as a result of substance use/abuse.

- "No matter what happens, my family will never go without food, clothing, or a home. I'll see to that."
- "I'll always make sure that my family is financially secure; I'm not worried about that."
- "I'm a good provider; that's all that matters."

Justifies use of alcohol/drugs (rationalization).

- "Everyone needs something to lift the spirits; life is rough sometimes."
- "The drink/drugs I take during lunch help me get through the rest of the day."
- "It's no fun to be the only sober one at a party."
- "I get a little shaky at work sometimes. A little drink/pill calms me down so I can do a better job."
- "The high feeling I get from alcohol/drugs makes me feel good and doesn't hurt anyone."

Blames others for use of alcohol/drugs *(projection)*.

- "I need to take alcohol/drugs. My employer/job is very demanding and stressful."
- "My kids are so noisy in the evening. After a day's work I can use a relaxing drink/drug."
- "If you think I'm bad, you should see Tim. He puts away a six-pack of beer before lunch, and I don't start drinking until I'm off work."
- "Being a wife and mother can be so unfulfilling sometimes. Taking a little 'nip/snort' helps me feel more important."
- "It's been lonely since my fiancé left me; an occasional drink/pill takes away the pain."

Blames sociocultural permissive attitude toward alcohol.

- "Our family always drank wine with meals. I've been drinking since I was young."
- "We always had cocktails before dinner at our house; it was a family ritual."
- "What good is a picnic or barbecue without beer?"
- "Drinking and drugs have always been part of important social gatherings."

Uses religion or culture as a means to sanction substance use.

- "Wine has long been used as a symbol during many religious ceremonies."
- "There's nothing wrong with drinking a little wine; it's part of our culture."

Reports need for increased amount of alcohol/drugs to reach same effect (increased tolerance; e.g., requires two drinks during lunch instead of one to get the same effect).

- "Pour me another drink, dear, the last one seemed so weak; it didn't do anything for me."

Continues to drink/use drugs despite obvious dangers; drinks or takes drugs inappropriately (e.g., driving while intoxicated; drinking/using drugs while at work or school).

Attempts unsuccessfully to abstain from psychoactive substances (going "on the wagon"); individual has recurrent/intermittent periods of abstinence but continually reverts to using substances.

- "I try to cut down on alcohol/drugs, but frankly, I really don't see the need."

Expresses suspiciousness toward others (paranoia).

- "I sometimes feel people are out to get me; they're always after me to stop using alcohol/drugs."
- "I'm tired of people hounding me about alcohol/drugs; they're all against me."

Verbalizes grandiose, omnipotent feelings.

- "I'm practically indestructible. A little alcohol/drugs can never hurt me."
- "Alcohol/drugs actually make me feel as if I can rule the world."

Relates underlying low self-esteem.

- "I feel more confident when I drink; what's wrong with that?"
- "I seem to be able to talk more easily after a few drinks/drugs; people like me better."

Denies that physical problems are associated with alcohol/drug use (e.g., individual continues to drink despite knowledge of enlarged liver, ulcers, cardiac problems, blackouts).

- "I actually feel better when I drink; my hands stop shaking" (withdrawal symptoms).
- "My wife/husband thinks that alcohol/drugs are causing my sleeping problems. Actually, insomnia runs in my family."

Minimizes alcohol/drug-related symptoms.

- "My stomachaches and morning headaches are from stress. I need to learn how to relax more."
- "My family and friends tell me I often do things I don't recall later, but I've never been in real trouble during those times" *(blackouts)*.

Displaces source of symptoms to other organs or conditions.

- "My physical ailments are not due to alcohol/drugs. I have a little ulcer and it gets irritated once in a while."
- "I always get shaky when I drink too much coffee; caffeine really makes my heart beat fast."

Makes dismissive gestures or comments when responding to others' concerns about alcohol/drug use (e.g., shrugs shoulders and changes the topic when confronted; makes jokes to diminish seriousness of problem).

- "I'm fine. I know just how much alcohol/drugs I can take. I've never been drunk/stoned to the point that I didn't know what I was doing."
- "Don't worry about me; I've never missed a day's work because of booze/drugs."

Seeks doctor's prescription for medication to "calm down" or "get a good night's sleep."

- "All I need from my doctor is a little tranquilizer to settle my nerves."
- "If I can just get my doctor to prescribe a little something to help me sleep, I'll be fine."

OUTCOME IDENTIFICATION AND EVALUATION

The client admits to alcohol/drug abuse problem.
- "I realize I have a problem with alcohol/drugs."
- "I can't control my intake of alcohol/drugs."
- "Once I start using alcohol/drugs, I'm not able to stop."

Seeks medical or psychologic treatment for alcohol/drug problem.
- "I need professional help for my dependence on alcohol/drugs."
- "I admitted myself for treatment because I can't quit using alcohol/drugs by myself."

Describes the negative effects of alcohol/drugs on body systems and emotional health and well-being.
- "Alcohol/drugs are ruining my health. If I don't stop, I could develop bleeding ulcers or have a stroke."
- "I realize the potential threat of contracting AIDS through the sharing of dirty needles."
- "I know about the possibility of fetal alcohol syndrome if I continue to use alcohol during pregnancy."
- "I'm aware that smoking cigarettes or marijuana can cause lung cancer or emphysema."
- "I've heard that cocaine use has been related to sudden death from heart failure."
- "Alcohol/drugs have made me a nervous wreck. I'm agitated, anxious, and suspicious."
- "When I use alcohol/drugs, I'm so preoccupied with my habit that I neglect myself emotionally and physically."

Explains the negative effects of alcohol/drugs on family, employment, and social life.
- "My alcohol/drug habit has caused my family a lot of heartache. I never have time for my spouse and kids."
- "My work is suffering because of my alcohol/drug habit. I can't seem to concentrate the way I used to."
- "I'm sure I act peculiar when I use alcohol/drugs; our friends hardly invite us anywhere anymore."

Verbalizes need for continued treatment for alcohol/drug dependency.
- "I realize that this is a lifelong problem for which I will always need help."
- "I'm going to continue attending alcohol/drug meetings when I leave the hospital."

Attends all therapeutic groups and meetings while in treatment facility.

Abstains from alcohol/drug use while in treatment facility. Expresses hope for an alcohol/drug-free future.
- "I want to enjoy my family, friends, and work as a sober/clean individual."
- "I'm eager to experience life without the effects of alcohol/drugs."

Uses effective coping methods and strategies to reduce stress and anxiety and build self-esteem.
- Engages in favorite sport or hobby (golf, tennis, dance, painting, sculpting).
- Exercises regularly (aerobics, walks, jogs, swims).
- Attends cognitive therapy and assertiveness training classes.
- Uses biofeedback, meditation, or relaxation tapes or strategies. (see Appendix B).
- Employs thought-stopping techniques.
- Continues to attend alcohol/drug community meetings.
- Learns to anticipate stress-producing situations and utilizes strategies to manage or avoid them (see Appendix B).

Reports positive changes in family, job, and social interactions as a result of abstinence from alcohol/drugs.
- "I have much more quality time now with my spouse and children. We're all much happier."
- "My employer says I'm doing so well that I may be up for a promotion. My coworker and I get along better, too."
- "I enjoy myself so much better now at social functions. I know people like me for myself."

Notifies alcohol/drug hotlines, counselors, or support groups (AA/NA) whenever he or she is anxious, fearful, or depressed or craves alcohol/drugs after discharge.

Participates in outpatient treatment centers, school programs (adolescents), and employee assistance programs (EAP) after discharge.

Abstains from alcohol/drug use after discharge.

PLANNING AND IMPLEMENTATION

Nursing Intervention	Rationale
Be aware of your own drinking/drug habits, biases, and attitudes before caring for clients with a diagnosis of alcohol/drug dependency.	Relying on your own thoughts, feelings, or behavior about chemical abuse/dependency as guidelines for judging and treating others may sabotage the nurse-client relationship and must be addressed before treatment. The nurse and other treatment team members need to remain objective.
Discuss your own feelings and biases regarding alcohol/drugs with qualified staff or therapists who can help promote objectivity.	Such discussion ensures objective, high-quality care for the client with a substance-abuse problem.

Continued

PLANNING AND IMPLEMENTATION—cont'd

Nursing Intervention	Rationale
Approach the client in a direct, matter-of-fact, nonjudgmental manner. • "I'm Kate, your nurse for the day shift. I'm part of the team who will help support you during your stay in the chemical dependency program."	A direct, nonjudgmental approach helps the nurse gain trust and establish a therapeutic relationship with the client.
Demonstrate concern and interest for the client as a worth-while individual who deserves help rather than using confrontation initially. **Therapeutic Responses** • "Jim, the staff cares about you, and everyone is committed to helping you succeed in the program." • "Joan, you deserve to have things go better in your life. This program will help you with that goal." **Nontherapeutic Responses** "Jim, the plain fact is you're an alcoholic, and treatment won't help until you admit it." "Joan, you're addicted to drugs, and we can only help you when you face your addiction."	Showing concern builds trust and enhances self-esteem. Use of confrontation too early in the client's treatment may result in the client's rejection of the nurse's efforts because the chemically dependent person has a low frustration tolerance and low self-esteem. Also, drugs and alcohol alter perceptions and cause memory deficits, especially in clients with a history of blackouts or sensory perceptual impairment. As the relationship evolves and the client gains more psychologic and physical strength, he or she will be better able to accept the chemical dependency diagnosis.
Continue to demonstrate a positive, supportive attitude toward the client while acknowledging the alcohol/drug problem. • "Tim, staff realizes it took courage to seek treatment for your alcohol/drug problem. We'll continue to do our part to help you achieve a substance-free life." • "Pat, we give you credit for admitting yourself to the chemical dependency program. We'll continue to help you work at eliminating alcohol/drugs from your life."	Letting the client know that he or she is not alone in the struggle, and that staff will help the client gradually overcome denial, confront the problem, and progress toward the goal, increases the client's trust, confidence, and self-esteem.
Assist the client to list the times, amounts, and situations related to alcohol/drug use in the form of a chart, log, or journal.	This strategy is especially useful in the early stages of substance abuse to help the client overcome denial, a common defense in clients with substance abuse problems.
Help the client identify critical times in which he or she is vulnerable to alcohol/drug use: midmorning when the children are most active; lunchtime in response to stressors at work; evenings after a difficult workday; before bedtime to sleep well.	Awareness of key times when the client is prone to drug/alcohol use can assist the client to avoid being alone during these times and to fill those times with learned stress-reducing strategies that replace alcohol/drug use (see Appendix B.)
Instruct the client to avoid social situations that trigger use of alcohol/drugs: watching TV, attending a sports event, eating in a restaurant that serves alcohol.	Avoidance of situations that may influence the client to use alcohol/drugs is a major factor in maintaining abstinence.
Help the client to develop an awareness of strengths and abilities. • "John, your coming here for treatment shows real strength of character." • "Pam, you have a real ability to get the group to attend to business; that's a strength."	The client will more readily accept his or her vulnerability (chemical dependency) and comply with the treatment plan if the nurse and other staff members point out the client's strengths and abilities.
Assess for nonverbal clues of substance abuse when the client persists in denying the problem: verbal and nonverbal inconsistencies, deterioration of physical appearance, ineffective work performance, impaired social skills.	This assessment helps the nurse and treatment team to substantiate the facts.

Gently feed back to the client the observed negative effects of drugs and alcohol.
- "Don, you say you always feel OK, but you also state that your stomach hurts and you have headaches every day."
- "Barbara, from your appearance it seems like you haven't felt well enough to care for yourself."
- "Jack, you said you haven't been able to go to work for several days. What happened?"
- "Joan, just before you were admitted, your family said you were extremely irritable and screamed at everyone."

Genuine, gentle feedback on the client's appearance and behavior by a trusted nursing staff helps the client gain clarity and discourages denial.

Teach the client, when receptive, that alcohol/drug dependence is an illness and not a moral problem.
- "Pat, chemical dependence is an illness that can be treated."
- "Tim, substance abuse is a treatable disorder."

Learning that alcohol/drug dependence is an actual disorder helps the client overcome denial and reduce guilt, both of which can be obstacles to treatment and recovery.

Engage the client in milieu activities that the client does well and will bring success and achievement.

The client who gains confidence by succeeding in the mental health setting may be able to transfer those same behaviors as the client attempts to overcome denial and eliminate use of drugs/alcohol.

Educate the client with information about the habitual nature of alcohol/drugs and the deleterious effects on all body systems.
Include information about HIV-related diseases, fetal alcohol syndrome, lung cancer, and cardiac dysrhythmias.
Inform the client about the negative effects on psychologic well-being and interpersonal relationships.
Use and suggest educational sources: films and documentaries; pamphlets, books, and articles; lectures and discussions; Internet resources.

Increased knowledge and awareness of the negative effects of drugs/alcohol are critical factors in encouraging the client to break through denial and choose to abstain from substance use.

Engage the client in therapeutic groups: role play and sociodrama, thought-stopping techniques, cognitive-behavioral therapy, assertiveness training, process or focus groups, alcohol/drug 12-step groups (see Appendix B).

Therapeutic groups help the client break through ineffective denial and learn alternative, effective coping strategies through the dynamics and universality of the group process.

Communicate staff's ongoing support and expectations that the client will overcome the substance abuse problem.
- "Pam, staff knows you can succeed as long as you continue to adhere to the treatment program."
- "Jay, you can do it. Others with chemical dependency problems have succeeded, and we feel positive about you, too."

Continued genuine support by nurses and the treatment team helps continue to instill confidence and hope for success in the client.

Engage the client and family in therapy groups with qualified family therapists, in collaboration with the client's psychiatrist.

A reliable, therapeutic group can help the client and family process the effects of alcohol/drugs on family interactions, devise methods to cope more effectively as a family unit, and assist the client to break through denial.

Encourage the client to attend several self-help groups, such as AA and NA, to choose the group with which the client is most comfortable.

Each self-help group is unique, and the client is more likely to succeed in a group to which the client can relate.

Teach the family the importance of joining companion groups such as Al-Anon and Alateen (refer to these groups in your community for more information).

These time-honored organizations can assist the client's family or significant others to better understand the concepts of codependency and enabling so that they are better able to change their responses and behaviors and define the boundaries between themselves and the chemically dependent member.

Continued

PLANNING AND IMPLEMENTATION—cont'd

Nursing Intervention	Rationale
Demonstrate continued patience with the client's progress and possible relapse.	Treatment of chemical dependence is a long, slow process, and the client may not always be in control. Loss of control and the need to use drugs are primary manifestations of the illness and require patience.
Assist the client to engage in activities that interest him or her and that promote satisfaction.	This process replaces time that was previously used for alcohol/drugs with rewarding, self-fulfilling activities.
Assist the client to set short-term, attainable goals, such as the "one day at a time" philosophy. • "Sam, plan to go one day without alcohol/drugs, and you will achieve your goal for today." • "Joy, if you're successful in abstaining from alcohol/drugs today, your goal for today will be attained." • "Pat, think about tomorrow when it gets here. Today you successfully abstained from alcohol/drugs." • "Jay, just stop using alcohol/drugs one day at a time rather than insisting you're going to give it all up forever."	Setting short-term goals and tackling them one day at a time helps prevent the client from becoming overwhelmed with unrealistic expectations and helps promote success.
Facilitate interactions between the client and other recovering persons.	Interactions with others who have similar problems as the client help to instill hope and offer support for continued abstinence.
Urge the client to avoid previous companions who use alcohol/drugs. • "John, it's necessary to break away from people who use alcohol and drugs if you want to remain alcohol/drug free." • "Dawn, it's best to make friends with people who are also recovering or who have never used alcohol or drugs." • "Mark, recovering alcoholics or drug users can be influenced by persons who drink or use drugs." • "Jill, people who have been successful in their recovery are those who have broken away from friends who drink or use drugs."	Breaking off relationships with previous drinking or drug-using companions is critical to recovery when the client is discharged; this helps to remove their negative influence on the client and facilitates an alcohol/drug-free life-style.
Help the client replace companions who drink/use drugs with nondrinking/nonusing friends and acquaintances. Introduce the client to members of AA or NA groups.	People who are recovering from alcohol/drugs have more opportunity for success if they associate with other recovering individuals who continually encourage and support them.
Direct the conversations with the client toward realistic concerns and thoughts: how to reenter the social and work world, how to say no to peers who apply pressure to use alcohol/drugs, how to cope with stressful situations rather than becoming trapped in denial.	This realistic approach helps the client overcome denial and concentrate efforts toward rebuilding a substance-free life.
Construct situations in which staff and client role-play ways to deal with concerns such as socialization, employment, and saying no to peers who use alcohol/drugs.	Role playing during nonstressful, nonthreatening times can help prepare the client to use learned strategies more easily in times of stress.
Offer positive feedback to the client whenever he or she socializes with others in the milieu, discusses problems related to drug use with staff and other clients, initiates conversations, and ceases to use ineffective denial, rationalization, projection, or intellectualization.	Praising the client for successful behaviors increases self-esteem and promotes repetition of positive behaviors.

Praise the client and family for acknowledgment of substance abuse and continued participation in self-help groups: AA/NA, Al-Anon, Alateen, Nar-Anon, Co-Dependents Anonymous (CODA), Adult Children of Alcoholics (ACA), school programs, employee assistance programs (EAPs). *Note:* The process of recovery for an individual with the diagnosis of chemical dependence is lifelong.

Positive feedback builds self-esteem, reinforces continued treatment, and promotes abstinence.

Care Plan
DSM-IV-TR Diagnosis | **Substance-Related Disorders**

NANDA Diagnosis: Disabled Family Coping

Behavior of significant person (family member or other primary person) disables his or her capacities and the client's capacities to effectively address tasks essential to either person's adaptation to the health challenge.

Focus:

For the family that is unable to cope effectively, has a history of destructive overt or covert behaviors, and adapts detrimentally to a stressor such as a substance-dependent member. Differs from the nursing diagnosis Dysfunctional Family processes: Alcoholism, which describes a family that generally functions well but whose functions have been altered by a stressor that has exceeded the family's ability to cope.

RELATED FACTORS (ETIOLOGY)

Family resistance to treatment for chemically dependent member
Enabling behaviors by family member(s) (see Glossary)
Inability of family to confront source of problem
Ambivalent family relationships
Codependent family member(s) (see Glossary)
Knowledge deficit regarding effective coping skills
Ineffective denial
Life-style of impaired family interactions
Destructive family patterns (e.g., domestic violence/abuse)
Self-esteem disturbance
Inadequate psychologic, physical, cognitive, or behavioral resources
Psychosocial stressors that exceed family's ability to cope
Antisocial personality traits demonstrated by family member(s)
Significant family member(s) with unexpressed feelings of guilt, shame, anger, anxiety, or despair
Biologic, genetic, or familial factors (e.g., family history of substance abuse)

DEFINING CHARACTERISTICS

Distortion of reality regarding the family member's substance abuse problem, including extreme denial about its existence or severity.

- Family ignores or defends against others' concerns about the member's chemical dependence.
- Family rejects others' attempts to help the chemically dependent member by denying the existence of the problem.
- Family demonstrates inappropriately excessive anger in response to questions about the chemically dependent member.

Demonstration of enabling behaviors toward chemically dependent member.

- Family makes excuses for member's substance abuse.
- Family member phones employer to say person is "too sick" to come to work; asks children to go to their rooms to play because parent needs to rest; explains to family and friends that spouse cannot attend a social function because of a previous commitment
- Family member assumes other role(s) in addition to own role (e.g., gets a second job to pay bills, runs all errands, makes home repairs, mother coaches son's Little League team).

Nontherapeutic family intervention patterns.

- The chemically dependent member (victim) deceives family member (rescuer) into believing that he or she (rescuer) is therapeutic and that they have a close relationship.
- The victim does not cut down on using alcohol/drugs, but the rescuer avoids telling him or her and becomes a "patsy" because confrontation could endanger their "close" relationship.
- When the victim gets drunk/high, he or she calls the rescuer, who gets angry and assumes the position of "persecutor." The victim then asserts that the rescuer "never really cared" and feels rejected and abandoned.
- The rescuer feels guilty and engages in self-blame.
- The victim feels guilty and repentant and returns to the rescuer, and the pattern continues.

Neglectful care of the chemically dependent person.

- Family/friend supplies person with alcohol/drugs; keeps liquor/pills in view of person or in unlocked cabinet/cupboard; drinks/uses drugs in presence of person.

Continued

Decisions are detrimental to family's economic
status.
- Allows money to be used to supply chemically
dependent individual's alcohol/drug habit so
that other family members go without food or
clothing.

Neglectful care of family member's social well-being.
- Family fails to attend to social needs of individuals:
misses PTA meetings, weddings; refuses invitations to
join social clubs; ceases to go shopping or golfing with
friends; stops inviting people home, including
friends of the children, because of shame or
embarrassment.

Impaired roles and relationships of family members (holds
family together in a paradoxical way); children assume
various "roles" to survive.
- Hero, caretaker, or "super kid"; takes care of family,
becomes little mom or dad; generally is an overachiever;
needs approval.
- Scapegoat: subject to anger, rage; will do anything for
attention; takes the blame for family problem; frequently
gets in trouble with the law or school authorities; gets
admitted to a psychiatric hospital.
- Mascot or "clown": uses humor to lighten up
seriousness.
- Lost child or "loner": shy, withdrawn, ignored, low
achiever.

(Refer to previous interventions for examples of enabling,
codependent, and rescuer behaviors of spouses/
significant adults.)

Note: Roles may overlap or interchange. Children may
reverse roles with parent: cook, clean, shop, remind them
of appointments, locate car keys, and care for them when
sick.

High rate of alcohol/drug use among family members.
- Spouse/children begin to abuse substances along with the
chemically dependent person.

Frequent loss or change of jobs directly related to substance
abuse.

Prolonged overconcern for or overprotection of chemically
dependent member, which promotes helplessness and
dependence.
- Drives individual home from bar or party after alcohol/
drug binge; attends to member's daily basic needs;
contacts family physician for "medication" to ease physical
and psychologic symptoms of substance abuse; hides
"family secret" from other relatives, friends, neighbors,
and coworkers.

Extreme agitation, aggression, or violence among family
members in response to frustration and anxiety.
Examples:
- Spousal or child abuse, neglect, or scapegoating.

History of chronic anxiety and depression and possible
suicide attempts by family members.

History of truancy from school or work or other legal
problems among family members.

OUTCOME IDENTIFICATION AND EVALUATION
Family

Admits alcohol/drug abuse problem of family member to a
trusted relative, friend, or professional person
(e.g., physician, psychiatrist, nurse, clergy, or members of
self-help group).

Attends self-help groups (e.g., Al-Anon, Alateen, Nar-Anon)
to educate self regarding relationship with chemically
dependent person.
- Does not defend against others' concerns or suspicions
about the person's substance abuse.
- Seeks or accepts help for chemically dependent
individual.
- Does not make excuses for alcohol/drug use (e.g., refuses
to call employer when person is "sick"); does not hide
problem from children, other relatives, friends, neighbors,
or coworkers.

Refuses to supply or make available alcohol/drugs for the
chemically dependent person.

Refuses to make finances available to replenish supplies of
alcohol/drugs; instead, allocates funds for needed food,
clothing, and recreation for other family members' needs.

Engages in social functions that benefit nonchemically
dependent members rather than hiding or retreating
because of fear or shame.
- Attends PTA meetings, weddings, and the like; socializes
with relatives, friends, coworkers; encourages children to
bring friends home.

Maintains appropriate family roles and relationships.
- Absence of children's roles (e.g., super kid, scapegoat,
mascot, lost child); no significant role reversal (e.g.,
"caretaking").
- Absence of enabling, codependent, or rescuing behavior
by spouse/significant adults.

Ceases to overprotect the chemically dependent person.
- Refuses to complete tasks, attend to daily needs, or hide
family "secret"; refrains from contacting physician or
emergency room for "medication" to bring "quick relief"
of symptoms related to alcohol/drug use.

Strongly encourages the chemically dependent member to
enter a treatment facility for the survival of the family
unit, as well as the impaired member.
- "John, your alcohol/drug habit is destroying you and
the entire family. It's urgent that you get into
treatment."
- "Barbara, your continued use of alcohol/drugs has
disabled all of us. It's time to get professional help."

Demonstrates significant reduction in anger, aggression,
violence, anxiety, or depression; instead manifests calm,
stable, cheerful, mature behavior patterns.

Utilizes effective coping strategies to deal with substance
abuse problem to vent feelings, share concerns, reduce
stress, and decrease isolation.
- Phones hotlines.
- Seeks supportive individuals (relatives, friends,
neighbors, clergy, counselors).

- Engages in positive social interactions and activities.
- Attends self-help and other support groups.

Replaces disabling behaviors with abling behaviors (begins with assisting chemically dependent member to enter into treatment while family also seeks help) to facilitate a healthy family system.

PLANNING AND IMPLEMENTATION

Nursing Intervention	Rationale
Assess the presence of factors that prevent the family from seeking or accepting help for the chemically dependent member. • Fear for safety of self and children (abuse problems) • Shame or embarrassment • Low self-esteem • Excessive guilt that justifies punishment • Ineffective denial ("Everything is OK.") • Family myth ("This family is different from any other.") • Deficient knowledge regarding the severity of problem, community resources, legal rights • Educational deficit regarding alcohol/drug dependence as a disease versus a moral problem • Lack of finances • Lack of support system • Loss of independence • Health problems	A thorough family assessment helps the nurse and treatment team determine the best approach and area of referral.
Provide opportunities for the family to discuss the disabling effects of substance abuse problem by asking questions when the family accompanies the client to the treatment facility. • "How do you cope with the stress of alcohol/drug use in your family?" • "Is anyone in the family depressed or suicidal?" (If "yes," proceed with suicide protocol. See care plan for Risk for Suicide, Chapter 3.) • "What are your thoughts about the disease of alcohol/drug dependency?" • "What are the family's most urgent concerns/fears?" • "How do family members argue?" • "Is there abuse/neglect in the home as result of alcohol/drugs?" (If "yes," notify appropriate authorities: child protective services, law enforcement agencies, social services.) • "What would the family like to see change?" • "How do you think change can occur?" • "What is the family's source of support?" • "Are you aware of self-help groups (AA, NA, ACA, CODA)?" • "How can staff help you cope more effectively?"	In-depth discussions with the client's family or significant others allow the family to validate their disabling coping methods in response to the stress of the client's substance abuse and to develop an awareness of how those coping patterns perpetuate the problem.
Discuss with the family the importance of regular social contacts with trusted, supportive individuals.	Such critical discussion helps the family/significant others share concerns, reduce stress, and prevent isolation.
Provide the family with a list of community services or agencies that offer information, education, and protection: telephone hotlines, counseling agencies, legal services, family shelters, self-help groups, child/adult/senior protective services, financial aid services, Internet resources.	This vital information ensures continued support that will strengthen the family's coping abilities and prevent disabling behaviors.

Continued

PLANNING AND IMPLEMENTATION—cont'd

Nursing Intervention	Rationale
Inform the family that alcoholism and drug dependence have deleterious effects on family systems.	This knowledge encourages the family to make a realistic appraisal of the situation and dispels myths and guilt.
Educate the family about the dangers of impaired roles and relationships among its members, especially the children.	Education helps to promote the knowledge that children from alcohol/drug-dependent families have a greater risk of becoming disabled adults (violent, suicidal, chemically dependent, antisocial, depressed, codependent).
Teach the family that violence is not normal for most families; violence may stop but usually becomes worse, and the victim is not responsible for the violence.	Learning about the risk for violence in most families helps to dispel myths and promotes the impetus for change through education.

Group Intervention or Confrontation Strategy for Individuals Who Resist Treatment

Facilitate group intervention or confrontation strategy with skilled intervention therapists to assist family members, friends, employers, and coworkers privately to confront the chemically dependent individual by stating facts objectively in a calm, direct manner, one at a time, without blaming, yelling, or nagging. • "Tom, your speech was slurred when you came home last night, and you didn't respond when I told you our son was injured at school today." • "Sue, you've been in your bathrobe all week and haven't made our daughter's school lunches." • "Ted, you have alcohol on your breath (*or* needle tracks on your arms)." • "Kay, I found a bottle of whiskey (*or* pills, syringe and vial) hidden in the bathroom hamper under the clothes." • "Dad, I was so embarrassed when you showed up drunk at my game." • "Liz, we used to have romantic times, but you haven't been able to engage in lovemaking for months."	Calm presentation of facts by significant persons helps the individual overcome denial and resistance by reinforcing awareness of the problem and its effects on others, whereas yelling, blaming, or nagging tends to reinforce the denial because the chemically dependent person has a low frustration tolerance and diminished self-esteem.
Proceed with the next step of the group confrontation process by having family, friends, and employer make clear, direct statements of consequences if substance abuse continues. • "Tom, either you enter a treatment program now, or you will have to leave your job." • "Sue, either you get help right away, or the children and I will move out." • "Ted, either you admit yourself to a treatment program, or I will leave your home." *Note:* The belief that chemically dependent individuals need to "hit bottom" before they admit their problem and seek help is no longer widely held. In many cases, interventions such as these can take place as soon as the problem is identified.	This powerful confrontation by caring family members and friends helps to facilitate the individual's entrance into treatment and offers hope for recovery.
Teach the family therapeutic skills. • Anxiety-reducing techniques • Assertive behaviors • Cognitive-behavioral skills • See Appendix B	Anxiety-reducing techniques decrease anxiety to a tolerable level. Assertive behaviors facilitate mature communication responses. Cognitive-behavioral skills increase self-esteem.
Praise the family for successful attempts to change disabling behaviors and use of effective coping methods to manage life stressors.	Positive feedback reinforces positive behaviors and builds confidence and self-esteem.

Care Plan

DSM-IV-TR Diagnosis   **Substance-Related Disorders**

NANDA Diagnosis: Risk for Injury

At risk for injury as a result of environmental conditions inter-acting with the individual's adaptive and defense resources.

Focus:

For the client who is at risk for injury or disease as a result of potentially damaging effects of alcohol/drugs on physical, physiologic, and psychologic systems related to psychoactive substance abuse, and potential for injury related to substance withdrawal behaviors.

RISK FACTORS

History of injury related to drug/alcohol use
- Car accidents
- Arguments, fights, provocative behavior
- Continues to drive while under influence of alcohol/drugs

Effects of alcohol/drugs on all body systems, organs, and functions, including mental status
- Nutritional, metabolic
- Neurologic
- Cardiorespiratory
- Gastrointestinal

Complications of withdrawal from alcohol/drugs
- Agitation, anxiety, irritability
- Disorientation, hallucinations
- Depression
- Paranoia
- Craving

Organic psychosis
- Dementia, delusions
- Hallucinations, illusions
- Altered spatial boundaries

Disinhibiting effects of alcohol/drugs on higher cortical centers
- Impulsive, aggressive behaviors

Sedative or depressive effects of substances on CNS
- Decreased sensorium

- Coma

Ataxia, unsteady gait, incoordination

Amnesia episodes or short-term memory lapses (blackouts)

Psychomotor agitation, hyperactivity, sensitivity, overreactivity

Perception of self as omnipotent, indestructible

Potential for fetal alcohol syndrome

Potential for HIV-related diseases as a result of contaminated needles

Susceptibility of ulcerated or perforated nasal septum related to drug inhalation

Susceptibility for physical disorders (e.g., lung cancer, emphysema, infections, cardiovascular diseases) associated with smoking cigarettes, marijuana

OUTCOME IDENTIFICATION AND EVALUATION

The client demonstrates absence of injuries as a result of alcohol/drug use.

Demonstrates absence of physical, physiologic, or psychologic symptoms related to alcohol/drug use.

Demonstrates absence of substance withdrawal behaviors.

Describes negative effects of alcohol/drugs on all body systems, organs, and functions.

Explains that driving under the influence of alcohol/drugs can result in accident, injury, chronic disability, or death.

Verbalizes potential psychologic effects of alcohol/drugs.

Explains damaging effects of alcohol, crack, and other substances on fetal life.

Abstains from use of alcohol/drugs.

Attends self-help groups and EAPs to maintain substance-free lifestyle.

Explains the danger of contracting HIV-related diseases and their life-threatening consequences.

Explains the danger of contracting lung cancer and other life-threatening diseases related to nicotine and cannabis use.

Describes the danger of sudden death because of cardiac dysrhythmias caused by cocaine use.

PLANNING AND IMPLEMENTATION

Nursing Intervention	Rationale
Alcohol (Withdrawal)	
Know that the severity of withdrawal symptoms is related to the length and extent of drinking before withdrawal, that complete abstinence from alcohol is not necessary for the development of withdrawal symptoms, and that decreased use of alcohol in people who have developed a high tolerance and physical dependence may precipitate withdrawal symptoms.	Knowledge regarding the symptoms and consequences of withdrawal from alcohol increases the nurse's awareness and promotes the client's safe withdrawal from alcohol.

Continued

PLANNING AND IMPLEMENTATION—cont'd

Nursing Intervention	Rationale
Alcohol (Withdrawal)—cont'd	
Assess the client for symptoms of withdrawal as early as 8 hours after abstinence from alcohol. Be aware that trauma victims (especially those with a history of head injury) and anyone suddenly admitted to the hospital or drug treatment facility must be observed for withdrawal symptoms.	A close and thorough nursing assessment of withdrawal-prone clients helps to protect them from injury, accident, or death.
Document observed behaviors and stages of withdrawal (see Box 9-3 on p. 273).	The nurse's keen assessment and documentation ensure that the client's early symptoms (stage 1) can be detected, treated, and controlled before the client's symptoms progress (stage 2).
Administer medications at the first sign of withdrawal symptoms.	Treating the client's early symptoms of withdrawal prevents progression to more serious symptoms (seizures) and maintains the client's health and safety.
Stay with the client if he or she is agitated or confused.	Remaining with the client ensures the client's safety and reduces the client's fear and anxiety, especially during early phases of withdrawal or detoxification.
Inform the client that symptoms represent the body's response to alcohol use and are temporary.	This information reassures the client that control over body functions will be regained.
Use restraints only if the client loses control and is a danger to self or others (see care plan for Risk for Self-Directed and Other-Directed Violence, Chapter 3, Mania).	Behavioral restraints are used as a least restrictive measure to protect the client and others from injury.
Inform the client and family that restraints are only temporary and will be removed as soon as the client regains control.	Explaining the reasons for restraint and its time-limited use helps to assure the client and family that immediate safety is the ultimate goal for the client and others.
Ambulate clients in stages 1 and 2 withdrawal as often as possible (see Box 9-3 on p. 275).	Gross motor movements such as walking help the client in early withdrawal to use the energy of anxiety through goal-directed physical activity.
Avoid ambulating clients in stages 3 and 4 withdrawal (see Box 9-3 on p. 275).	Increased activity and stimulation in later stages of withdrawal can promote confusion and hallucinations; also, the client is prone to convulsions or seizure activity and may sustain an injury.
Reinforce reality if the client is disoriented, confused, or experiencing hallucinations or illusions. • "Tim, I'm Kathy, your nurse. You're in the hospital. That shadow is from the curtain on the window." • "Pam, your family is right outside. That noise is coming from people in the waiting room."	Giving the client clear, basic factual information in a matter-of-fact way helps to promote reality orientation and reduce fear and confusion.
Speak to the client in a calm manner with short, concrete statements. • "Tim, this medication will help you feel less anxious." • "Susan, I'll be back to check on you in 10 minutes."	Brief concrete statements by a calm nurse help to decrease the client's anxiety and reinforce understanding. Clients in withdrawal are generally agitated and confused, and calm, concrete responses are helpful.
Reduce all unnecessary stimulation (e.g., lights, noise, movement).	A quiet environment helps to calm the client, promotes orientation, reduces confusion, and diminishes the incidence of illusions from lights, shadows, sounds, and touch.
Remain with the client, especially during times of restraint, confusion, agitation, disorientation, and hallucinations.	Staying with the client when he or she is anxious, frightened, or confused helps to reduce debilitating symptoms, diminish fear, and promote comfort and trust.

Alcohol (Fluid and Electrolyte Balance)	
Monitor intake and output every 8 hours, and ensure a daily fluid intake of 2500 ml orally (unless contraindicated). Offer juices every 2 hours while awake. Discuss intravenous therapy with physician if intake is reduced or dehydration increases.	Monitoring fluid and electrolytes on a regular basis helps to ensure fluid/electrolyte balance and meet hydration needs. Dehydration of brain tissue can result in alcoholic "blackouts." Hypomagnesemia (low magnesium) may contribute to blackouts. Hypokalemia (low potassium) is also a danger and can produce cardiac dysrhythmias.

Drugs	
Assess the client's level of consciousness (see Box 9-5 on p. 276).	Assessment ensures that the nurse intervenes early in the process, which may prevent respiratory failure, cardiac dysrhythmias, irreversible coma, and death due to drug toxicity or overdose.
Document level of consciousness, and report significant changes to the physician.	Documentation maintains the client's safety, prevents progressive decrease in levels of consciousness, and can prevent coma and death.
Check vital signs and neurologic functions every 15 minutes until full consciousness returns.	Assessing vital signs and neurologic functions frequently helps to maintain the client's vital functions, which can prevent irreversible coma, neurologic dysfunction, and death.
Assess the client's airway for patency and adequate ventilation and breathing patterns; assess respiratory tract for obstructions (mucus plugs, vomitus, tongue); turn head to side and have suction equipment available.	Frequent assessment of airway patency, ventilation, and breathing patterns can prevent aspiration and facilitate adequate respiratory function.
Monitor the the client for symptoms of abnormal respiratory patterns: wheezes, crowing respiration, apnea, sternal retractions. Notify physician immediately if symptoms occur.	Monitoring of respiratory function is critical in the event that the nurse needs to notify the physician and initiate intubation or ventilation therapy as soon as possible.
Have life support systems available in accordance with the facility's protocol.	Life support equipment may be needed to sustain and maintain vital functions and prevent death as a result of respiratory failure or cardiovascular collapse.
Monitor electrocardiographic (ECG) patterns; if necessary, initiate standard emergency life support systems, and notify physician and code team stat (according to hospital protocol).	Emergency measures may be needed to prevent cardiovascular collapse and death.
Catheterize client as indicated; assess intake and output; obtain urinalysis, blood urea nitrogen (BUN), and other relevant laboratory studies.	Urinalysis and renal function tests help to determine toxic effects on kidneys due to psychoactive substances and prescription drugs and to evaluate possible need for dialysis.
Administer appropriate IV fluids, progressing to oral fluids when condition permits; continue to monitor intake and output.	Adequate hydration and monitoring intake/output help to maintain fluid/electrolyte balance and to evaluate kidney function.
Administer appropriate drugs (benzodiazepines, antipsychotics) as ordered.	Specific drugs are given to treat withdrawal symptoms or to prevent or treat psychosis related to drug toxicity.
When the client is physically stable, assess for symptoms of organic mental syndrome (disorientation, aphasia, dementia).	Assessing the client for organicity and disorientation helps the nurse determine the degree of cognitive-perceptual dysfunction due to the effects of drugs on the central nervous system and to develop an appropriate treatment plan.
Communicate with the client in a calm, low-key manner, using low to moderate voice tones and short, simple statements.	A calm, brief communication style by staff helps to promote orientation, reinforce cognitive-perceptual functions, and decrease anxiety and agitation.

Continued

PLANNING AND IMPLEMENTATION—cont'd

Nursing Intervention	Rationale
Drugs—cont'd	

Avoid using abstractions or proverbs; instead, speak in concrete terms when communicating with the client.	Individuals with cognitive-perceptual impairment have difficulty conceptualizing and require clear, concrete statements to enhance understanding and decrease frustration.

Therapeutic Response
- "Jack, you're in the hospital because you have a drug problem. I'm Joan, one of the nurses who will help you."

Nontherapeutic Response
"Susan, you're here to 'get clean.' I'm one of the nurses who will help you beat the drug habit."

Assess the client for behaviors that reflect thought disorders (e.g., delusions, confabulation, ideas of reference, paranoia).	Assessing the client's thought processes and cognition helps the nurse determine the extent of the client's illogical thinking and develop a treatment plan that promotes logic and trust.
Avoid challenging the client's delusional system too early in the treatment regimen; instead, try to determine the fears and concerns that may underlie the client's behaviors.	This therapeutic approach helps reduce incidents of aggression; clients may become extremely agitated in the early stages of withdrawal because of misinterpretation of the environment. If the client's perceived concerns and threats are addressed, trust and cooperation are more likely to occur.

Therapeutic Response
- "Don, it's not unusual to have uncomfortable thoughts now. What are your concerns when you say 'nothing can hurt you,' and how can staff help you feel more comfortable?"

Nontherapeutic Response
"Barbara, what you're thinking just isn't true. You're not indestructible, and you need to trust the staff so we can help you."

This nontherapeutic response strongly negates the person's thoughts, ignores the underlying concerns, and defends the staff (by intimating that the client cannot be helped unless he or she trusts and complies). This type of response may promote the client's self-doubt, diminish self-esteem, and increase perceived threats, which can perpetuate mistrust, resistance, and aggression.

When the client is receptive, reinforce reality with simple, concrete statements in a calm, nonthreatening manner.	

Therapeutic Responses
- "Paul, you're saying that drugs can't hurt you because you're indestructible. Actually, you're here because drugs have been harmful to you."
- "Sarah, I know you believe the clients acted as if they were all against you in group today. In reality, they were offering you some honest feedback about your denial."

Therapeutic responses promote logical thinking and decrease risk of injury.

Nontherapeutic Responses
"Paul, why would you be here if drugs can't hurt you?"
"Sarah, it's not going to help you to think everyone's against you. You need to learn to accept the truth."

Nontherapeutic responses challenge the client in a condescending manner, which may reduce self-esteem and result in more mistrust and denial.

Assess the client for sensory-perceptual alterations (e.g., hallucinations, illusions).	Psychoactive substances are capable of crossing the blood-brain barrier and altering neurotransmitters such as dopamine, which can result in sensory-perceptual disturbances.
Present a nonthreatening reality to the client who experiences sensory-perceptual disturbances.	This presentation helps to correct the distortion without provoking agitation or aggression. Hallucinations or illusions can be very frightening to a client and cause misinterpretation of the environment, which can lead to injury.

Assess the client (both adolescents and adults) for symptoms of depression and evaluate for suicidal ideation, gestures, attempts, or plans (see care plan for Risk for Suicide, Chapter 3, Depression).

A suicide assessment may help to interrupt suicide and maintain client safety until he or she no longer demonstrates suicidal behaviors.

Facilitate seclusion/restraint if the client verbalizes or demonstrates a risk for injury toward others because of the adverse effects of substance use/withdrawal (see care plan for Risk for Self-Directed Other-Directed Violence, Chapter 3, Mania).

Seclusion/restraint may be necessary as least restrictive measure to protect others in the environment from injury and to maintain safety for the client and others.

Help the client replace drug use with functional, healthy behaviors and activities.
- The client develops sports, hobbies, or activities of interest.
- Acquires friends who abstain from drugs.
- Avoids friends who use or encourage drugs and situations that may lead to drug use.
- Attend therapeutic and self-help groups (e.g., NA, CA, EAPS, refer to these organizations in your community or workplace).

Engaging in healthy activities helps to prevent injury, illness, and destruction and assists the client to maintain a drug-free lifestyle.

Alcohol/Drug Education

Teach the client/family about the physical, physiologic, and psychologic effects of alcohol/drugs.

Educating the client/family about the potential for injury, illness, and disability as a result of substance use promotes treatment compliance and recovery.

Educate the client/family about the potential for injury, disability, or death as a result of driving an automobile while under the influence of alcohol/drugs.

Informing the client/family about the serious risks of driving while under the influence of drugs or alcohol helps deter the client from driving after drinking or using psychoactive substances.

Explain to the client/family about the potential for injury to and death of a fetus as a result of the ingestion of alcohol or drugs during pregnancy (e.g., fetal alcohol syndrome, "crack" babies).

Educating the client/family about the risks of taking drugs or alcohol during pregnancy discourages the client from using psychoactive substances during pregnancy and encourages her to educate others.

Discuss with the client/family the dangers of impulsive, aggressive behaviors as a result of the disinhibiting effects of alcohol/drugs on the higher cortical centers of the brain.

Increased knowledge about the potential of injury to self and others as a result of alcohol/drugs helps deter the client from using or abusing substances in the future.

Educate the family about the importance of their continued support, encouragement, and attendance at family self-help groups (e.g., Al-Anon, Nar-Anon).

Use of available community resources helps to promote the individual's continued recovery and prevent injury and illness related to drug use.

Teach the client/family about the dangers of contracting AIDS and other blood-related diseases through dirty needle sharing, reinforcing that AIDS is a life-threatening illness.

Educating the client/family about the risk of contracting a life-threatening illness by sharing dirty needles helps deter the client from drug use.

Alcohol (Nutrition)

Eliminate caffeine from the client's diet (e.g., coffee, tea, cocoa, colas, chocolate).

Caffeine is a stimulant that results in tachycardia, which provokes feelings of anxiety and agitation. Withdrawal from any psychoactive substance produces the opposite effect of the drug itself. Because alcohol depresses higher cortical functions and has a disinhibiting, sedative effect on the CNS, withdrawal conversely produces anxiety, which would be increased by ingestion of caffeine products.

Continued

PLANNING AND IMPLEMENTATION—cont'd

Nursing Intervention	Rationale
Alcohol (Nutrition)—cont'd	

Nursing Intervention	Rationale
Offer the client frequent high-protein foods and snacks and mineral/multivitamin supplements, especially B vitamins. Include thiamine replacement.	The person who craves alcohol is generally uninterested in a well-balanced diet and is therefore nutritionally depleted. Vitamin and mineral supplements help to the client' meet dietary requirements. The B vitamins help to calm the agitated CNS and prevent anemia and peripheral neuropathy. Thiamine deficiency can produce Wernicke-Korsakoff syndrome, which is usually associated with alcoholism and characterized by confusion, disorientation, amnesia, and confabulation.
Teach the client/family about the need for a nutritionally balanced diet that includes foods high in protein and rich in B vitamins.	This information helps the client/family plan meals that will increase the client's health status and develop a stronger immune system as a defense against disease and disability.

Alcohol (Physical Care)	
Provide the physical care necessary for clients with diseases, disabilities, or impairment as a result of the deleterious effects of alcohol on all body systems.	Good physical care, including hygiene and grooming, helps the client maintain health, safety, and comfort and prevents progression of injury and disease.

Alcohol (Depression)	
Assess the client for signs of depression that may be experienced as a result of alcoholic life-style *(secondary depression)* or that may have been present all along and preceded alcohol abuse *(primary depression)*. In either case, symptoms such as loss of energy, anorexia, feelings of worthlessness or hopelessness (adults) or apathy, acting-out behaviors, and trouble with the law (adolescents) must be addressed and treated.	Assessing the client for depression helps to prevent destructive behaviors, including suicide, and promotes the client's health and safety.
Assess the client for suicidal ideation, gestures, attempts, or plans; seclude/restrain the client, if necessary (see care plan for Risk for Suicide, Chapter 3, Depression).	Assessment and prevention of suicide is critical because it may save the client's life.
Proceed with other measures if the client has no specific suicidal plans but requires close observation. • Remove all sharp objects from patient areas. • Initiate other suicidal precautions as indicated by facility protocol.	Maintaining a safe environment and initiating suicidal precautions are critical to the safety and well-being of the client and others in the therapeutic milieu.

Alcohol//Drug Education	
Teach the client/family to replace alcohol/drug use with more functional, healthy activities and learning opportunities. • The client/family participates in sports, hobbies, and other recreational activities. • Attains alcohol/drug-free social life. • Uses "say no" strategy. • Attends self-help groups, employee treatment programs, and drunk-driving classes and seminars, as needed, and reads about potential critical problems (fetal alcohol syndrome).	Engaging in satisfying activities and attending time-honored, reliable community organizations help the client/family to prevent the client's self-destructive behaviors and promote the client's health and safety and a fulfilling, alcohol-free and drug-free lifestyle.

Care Plan

NANDA Diagnosis: Risk for Self-Directed and Other-Directed Violence

At risk for behaviors in which an individual demonstrates that he or she can be physically, emotionally, and sexually harmful to self or others.

Focus:

For the client whose use/abuse of alcohol/drugs may lead to violent/destructive behaviors as a result of the disinhibiting effects of psychoactive substances, complications of withdrawal (agitation, excitement, irritability), flashbacks, depressed state, and psychoses (hallucinations, illusions, delusions).

RISK FACTORS

History of violence related to drug/alcohol use

Complications of withdrawal from alcohol/drugs (agitation, excitement, suspicion, paranoia, euphoria, mania)

Psychotic symptoms (hallucinations, illusions, delusions)

Disinhibiting effects on higher cortical centers, leading to impulsive, aggressive, or violent acts

Hyperactivity, extreme sensitivity, overreactivity, psychomotor agitation

Argumentative, provocative, boisterous behavior, verbal threats, threatening gestures (kicks furniture, slams doors, punches hand with first).

Panic anxiety

Flashbacks

Low self-esteem

Hopelessness

Depressed state

Suicidal ideation, gestures, plans

OUTCOME IDENTIFICATION AND EVALUATION

The client demonstrates absence of suicidal behaviors.

Demonstrates absence of violence directed toward others.

Abstains from substance use.

Explains potential violent effects of alcohol/drug use.

Demonstrates no substance-withdrawal behaviors.

Manifests no hallucinations, illusions, delusions, paranoia.

Demonstrates absence of depressive behaviors.

Exhibits increased sense of hope (makes future plans).

Exhibits increased self-esteem.

Demonstrates good impulse control.

Exhibits no signs of agitation, excitement, irritability.

Demonstrates absence of sensitivity, overreactivity, verbal threats.

Replaces substance use with functional activities, hobbies.

Attends therapeutic groups to maintain substance-free lifestyle and eliminate potential for violence.

PLANNING AND IMPLEMENTATION

Nursing Intervention	Rationale
Assess the client's history for violent or self-destructive behaviors as a result of alcohol or drug use.	A history of violence is the best predictor of violence, and prediction is the most effective means of prevention.
Assess the client for symptoms of withdrawal from alcohol and drugs. (See care plan on Risk for Injury for more specific information on client withdrawal from alcohol or drugs.)	Assessing early for withdrawal symptoms helps to protect the client and others from destructive behaviors as a result of agitation, irritability, excitement, paranoia, euphoria, or mania.
Administer appropriate prn medications to individuals who demonstrate withdrawal behaviors.	Administering appropriate medications for withdrawal helps to relieve symptoms, maintain health and safety, and prevent destructive acts.
Assess the client for symptoms of organic psychosis (e.g., dementia, hallucinations, illusions, delusions).	Assessment helps the nurse and staff evaluate the extent of the client's reality orientation and intervene to prevent aggression or violence.
Present a calm, nonthreatening reality to clients who demonstrate psychotic features (see care plan for Risk for Injury).	Presenting reality without challenging or angering the client helps to prevent violence or aggression while reinforcing reality.
Decrease stimulation when the client's behavior reflects a risk for violence (e.g., reduce noise, movement, lights, TV, radio), or accompany the client to a quieter area.	Reducing stimulation helps to promote a quiet, soothing environment that will calm the client's internal stimulation and reduce or eliminate the risk of aggression or violence.

Continued

PLANNING AND IMPLEMENTATION—cont'd

Nursing Intervention	Rationale
Avoid challenging the client who exhibits psychomotor agitation, hypersensitivity, overreactivity, low impulse control, flashbacks, verbal threats, threatening gestures (especially with approach-avoidance behaviors), and pacing with escalating aggression.	The client with these behaviors may need to be allowed to "run self down" in a large, secured environment, while being closely observed by the team, or may require medication/seclusion/restraint to prevent violence and harm to self or others.
Administer appropriate prn medications for the client who experiences aggressive or destructive behaviors as a result of flashbacks, psychosis, or low impulse control (refer to the facility's policy for administration of emergency medications; see pharmacotherapy box in this chapter).	Offering medications during the early stages of agitation often can prevent harmful behaviors from escalating to violence and avoid the need for seclusion/restraint.
Assess the client for symptoms of hopelessness, despair, or depression and for suicidal thoughts, gestures, or plans (see care plan for Risk for Suicide, Chapter 3).	Assessment helps to protect the client from self-destructive behaviors.
Seclude/restrain the client who is potentially dangerous to self or others (uses verbal threats; exhibits suicidal ideations, gestures, or plans; perceives the environment as hostile and dangerous; demonstrates angry, impulsive outbursts toward others; experiences frightening flashbacks or psychoses) (see care plan for Risk for Self-Directed and Other-Directed Violence, Chapter 3).	Seclusion/restraint is used as a least restrictive measure to protect the client and others from violence or harm when other methods fail (see care plan for Seclusion and Restraint, Chapter 3).
Engage the client in short, simple, concrete interactions during the day, in a calm, low-key manner.	Brief, frequent, calm, concrete interactions help the nurse and staff to assess continually the client's potential for self-destructive behaviors and violence directed toward others, with minimal distraction and stimulation.
Provide frequent quiet times, especially when the client appears more aggravated, highly sensitive, and overreactive and after a stimulating experience or intense encounter with staff, group, or psychiatrist. *Note:* A client may request a quiet time or "alone time," or a nurse may suggest it while the client is able to comply.	Initiating quiet time when the client's behavior warrants it helps to calm the client and minimize opportunities for escalating behaviors and violence by providing rest and relaxation.
Engage the client in activities that involve gross motor movements: walking, running, stationary bicycles, Ping-Pong, volleyball.	Physical and motor activities help the client to expend and redirect energy toward functional, rewarding exercises rather than use energy to generate aggressive, violent acts.
Assign the client to groups in which members discuss with each other concerns and feelings regarding alcohol/drugs: focus or process groups, relationship groups, family/friends, AA/NA, "step groups" (the 12-step program is discussed in a progressive manner; see Box 9-4 on p. 276).	Therapeutic group discussion facilitated by experienced staff helps the client gain a better understanding of the risk for aggression and violence due to the disinhibiting and psychoactive effects of alcohol/drugs. People who abuse substances learn best to control themselves by identifying with each other's similar experiences. Dealing with anger in a safe group setting can prepare clients to manage volatile emotions in other situations.
Engage the client in a variety of therapeutic strategies and group exercises. • Deep-breathing exercises • Relaxation techniques • Visual imagery • Cognitive-behavioral therapy • Assertive response behaviors • See Appendix B.	These exercises and strategies tend to reduce anxiety and tension. Deep-breathing oxygenates the blood and slows the heart rate. Relaxation reduces muscle tension and promotes relaxation. Visual imagery creates a calm mental state. Cognitive-behavioral therapies minimize negative self-concept and increase self-esteem. Assertiveness training reduces the incidence of aggression and violence.

Praise the client and family for efforts made toward managing uncontrolled anger and aggression.

Teach the client/family the importance of abstaining from alcohol/drugs and the relationship between psychoactive substances and violence.

Genuine praise for efforts made to control anger and aggression help to reinforce positive behaviors and reduce or eliminate the risk of violence. Reinforcement tends to promote repetition.

Educating the client/family about the link between alcohol/drugs and violence helps to reinforce abstinence and eliminate the risk of violence by teaching cause and effect.

## chapter 10

Eating Disorders

Eating disorders are serious and potentially life threatening when interventions are nonexistent, delayed, or unsuccessful. In the 1970s, eating disorders began to receive closer public and clinical attention as a result of the hospitalizations and deaths of high-profile celebrities whose eating problems were disclosed.

During that time a national trend toward adoration and emulation of unnaturally slender bodies gained momentum. Television, magazines, films, and clothing stores projected the thin image everywhere. Enmeshed in this trend were many people who seemed obsessed with being excessively thin. Normal-sized, healthy individuals were starving themselves or purging their food in an effort to fulfill the image. As a result, the number of eating disorders grew rapidly. Other causes for eating disorders are discussed next.

ETIOLOGY

Eating behaviors and related issues are multiple and complex. Research on psychologic and psychosocial etiology is more available than research on biologic causes, largely because many identifiable biologic changes in clients with eating disorders may result from the disorder rather than being the cause (Box 10-1). As with other disorders, the combination or convergence of biopsychosocial factors is probable. Another problem arises in attempting to describe causation for eating disorders because of coexisting disorders with similar symptoms.

Box 10-1 Etiology of Eating Disorders

BIOLOGIC
Genetic (no marker implicated to date)
Neuroendocrine dysfunction
Neurotransmitter dysregulation
Neuropathology (enlargement of ventricules and sulci in cortex)
Gastrointestinal enzymes

PSYCHOLOGIC/DEVELOPMENTAL
Psychoanalytic (interrupted autonomy/individuation/separation)
Gender identity disturbance
Emerging sexuality (fears related to roles, expectations)
Comorbid disorders (depression)
Perception of failure (resultant low self-esteem)
Need for control
Obsessive-compulsive disorder

SOCIAL
- Image comparison (TV, films, magazines, models)
- Body dissatisfaction
- Unrealistic body proportions as play things (dolls, figurines)
- Exercise/beauty myth
- Family dysfunction (rigid, enmeshed, overprotective; parents fear child's development)
- Sexual abuse

EPIDEMIOLOGY

Eating disorders usually begin in adolescence and affect females more than males by a ratio of 10:1. (*Note:* Fewer samples of males have been researched.) Age of onset is usually 14 to 16 years for anorexia and 18 to 24 years for bulimia, but bulimia occurs in all age groups. Statistics are similar in the United States and in all other industrialized countries. Lifetime occurrence for anorexia nervosa in young women is 0.5% to 1%, and 1% to 3% have bulimia nervosa. White and Hispanic women have a higher prevalence than Asian- or African-Americans. Prevalence in first-degree relatives is high for both disorders.

Comorbidity

Other mental disorders may coexist with eating disorders. With anorexia nervosa, dysthymia and major depression are prevalent, as well as anxiety disorders, particularly obsessive-compulsive disorder (OCD). OCD occurs in approximately one half or more of those with anorexia and exists before the eating disorder in most clients. The most common disorders with bulimia are depression, substance-related disorders, and OCD. Personality disorders also are often diagnosed in clients with eating disorders.

ASSESSMENT AND DIAGNOSTIC CRITERIA

Anorexia Nervosa

Defining characteristics of anorexia nervosa are (1) refusal to attain or maintain minimal normal body weight for age and height, (2) extreme fear of gaining weight, (3) perceptual disturbance (sees self as "fat," even when grossly underweight), and (4) amenorrhea (after menarche, females miss at least three consecutive menstrual periods; before menarche, menstrual cycle is delayed).

Weight loss is caused primarily by food intake reduction as the diet becomes more and more restricted, eliminating high-caloric foods. The term *anorexia* is a misnomer because there is seldom a loss of appetite until the individual is extremely malnourished and near death. Death occurs in more than 10% of those individuals who require hospitalization and usually results from starvation, suicide, or electrolyte imbalance.

Other methods the individual uses to lose weight are *purging* (excessive use of diuretics or laxatives and self-induced vomiting) and increased and excessive exercise. Often the voluntary food restriction cannot be maintained, and eating binges occur, followed by the purging. Usually, food is thought about constantly, and unusual behaviors may develop, such as passionately collecting recipes and cookbooks, preparing voluminous meals for other people but not eating them, or secretly hiding food throughout the house.

With the intense fear of weight gain comes a distorted self-image, and a very thin body is still perceived as fat. If the individual perceives herself as thin, the perception of "fat parts" (buttocks, thighs, abdomen) remains where none exists. Denial of any accompanying medical disturbances is strong among individuals with anorexia nervosa.

Amenorrhea occurs in postmenarcheal females. Also, menarche may be delayed in anorexia nervosa because of failure of the pituitary to secrete follicle-stimulating and luteinizing hormones (FSH and LH) that in turn stimulate estrogen production.

Associated disturbances most frequently found with anorexia nervosa are (1) symptoms of depression (major depression may be diagnosed, but determinants are necessary regarding depression as a secondary result of physiologic starvation); (2) obsessive-compulsive characteristics both in relation to food and unrelated to food and eating; (3) somatic complaints; and (4) other characteristics such as compulsive stealing, excessive need to control the environment, limited sociability, and feelings of ineffectiveness.

Bulimia Nervosa

Defining characteristics of bulimia nervosa are binge eating coupled with methods to prevent weight gain. Diagnosis is made when bingeing and associated weight loss methods occur at least twice a week for 3 months.

A *binge* refers to consumption of an amount of food that is much larger than most individuals can eat, with the eating done in usually less than 2 hours. Typically the type of food is soft, easy to swallow, sweet, and high in calories (ice cream, pastries, cakes), but many individuals eat foods other than sweets. Often the eating is done inconspicuously or secretively, and the individual feels a lack of control over the behavior. Snacking throughout the day, even though a large volume of food is consumed, is not considered binge eating.

Compensatory techniques are used by individuals with bulimia to prevent weight gain after binges. The most common method is *self-induced vomiting*, which is done by 80% to 90% of binge eaters. Most often a person sticks fingers down the throat to stimulate a gag reflex, but implements may be used, or rarely, individuals use syrup of ipecac to induce vomiting. Another method of purging the system is through laxatives and diuretics; rarely a person uses enemas for catharsis. Usually the person reaches a point of being able to vomit at will. Vomiting decreases weight gain but also decreases bloating and feelings of being full so that eating can continue. Many individuals describe a sense of relief or release of tension and anxiety after vomiting, but depression follows the episode as the person deals with postbinge remorse or despair.

As with anorexia nervosa, individuals with bulimia may employ excessive exercise methods to control weight, but this method is not usually utilized as vigorously as in anorexia nervosa. Fasting also may be used to control weight.

Control is a major issue in bulimia nervosa, and a sense of lack of control predominates. A state of frenzy may exist during the eating binge, or the individual may describe feelings of dissociation during the episode. In either case, affected individuals say they lose an internal locus of control over the situation.

DSM-IV-TR Categories

Diagnostic and Statistical Manual of Mental Disorders (DSM-IV-TR) categories for eating disorders provide subtypes for anorexia and bulimia (see box below and Appendix A).

Subtypes assigned to the diagnosis of anorexia nervosa are as follows:

- *Restricting type:* Weight loss primarily results from dieting, fasting, or excessive exercise.
- *Binge-eating/purging type:* Weight loss results from regular binge eating and purging during the current episode.

Subtypes of bulimia nervosa are the following:

- *Purging type:* Person regularly uses self-induced vomiting and misuses laxatives, diuretics, enemas during the episode.
- *Nonpurging type:* Person uses methods other than purging, such as fasting and excessive exercise.

▌ INTERVENTIONS

Primary prevention is key in eating disorders. Advocates for eating disorder awareness can do much to educate parents, teachers, and students about the pitfalls and dangers related to dysfunctional eating. Each group can learn to assess behaviors and potential problems and intervene to help the client before the problem is beyond control.

The first line of treatment for clients with acute eating disorders is safety and health. This may include suicide intervention (usually in the case of existing comorbid diagnoses) and interruption of self-destructive behaviors directed at starvation or purging of food. When it is determined that the client is free from self-harm, the focus shifts to reestablishing nutritional balance and, by learning new techniques, substituting healthy behaviors for existing harmful ones.

DSM–IV–TR Eating Disorders

Anorexia Nervosa
- Restricting Type
- Binge-Eating/Purging Type

Bulimia nervosa
- Purging Type
- Nonpurging Type

Therapies

Therapeutic nurse-client relationship

The nurse-client relationship can be an effective vehicle for behavior change in clients who have eating disorders (see Chapter 1). The client with anorexia nervosa will probably defy the alliance because of habitual avoidance behaviors, anger, and mistrust that have developed as others, in the client's perception, have "forced" the client to eat. The nurse performs a thorough autodiagnosis to avoid judging or becoming angry at the client or in the worst case, take the client's rejection personally and abandon interactions. These clients pose a challenge to the nurse who is not prepared for opposition and rejection of help.

Clients with bulimia require the nurse's careful attention to modeling mature interactions, tolerating the client's superficial approach to treatment, and being patient while the client learns and practices alternatives to binge-purging behaviors. The care plans assist with specific nursing interventions and rationale.

General interventions involve relational, cognitive, behavioral, and medical techniques and include the following:
- Monitor meals, weight, and exercise.
- Stay with client for 1 hour after eating to prevent purging.
- Maintain adequate calories as determined for the client.
- Avoid manipulation and power struggles over type and amount of food.
- Educate about real versus idealized body weight/size and importance of fat in diet.
- Encourage activities and interactions that increase self-esteem.
- Encourage discussion of perceptions, thoughts, and feelings.
- Refute irrational ideas respectfully, and teach substitution of rational, positive thinking. (Cognitive therapy has proved to be more effective than relational therapies for some clients.)
- Encourage the client to engage in mature peer interactions.
- Teach assertiveness, and assist the client to practice in role play.
- Support and praise all efforts to succeed in becoming healthy.
- Support the client and family working together to achieve wellness.

Safety

Clients may enter the hospital with suicidal ideation, threats, gestures, or attempts and must be protected from self-harm. The nurse follows guidelines as outlined in the care plans (see Chapter 3).

Cognitive-behavioral therapies

Behavior modification programs and cognitive-behavioral therapies, both in individual and group settings, have shown promise. Behavioral interventions focus on interruption of the dysfunctional eating patterns. Psychologic approaches strive to (1) increase insight into the complex dynamics of the disorder and (2) improve communication and coping skills (see Appendix B).

Family Therapy

Dynamics are frequently dysfunctional in families in which a member has an eating disorder. Education regarding the disorder and establishing healthy interactions is essential.

Medications

First-line medications used to treat eating disorders with concomitant depression are the atypical antidepressants or selective serotonin reuptake inhibitors (SSRIs), such as fluoxetine (Prozac) and paroxetine (Paxil). Fluoxetine and paroxetine inhibit neuronal reuptake of serotonin in the central nervous system (CNS) but not reuptake of norepinephrine. They provide relief from depression and have less intense side effects than the typical antidepressants. They may also relieve OCD behaviors such as rituals of binge-purge episodes. The SSRIs may be augmented with low-dose atypical antipsychotic medications to treat mild psychosis, obsessive thoughts, or ruminations. Benzodiazepines are not recommended because of their addicting qualities; therefore fluoxetine and paroxetine are also used to treat mild anxiety, induce relaxation, and promote a restful sleep (see Pharmacotherapy box below for doses).

PROGNOSIS AND DISCHARGE CRITERIA

The prognosis for bulimia is better than for anorexia nervosa. For both disorders, early intervention increases probability of successful outcomes. Approximately 80% of clients who receive treatment for bulimia within the first few years recover, whereas only 69% to 70% recover if longer periods elapse before treatment occurs (Reas, 2000). Outcomes for anorexia nervosa are more guarded because of multiple interacting factors. When treated early, and when the client's weight is not too low, outcome is more favorable.

Other important factors include (1) presence or absence of existing comorbid diagnoses, (2) degree of involvement and healthy support from family and significant others, (3) degree to which distorted thinking has been eliminated or modified, and (4) time of discharge. The last factor refers to clients being discharged before all their desired weight is regained and before they have practiced healthy techniques for a sufficient time. When intensive follow-up treatment is provided, clients with anorexia usually have a more favorable prognosis.

Discharge criteria are as follows:
- The client maintains adequate nutrition.
- Maintains weight range as determined by nutritionist.
- Describes alternative behaviors for disruptive eating patterns.
- Maintains attendance in eating disorder support group.
- Verbalizes realistic goals.
- Verbalizes positive self-esteem.
- Describes realistic appraisal of body.
- Demonstrates internal locus of control.
- Expresses adequate knowledge about disorder.
- Describes triggers for disruptive eating behavior.
- Explains medication required: dose, frequency, time, side effects.
- Participates in "no harm" contract.
- Demonstrates appropriate family and social interactions. States resources to contact when feeling out of control.

The box on p. 306 provides guidelines for client and family teaching in the management of eating disorders.

PHARMACOTHERAPY   **Eating Disorders**

FLUOXETINE (PROZAC)

Initially 20 mg/day orally in morning for 4 weeks; may be increased to 20 mg twice daily for optimal relief; *not to exceed* 80 mg/day.

PAROXETINE (PAXIL)

Initially 20 mg/day orally in morning for 4 weeks; may be increased by 10 mg/day every week to desired response; *not to exceed* 50 mg/day.

METOCLOPRAMIDE (REGLAN)

May be used in bulimia to help empty the stomach contents, thus reducing the feeling of fullness. This may discourage vomiting or purge episodes.

The nurse should inform the client taking SSRIs to do the following:
- Discuss medication effects with physician and pharmacist before taking medication.
- Contact physician for any unexpected side effects.
- Call emergency services for any allergic, unusual, or adverse effects.

CLIENT AND FAMILY TEACHING   **Eating Disorders**

Nurse Needs to Know

- Clients with an eating disorder often struggle with long-term maladaptive eating patterns and food-related behaviors.
- Clients often mistakenly appear to be well-adjusted, successful, and happy.
- Clients use food and food-related behaviors in a destructive way to deal with painful emotions and life conflicts and to gain a sense of control.
- Behaviors and problems related to eating disorders may often appear in other disorders, such as depression, schizophrenia, or personality disorders.
- The client's nutritional state is directly related to physical health and may influence or be influenced by psychiatric problems as well.
- Eating disorders are complex problems that may be treated in a variety of settings and often require both medical and psychiatric interventions.
- The hospital setting offers the client a controlled environment in which food, fluid intake/output, weight, medication, and activities can be monitored.
- Hospitalization also separates the client from the family, which may be a contributing factor in the client's problems.
- Anorexia nervosa and bulimia nervosa are two frequently treated eating disorders that often require periods of hospitalization.
- Major factors related to anorexia nervosa are self-starvation, body image disturbance, morbid fear of weight gain, and denial of danger to health.
- Major factors related to bulimia nervosa are bingeing and purging, use of laxatives or enemas, strict dieting patterns, and vigorous exercise regimen.
- Clients with both types of eating disorders often have histories of dysfunctional family patterns, depression, and powerlessness.
- Clients with anorexia nervosa may lose a critical amount of weight and require tube feeding or parenteral methods to regain lost nutrients.
- Clients with anorexia nervosa should not be forced to eat or punished for not eating because these methods only make them fight more for control.
- The nurse needs to remain with these clients from 1½ to 2 hours after meals, including bathroom supervision, because they tend to vomit or discard food.
- A calm, matter-of-fact approach works best with these clients; disapproval or judgmental behavior may remind them of family power struggles.
- Behavior modification programs that offer structure and limit setting and goals have been successful for clients with eating disorders.

Teach Client and Family

- Educate the client/family about anorexia nervosa and bulimia nervosa.
- Explain to the family that although the client may appear well adjusted at times, she may be self-destructive or suicidal and need hospitalization.
- Teach the family that the client uses food and food-related behaviors in a self-injurious way to gain control and deal with painful conflicts and emotions.
- Teach the family to develop an alliance with the client to promote trust.
- Caution the family to look for signs of depression or other underlying disorders that could lead to suicidal behaviors.
- Tell the family that the client may have a significant body image disturbance that distorts self-image and promotes self-starvation.
- Teach the client/family the dangers of self-starvation to the client's physical health and that a weight less than 90 pounds can be life-threatening.
- Educate the client/family about the possibility of family power struggles, and caution the family not to use force or threats when the client refuses to eat.
- Teach the family to use a matter-of-fact approach when serving or removing the client's food and to establish a predictable mealtime routine.
- Caution the family about the client's tendency to hoard, discard, or vomit food, and advise the family to remain with client 1½ to 2 hours after meals.
- Caution the family that the client may resist urinating and may drink large amounts of water to cover up actual weight, and that a bulimic client may use laxatives, enemas, or purging to maintain weight or lose unwanted weight.
- Teach the family basic behavior modification and limit-setting strategies.
- Instruct the family to set limits on the client's daily exercise regimen as necessary because the client may exercise until physically exhausted to remain thin.
- Instruct the family to allow the client to retain power and control over daily tasks as much as possible so that the client will not need to use food to control his or her life.
- Educate the client/family about medication, and reinforce compliance.
- Inform the family that progress is often slow because eating disorders are complex, long-standing problems that did not develop overnight.
- Teach the client/family to identify psychosocial and family stressors that lead to dysfunctional eating patterns and how to manage and prevent them.
- Instruct the family to praise the client for efforts made to gain weight, eat adequate nutrients, and develop healthier eating patterns.

- The client should initially eat meals with the nurse or staff member; other clients' comments during meals may remind the client of family power struggles.
- When client is ready to eat with other clients, the nurse and dietitian should work with the client to select nutritious meals.
- Reinforce the client's progress in regaining nutritional health and adequate weight, and praise the client/family for efforts to reduce power struggles.
- Reinforce medication compliance both in the hospital and at discharge.
- Provide information on community groups and resources to help the client and family after discharge (client may continue therapy in outpatient setting).
- Access current educational resources on the Internet and in the library.

- Tell the family to praise the client for signs of independence and a more realistic perception of body image.
- Educate the client/family about the importance of individual and family therapy in helping them maintain a healthy relationship.
- Inform the client/family about community groups available after discharge.
- Teach the client/family how to access current Internet and library resources.

Care Plans

- Imbalanced Nutrition: Less Than Body Requirements
- Disturbed Body Image

Care Plan
DSM-IV-TR Diagnosis | **Anorexia Nervosa; Bulimia Nervosa**

NANDA Diagnosis: Imbalanced Nutrition: Less Than Body Requirements

Intake of nutrients insufficient to meet metabolic needs.

Focus:
For the client whose nutritional state is severely compromised as a result of anorexia nervosa or bulimia nervosa, characterized by gross disturbances in eating behaviors (self-starvation, binge-purge cycles).

RELATED FACTORS (ETIOLOGY)

Anorexia Nervosa

Self-starvation: Inadequate nutritional intake for age, height, and metabolic need

Body image disturbance: Inability to perceive body size and shape realistically

Denial of severity or consequences of starvation on the body's physical and psychologic functions

Extreme regimen of physical exercise in an effort to burn unwanted calories

Extreme fear of weight gain, even if obviously underweight or emaciated, which does not diminish as weight loss progresses

Enmeshed family patterns (power struggles, overcontrolling mothers, lack of open affection among members)

Multifaceted etiology (biologic, psychologic, developmental, sociocultural, behavioral)

Powerlessness

Bulimia Nervosa

Self-induced vomiting (purging) generally after consuming large amounts of food (bingeing)

Use of laxatives or diuretics in an effort to lose weight

Strict dieting or fasting to prevent weight gain

Vigorous exercise regimen in an effort to lose weight

Persistent overconcern with body weight and shape (need to be "perfect")

History of depression

Disruptive family behavior patterns (overcontrolling mother; powerful, distant father)

Knowledge deficit regarding possible dire consequences of binge-purge behaviors

Multifaceted etiology (biologic, psychologic, sociocultural, behavioral)

Powerlessness

DEFINING CHARACTERISTICS

Anorexia Nervosa

The client is 15% or more under ideal body weight.

Refuses to eat nutrients sufficient to maintain body weight for age, height, and stature (self-starvation).

Reports nutritional intake less than recommended dietary allowance (RDA).

Verbalizes intense fear of weight gain or becoming fat, even though emaciated or grossly underweight and desirous of food.

Expresses disturbance in the way body weight, size, or shape is experienced or viewed; claims to "feel fat" even when emaciated.

States that one or more areas of the body are "too fat," even if obviously underweight.

Perceives reflection of self in mirror as "fat," although grossly underweight.

Absence of three or more menstrual cycles (amenorrhea) not caused by any other condition or disorder.

Uses laxatives, enemas, suppositories, or diuretics to lose weight (more often done by clients with bulimia nervosa).

Hoards, conceals, crumbles, or throws own food away; dawdles over meals.

Continued

Verbalizes that life is viewed as a "constant struggle with weight."

Prepares elaborate meals for others, often forcing them to eat, but eats only a narrow selection of low-calorie foods.

Demonstrates preoccupation with food, nutrients, food preparation, and serving food to others.

Denies thinness, hunger, need for treatment, or probability of illness or death as a result of starvation.

Manifests compulsive or bizarre behavior patterns: frequent handwashing; hoarding food, linen, utensils; calorie counting and preoccupation.

Exhibits significantly delayed psychosexual development (adolescent clients).

Displays marked lack of interest in sex (adult clients).

Exhibits fluid and electrolyte imbalance.

Has slow pulse; decrease in body temperature.

Has marked constipation.

Demonstrates hollow face with sunken eyes, growth of lanugo on skin, yellow tinge of skin, and dry hair, which may fall out.

Expresses loss of appetite (late stage of anorexia nervosa).

Expresses depression and suicidal thoughts and attempts, especially after forced weight gain.

Experiences episodes of overeating followed by vomiting (more common in bulimia nervosa).

Uses self-starvation as an attempt to strive for control and "perfection."

Bulimia Nervosa

The client experiences recurrent episodes of binge eating (rapid consumption of large amounts of food in discrete period) with feeling a lack of control during binge episode, followed by self-induced vomiting (purge).

Reports use of laxatives, enemas, or diuretics in an effort to lose weight.

Demonstrates vigorous exercise regimen to lose weight.

Engages in strict dieting or fasting to prevent weight gain.

Verbalizes persistent concern about body shape and weight gain, with frequent fluctuations in weight due to alternating binges and fasts.

Exhibits weight that ranges from normal to slightly underweight or slightly overweight.

Reports eating sweet-tasting, high-calorie foods with smooth texture that can be rapidly consumed and easily vomited (e.g., ice cream, pastries).

Demonstrates attempts to conceal binge-purge behaviors or to eat as inconspicuously as possible.

Expresses frequent disparaging self-criticism, guilt, and depressed mood after bingeing episodes.

Demonstrates dental erosion as a result of acidic gastric secretions from frequent vomiting episodes.

Exhibits fluid and electrolyte imbalance (in more serious episodes).

OUTCOME IDENTIFICATION AND EVALUATION

Anorexia Nervosa

The client consumes adequate daily calories per kilogram of body weight (cal/kg).

Demonstrates and maintains ideal body weight for age, height, and stature.

Maintains normal fluid and electrolyte levels.

Demonstrates skin turgor and muscle tone that reveal nutritional state commensurate with physiologic and metabolic needs.

Perceives ideal body weight and shape as normal, with absence of distorted self-image.

Resumes and maintains normal menstrual cycles.

Expresses absence of persistent fear of weight gain.

Ceases to engage in overly strenuous exercise regimen to lose weight.

Resumes and maintains psychosexual development commensurate with age (adolescents).

Resumes and maintains sexual interests and behaviors appropriate for age (young adults)

Demonstrates absence of preoccupation with food (preparing, arranging, and serving food while eating little or none).

Ceases to hoard, conceal, crumble, or throw food away.

Verbalizes feeling "in control" of life functions and no need to withhold food to feel in control.

Assists in resolution or management of family enmeshment issues that perpetuate the disorder.

Bulimia Nervosa

The client maintains weight that is normal for age, height, and stature.

Ceases binge-purge episodes.

Demonstrates absence of use of laxatives or diuretics to lose weight.

Ceases to exercise vigorously in an effort to lose weight.

Stops dieting or fasting to prevent weight gain.

Verbalizes feeling comfortable and satisfied with body weight, shape, and image.

Demonstrates normal social eating patterns without attempts to conceal food or eat in isolation.

Eats nutritionally balanced meals.

Maintains normal fluid and electrolyte balance.

Verbalizes feeling more "in control" of life functions without the need to control life through binge-purge episodes.

Verbalizes resolution or management of control issues surrounding client and family interactions.

PLANNING AND IMPLEMENTATION

Nursing Intervention	Rationale
Anorexia Nervosa	
Assess the client's history of menstrual patterns (amenorrhea), diet/nutrition regimen (self-starvation, negative nitrogen balance) weight (15% or more under ideal body weight), skin tone, skin turgor (triceps skinfold, midarm muscle circumference less than 60% standard measurement), muscle tone (weakness, tenderness), diagnostic studies (abnormal hemoglobin, serum albumin, serum transferrin/iron-binding capacity, lymphocytes, thyroid/hormonal function, fluid/electrolyte balance), cardiac function (tachycardia on minimum exercise, bradycardia at rest), exercise regimen (excessive for weight and condition), mental status (irritability, confusion, anxiety, depression, obsessive-compulsive behaviors), emotional state (negative self-concept, distorted body image), and social/developmental tasks (congruent/incongruent with age and status).	Individuals with anorexia nervosa require in-depth physical, mental, emotional, social, and developmental assessments because this disorder affects multiple systems and dimensions. Early assessment and interventions prevent further deterioration and promote restoration of health and function.
Explain to the client/family the hospital procedures, regulations, and expectations regarding nutritional therapy.	The hospital setting provides a controlled environment in which food and fluid intake and output, medication, and activities can be monitored. Hospitalization also separates the client from the family (which may be a contributing factor) and provides interactions with others with the same diagnosis so that problems can be shared. Management of the client's underlying conflicts cannot be formally addressed until nutritional status is improved and the client is out of danger.
Client Who Is Critically Malnourished	
Hyperalimentation (parenteral nutrition) or total parenteral nutrition (TPN) may be given through central venous or right atrial catheter. Monitor the client closely for signs of infection (redness at site, fever).	Parenteral nutrition can provide adequate nutrition, electrolytes, and other nutritional requirements when the client's immune system and overall health are severely compromised. The client has no opportunity to vomit nutrients with this method.
Provide tube feedings of liquid nutrients, if indicated, making sure first to give the client a choice between oral nutrients and tube feedings. Use of a nasoduodenal tube may be effective. *Note:* Tube feedings may be used alone or with oral or parenteral nutrition and may be decreased as oral consumption becomes adequate.	Tube feedings are indicated if the client has been unable to maintain or increase weight adequately through oral methods, or if a medical condition (electrolyte or acid-base problem) needs immediate correcting and may be a threat to physical health. Offering the client a choice avoids a power struggle, as long as the nurse emphasizes that the client's health is the priority. Nasoduodenal feeding reduces the chance of vomiting and siphoning feedings.
When tube feeding is indicated, insert the tube immediately, and begin feeding in a nonpunitive, matter-of-fact way, without engaging in bargaining.	Setting limits in a direct, calm manner is essential in avoiding a power struggle; especially at this critical time when the client's health is an issue. The nurse's behavior lets the client know that this is a medical treatment and not a punishment.
Tube feedings and TPN may be best administered during the night.	Administering these treatments at night may reduce the amount or sympathy given to the client by other clients or the family and may minimize the client's use of secondary gains (e.g., attention seeking) that may accompany tube feeding. Also, such treatment is less likely to interfere with client's daytime activities.

Continued

PLANNING AND IMPLEMENTATION—cont'd

Nursing Intervention	Rationale
Client Who Is Critically Malnourished—cont'd	
Directly observe the client for a specified period (initially 90 minutes, gradually decreasing to 30 minutes), or remove nasogastric tube after the feeding.	Direct observation during critical times reduces the client's chances of vomiting or siphoning feedings.
Approach the client in a calm, nonjudgmental, professional manner during administration of hyperalimentation or tube feedings.	A calm, nonjudgmental approach helps the client view replacement therapy as a medical treatment versus a punitive action, which may minimize guilt and shame and support compliance. A hurried, overzealous approach may terrify the client who is not ready to accept body rebuilding and may force the client to lose more weight. This approach may also remind the client of family power struggles, which may promote feelings of anger, frustration, and helplessness.
Assess the client for possible suicidal behavior (e.g., ongoing resistance to treatment, hopelessness, depressed mood, suicidal or self-destructive statements or gestures), and intervene in a nonjudgmental way. (see care plan for Risk for Suicide, Chapter 3).	Clients with anorexia nervosa have been known to attempt suicide after rapid or forced weight gain, especially if they perceive disapproval from others.
Client Who Is Not Critically Malnourished	
Initiate a structured, supportive environment, especially during mealtimes. • Establish routine tasks and activities. • Serve meals at the same time each day.	Clients with anorexia nervosa feel out of control and vulnerable. A structured, supportive environment provides external safety and comfort and helps the client establish internal control. A client who feels empowered is less likely to use self-starvation as a way to gain control of life.
Develop a contract regarding the treatment regimen, if client agrees and is emotionally capable to fulfill its terms. Collaborate with the physician and treatment team.	A contract promotes the client's sense of responsibility and control and helps to establish treatment goals. A team approach provides consistency.
Initially, sit with the client calmly and consistently during meals, and restrict the client from eating with other clients or visitors.	Other clients or visitors may demonstrate family patterns (urging the client to eat, paying too much attention to the client for not eating). The client will detect the sense of urgency and react negatively to the pressure. Because food is an area of control for the client, consistent calm behaviors by staff allow the client to trust staff and resist withholding food to gain control.
Serve and remove the client's food in a calm manner, avoiding requests to "eat more" or similar directives. Staff should be aware of facial expressions and gestures that indicate disapproval of the client's insufficient food consumption.	Forcing or coercing the client to eat when the client is not ready may remind the client of authoritative family patterns and invoke guilt, shame, and helplessness, which could lead to further withholding of food. Serving and removing food when mealtime is over sets limits and informs the client about what to expect.
Avoid the use of trickery, bribery, cajoling, coaxing, or threats to encourage the client to eat.	This type of behavior may encourage the client to resort to manipulation and deceit because it may remind the client of family power struggles.
Give the client one-to-one supervision during meals and for 90 minutes after meals, gradually decreasing the time. Restrict the client from using the bathroom for at least 30 minutes after each meal. When there is evidence of vomiting, remain with the client and supervise bathroom use for at least 2 hours after meals.	The client may use unsupervised time to hide or discard food and may use the bathroom to vomit or dispose of hidden food.

Promote a pleasant, relaxing environment during the client's mealtimes. Minimize distractions and encourage use of relaxation techniques (deep breathing, reduction of muscle tension) just before the meal. (see Appendix B for therapeutic activities).

Eating is an anxiety-provoking activity for the client, and simple stress reduction activities and a quiet atmosphere may help relax the client and promote food consumption and easier digestion.

Design with the client a behavior modification program that provides rewards for weight gain and does not punish or harass the client for weight loss (grant and restrict privileges based on weight gain or loss) as a way to help the client gain control. Do not focus on eating, mealtimes, calorie counts, or physical activity. Talk with the client about feelings and situations that may have contributed to weight loss, and discuss ways to modify behavior and reduce the trend.

Behavior modification programs provide structured eating situations that allow select clients some control in choosing their food. These programs tend to facilitate short-term weight gain without using rigid rules that provoke power plays between the client and staff. This approach forces the client to deal with feelings and emotions rather than focus on food and eating.

Provide liquid diets of 1400 to 1800 calories by mouth in the initial stages of treatment.

Some clients with anorexia nervosa have a morbid fear of solid foods, especially in the early stages of treatment, and may benefit from an oral liquid diet.

Help the client maintain a weight of at least 90 to 95 pounds. Work with the physician, dietitian, and treatment team.

The client initially cannot tolerate a normal weight without feeling "too fat"; 90 to 95 pounds is considered the "out of danger" weight for most clients and is generally an acceptable compromise for clients after a brief period of therapy.

Monitor the client's vital signs, including pain as a fifth vital sign. Monitor laboratory values (fluid and electrolytes, acid-base balance, liver enzymes, albumin) as ordered by the physician.

The client's ongoing physical health, safety, and comfort are priorities and critical factors in determining safe, effective nursing interventions.

Monitor the client's intake and output, and maintain the record at the nurses' station rather than in the client's room. Intake and output results should be recorded as quietly as possible.

The client may be tempted to give inaccurate information about intake and output and may become overly emotional with the results, which could interfere with the treatment focus and goals.

Weigh the client daily, at the same time every day, before voiding and before mealtime. The client should wear the same attire, preferably a hospital gown. Weigh the client in a calm, matter-of-fact way, without signs of either disapproval or elation.
Note: Reasonable weight gain is less anxiety producing and more likely to be maintained.

A consistent weighing pattern is critical for accurate weight comparison over time. The client may resist voiding and hold urine or even hide weighted objects on the body to increase weight. A calm, matter-of-fact approach without extremes of emotion helps the client separate emotions from this important medical measurement.

Assess the client's patterns of elimination, and consult with the dietitian to provide adequate amounts of fiber and fluid in the client's diet.

The client can become constipated, which can be treated with increased fiber and fluids.

Avoid the use of laxatives, suppositories, or enemas to relieve constipation.

The client may abuse laxatives, suppositories, or enemas as a means to control weight; therefore using them as a medical treatment may justify the client's continued abuse.

Focus on the client's strengths and capabilities: seeking help for problems, attending groups and activities, participating in the treatment program.

This focus helps to build self-confidence and offers the client hope for progress and success in regaining nutritional health.

Have the client eventually eat with other clients in the hospital dining room.

Eating with others promotes normal social interactions during mealtimes, prevents hoarding, and demonstrates trust by the staff.

Avoid responding to or focusing on the client's continuing preoccupation with food.

Clients with anorexia nervosa are often obsessed with food and food topics. As the client's condition improves, the preoccupation will diminish.

Continued

PLANNING AND IMPLEMENTATION—cont'd

Nursing Intervention	Rationale
Client Who Is Not Critically Malnourished—cont'd	

Offer the client a choice of food from the hospital menu, working with the dietician and physician.	The client experiences more control when given a choice of foods and nutrients, with the support and expertise of the treatment team.
Be alert to the client's possible choices of low-calorie foods or beverages, hoarding food, and disposing of food in places such as pockets or wastebaskets.	The client may need guidance initially to select foods that are nutritionally adequate and may be tempted to resort to previous habits to avoid eating high-calorie foods.
Collaborate with the dietitian and client to select and prepare a tray with an adequate amount of food that suits the client's taste and fulfills nutritional requirements.	This collaboration includes the client as an important member of the treatment team and encourages self-responsibility in progress and recovery.
Praise the client when she consumes an adequate amount of food within a prescribed time.	Positive reinforcement builds self-esteem and promotes repetition of functional behaviors.
Discuss with the client any fears she may have about physical development and how such fears may lead to self-starvation as a means to slow down developmental and maturational processes. Inform the client of the dangers of self-starvation as a solution.	Discussing the client's fears and giving information about the anxieties of growth and development shared by many clients with anorexia nervosa help increase the client's awareness that self-starvation is a dangerous way to avoid normal growth and development.
Administer prescribed medications (see section on medications).	Medications may be prescribed to treat symptoms of anxiety, depression, and other conditions that may accompany eating disorders.
Teach the client and family about electroconvulsive therapy (ECT), if prescribed, and explain to the client that it is not a punishment.	ECT may be prescribed in extremely difficult cases when malnutrition is severe and life threatening. A brief series of ECT may stimulate the client's appetite and make her more amenable to treatment. ECT should always be explained to the client and family to assuage fear and guilt.
Help the client express feelings and fears about sexuality and intimacy, if appropriate, and relate those feelings and fears to self-starvation.	The client can develop an awareness of feelings and fears about sexuality and intimacy through discussions with a trusted staff person. In time the client may be able to understand that self-starvation is a dysfunctional attempt to avoid sexual maturity and resist the transition from adolescence to intimacy.
Confront the client with the fact that self-starvation is self-destructive behavior that could lead to death.	Such confrontation, when the client is ready, helps the client realize the potentially serious consequences of self-starvation and break through maladaptive denial to avoid possibly lethal results.
Respond assertively to the client who uses manipulative behaviors to distract from their eating disorder. *Client:* "How can you talk to me about being too thin? You're thin yourself."	Clients benefit from direct communication, as they are often in a state of maladaptive denial regarding their problem, and need kind but firm confrontation.

Therapeutic Response

- *Nurse:* "I may be thin, but you have an eating disorder problem, and we're here to help you with your problem."

This therapeutic response by the nurse reflects kind, firm confrontation.

Nontherapeutic Responses

Nurse: "My thinness is not your concern. I'm not the one with the eating disorder."
Nurse: "OK, let's discuss your feelings about my thinness before we talk about your problem."

The first nontherapeutic response is more aggressive than assertive, which may put the client on the defensive and block the therapeutic process.
The second nontherapeutic response encourages the client to focus on the nurse's thinness, which distracts from the client's problem and crosses professional boundaries.

Develop with the client a realistic exercise program.

Nursing staff must prevent excessive exercise by the client to prevent weight loss.

Discuss with the client unrealistic or irrational perceptions of body shape and size.

Challenge the client's beliefs about his or her body shape and size in a realistic, nonthreatening manner to promote a healthier self-perception.

Communicate to the client the staff's expectations of behaviors that are congruent with client's developmental stage.

Promote healthy, age-appropriate functioning rather than regression, and encourage more mature behaviors.

Discuss with the client the irrational need to be "perfect."

Give the client permission to talk about possible sources of irrational desires about "perfection." Some clients with eating disorders have experienced the need to achieve perfection early in life and thus starve themselves as a way to accomplish a "perfect" image and sense of worth.

Help the client, in individual and group settings, to develop realistic beliefs about food, weight, and physical attractiveness.
- The client engages in individual therapeutic interactions.
- Attends cognitive-behavioral therapy and assertiveness training classes.
- Participates in group therapy with other clients who have anorexia nervosa.
- Participates in family therapy sessions.
- See Appendix B.

Communicating with the client individually or in therapeutic groups is essential to break the vicious cycle of anorexia nervosa, reduce or eliminate the preoccupation with food and weight, and promote healthy eating habits and a productive life-style.

Engage the client in individual therapy.

Help the client understand self and illness and receive continuous feedback on progress and behavior from a trusted, knowledgeable, supportive person.

Provide family therapy regarding family enmeshment, which consists of overinvolved family members.

Some clients with anorexia nervosa may be members of an "enmeshed family" and may use self-starvation to gain control against an overcontrolling mother, family member, or family system. The family of the client is concerned with power and control, in addition to massive denial of parental conflicts. Family therapy approaches these conflicts, and parents are asked to focus on their problems and recognize their need for persistent control.

Provide cognitive-behavioral therapy and assertiveness training for the client (see Appendix B).
Note: Premorbid personalities of some clients (characteristics developed before disease onset) consist of compliance, obedience, passivity, dependence, and the need to be perfect and "make the family proud."

Some clients with anorexia nervosa have been overly criticized, corrected, or invalidated by dominant, overcontrolling mothers during the formative years. Assertive response behaviors can help the client express feelings openly and directly and break the cycle of self-starvation as a means of gaining control of life situations. Cognitive-behavioral therapy can help the client replace erroneous, self-defeating thoughts with more realistic ones and thus build confidence and self-control.

Engage the client in supportive, fact-finding interpersonal psychotherapy in which the client is primarily responsible for exploring and examining needs, impulses, and feelings that originate from within the self. Avoid a psychoanalytic approach that consists of interpreting repressed motives and conflicts.

Use fact-finding therapy to allow the client to discover her own needs, impulses, and feelings through the various therapeutic modalities. Learning more about the self helps the client better understand cognitive and perceptual difficulties that originate in childhood so that growth and healing can occur. Conversely, the analytic, interpretive method is not recommended because the client may either incorporate the therapist's interpretations into her own identity or she may become suspicious because the interpretations came from outside the self.

Continued

PLANNING AND IMPLEMENTATION—cont'd

Nursing Intervention	Rationale

Client Who Is Not Critically Malnourished—cont'd

Nursing Intervention	Rationale
Staff should participate in daily multidisciplinary team conferences to discuss, evaluate, and support each other.	When staff meet regularly, they can provide consistent, effective client care with confidence and avoid splitting of staff by clients.
Include the client in her own care planning process.	It is important to elicit the client's approval of and adherence to the treatment plan and to promote the client's autonomy and independence.

Bulimia Nervosa

Nursing Intervention	Rationale
Ensure completion of a thorough physical assessment and laboratory workup. Assess the client's history of binge-purge patterns; weight fluctuations; use of laxatives, enemas, or diuretics; dieting and fasting behaviors; exercise and activity regimen; fluid and electrolyte status; cardiac and gastrointestinal systems; dental and parotid condition; thyroid function; mood and affect (depressed, suicidal); guilt, shame, or self-contempt, especially following binges; self-esteem/perceptual disturbances; social relationships; abuse of drugs or alcohol; family behavior patterns; life stressors; and background of medical or psychiatric disorders related to self or close family members. • Abnormal dexamethasone suppression test (DST) may indicate major depression, which generally occurs a year before onset of bulimic symptoms. • Note a delayed thyroid-stimulating hormone (TSH) response to thyroid-releasing hormone (TRH). • A reduced intake of potassium and loss of potassium are common in clients who abuse diuretics and laxatives and engage in vomiting. Cardiac dyshythmias or cardiac arrest can result from reduced serum potassium, or hypokalemia (most common cause of death in bulimia). • Note especially any family history of major depression or bipolar disorder, a need to be "perfect" to please controlling mothers and powerful distant fathers, and signs of suicidal behavior (see care plan for Risk for Suicide, Chapter 3).	Clients with bulimia nervosa require an indepth, multisystem assessment and laboratory workup. This disorder has a multifaceted etiology, and early assessment and interventions will prevent further deterioration and complications by promoting functional healthy eating patterns. Problems can include extensive dental decay and irreversible perimolysis on lingual surfaces of incisors caused by frequent contact with gastric secretions from emesis and sugary foods; parotid gland swelling; stomach ulcers; involuntary vomiting; sore throats; esophageal or rectal bleeding; myocardial contractility problems; low serum phosphate from massive laxative abuse; low serum chloride; low serum potassium and metabolic acidosis (renal effect of chronic vomiting); muscle weakness and contractility problems from hypokalemia; and acute gastric dilation and rupture of the stomach. Clients may be preoccupied with food, weight, and body image. Clients may have faulty perceptions of "feeling fat," even when weight is normal, and overwhelming feelings of guilt, shame, and self-contempt after binges, as well as fear of losing control. Clients may also exhibit obsessive-compulsive behaviors, such as binge eating and/or compulsive shoplifting (usually involving food, laxatives, or other affordable items). Social sensitivity may lead to secretive eating to satisfy binge-purge patterns. These clients have been known to attempt suicide due to an underlying depression that may or may not be obvious.
Initiate with the client and family hospitalization for nutritional therapy as indicated, as well as treatment directed toward underlying conflicts that contribute to binge-purge behaviors: life stressors, need to be "perfect," negative self-concept. *Note:* Some clients with bulimia nervosa may be treated for nutritional, physical, and emotional problems on an outpatient basis if their condition is stable and no emergency exists. Families should also be counseled with the client to resolve conflicts surrounding the eating disorder (see Appendix B).	The hospital setting provides a controlled environment in which clients can be observed during and after meals to prevent binge-purge behavior. A safe, supportive setting also exposes the client to a therapeutic environment in which individual, group, and other interactive therapies can take place with other clients who have bulimia. This setting, as well as outpatient treatment, gives clients the opportunity to share problems and discuss strategies for management of symptoms.
Weigh the client (as ordered) in the same amount of attire and on the same scale.	Staff must ensure accurate weight.

Offer structure and support during mealtimes (with an appropriate staff/client ratio) by creating a calm, pleasant environment and providing nutritionally balanced, attractive meals.	Staff should work to gain the client's trust and cooperation while providing adequate nutrition and staff guidance and supervision.
Observe the client for 2 hours after meals. Contracts may stipulate agreed-on behaviors.	Observation is necessary to prevent self-induced vomiting or regurgitation and is part of the therapeutic process.
Participate in interdisciplinary group meetings.	The nurse's interdisciplinary participation allows the nurse to help the client plan goals and assist in the management of her own care and ensures consistency among staff members.
Designate one staff member each day, when possible, as the client's primary therapist.	Designating a daily therapist helps to avoid manipulation and splitting behaviors by the client.
Involve the client in her own care-planning process, whenever possible.	Involvement helps promote the client's accountability for her own treatment and foster autonomy and self-confidence.
Prevent the client's use of laxatives, suppositories, enemas, and diuretics.	This intervention is essential to prevent potassium loss through urine and stool and serious complications from potassium and other electrolyte depletion.
Administer fluids and high-fiber foods as ordered.	Fluids and fiber prevent constipation and the resulting temptation to use laxatives and enemas.
Act as a role model both in and out of the hospital by practicing good nutrition and weight control.	Role modeling is important for the client's healthy, mature development.
Educate the public through community groups and middle schools, high schools, and colleges about the importance of well-balanced nutrition for a person's physical and mental capacities and the deleterious effects of bulimia nervosa.	Increased knowledge prevents dysfunctional eating patterns and promotes healthy nutritional habits in high-risk and future high-risk populations.
Counsel clients and nonhospitalized persons about the benefits of sensible daily exercise, in accordance with the physician's orders.	Moderate exercise increases metabolism and produces safe, sensible weight loss. Exercise may also improve the person's mood by activating endorphins and promoting a healthier, more attractive physical appearance, which discourages binge-purge cycles.
Approach the client with a nonjudgmental, caring attitude.	This approach bolsters self-esteem and helps modify the client's perfectionist approach to life.
Administer prescribed antidepressant medications as ordered, including selective serotonin reuptake inhibitors (SSRIs) and antipsychotics (see section on Medications).	Atypical SSRI antidepressants, such as fluoxetine (Prozac) and paroxetine (Paxil), are now the preferred medications for eating disorders in clients with depression. SSRIs are also used to promote sleep in clients with anxiety. Atypical antipsychotics may be used to manage obsessive-compulsive psychosis.
Administer metoclopramide (Reglan), as ordered.	Reglan may be used to promote or hasten gastric emptying. Frequent vomiting (purging) decreases the stomach's ability to effectively empty all its contents. When gastric emptying is delayed, the client with bulimia experiences a constant sense of "fullness" that promotes more vomiting (purging) and the fear that nothing, not even vomiting, can prevent the feeling of fullness. Reglan empties the stomach's contents more efficiently and reduces or eliminates the sense of fullness, which may discourage vomiting or purge episodes.
Allow the client to create her own menus from a selection of available, nutritious foods.	The client needs to gain confidence in self and feel that she is in control of the environment.

Continued

PLANNING AND IMPLEMENTATION—cont'd

Nursing Intervention	Rationale
Bulimia Nervosa—cont'd	
Be alert to the client's choices of sweet, soft, or sugary foods that can be easily binged and purged, and guide the client toward more balanced nutritional selections.	This focus on healthy food choices can prevent the client's temptation to binge and purge.
Instruct the family about the visitation policy, and advise them to avoid discussing food and weight issues with the client.	The client needs to become responsible for food management while in the hospital and continue the behavior on discharge.
Discuss with the client who is over 18 years of age optional living arrangements other than returning to live in the family home, if the family is dysfunctional and/or controlling (include therapist and physician).	Such discussion encourages the client's independence and separation from parental conflicts that often perpetuate the binge-purge cycle.
Teach the client that binge-purge episodes are self-destructive acts and a dysfunctional attempt to control one's life, which could lead to serious physical and emotional complications and even death.	Education helps to promote awareness of the harsh realities of life and death and assists the client to control life in areas of work, play, and love rather than through harmful binge-purge episodes. The client is better able to deal with confrontation when trust is built and self-esteem reestablished.
Facilitate a behavior modification program that involves the client's input in the program.	Behavior modification provides a structured eating situation while allowing the client some control in the program, although it may be effective only in mild cases or for short-term weight gain.
Engage the client in social milieu activities, including meals.	Involving the client in the milieu discourages social isolation, minimizes secret binge-purge episodes, and increases healthy social interactions consistent with the client's developmental level.
Focus on the client's strengths, talents, and capabilities.	This focus helps build self-esteem and discourages guilt and self-criticism, especially after binge episodes.
Provide cognitive-behavioral therapy for the client (see Appendix B).	Through cognitive-behavioral therapy, clients learn to replace spontaneous, erroneous thoughts and beliefs about self with more realistic perceptions and to reduce guilty thoughts and perfectionist desires that lead to binge-purge cycles.
Engage the client in group therapy sessions with other clients of approximate weight and stature.	Group therapy allows the client to compare her own normal weight with others with similar weight and stature, gain a healthier perspective of actual physical appearance, and stop "feeling fat."
Discuss with the client his or her feelings of intimacy (see section on anorexia nervosa) and sexuality, if warranted.	This discussion helps the client "get in touch" with developmental needs and promotes interpersonal relationships. Clients with bulimia generally are distracted from social tasks because of their obsession with binge-purge behaviors, which in turn drive others away. The resultant loneliness or isolation leads to more binge-purge episodes.
Discuss with the client irrational beliefs about needing to be "perfect."	Determining sources of irrational beliefs gives the client permission to be less than "perfect" and still be a worthwhile person.
Help the client develop realistic beliefs about food, weight, and attractiveness.	Developing healthier beliefs can break the binge-purge cycle; lessen obsessions with food, weight, and physical appearance; and promote a healthier, more productive life-style.

Provide assertiveness training (see Appendix B).

Assertiveness training helps the client learn to ask for wants and needs directly, thus gaining more self-control.

Explore with the client any irrational aspects of the culture's preoccupation with thinness.
- Fashion advertisements tend to prey on the vulnerability of young women, who learn to equate thinness with self-worth.

Such exploration encourages the client to think about her own values independent of society.

Conduct a suicide assessment if the client expresses thoughts, behaviors, or plans for suicide (see care plan for Risk for Suicide, Chapter 3.)

A suicide assessment, when warranted, can prevent harm or injury and protect the client from uncontrollable impulses.

Suggest that the client attend self-help groups: bulimia nervosa groups (preferred), Overeaters Anonymous (if appropriate), chemical dependency groups (if warranted).

A self-help group can broaden the client's support system and introduce the client to a source of strength, empathy, support, and encouragement.

Praise the client throughout the treatment program for efforts made in dealing successfully with family and in managing conflicts that lead to binge-purge behaviors.

Frequent positive feedback, when warranted, increases the client's self-esteem, builds confidence, and reinforces continued successful eating behaviors.

Praise the client and family for progress made in dealing successfully with family conflicts and helping the client manage binge-purge behaviors.

Positive feedback reinforces continued functional behavior patterns.

Care Plan
DSM-IV-TR Diagnosis   **Anorexia Nervosa; Bulimia Nervosa**

NANDA Diagnosis: Disturbed Body Image
Confusion in mental picture of one's physical self.

Focus:
For the client with anorexia nervosa who experiences disturbances in body weight, size, or shape ("feels fat," perceives physical self as "looking fat" even when emaciated) and for the client with bulimia nervosa who is overconcerned with body shape and weight and often "feels fat," even when maintaining ideal weight, but does not experience the severe perceptual distortions of the client with anorexia nervosa.

RELATED FACTORS (ETIOLOGY)

Anorexia Nervosa
Cognitive-perceptual disturbances

Bulimia Nervosa
Persistent overconcern with body weight and physical shape

DEFINING CHARACTERISTICS

Anorexia Nervosa
The client demonstrates inability to perceive body size, body functions, and physical needs realistically.
Displays maladaptive denial of body image and physical experience of body weight and stature.
- States, "I'm fat," while looking in the mirror at physically thin or emaciated body.

Bulimia Nervosa
The client experiences "feeling fat," even when ideal weight is maintained.

OUTCOME IDENTIFICATION AND EVALUATION

Anorexia Nervosa
The client demonstrates realistic perceptions of body image, weight, and physical appearance.
Experiences realistic feelings about body size, needs, and functions.
Demonstrates absence of cognitive-perceptual distortions related to body size, weight, appearance, and physical functions.
Exercises within limits of endurance to maintain physical and emotional wellness.

Bulimia Nervosa
The client demonstrates absence of overconcern or obsessive thoughts regarding body weight, shape, or size.
Expresses satisfaction with maintained ideal weight versus "feeling fat."
Maintains reasonable exercise regimen consistent with age, weight, and physical needs.
Discusses body size, shape, and appearance in positive terms.

PLANNING AND IMPLEMENTATION

Nursing Intervention	Rationale
Anorexia Nervosa	
Assess the client's degree of body image disturbance: distortions regarding body size/weight, appearance, body functions, and physical needs.	A thorough assessment of the client's obsession with body image disturbance helps the nurse determine the extent of the client's denial and cognitive-perceptual disturbance to plan appropriate interventions.
Help the client express feelings and concerns about self, body image, body size/weight, body function, and physical needs.	The client's ventilation of perceptions and distortions helps clarify areas of conflict and concern that must be addressed in the treatment plan.
Point out verbalized misperceptions of body image in a calm, direct, nonthreatening manner. • *Client:* "My legs are fat; they're awful." • *Nurse:* "Your legs are beginning to look strong and healthy since you're almost at your ideal weight." • *Client:* "But I'm afraid they look too fat." • *Nurse:* "Your daily walks will help tone your legs and all your body. Let's talk about how your body will change for the better."	Pointing out the client's misperceptions in a calm, factual way helps correct the client's distortions without challenging her belief system and inciting anger, guilt, or shame.
Teach the client to visualize and verbalize realistic thoughts and affirmations about her body. • "I am healthy when I'm at my ideal weight." • "I have more energy at my ideal weight." • "I can choose healthy foods to eat." • "My body looks healthy when I'm at my ideal weight." • See Appendix B for visualization and cognitive strategies.	Affirmations help the client replace negative beliefs and distortions with realistic perceptions.
Have the client create own statements and affirmations to practice and use throughout the day, especially during stressful times such as mealtimes and visiting with family.	Affirming self-created statements empowers the client to use own tools independently.
Help the client view self in a full-sized mirror with little clothing, and ask the client to describe what she sees and how she would like to look.	This therapeutic exercise helps the client realistically appraise her body while progressing throughout the treatment program. In the early stages of anorexia nervosa, clients view their physical image as "fat" even when they are emaciated. A more accurate perception of the body indicates progress.
Engage the client in exercises that include touch or massage (if not contraindicated). *Note:* This exercise may require an order.	Touch and massage exercise are used therapeutically to help the client "get in touch" with body boundaries, minimize feelings of depersonalization, and promote realistic perceptions of physical self.
Advise the client to wear clothing one size larger than the current size.	Wearing slightly larger clothing provides motivation for weight gain and a healthier, more appropriate shape for age and stature.
Verbalize recognition of the client's attempts to communicate perceptions, feelings, and concerns in individual and group interactions.	Recognizing the client's efforts to communicate body-image perceptions reinforces the client's continued expressions of body image and functions.
Provide support and praise for the client's accurate perceptions of body size, body image, and body functions, as well as for demonstration of more adaptive eating patterns and a reasonable exercise regimen.	Positive feedback reinforces the client's self-esteem and promotes more realistic self-perceptions and healthier eating and exercise behaviors.

Provide sexuality education classes as necessary with a qualified therapist.
Note: This teaching may require physician order and parental permission.

The major physical and physiologic changes of adolescence can contribute to anorexia nervosa. Feelings of powerlessness and loss of control of feelings (particularly sexual), sensations, and physical development often lead to an unconscious effort to desexualize the self. The client may try to overcome these fears by taking control of bodily appearance, development, and function. Sexuality education may help the client confront sexual fears and give up "childlike" appearance and image.

Educate the family to relinquish control and responsibility for the client and to allow the client to take control and responsibility for her own life.

This responsibility gives the client the opportunity to grow, develop, and take charge of her own life. As the client makes more independent decisions, emotional growth can occur, and the client will develop a more positive, mature self-concept.

Bulimia Nervosa

Discuss with the client feelings and obsessions concerning weight gain and body shape/size.

This discussion helps to clarify the extent of the client's concerns and allows the client to ventilate feelings about body shape/size.

Focus on areas of the client's strengths and areas of control (entering hospital to seek help voluntarily, participation in the treatment program).

Focusing on strengths increases the client's self-esteem and feelings of self-control. Most patients with bulimia nervosa have a negative self-concept and feel a lack of control over body, self, and life situations.

Respond to the client's erroneous statements about body image with realistic, nonjudgmental comments.
- *Client:* "I'm not underweight, so there's nothing really wrong with me."
- *Nurse:* "Your weight is ideal for your height. Bingeing and purging are harmful to your body functions."
- *Client:* "I'm feeling fat and shapeless. I vomit occasionally to control my weight."
- *Nurse:* "Although you feel fat, your weight is ideal for your height. Vomiting will not reshape your body, but it will cause other problems."

Factual, realistic statements by nursing and the therapeutic team help to correct the individual's perceptions without challenging her right to express thoughts and feelings.

Discuss with the client irrational beliefs about needing to be "perfect" and resorting to binge-purge behaviors as a means of gaining "perfection."

This discussion helps the nurse and therapeutic team determine possible sources of irrational beliefs and gives the client permission to be less than perfect and still be a worthwhile individual. Clients with bulimia nervosa often judge "perfection" by physical appearance.

Help the client gain control in areas other than dieting/fasting and bingeing/purging, such as managing her own daily activities, work, leisure time, and social functions.

Helping individuals concentrate on neglected areas of life increases feelings of control, promotes a more positive self-concept, and minimizes dysfunctional behaviors. Clients often focus on food, weight, and self-image to control areas in life in which they feel helpless or powerless.

Be aware of your own reactions toward the client's dysfunctional behaviors.

Feelings of anger, impatience, and irritation are not uncommon responses by staff because clients with bulimia nervosa may continue to see themselves as "fat." Also, depression, social phobias, obsessive-compulsive symptoms, drug abuse, and psychosexual dysfunctions often affect the client's perceptions and can inhibit progress.

Continued

PLANNING AND IMPLEMENTATION—cont'd

Nursing Intervention	Rationale
Bulimia Nervosa—cont'd	
Engage the client in social situations and activities in the therapeutic milieu.	Milieu therapy provides role models of both sexes who can relate to the client and offer approval and positive feedback in a controlled social context. Peer interactions and approval can help increase the client's self-concept and promote more realistic perceptions of physical body and body image.
Praise the client for statements that reveal the client's positive feelings about self and body and the client's belief that she is attractive and healthy at her ideal weight.	Positive feedback reinforces a positive self-concept and repetition of functional behaviors.

chapter **11**

Sexual and Gender Identity Disorders

F or humans, sexuality is one form of self-expression that encompasses biologic, perceptual, cognitive, emotional, and social uniqueness. Sexuality has been researched, defined, and described for decades. The following developmental terms help to define and explain sexuality:

- **Sexual identity** is the state of being male or female as defined by anatomy and physiology.
- **Gender identity** is the individual's perception and understanding of self as male or female. The person's perception of his or her sexual identity is shaped and reinforced through socialization and is usually fixed by 3 years of age.
- **Gender role** is the person's expression of his or her gender identity by way of behaviors, attitudes, and emotions appropriate for the gender.
- **Sexual orientation** is sexual preference, or feelings and attraction to the male or female gender. *Heterosexuality* refers to sexual preference, arousal, and activity toward the opposite gender. *Homosexuality* refers to sexual preference, arousal, and activity toward the same gender. Sexual orientation is thought to be fixed before pubescence. Homosexuality is not listed as a disorder in the Diagnostic and Statistical Manual of Mental Disorders (DSM-IV-TR). Sexual disorders manifest in physical or mental symptoms, or a combination of the two.

ETIOLOGY

Cause is sometimes established for sexual disorders due to medical conditions(s) or those that are substance induced. In general, although several theories are presented, definitive cause and effect for most sexual disorders is still

---

Box 11-1   **Biologic Factors That Contribute to Sexual Disorders**

DISEASES
Cancer
Genital infections
Degenerative diseases

NEUROLOGIC DYSFUNCTION
Spinal cord injury
Cerebrovascular accident
Head injury

ENDOCRINE DYSFUNCTION
Diabetes mellitus
Hormone dysregulation

VASCULAR DISORDERS
Cardiac disease
Peripheral circulatory disorders

MEDICATIONS/SUBSTANCES
Antipsychotics
Antihypertensives
Sedatives
Narcotics
Antidepressants
Alcohol

speculative. Box 11-1 lists known biologic factors that contribute to sexual disorders. With many other mental disorders, etiology most likely evolves from the convergence of biologic, psychologic, social, and environmental factors.

Other etiologic factors that relate to sexual disorders are heredity, familial and cultural origins (transmission of paraphiliac disorders or female circumcision and genital mutilation), or psychologic and psychosocial causes. Early childhood exposure to sex acts is often emotionally, psychologically, or physically traumatic for the child and frequently results in sexuality problems or other mental disorders. Examples include (1) response to stress and anxiety, (2) sexual abuse, (3) failure to achieve the developmental task of intimacy, (4) excessively repressive and restrictive environments (religious, cultural, familial), (5) oppressive or hindering attitudes and myths about male and female roles, (6) ignorance about anatomy or sexual arousal and behaviors patterns that perpetuate or interfere with interest and performance during sexual activity, and (7) couples criteria (common sexual activity interests, compatible sex drives, communication ability/willingness, idealized versus real mate, boredom/disinterest).

Human sexuality is a complex interplay of many factors. Norms for sexual activity are defined and refuted continuously. This chapter uses the widely accepted classification of sexual disorders presented in the *DSM-IV-TR* (see Appendix A).

EPIDEMIOLOGY

Sex is a popular topic that permeates daily life in newspapers, fiction and nonfiction books, magazines, textbooks, films, television, on the beach, on the street, in the parks, in neighboring yards, and in the home. However, sexuality remains a subject that has relatively low research activity. Research directed at sexual disorders is influenced by the underreporting of sexual problems, even though they are common.

The most common sexual dysfunctions in males are erectile dysfunction and premature ejaculation; in females, orgasmic dysfunction is most common. Age of onset for sexual disorders is typically in early adulthood, late 20s, or early 30s. Sexual disorders usually occur during sexual activity with a partner but are also reported during masturbation. For a dysfunction to be diagnosed as a sexual disorder, the criteria described next should not occur only during other Axis I disorders, such as major depression, substance abuse, or obsessive-compulsive disorder, and should not result from these disorders.

Some sexual disorders may put the individual or others in danger. For example, the person with pedophilic fantasies may act on them and endanger a child or children and may place himself in jeopardy for incarceration. Sexually masochistic and sadistic disorders may put the seeker or perpetrator in danger for injury and/or incarceration. The highest proportion of sex offenses occur against children, and the majority of sex offenders commit acts in conjunction with pedophilia, voyeurism, or exhibitionism.

Sexual disorders jeopardize social and intimate relationships and frequently cause disrupted relations when not addressed, go untreated, or do not respond to treatment.

Paraphilias (except for masochism; see next section) are 20 times more prevalent in males and are seldom seen in females. Approximately one half of the individuals treated for paraphilias are married. Usually the disorder occurs in childhood or adolescence and may last a lifetime, becoming more intense under stress. The fantasies and urges may weaken or abate in older age groups.

ASSESSMENT AND DIAGNOSTIC CRITERIA

The *Diagnostic and Statistical Manual of Mental Disorders (DSM-IV-TR)* lists three distinct categories representing sexual disorders: sexual dysfunctions, paraphilias, and gender identity disorders (see box below; see also Appendix A).

Sexual Dysfunctions

Defining characteristics for sexual dysfunctions are disturbance of sexual desire and the psychophysiologic changes that occur during the sexual response cycle (see box on opposite page). Regardless of type, the dysfunction causes disturbed interpersonal relationships and marked distress for the individual, the partner, or both.

DSM-IV-TR Sexual and Gender Identity Disorders

Sexual Dysfunctions
Sexual desire disorder
Sexual arousal disorder
Orgasmic disorder
Sexual pain disorder
Sexual dysfunction due to a general medical condition

Paraphilias
Exhibitionism
Fetishism
Frotteurism
Pedophilia
Sexual masochism
Sexual sadism
Transvestic fetishism
Voyeurism
Paraphilia NOS

Gender Identity Disorders
Gender identity disorder
• In children
• In adolescents or adults
Gender identity disorder NOS
Sexual disorder NOS

NOS, Not otherwise specified.

DSM–IV–TR Sexual Dysfunctions

All Primary Sexual Dysfunctions
Lifelong type/acquired type
Generalized type/situational type
Due to psychologic factors/combined factors

Sexual Desire Disorders
Hypoactive sexual desire disorder
Sexual aversion disorder

Sexual Arousal Disorders
Female sexual arousal disorder
Male erectile disorder

Orgasmic Disorders
Female orgasmic disorder
Male orgasmic disorder
Premature ejaculation

Sexual Pain Disorders
Dyspareunia (not due to a general medical condition)
Vaginismus (not due to a general medical condition)

Sexual Dysfunction due to a General Medical Condition
Female hypoactive sexual desire disorder
Male hypoactive sexual desire disorder
Male erectile disorder
Female dyspareunia
Male dyspareunia
Other female sexual dysfunction
Other male sexual dysfunction

Substance-Induced Sexual Dysfunction*
Sexual dysfunction not otherwise specified

*See Chapter 9 and Appendix A.

The *human sexual response cycle* refers to a neurobiologic process first described by the researchers Masters and Johnson in the 1960s. Subsequent research on the response cycle supports the findings of Masters and Johnson, stating that women and men have different response patterns that may interfere with sexual activity when differences are not known or not considered by two partners of the opposite gender. The human sexual response cycle includes the following four phases:

1. **Sexual desire** is described as increased interest, intention, and willingness to move forward into intimate sexual interaction. It may be stimulated by characteristics of the other person, environmental cues, or the individual's own neurophysiologic stimulus.
2. **Excitement,** or the *arousal phase,* results in dramatic neurologic and vascular changes in both men and women, in addition to cognitive and emotional changes that further stimulate the partners to continue engagement. The male penis becomes and remains erect and elongated as it fills with blood. Female changes include pelvic congestion; vaginal lubrication; enlargement of the clitoris, labia, and breasts; and other internal vaginal and uterine changes.
3. **Orgasm** occurs at the height of the arousal phase and is manifested by strong rhythmic contractions in the pelvis that may affect the entire body; release of sexual tension that occurred in the first two phases; and a peak sensation of pleasurable release. Semen is emitted by the male penis, and many internal changes occur in both partners.
4. **Resolution** is a sense of general relaxation, well-being, and muscle relaxation. The male is physiologically refractory to further erection and orgasm for a variable time. The female may be able to respond immediately to additional stimulation.

Inhibitions may occur at one or more of these phases in the response cycle, although inhibition in the resolution phase rarely indicates clinical pathology. In most cases of sexual dysfunction, there is a disturbance in both the subjective sense of pleasure or desire and the objective performance.

Sexual desire disorders

Hypoactive sexual desire disorder
Persistent or recurrent absent or deficient sexual fantasies and desire for sexual activity, taking into account age, sex, and the context of the person's life.

Sexual aversion disorder
Persistent or recurrent extreme aversion to and avoidance of all or nearly all genital sexual contact with a sexual partner.

Sexual arousal disorders

Female sexual arousal disorder
Persistent or recurrent partial or complete failure to attain or maintain lubrication or swelling response of sexual excitement until completion of sexual activity, *or* persistent or recurrent lack of subjective sense of sexual excitement and pleasure during sexual activity.

Male erectile disorder
Persistent or recurrent partial or complete failure to attain or maintain erection until completion of sexual activity, *or* persistent or recurrent lack of subjective sense of sexual excitement and pleasure during sexual activity.

Orgasmic disorders

Female orgasmic disorder
Persistent or recurrent delay in or absence of orgasm following a normal sexual excitement phase. Some females may experience orgasms during noncoital clitoral stimulation but are unable to experience it during coitus in the absence of manual clitoral stimulation. The judgment of

whether this condition justifies this diagnosis is made by thorough sexual evaluation and trial of treatment by a qualified expert. Age, experience, and adequacy of stimulation are considered.

Male orgasmic disorder

Persistent or recurrent delay in or absence of orgasm following a normal sexual excitment phase, considering the person's age and other factors. Failure to achieve orgasm is generally restricted to an inability to reach orgasm in the vagina, with orgasm possible with other types of stimulation such as masturbation.

Premature ejaculation

Persistent or recurrent ejaculation with minimal sexual stimulation, or before, on, or shortly after penetration, and before the person desires it, considering the person's age, newness of the sex partner or situation, and frequency of the sexual activity.

Sexual pain disorders

Dyspareunia

Persistent or recurrent genital pain in either a male or female before, during, or after sexual intercourse, not caused solely by lack of lubrication or vaginismus.

Vaginismus

Persistent or recurrent involuntary spasm of the musculature of the outer third of the vagina, which interferes with coitus.

Substance-induced sexual dysfunction

The defining characteristic of this diagnosis is significant sexual dysfunction causing distress and interference with interpersonal relationships. Symptoms of dysfunction are substance-specific physiologic effects as a result of intake of drugs of abuse, medications, or toxic exposure. Manifestations of dysfunction include the following:
• With impaired desire—absent or deficient sexual desire
• With impaired arousal—impaired sexual arousal (impaired lubrication, erectile dysfunction)
• With impaired orgasm—orgasmic impairment
• With sexual pain—pain associated with intercourse

Sexual dysfunction not otherwise specified

Dysfunctions that do not meet criteria for any of the specific sexual dysfunctions listed above, such as the following:
• No erotic sensation or even complete anesthesia, despite normal physiologic component of orgasm
• The female analog of premature ejaculation
• Genital pain occurring during masturbation

Sexual disorder

Sexual dysfunction not classified in any of the previous categories may be classified as a general "sexual disorder." This category rarely may be used concurrently with one of the specific diagnoses when both are necessary to explain or describe the clinical condition, as in the following examples:

• Marked feelings of inadequacy regarding body habitus, size and shape of sex organs, sexual performance, or other traits related to self-imposed standards of masculinity or femininity
• Distress about a pattern of repeated sexual conquests or other form of nonparaphilic sexual addictions involving a succession of people who exist only as "things to be used"
• Persistent and marked distress about the individual's sexual orientation

Treatment

Individuals who experience sexual dysfunctions as described in the *DSM-IV-TR* may benefit from intervention with a qualified sex therapist. We have elected to construct a care plan based on common problems related to physiologic and psychologic stressors (e.g., effects of prescribed medication, chronicity of the mental or emotional disorder, long-term institutionalization) that interfere with sexual function, performance, and gratification of the client with a mental or emotional disorder. Thus this chapter's care plan is based on sexuality problems experienced by psychiatric clients that are best addressed by nurses.

Paraphilias

The defining characteristics for the paraphilias are persistent, intense, and recurrent sexual urges, fantasies, or behaviors that involve nonliving objects, other nonconsenting persons (children or adults), or humiliation or pain and that occur over at least a 6-month period (see box below). The disorders interfere with reciprocal intimate sexual relationships. A diagnosis for pedophilia, exhibitionism, frotteurism, or voyeurism is made only if the person has acted on the urges and fantasies or if they cause extreme distress.

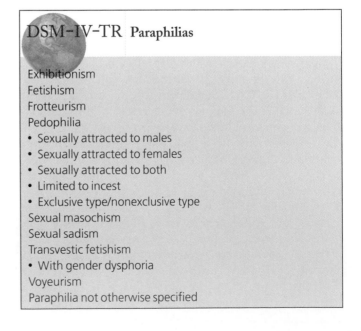

DSM-IV-TR Paraphilias

Exhibitionism
Fetishism
Frotteurism
Pedophilia
• Sexually attracted to males
• Sexually attracted to females
• Sexually attracted to both
• Limited to incest
• Exclusive type/nonexclusive type
Sexual masochism
Sexual sadism
Transvestic fetishism
• With gender dysphoria
Voyeurism
Paraphilia not otherwise specified

Individuals with paraphilias may be driven to be near their fantasy. Therefore they may select work, volunteer, or become involved in hobbies that bring them near to the object of their fantasy (e.g., teacher's aide, salesperson for ladies underwear). They often collect pictures, films, and artwork that depict the object of their disorder. They may not find or be able to keep partners who share their disorder, so they may use prostitutes to act out the fantasy or urge. Various responses by the individuals are the consequence of these disorders. Some persons with a paraphilia have no remorse, whereas others express guilt, shame, remorse, and depression.

The diagnoses of paraphilia include the following:

- **Exhibitionism.** Exposure of one's genitals to unsuspecting stranger(s), followed by sexual arousal.
- **Fetishism.** Use of objects (e.g., female underpants, bras, stockings; shoes; feathers; fur) for purpose of sexual arousal and during sexual activity.
- **Frotteurism.** Touching or rubbing against a nonconsenting person, to stimulate sexual arousal.
- **Pedophilia.** Sexual activity with a prepubescent child or children 13 years of age or younger; offender generally is at least 16 years of age and at least 5 years older than the child/children and may be homosexual, heterosexual, or bisexual; may be limited to incest, exclusive type (attracted only to children), or nonexclusive type (also attracted to adults of either gender).
- **Sexual masochism.** The act of being humiliated, beaten, bound, or otherwise made to suffer while alone (masturbating) or with others. One dangerous form of masochism called *hypoxyphilia* involves oxygen deprivation (plastic bags, nooses, chemical substances) in the brain; may cause death.
- **Sexual sadism.** Acts in which physical (whipping, restraint) or psychologic suffering (humiliation) of the victim is sexually arousing to the perpetrator. Seriousness of sadistic acts usually increases over time, raising potential for injury or death of partner.
- **Transvestic fetishism.** The act of cross-dressing in a heterosexual male (wears female clothing to achieve sexual arousal) that does not meet the criteria for gender identity disorder, nontranssexual type, or transsexualism.
- **Voyeurism.** The act of observing an unsuspecting person who is naked, in the process of disrobing, or engaging in sexual activity to achieve sexual arousal.
- **Paraphilias not otherwise specified.** Disorders that do not meet criteria for the specific categories, such as the following:

  Telephone scatologia. Lewdness; obscene phone calling, sex line telephoning.

  Necrophilia. Sexual activity with corpses.

  Partialism. Exclusive focus on body part that generates sexual arousal (breasts, buttocks, feet).

  Zoophilia. Sexual activity with animals; also known as *bestiality.*

  Coprophilia. Sexual arousal on contact with feces.

  Klismaphilia. Sexual arousal generated by the use of enemas.

  Urophilia. Sexual arousal on contact with urine.

  Ephebophilia. Fondling and other types of sexual activities with children who are developing secondary sexual characteristics (pubic hair, breasts); children generally 13 to 18 years of age.

  Paraphilic coercive disorder. Rape; aggressive sexual assault involving an act of sexual intercourse with a female against her will and without her consent.

Gender Identity Disorder

Defining characteristics of gender identity disorder are (1) the persistent, strong desire to be the opposite sex or insistence that one is the opposite sex (cross-gender identification) and (2) persistent discomfort with own sex (male or female) and feelings of inappropriateness in the gender role of the assigned sex (see box below).

Cross-gender identification surpasses merely wanting to be the opposite sex for cultural advantages and instead is manifested as significant preoccupation with activities that are traditionally reserved for the opposite sex. Individuals prefer dressing in clothing of the opposite sex (cross-dressing), have persistent fantasies of being the opposite sex or show preference for cross-sex roles in make-believe play, participate in stereotypic games of the other sex, and prefer playmates of the opposite sex.

Discomfort with the individual's own sex or gender role manifests as (1) disgust with his or her genitals, (2) rejection of usual assigned position for urination (boys, standing; girls, sitting), and (3) insistence by the girl that she will not menstruate or have larger breasts and by the boy that he will not have a penis when he grows up.

In both sexes, homosexuality is often an outcome, occurring in one third to two thirds of those who have gender identity disorder, although fewer girls than boys become homosexual. Parents may become alarmed when one of their children displays behaviors they believe are stereotypically associated with the opposite sex, but they need to be reassured in many cases that their child's

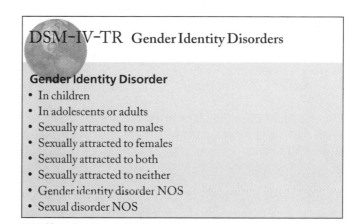

DSM–IV–TR **Gender Identity Disorders**

Gender Identity Disorder
- In children
- In adolescents or adults
- Sexually attracted to males
- Sexually attracted to females
- Sexually attracted to both
- Sexually attracted to neither
- Gender identity disorder NOS
- Sexual disorder NOS

NOS, Not otherwise specified.

nonconformity may not represent the profound disturbance of sexual identity defined in this disorder. Marked distress or impairment of function in the affected person must also be present to make a diagnosis.

INTERVENTIONS

Nurses must first be comfortable with their own sexuality. They also must be knowledgeable about normal sexual function, open to discussion with clients about their disorder, and able to discuss all aspects of the problem. If nurses appear embarrassed or repulsed by the subject of sex, clients' responses to the assessment will be superficial and untruthful because of their own guilt, embarrassment, or conflict about their disorder.

Treatment Settings

Sexual disorders are often treated in clinics that focus on the specialty or in the offices of sex therapists. Nurses frequently treat clients with sexual disorders who have been admitted for a comorbid disorder (depression, obsessive-compulsive disorder, substance use disorder), when the underlying sex disorder is subsequently discovered.

Therapies

Therapeutic nurse-client relationship

Development of trust and rapport is an essential precursor to the treatment of clients with sexual disorders. Clients may also be at risk for or have coexisting medical conditions or disorders (HIV, AIDS), so the nurse's sensitivity in the relationship will facilitate the extensive work that the client must do. The nurse always discusses and maintains confidentiality and privacy with the client, being sure to disclose information that will need to be shared with the treatment team. Principles of the nurse-client relationship are modified to fit the client's needs and problems (see Chapter 1).

Cognitive-behavioral therapy

Cognitive-behavioral therapy may be employed to assist the client to refute irrational thoughts and endangering behaviors. Clients with sexual disorders often "catastrophize" their situations or conditions, and they are able to come to rational conclusions and begin to problem-solve using techniques and methods from cognitive therapy. Thought stopping and thought substitution are helpful exercises to practice. Values clarification exercises also assist the client to gain insight. Behavioral techniques that may be employed are role playing with the client, systematic desensitization, and exposure-response prevention (See Appendix B for explanations of these therapeutic interventions).

Medications

Medication, as with other therapeutic modalities that treat these complex disorders, is generally administered on an outpatient basis. One of the goals of medication is to provide the client with relief from the anxiety and depression that often accompany the trauma of sexual dysfunction and diagnostic testing. Clients with sexual disorders may use alcohol, street drugs, and other substances, which often contribute to their problems. Other sexual issues include fear of intimacy, guilt and shame, cultural and spiritual concerns, and other deeper pathologic problems. These issues may require long-term psychotherapy, physical or medical interventions, and even legal involvement, all of which threaten to change the client's life or life-style.

Both first- and second-generation drugs may adversely affect a person's libido or sexual activity, which may exacerbate the client's existing problems in both inpatient and outpatient settings. A client who is already experiencing low self-esteem associated with a psychiatric diagnosis may be further traumatized from sexual problems resulting from medication. For example, male clients being treated for depression may develop impotence or priapism (painful, sustained erection). All categories of medications prescribed for psychiatric disorders need to be diligently monitored by physicians, clinical pharmacists, nurses, clients, and families for adverse effects on the client's libido and sexual functioning (both men and women are affected).

PROGNOSIS AND DISCHARGE CRITERIA

The prognosis for clients with sexual disorders depends on many factors, including the client's ability to tolerate intimacy, motivation to correct dysfunction, willingness to engage in therapy, and commitment to the couple's relationship. With couples therapy, prognostic factors include the couple's readiness to make changes, recognition of each other's needs and the priority of this problem in their daily lives, and ability to remain realistic. The paraphilias are often difficult to change, and couples who remember this are less frustrated with setbacks. Time and the couple's intention help them make the changes.

Other factors that influence prognosis are the type and severity of the disorder. Some paraphilias may not be perpetrated on others, whereas other diagnoses in this category have the potential for threat of injury to others, problems with the law, or worse consequences (pedophilia, sexual sadism, frotteurism, exhibitionism).

Discharge criteria are as follows:
- The client verbalizes knowledge regarding the sexual disorder and sexual activity and their relationship to mental disorder, hospitalization, and the medication regimen.
- Verbalizes the desire to engage in a satisfying sexual relationship within capacity.
- Develops age-appropriate intimacy with a significant person within the client's capacity.
- Demonstrates interest and energy in satisfying sexual activity, with significant reduction in sexual limitations, or dysfunctions, within capacity.

- Expresses need for ongoing therapy with qualified sex therapist if necessary or appropriate.
- Expresses desire for community involvement to enhance socialization, intimacy, and alternate satisfying activities.

The box below provides guidelines for client and family teaching in the management of sexual and gender identity disorders.

CLIENT AND FAMILY TEACHING   **Sexual and Gender Identity Disorders**

Nurse Needs To Know

- The nurse must develop awareness of own sexuality and sexual biases before helping clients with sexual problems.
- A client's sexuality and sexual health consist of emotional, social, cultural, spiritual, and intellectual aspects, as well as sexual factors.
- Sexual dysfunction or disorder is defined as a physical disorder, such as a problem with an orgasm or erection.
- Sexual apathy or aversion is considered a "nondysfunction" and results from a lack of sexual desire or arousal.
- Sexual problems such as impotence or priapism may result from medication prescribed for a psychiatric diagnosis and may be temporary but traumatic.
- Close monitoring of adverse effects on a client's libido or sexual functioning is an important part of drug therapy.
- Substances such as alcohol or street drugs can also cause sexual dysfunction.
- Sexual disorder or apathy can result in marked distress or difficulty for the client with interpersonal relationships, no matter what the cause.
- Clients with a long history of psychiatric problems often find it difficult to maintain relationships that lead to intimacy and healthy sexual activity.
- Clients and families need information about the possible adverse effects of prescribed medication on the client's sexual functioning so that they will not be frightened or alarmed. Medication adjustment may be necessary.
- Clients and families can be helped to develop alternate expressions of intimacy and closeness if they desire, with the help of a qualified therapist.
- Gender identity disorder is often a complex, long-standing problem that requires empathy, understanding, and specialized counseling.
- Homosexuality occurs in one to two thirds of those with gender identity disorder, and fewer girls than boys become homosexual.
- Cross-gender identification is manifested as significant preoccupation with activities traditionally reserved for the opposite sex.
- Discomfort or disgust with a person's own sex, gender role, or genitals is a signal that the person is disturbed about sexual identity and needs therapy.

Teach Client and Family

- Educate the client/family about the client's disorder, symptoms, behaviors, treatment, and management strategies.
- Teach the client/family about healthy, human sexuality and function and the influence of culture, ethnicity, and spirituality.
- Explain to the client/family that some sexual problems may be related to the client's prescribed medication and may be temporary.
- Advise the client to speak to the physician about sexual problems to determine if medication adjustment is possible.
- Teach the client about the relationship among alcohol, street drugs, and sexual problems, if warranted.
- Educate the client/family to identify stressors or situations that may contribute to the client's sexual problems (apathy or aversion).
- Instruct the client/family to identify situations or objects that may arouse the client to engage in adverse sexual behaviors (paraphilias).
- In collaboration with the physician, suggest that the client consult with a qualified sex therapist for problems that require ongoing intense therapy.
- Inform the client/family that some sexual disorders require long-term treatment and that patience and tolerance are necessary.
- Teach the client to use therapeutic milieu activities to express emotions in a socially acceptable way.
- Instruct the client to discuss feelings in groups in an appropriate manner.
- Inform the client that engaging in interpersonal interactions with peers promotes healthy social functioning.
- Teach the client that physical activities such as running or exercising are healthy alternatives for venting pent-up emotions and frustrations.
- Suggest to the family that counseling, if warranted, may help them cope with the client's disorder.
- Teach the family how to use firm, direct communication and other assertive skills if the client acts out in a sexually inappropriate way.
- Instruct the family to use emergency resources and phone numbers if the client requires urgent clinical or legal interventions.

Continued

| CLIENT AND FAMILY TEACHING | Sexual and Gender Identity Disorders—cont'd |

- Paraphilias include a wide range of sexual behaviors in which the individual is aroused in response to sexual objects or situations not considered typical.
- The arousal source in a person with paraphilia may be so bizarre that it can interfere with the capacity for healthy, reciprocal sexual activity.
- Persons with paraphilia often suffer from other mental, substance-related, and personality disorders and often do not think they are ill.
- Persons with paraphilia often come in contact with the legal system because of their antisocial, atypical sexual behavior and often require long-term therapy.
- The focus of therapy for these complex disorders is multifaceted and includes education about human sexuality and sexual function by a qualified therapist.
- The family may also need special counseling to deal with the client's disorder.
- Provide opportunities for the client to express emotions through milieu groups and activities.
- Praise the client for engaging in conventional social relationships with other clients and for respecting the rights and needs of others.
- Direct the client in a firm but kind manner when he or she uses inappropriate sexual remarks or behaviors in the psychiatric milieu.
- Reinforce the client's strengths, capabilities, and healthy nurturing behavior.
- Provide mature, assertive, healthy expressions and role modeling for the client.
- Provide the client and family with emergency phone numbers if the client's sexual problems require immediate clinical or legal interventions.
- Reinforce treatment and medication compliance as needed.
- Provide information on community groups and resources to help the client and family after discharge (client may require ongoing sexual therapy).
- Access current educational resources available on the Internet and in the library.

- Teach the client/family about the importance of treatment and medication compliance.
- Instruct the family to praise the client for appropriate sexual expression and behaviors.
- Inform the client/family about local community support groups that may help them after discharge.
- Educate the client/family about current resources in the library and on the Internet.

Care Plan

- Sexual Dysfunction

Care Plan
DSM-IV-TR Diagnosis **Sexual Dysfunction**

NANDA Diagnosis: Sexual Dysfunction

Change in sexual function that is viewed as unsatisfactory, unrewarding, or inadequate.

Focus:

For the client who experiences a change in sexual function as a result of the effects of a chronic mental disorder; nontherapeutic effects of psychotropic drugs that may inhibit sexual drive, function, or performance; and institutionalization that interferes with the person's progression toward intimacy and sexual gratification. (Physical disease/dysfunction can also contribute to sexual disorders; see Box 11-1.)

RELATED FACTORS (ETIOLOGY)

Biopsychosocial alteration of sexuality
- Medication effects
- Chronic mental disorder/developmental lag
- Institutionalization

Ineffectual role models

Dependent, ineffective relationships

Lack of emotionally stable significant other

Inability to attain or maintain a successful intimate relationship

Knowledge deficit regarding sex and sexual practices

DEFINING CHARACTERISTICS

The client verbalizes loss of interest in and energy for sexual activity since taking prescribed psychotropic medications.
- "I just don't have the stamina or desire for sex since I began taking this medication."

Reports actual or perceived sexual limitations imposed by mental disorder or physical dysfunction.

- "This mental problem has really ruined my sex life."
- "No one wants to make love with somebody who has a mental illness."
- "This physical illness has really taken a toll on my sex life."

Seeks relations with equally vulnerable clients in mental health facility.

Demonstrates difficulty in achieving perceived sex role throughout chronic mental disorder.

- Fails to achieve chronologic developmental task of intimacy.
- Demonstrates inability to engage in sexual activity with another person or significant partner.

Expresses lack of knowledge regarding ability to find satisfactory sexual expression or alternate gratifying activities alone or with a partner.

- "I just don't know how to have a sexual experience with anyone."
- "I wish I could at least find some friend or hobbies to make me happy even if I can't have sex."

Reports absent or dysfunctional role models during critical developmental stages.

OUTCOME IDENTIFICATION AND EVALUATION

The client demonstrates ability to attain and maintain ongoing intimate relations with age-appropriate partner.

Works with psychiatrist/therapist to adjust prescribed dosage of psychotropic medication to achieve maximum sexual potency and performance.

Verbalizes achievement of sexual gratification in accordance with developmental capacity, effects of medication, and mental/emotional functions.

Demonstrates ability to engage in alternative satisfying friendships, hobbies, and activities instead of sexual activities during periods of institutionalization.

PLANNING AND IMPLEMENTATION

Nursing Intervention	Rationale
Assess through the interview process the client's degree of sexual frustration and dysfunction, beginning with less personal therapeutic statements and progressing to more personal statements.	This type of thoughtful, progressive interview helps the nurse build trust and rapport with the client and determine the extent of the client's sexual problems to plan relevant interventions.

Less Personal: Interview

Reflect the client's statements. • "John, you've expressed concern about your lack of energy and interest lately, and you've been avoiding other clients and activities." Voice concerns. • "The staff and I are concerned that you don't seem to want to take your medication. What seems to be the problem?" • Sit in silence for awhile, and use active listening (the client needs an opportunity to vent concerns). Elicit feelings with open-ended statements. • "What is it about your medication and illness that is troubling to you?" • Allow the client sufficient time to respond.	This type of nonthreatening interview builds trust and rapport and sets the stage for a more indepth interview in the future, if necessary.

More Personal: Interview

Offer information when appropriate. • "John, medication such as yours can affect sexual drive and activity." Use direct questioning. • "Has your illness or medication affected your sexual activities and relationships?" If answer is "yes," reassure the client that although symptoms are troubling, they are not unique (to decrease fear or embarrassment). • "Other clients with mental disorders who take medication similar to yours have experienced some of the same sexual problems." Offer suggestions that may bring relief and hope. • "John, you could discuss your problem with your doctor, who may be able to adjust your medication or provide other ways to relieve your problem." *Note:* Modify interview according to each client's developmental stage and cognitive, affective, and social capabilities. Be careful not to offer false hope. Be sure to assess for pain, physical problems, or disease and refer as necessary.	This type of interview is more in-depth and will elicit more personal information from the client who already trusts the nurse to be professional and discreet.
Construct a list of the client's medications that are most likely responsible for altering or decreasing libido, sexual performance, or sexual activity. Refer to the list for effects on sexual function and performance (see section on medications).	A list of medications helps to reinforce that the physician's adjustment of the dose of some drugs may correct or ameliorate the problem.
Suggest alternative activities to sublimate or substitute overt sexual activity and gratification. • The client plays a musical instrument. • Engages in physical exercise, activity, or sport: walks briskly, pounds pillows/batakas, plays volleyball.	Satisfying nonsexual activities may help the client experience pleasure while he or she is unable to engage in intimate relationships or direct sexual activity during hospitalization.

- Participates in games that require mental energy (e.g., chess, Scrabble).

Note: Supplemental activities should correlate with each client's developmental stage and physical, mental, emotional, and social functioning.

Engage the client in sexuality education classes with a qualified sex therapist, as needed, in collaboration with the client's psychiatrist.	Education about sexual issues from a reliable source can increase the client's knowledge of sexuality and provide alternative means to enhance interpersonal relationships and sexual performance/gratification.
Enroll the client in an education class with a registered hospital pharmacist who, in collaboration with a nurse, will teach the effects of prescribed medications. (A physician is generally a consultant for medication education affecting his or her clients.)	Medication education increases the client's knowledge regarding the effects of medication on libido, sexual performance, and sexual activity and gives the client an opportunity to voice concerns with other clients who may have similar problems.
Help the client meet age-appropriate sleep/rest needs.	Sufficient sleep helps the client conserve energy stores required for interpersonal relationships that could lead to intimacy and healthy sexual expression.
Decrease noise and stimulation in the client's immediate environment before and at bedtime. Provide time for daytime nap(s), if necessary. Engage the client in appropriate milieu activities with same-age clients. *Note:* In most psychiatric settings, sexual activity is not encouraged or permitted.	These interventions encourage active socialization as a prelude to intimate relationships and healthy sexual expression compatible with the client's developmental age and preference.

Discharge Plan

Refer the client to a therapist who specializes in sexual dysfunctions related to mental disorders, institution-alization, developmental lag, medication effects, and physical dysfunction in collaboration with the client's psychiatrist.	A qualified therapist will ensure that the client receives ongoing professional help for sexual problems. Physical intervention by a medical doctor may be warranted, in which case appropriate referral should be made.
Encourage the client to join community groups or organizations and use community resources. • Church group or affiliations • Youth or adult recreation center Include the family, with the client's permission.	Community resources help to support the client's continuing interpersonal interactions and relationships that could foster intimacy and healthy, satisfying sexual activity and experiences.

DSM-IV-TR Classification

NOS – Not Otherwise Specified.

An *x* appearing in a diagnostic code indicates that a specific code number is required.

An ellipsis (. . .) is used in the names of certain disorders to indicate that the name of a specific mental disorder or general medical condition should be inserted when recording the name (e.g., 293.0 Delirium Due to Hypothyroidism).

If criteria are currently met, one of the following severity specifiers may be noted after the diagnosis:

- Mild
- Moderate
- Severe

If criteria are no longer met, one of the following specifiers may be noted:

- In Partial Remission
- In Full Remission
- Prior History

DISORDERS USUALLY FIRST DIAGNOSED IN INFANCY, CHILDHOOD, OR ADOLESCENCE

Mental Retardation

Note: These are coded on Axis II.

317	Mild Mental Retardation
318.0	Moderate Mental Retardation
318.1	Severe Mental Retardation
318.2	Profound Mental Retardation
319	Mental Retardation, Severity Unspecified

Learning Disorders

315.00	Reading Disorder
315.1	Mathematics Disorder
315.2	Disorder of Written Expression
315.9	Learning Disorder NOS

From American Psychiatric Association: *Diagnostic and statistical manual of mental disorders*, ed 4, third revision, Washington, DC, 2000, The Association.

Motor Skills Disorder

315.4	Developmental Coordination Disorder

Communication Disorders

315.31	Expressive Language Disorder
315.32	Mixed Receptive-Expressive Language Disorder
315.39	Phonological Disorder
307.0	Stuttering
307.9	Communication Disorder NOS

Pervasive Developmental Disorders

299.00	Autistic Disorder
299.80	Rett's Disorder
299.10	Childhood Disintegrative Disorder
299.80	Asperger's Disorder
299.80	Pervasive Developmental Disorder NOS

Attention-Deficit and Disruptive Behavior Disorders

314.xx	Attention-Deficit/Hyperactivity Disorder
.01	Combined Type
.00	Predominantly Inattentive Type
.01	Predominantly Hyperactive-Impulsive Type
314.9	Attention-Deficit/Hyperactivity Disorder NOS
312.xx	Conduct Disorder
.81	Childhood-Onset Type
.82	Adolescent-Onset Type
.89	Unspecified Onset
313.81	Oppositional Defiant Disorder
312.9	Disruptive Behavior Disorder NOS

Feeding and Eating Disorders of Infancy or Early Childhood

307.52	Pica
307.53	Rumination Disorder
307.59	Feeding Disorder of Infancy or Early Childhood

Tic Disorders

307.23	Tourette's Disorder
307.22	Chronic Motor or Vocal Tic Disorder
307.21	Transient Tic Disorder

Specify if: Single Episode/Recurrent

307.20   Tic Disorder NOS

Elimination Disorders

—.-   Encopresis
787.6   With Constipation and Overflow Incontinence
307.7   Without Constipation and Overflow Incontinence
307.6   Enuresis (Not Due to a General Medical Condition)

> *Specify type:* Nocturnal Only/Diurnal Only/Nocturnal and Diurnal

Other Disorders of Infancy, Childhood, or Adolescence

309.21   Separation Anxiety Disorder

> *Specify if:* Early Onset

313.23   Selective Mutism
313.89   Reactive Attachment Disorder of Infancy or Early Childhood

> *Specify type:* Inhibited Type/Disinhibited Type

307.3   Stereotypic Movement Disorder

> *Specify if:* With Self-Injurious Behavior

313.9   Disorder of Infancy, Childhood, or Adolescence NOS

DELIRIUM, DEMENTIA, AND AMNESTIC AND OTHER COGNITIVE DISORDERS

Delirium

293.0   Delirium Due to . . . *[Indicate the General Medical Condition]*
—.-   Substance Intoxication Delirium *(refer to Substance-Related Disorders for substance-specific codes)*
—.-   Substance Withdrawal Delirium *(refer to Substance-Related Disorders for substance-specific codes)*
—   Delirium Due to Multiple Etiologies *(code each of the specific etiologies)*
780.09   Delirium NOS

Dementia (147)

294.xx* Dementia of the Alzheimer's Type, With Early Onset *(also code 331.0 Alzheimer's disease on Axis III)*
 .10   Without Behavioral Disturbance
 .11   With Behavioral Disturbance
294.xx* Dementia of the Alzheimer's Type, With Late Onset *(also code 331.0 Alzheimer's disease on Axis III)*
 .10   Without Behavioral Disturbance

 .11   With Behavioral Disturbance
290.xx   Vascular Dementia
 .40   Uncomplicated
 .41   With Delirium
 .42   With Delusions
 .43   With Depressed Mood

> *Specify if:* With Behavioral Disturbance

Code presence or absence of a behavioral disturbance in the fifth digit for Dementia Due to a General Medical Condition:

0 = Without Behavioral Disturbance
1 = With Behavioral Disturbance

294.1x* Dementia Due to HIV Disease *(also code 042 HIV on Axis III)*
294.1x* Dementia Due to Head Trauma *(also code 854.00 head injury on Axis III)*
294.1x* Dementia Due to Parkinson's Disease *(also code 332.0 Parkinson's disease on Axis III)*
294.1x* Dementia Due to Huntington's Disease *(also code 333.4 Huntington's disease on Axis III)*
294.1x* Dementia Due to Pick's Disease *(also code 331.1 Pick's disease on Axis III)*
294.1x* Dementia Due to Creutzfeldt-Jakob Disease *(also code 046.1 Creutzfeldt-Jakob disease on Axis III)*
294.1x* Dementia Due to . . . *[Indicate the General Medical Condition not listed above] (also code the general medical condition on Axis III)*
—.–   Substance-Induced Persisting Dementia *(refer to Substance-Related Disorders for substance-specific codes)*
—.–   Dementia Due to Multiple Etiologies *(code each of the specific etiologies)*
294.8   Dementia NOS

Amnestic Disorders

294.0   Amnestic Disorder Due to . . . *[Indicate the General Medical Condition]*

> *Specify if:* Transient/Chronic

—.–   Substance-Induced Persisting Amnestic Disorder *(refer to Substance-Related Disorders for substance-specific codes)*
294.8   Amnestic Disorder NOS

Other Cognitive Disorders

294.9   Cognitive Disorder NOS

MENTAL DISORDERS DUE TO A GENERAL MEDICAL CONDITION NOT CLASSIFIED ELSEWHERE

293.89   Catatonic Disorder Due to . . . *[Indicate the General Medical Condition]*

*ICD-9-CM code valid after October 1, 2000.

310.1   Personality Change Due to . . . *[Indicate the General Medical Condition]*

        Specify type: Labile Type/Disinhibited Type/ Aggressive Type/Apathetic Type/Paranoid Type/ Other Type/ Combined Type/Unspecified Type

293.9   Mental Disorder NOS Due to . . . *[Indicate the General Medical Condition]*

SUBSTANCE-RELATED DISORDERS

The following specifiers apply to Substance Dependence as noted:

[a]With Physiological Dependence/Without Physiological Dependence
[b]Early Full Remission/Early Partial Remission/Sustained Full Remission/Sustained Partial Remission
[c]In a Controlled Environment
[d]On Agonist Therapy

The following specifiers apply to Substance-Induced Disorders as noted:

[I]With Onset During Intoxication/[W]With Onset During Withdrawal

Alcohol-Related Disorders

Alcohol Use Disorders

303.90   Alcohol Dependence[a,b,c]
305.00   Alcohol Abuse

Alcohol-Induced Disorders

303.00   Alcohol Intoxication
291.81   Alcohol Withdrawal

        Specify if: With Perceptual Disturbances

291.0   Alcohol Intoxication Delirium
291.0   Alcohol Withdrawal Delirium
291.2   Alcohol-Induced Persisting Dementia
291.1   Alcohol-Induced Persisting Amnestic Disorder
291.x   Alcohol-Induced Psychotic Disorder
  .5   With Delusions[I,W]
  .3   With Hallucinations[I,W]
291.89   Alcohol-Induced Mood Disorder[I,W]
291.89   Alcohol-Induced Anxiety Disorder[I,W]
291.89   Alcohol-Induced Sexual Dysfunction[I]
291.89   Alcohol-Induced Sleep Disorder[I,W]
291.9   Alcohol-Related Disorder NOS

Amphetamine (or Amphetamine-Like)–Related Disorders

Amphetamine Use Disorders

304.40   Amphetamine Dependence[a,b,c]
305.70   Amphetamine Abuse

Amphetamine-Induced Disorders

292.89   Amphetamine Intoxication
        Specify if: With Perceptual Disturbances

292.0   Amphetamine Withdrawal
292.81   Amphetamine Intoxication Delirium
292.xx   Amphetamine-Induced Psychotic Disorder
  .11   With Delusions[I]
  .12   With Hallucinations[I]
292.84   Amphetamine-Induced Mood Disorder[I,W]
292.89   Amphetamine-Induced Anxiety Disorder[I]
292.89   Amphetamine-Induced Sexual Dysfunction[I]
292.89   Amphetamine-Induced Sleep Disorder[I,W]
292.9   Amphetamine-Related Disorder NOS

Caffeine-Related Disorders

Caffeine-Induced Disorders

305.90   Caffeine Intoxication
292.89   Caffeine-Induced Anxiety Disorder[I]
292.89   Caffeine-Induced Sleep Disorder[I]
292.9   Caffeine-Related Disorder NOS

Cannabis-Related Disorders

Cannabis Use Disorders

304.30   Cannabis Dependence[a,b,c]
305.20   Cannabis Abuse

Cannabis-Induced Disorders

292.89   Cannabis Intoxication
        Specify if: With Perceptual Disturbances

292.81   Cannabis Intoxication Delirium
292.xx   Cannabis-Induced Psychotic Disorder
  .11   With Delusions[I]
  .12   With Hallucinations[I]
292.89   Cannabis-Induced Anxiety Disorder[I]
292.9   Cannabis-Related Disorder NOS (241)

Cocaine-Related Disorders

Cocaine Use Disorders

304.20   Cocaine Dependence[a,b,c]
305.60   Cocaine Abuse

Cocaine-Induced Disorders

292.89   Cocaine Intoxication
        Specify if: With Perceptual Disturbances

292.0   Cocaine Withdrawal
292.81   Cocaine Intoxication Delirium
292.xx   Cocaine-Induced Psychotic Disorder
  .11   With Delusions[I]
  .12   With Hallucinations[I]
292.84   Cocaine-Induced Mood Disorder[I,W]
292.89   Cocaine-Induced Anxiety Disorder[I,W]
292.89   Cocaine-Induced Sexual Dysfunction[I]
292.89   Cocaine-Induced Sleep Disorder[I,W]
292.9   Cocaine-Related Disorder NOS

Hallucinogen-Related Disorders

Hallucinogen Use Disorders

304.50 Hallucinogen Dependence[b,c]
305.30 Hallucinogen Abuse

Hallucinogen-Induced Disorders

292.89 Hallucinogen Intoxication
292.89 Hallucinogen Persisting Perception Disorder (Flashbacks)
292.81 Hallucinogen Intoxication Delirium
292.xx Hallucinogen-Induced Psychotic Disorder
  .11   With Delusions[I]
  .12   With Hallucinations[I]
292.84 Hallucinogen-Induced Mood Disorder[I]
292.89 Hallucinogen-Induced Anxiety Disorder[I]
292.9 Hallucinogen-Related Disorder NOS

Inhalant-related disorders

Inhalant Use Disorders

304.60 Inhalant Dependence[b,c]
305.90 Inhalant Abuse

Inhalant-Induced Disorders

292.89 Inhalant Intoxication
292.81 Inhalant Intoxication Delirium
292.82 Inhalant-Induced Persisting Dementia
292.xx Inhalant-Induced Psychotic Disorder
292.11 With Delusions[I]
292.12 With Hallucinations[I]
292.84 Inhalant-Induced Mood Disorder[I]
292.89 Inhalant-Induced Anxiety Disorder[I]
292.9 Inhalant-Related Disorder NOS

Nicotine-Related Disorders

Nicotine Use Disorder

305.1 Nicotine Dependence[a,b]

Nicotine-Induced Disorder

292.0 Nicotine Withdrawal
292.9 Nicotine-Related Disorder NOS

Opioid-Related Disorders

Opioid Use Disorders

304.00 Opioid Dependence[a,b,c,d]
305.50 Opioid Abuse

Opioid-Induced Disorders

292.89 Opioid Intoxication

Specify if: With Perceptual Disturbances

292.0 Opioid Withdrawal
292.81 Opioid Intoxication Delirium
292.xx Opioid-Induced Psychotic Disorder
  .11   With Delusions[I]
  .12   With Hallucinations[I]

292.84 Opioid-Induced Mood Disorder[I]
292.89 Opioid-Induced Sexual Dysfunction[I]
292.89 Opioid-Induced Sleep Disorder[I,W]
292.9 Opioid-Related Disorder NOS

Phencyclidine (or Phencyclidine-Like)–Related Disorders

Phencyclidine Use Disorders

304.60 Phencyclidine Dependence[b,c]
305.90 Phencyclidine Abuse

Phencyclidine-Induced Disorders

292.89 Phencyclidine Intoxication

Specify if: With Perceptual Disturbances

292.81 Phencyclidine Intoxication Delirium
292.xx Phencyclidine-Induced Psychotic Disorder
  .11   With Delusions[I]
  .12   With Hallucinations[I]
292.84 Phencyclidine-Induced Mood Disorder[I]
292.89 Phencyclidine-Induced Anxiety Disorder[I]
292.9 Phencyclidine-Related Disorder NOS

Sedative-, Hypnotic-, or Anxiolytic-Related Disorders

Sedative, Hypnotic, or Anxiolytic Use Disorders

304.10 Sedative, Hypnotic, or Anxiolytic Dependence[a,b,c]
305.40 Sedative, Hypnotic, or Anxiolytic Abuse

Sedative-, Hypnotic-, or Anxiolytic-Induced Disorders

292.89 Sedative, Hypnotic, or Anxiolytic Intoxication
292.0 Sedative, Hypnotic, or Anxiolytic Withdrawal

Specify if: With Perceptual Disturbances

292.81 Sedative, Hypnotic, or Anxiolytic Intoxication Delirium
292.81 Sedative, Hypnotic, or Anxiolytic Withdrawal Delirium
292.82 Sedative-, Hypnotic-, or Anxiolytic-Induced Persisting Dementia
292.83 Sedative-, Hypnotic-, or Anxiolytic-Induced Persisting Amnestic Disorder
292.xx Sedative-, Hypnotic-, or Anxiolytic-Induced Psychotic Disorder
292.11 With Delusions[I,W]
292.12 With Hallucinations[I,W]
292.84 Sedative-, Hypnotic-, or Anxiolytic-Induced Mood Disorder[I,W]
292.89 Sedative-, Hypnotic-, or Anxiolytic-Induced Anxiety Disorder[W]
292.89 Sedative-, Hypnotic-, or Anxiolytic-Induced Sexual Dysfunction[I]
292.89 Sedative-, Hypnotic-, or Anxiolytic-Induced Sleep Disorder[I,W]

292.9   Sedative-, Hypnotic-, or Anxiolytic-Related Disorder NOS

Polysubstance-Related Disorder

304.80   Polysubstance Dependence[a,b,c,d]

Other (or Unknown) Substance–Related Disorders

Other (or Unknown) Substance Use Disorders

304.90   Other (or Unknown) Substance Dependence[a,b,c,d]
305.90   Other (or Unknown) Substance Abuse

Other (or Unknown) Substance–Induced Disorders

292.89   Other (or Unknown) Substance Intoxication

   Specify if: With Perceptual Disturbances

292.0   Other (or Unknown) Substance Withdrawal

   Specify if: With Perceptual Disturbances

292.81   Other (or Unknown) Substance–Induced Delirium
292.82   Other (or Unknown) Substance–Induced Persisting Dementia
292.83   Other (or Unknown) Substance–Induced Persisting Amnestic Disorder
292.xx   Other (or Unknown) Substance–Induced Psychotic Disorder
   .11   With Delusions[I,W]
   .12   With Hallucinations[I,W]
292.84   Other (or Unknown) Substance–Induced Mood Disorder[I,W]
292.89   Other (or Unknown) Substance–Induced Anxiety Disorder[I,W]
292.89   Other (or Unknown) Substance–Induced Sexual Dysfunction[I]
292.89   Other (or Unknown) Substance–Induced Sleep Disorder[I,W]
292.9   Other (or Unknown) Substance–Related Disorder NOS

SCHIZOPHRENIA AND OTHER PSYCHOTIC DISORDERS

295.xx   Schizophrenia
   The following Classification of Longitudinal Course applies to all subtypes of Schizophrenia:

Episodic With Interepisode Residual Symptoms (*specify if:* With Prominent Negative Symptoms)/Episodic With No Interepisode Residual Symptoms
Continuous (*specify if:* With Prominent Negative Symptoms)
Single Episode In Partial Remission (*specify if:* With Prominent Negative Symptoms)/Single Episode In Full Remission
Other or Unspecified Pattern

295.30   Paranoid Type
295.10   Disorganized Type

295.20   Catatonic Type
295.90   Undifferentiated Type
295.60   Residual Type
295.40   Schizophreniform Disorder

   Specify if: Without Good Prognostic Features/With Good Prognostic Features

295.70   Schizoaffective Disorder

   Specify type: Bipolar Type/Depressive Type

297.1   Delusional Disorder

   Specify type: Erotomanic Type/Grandiose Type/Jealous Type/Persecutory Type/Somatic Type/Mixed Type/ Unspecified Type

298.8   Brief Psychotic Disorder

   Specify if: With Marked Stressor(s)/Without Marked Stressor(s)/With Postpartum Onset

297.3   Shared Psychotic Disorder
293.xx   Psychotic Disorder Due to . . .

   [Indicate the General Medical Condition]

   .81   With Delusions
   .82   With Hallucinations
—.–   Substance-Induced Psychotic Disorder *(refer to Substance-Related Disorders for substance-specific codes)*

   Specify if: With Onset During Intoxication/With Onset During Withdrawal

298.9   Psychotic Disorder NOS

MOOD DISORDERS

Code current state of Major Depressive Disorder or Bipolar I Disorder in fifth digit:

   1 = Mild
   2 = Moderate
   3 = Severe Without Psychotic Features
   4 = Severe With Psychotic Features
       Specify: Mood-Congruent Psychotic Features/Mood-Incongruent Psychotic Features
   5 = In Partial Remission
   6 = In Full Remission
   0 = Unspecified

The following specifiers apply (for current or most recent episode) to Mood Disorders as noted:

[a]Severity/Psychotic/Remission Specifiers/[b]Chronic/[c]With Catatonic Features/[d]With Melancholic Features/[e]With Atypical Features/[f]With Postpartum Onset

The following specifiers apply to Mood Disorders as noted:

[g]With or Without Full Interepisode Recovery/[h]With Seasonal Pattern/[i]With Rapid Cycling

Depressive Disorders

296.xx   Major Depressive Disorder
296.2x   Single Episode[a,b,c,d,e,f]
296.3x   Recurrent[a,b,c,d,e,f,g,h]
300.4   Dysthymic Disorder

> *Specify if:* Early Onset/Late Onset
> *Specify if:* With Atypical Features

311   Depressive Disorder NOS

Bipolar Disorders

296.xx   Bipolar I Disorder
296.0x   Single Manic Episode[a,c,f]

> *Specify if:* Mixed

296.40   Most Recent Episode Hypomanic[g,h,i]
296.4x   Most Recent Episode Manic[a,c,f,g,h,i]
296.6x   Most Recent Episode Mixed[a,c,f,g,h,i]
296.5x   Most Recent Episode Depressed[a,b,c,d,e,f,g,h,i]
296.7   Most Recent Episode Unspecified[g,h,i]
296.89   Bipolar II Disorder[a,b,c,d,e,f,g,h,i]

> *Specify (current or most recent episode):* Hypomanic/
> Depressed

301.13   Cyclothymic Disorder
296.80   Bipolar Disorder NOS
293.83   Mood Disorder Due to . . .

> [Indicate the General Medical Condition]
> *Specify type:* With Depressive Features/With Major
> Depressive–Like Episode/With Manic
> Features/With Mixed Features

293.83   Substance-Induced Mood Disorder *(refer to*
> *Substance-Related Disorders for substance-specific codes)*

> *Specify type:* With Depressive Features/With Manic
> Features/With Mixed Features
> *Specify if:* With Onset During Intoxication/With
> Onset During Withdrawal

296.90   Mood Disorder NOS

ANXIETY DISORDERS

300.01   Panic Disorder Without Agoraphobia
300.21   Panic Disorder With Agoraphobia
300.22   Agoraphobia Without History of Panic Disorder
300.29   Specific Phobia

> *Specify type:* Animal Type/Natural Environment
> Type/Blood-Injection-Injury Type/Situational Type/
> Other Type

300.23   Social Phobia

> *Specify if:* Generalized

300.3   Obsessive-Compulsive Disorder

> *Specify if:* With Poor Insight

309.81   Posttraumatic Stress Disorder

> *Specify if:* Acute/Chronic
> *Specify if:* With Delayed Onset

308.3   Acute Stress Disorder
300.02   Generalized Anxiety Disorder
293.84   Anxiety Disorder Due to . . .

> [Indicate the General Medical Condition]
> *Specify if:* With Generalized Anxiety/With Panic
> Attacks/With Obsessive-Compulsive Symptoms

—.—   Substance-Induced Anxiety Disorder *(refer to*
> *Substance-Related Disorders for substance-specific*
> *codes)*

> *Specify if:* With Generalized Anxiety/With Panic
> Attacks/With Obsessive-Compulsive Symptoms/
> With Phobic Symptoms
> *Specify if:* With Onset During Intoxication/With
> Onset During Withdrawal

300.00   Anxiety Disorder NOS

SOMATOFORM DISORDERS

300.81   Somatization Disorder
300.82   Undifferentiated Somatoform Disorder
300.11   Conversion Disorder

> *Specify type:* With Motor Symptom or Deficit/With
> Sensory Symptom or Deficit/With Seizures or
> Convulsions/With Mixed Presentation

307.xx   Pain Disorder
   .80   Associated With Psychological Factors
   .89   Associated With Both Psychological Factors and
           a General Medical Condition

> *Specify if:* Acute/Chronic

300.7   Hypochondriasis *Specify if:* With Poor Insight
300.7   Body Dysmorphic Disorder
300.82   Somatoform Disorder NOS

FACTITIOUS DISORDERS

300.xx   Factitious Disorder
300.16   With Predominantly Psychological Signs and
           Symptoms
300.19   With Predominantly Physical Signs and
           Symptoms
300.19   With Combined Psychological and Physical
           Signs and Symptoms
300.19   Factitious Disorder NOS

DISSOCIATIVE DISORDERS

300.12   Dissociative Amnesia
300.13   Dissociative Fugue

300.14   Dissociative Identity Disorder
300.6   Depersonalization Disorder
300.15   Dissociative Disorder NOS

SEXUAL AND GENDER IDENTITY DISORDERS

Sexual Dysfunctions

The following specifiers apply to all primary Sexual Dysfunctions:

Lifelong Type/Acquired Type
Generalized Type/Situational Type
Due to Psychological Factors/Due to Combined Factors

Sexual desire disorders

302.71   Hypoactive Sexual Desire Disorder
302.79   Sexual Aversion Disorder

Sexual arousal disorders

302.72   Female Sexual Arousal Disorder
302.72   Male Erectile Disorder

Orgasmic disorders

302.73   Female Orgasmic Disorder
302.74   Male Orgasmic Disorder
302.75   Premature Ejaculation

Sexual pain disorders

302.76   Dyspareunia (Not Due to a General Medical Condition)
306.51   Vaginismus (Not Due to a General Medical Condition)

Sexual dysfunction due to a general medical condition

625.8   Female Hypoactive Sexual Desire Disorder Due to . . . *[Indicate the General Medical Condition]*
608.89   Male Hypoactive Sexual Desire Disorder Due to . . . *[Indicate the General Medical Condition]*
607.84   Male Erectile Disorder Due to . . . *[Indicate the General Medical Condition]*
625.0   Female Dyspareunia Due to . . . *[Indicate the General Medical Condition]*
608.89   Male Dyspareunia Due to . . . *[Indicate the General Medical Condition]*
625.8   Other Female Sexual Dysfunction Due to . . . *[Indicate the General Medical Condition]*
608.89   Other Male Sexual Dysfunction Due to . . . *[Indicate the General Medical Condition]*
——.—   Substance-Induced Sexual Dysfunction *(refer to Substance-Related Disorders for substance-specific codes)*

Specify if: With Impaired Desire/With Impaired Arousal/With Impaired Orgasm/With Sexual Pain
Specify if: With Onset During Intoxication

302.70   Sexual Dysfunction NOS

Paraphilias

302.4   Exhibitionism
302.81   Fetishism
302.89   Frotteurism
302.2   Pedophilia

Specify if: Sexually Attracted to Males/Sexually Attracted to Females/Sexually Attracted to Both
Specify if: Limited to Incest
Specify type: Exclusive Type/Nonexclusive Type

302.83   Sexual Masochism
302.84   Sexual Sadism
302.3   Transvestic Fetishism

Specify if: With Gender Dysphoria

302.82   Voyeurism
302.9   Paraphilia NOS

Gender Identity Disorders

302.xx   Gender Identity Disorder
   .6   in Children
   .85   in Adolescents or Adults

Specify if: Sexually Attracted to Males/Sexually Attracted to Females/Sexually Attracted to Both/Sexually Attracted to Neither

302.6   Gender Identity Disorder NOS
302.9   Sexual Disorder NOS

EATING DISORDERS

307.1   Anorexia Nervosa

Specify type: Restricting Type; Binge-Eating/Purging Type

307.51   Bulimia Nervosa

Specify type: Purging Type/Nonpurging Type

307.50   Eating Disorder NOS

SLEEP DISORDERS

Primary Sleep Disorders

Dyssomnias

307.42   Primary Insomnia
307.44   Primary Hypersomnia

Specify if: Recurrent

347   Narcolepsy
780.59   Breathing-Related Sleep Disorder
307.45   Circadian Rhythm Sleep Disorder

Specify type: Delayed Sleep Phase Type/Jet Lag Type/Shift Work Type/Unspecified Type

307.47   Dyssomnia NOS

Parasomnias

307.47 Nightmare Disorder
307.46 Sleep Terror Disorder
307.46 Sleepwalking Disorder
307.47 Parasomnia NOS

Sleep Disorders Related to Another Mental Disorder

307.42 Insomnia Related to . . . *[Indicate the Axis I or Axis II Disorder]*
307.44 Hypersomnia Related to . . . *[Indicate the Axis I or Axis II Disorder]*

Other Sleep Disorders

780.xx Sleep Disorder Due to . . . *[Indicate the General Medical Condition]*
780.52 Insomnia Type
780.54 Hypersomnia Type
780.59 Parasomnia Type
780.59 Mixed Type
—.–   Substance-Induced Sleep Disorder *(refer to Substance-Related Disorders for substance-specific codes)*

Specify type: Insomnia Type/Hypersomnia Type/Parasomnia Type/Mixed Type
Specify if: With Onset During Intoxication/With Onset During Withdrawal

IMPULSE-CONTROL DISORDERS NOT ELSEWHERE CLASSIFIED

312.34 Intermittent Explosive Disorder
312.32 Kleptomania
312.33 Pyromania
312.31 Pathological Gambling
312.39 Trichotillomania
312.30 Impulse-Control Disorder NOS

ADJUSTMENT DISORDERS

309.xx Adjustment Disorder
.0   With Depressed Mood
.24   With Anxiety
.28   With Mixed Anxiety and Depressed Mood
.3   With Disturbance of Conduct
.4   With Mixed Disturbance of Emotions and Conduct
.9   Unspecified

Specify if: Acute/Chronic

PERSONALITY DISORDERS

Note: *These are coded on Axis II.*
301.0   Paranoid Personality Disorder
301.20 Schizoid Personality Disorder

301.22 Schizotypal Personality Disorder
301.7   Antisocial Personality Disorder
301.83 Borderline Personality Disorder
301.50 Histrionic Personality Disorder
301.81 Narcissistic Personality Disorder
301.82 Avoidant Personality Disorder
301.6   Dependent Personality Disorder
301.4   Obsessive-Compulsive Personality Disorder
301.9   Personality Disorder NOS

OTHER CONDITIONS THAT MAY BE A FOCUS OF CLINICAL ATTENTION

Psychological Factors Affecting Medical Condition

316   . . . *[Specified Psychological Factor] Affecting . . . [Indicate the General Medical Condition]*
Choose name based on nature of factors:
Mental Disorder Affecting Medical Condition
Psychological Symptoms Affecting Medical Condition
Personality Traits or Coping Style Affecting Medical Condition
Maladaptive Health Behaviors Affecting Medical Condition
Stress-Related Physiological Response Affecting Medical Condition
Other or Unspecified Psychological Factors Affecting Medical Condition

Medication-Induced Movement Disorders

332.1   Neuroleptic-Induced Parkinsonism
333.92 Neuroleptic Malignant Syndrome
333.7   Neuroleptic-Induced Acute Dystonia
333.99 Neuroleptic-Induced Acute Akathisia
333.82 Neuroleptic-Induced Tardive Dyskinesia
333.1   Medication-Induced Postural Tremor
333.90 Medication-Induced Movement Disorder NOS

Other Medication-Induced Disorder

995.2   Adverse Effects of Medication NOS

Relational Problems

V61.9   Relational Problem Related to a Mental Disorder or General Medical Condition
V61.20 Parent-Child Relational Problem
V61.10 Partner Relational Problem
V61.8   Sibling Relational Problem
V62.81 Relational Problem NOS

Problems Related to Abuse or Neglect

V61.21 Physical Abuse of Child
(code 995.54 if focus of attention is on victim)
V61.21 Sexual Abuse of Child
(code 995.53 if focus of attention is on victim)

V61.21   Neglect of Child
         (code 995.52 if focus of attention is on victim)
—.—   Physical Abuse of Adult
V61.12   (if by partner)
V62.83   (if by person other than partner)
         (code 995.81 if focus of attention is on victim)
—.—   Sexual Abuse of Adult
V61.12   (if by partner)
V62.83   (if by person other than partner)
         (code 995.83 if focus of attention is on victim)

Additional Conditions That May be a Focus of Clinical Attention

V15.81   Noncompliance with Treatment
V65.2   Malingering
V71.01   Adult Antisocial Behavior
V71.02   Child or Adolescent Antisocial Behavior
V62.89   Borderline Intellectual Functioning

> *Note:* This is coded on Axis II.

780.9   Age-Related Cognitive Decline
V62.82   Bereavement
V62.3   Academic Problem
V62.2   Occupational Problem

313.82   Identity Problem
V62.89   Religious or Spiritual Problem
V62.4   Acculturation Problem
V62.89   Phase of Life Problem

ADDITIONAL CODES

300.9   Unspecified Mental Disorder
         (nonpsychotic)
V71.09   No Diagnosis or Condition on Axis I
799.9   Diagnosis or Condition Deferred on Axis I
V71.09   No Diagnosis on Axis II
799.9   Diagnosis Deferred on Axis II

MULTIAXIAL SYSTEM

Axis I   Clinical Disorders
          Other Conditions That May Be a Focus of
          Clinical Attention
Axis II   Personality Disorders
          Mental Retardation
Axis III General Medical Conditions
Axis IV   Psychosocial and Environmental Problems
Axis V   Global Assessment of Functioning

Psychiatric/ Psychosocial Therapies

Behavior therapy Type of therapy that focuses on modifying observable behavior, emotions, and verbalizations by manipulating the environment, the behavior, or the consequences of the behavior. In contrast to *psychoanalytic therapy,* which focuses on repressed, intrapsychic conflicts, behavioral approaches focus on the effects rather than the cause. They include the works of Ivan Pavlov (classic conditioning) and B.F. Skinner (operant conditioning) but have also been applied to many other types of therapies, including *rational-emotive therapy,* a type of cognitive therapy developed by Ellis, and the *cognitive therapy* developed later by Beck, both listed separately. Behavioral strategies are also used in behavioral contracts to reinforce positive behaviors and diminish maladaptive behaviors.

Cognitive therapy Form of therapy (developed by Aaron Beck) most often used in depression and currently being used for other nonpsychotic disorders that stem from the individual's negative self-concept or exaggerated, prolonged guilt and the consequent automatic thoughts of self-deprecation.

The goal of cognitive therapy is to diminish depressive symptoms by helping the individual recognize, challenge, and invalidate distorted automatic thoughts through a series of mental exercises and ultimately to replace them with appropriate, realistic thoughts based on more accurate evaluations. In practice, cognitive and behavioral therapeutic concepts are often used together.

Beck, however, places much more importance on the internal or mental experiences of his clients than does behaviorism. He emphasizes that behavioral techniques are used to supplement the cognitive work. One of the main reasons for using a behavioral technique is to demonstrate to the client that the negative assumptions and conclusions are incorrect, thus paving the way for improved performance in aspects of life that are important to the client.

Thought stopping Cognitive strategy used to treat individuals with depression characterized by irrational, anxiety-provoking, and brooding behaviors. The goal of thought stopping is to inhibit these maladaptive behaviors by instructing the client to shout "stop" after he or she expresses the illogical behavior. In this way the client learns to control the thoughts and thus control the maladaptive behavior. Thought stopping has been reported to be useful in the treatment of obsessive-compulsive disorders; the word "stop" is initiated by the nurse-therapist, followed by an exaggerated stimulus, such as a loud noise, or by the client loudly echoing the word "stop." Consequently, the troublesome thought is interrupted or blocked by principles of counterconditioning, and the behavior is inhibited as well.

Thought substitution Cognitive approach (developed by Wolpe) in which the client is instructed to substitute a positive or rational thought for a negative, distorted thought.

Reframing/relabeling Cognitive technique in which the nurse-therapist renames or relabels seemingly dysfunctional behavior as reasonable and understandable behavior to take away the negative motive for the act. The goal of renaming or relabeling is to emphasize the positive aspects of interpersonal feelings and behaviors.

- The client who is scheduled to lead the morning community meeting may repeatedly refer to herself as "anxious." The nurse, knowing the client is well prepared, relabels "anxious" as "enthusiastic."
- The client may continually refer to a nurse's action as "hovering." The nurse, realizing the client needs to be closely watched, renames "hovering" as "caring."

Rational-emotive therapy (RET) Type of cognitive therapy (developed by Albert Ellis) that preceded Beck's work, based on the premise that an individual's values and beliefs control his or her behavior. Many beliefs and assumptions are irrational and self-defeating, and people often evaluate their behavior by using these faulty thoughts. Some false assumptions include the following:

1. A person should be loved and approved of by everyone.
2. A person should be competent and talented to prove that he or she is adequate.
3. A person has little control over his or her life, and pressures make one feel angry, hostile, and depressed.

4. Past experiences are the most important influence on present behavior and cannot be changed.

5. Order and understanding of the world are necessary for happiness and well-being.

6. One should not question society's beliefs, or one may be punished.

RET helps individuals or groups examine irrational thoughts and behaviors through verbal discussions and written assignments, followed by activities that allow individuals to challenge their faulty beliefs by directly confronting the feared situations and noting that the results are not devastating. Individuals can thus rid themselves of irrational thoughts and self-defeating behaviors and replace them with rational beliefs and healthy behaviors. RET is useful in mild to moderate anxiety, when insight and reasoning can overcome the physiologic symptoms of anxiety; this therapy is useful for high-functioning individuals. *Rational-emotive behavior therapy (REBT)* expands on the original work (see Ellis, 2001, in References).

Deep-breathing exercises Simple, adaptive therapeutic technique for reducing anxiety in individuals with mild to moderate levels of anxiety. Deep-breathing exercises may be used in conjunction with relaxation exercises. The person is instructed as follows:

1. Sit in a quiet place.

2. Breathe slowly and deeply through the nose (may close eyes).

3. Allow the breathing to become natural and set its own pace.

4. Concentrate on the breathing: the air coming in, slowly filling the lungs with oxygen, expanding the chest cavity, and slowly being exhaled.

5. Count silently during inhalations, then exhale.

6. Disregard distracting thoughts or stimuli, and focus back on the slow, rhythmic breathing patterns.

7. Accept whatever thoughts, feelings, or sensations arise, and redirect attention back to the breathing.

Deep-breathing exercises reduce the physiologic effects of anxiety by slowing the heart rate, which positively influences the person's emotional state.

Benson's relaxation response Simple, basic procedure (developed by H. Benson) for eliciting relaxation in persons experiencing tension and mild to moderate levels of anxiety. The person is instructed as follows:

1. Sit in a quiet place in a position of comfort.

2. Close eyes.

3. Relax all muscles as deeply as possible, beginning at the feet and progressing slowly up to the face.

4. Keep all the muscles relaxed.

5. Breathe through the nose with awareness of the breathing.

6. Say the word "one" silently, when breathing out.

7. Breathe easily and naturally, not forcefully.

8. Continue the exercise for 10 to 20 minutes, opening eyes to check time periodically; do not use alarm clock.

9. Sit quietly for several minutes on completion of exercise, first with eyes closed, then with eyes open.

10. Do not stand up for several minutes after exercise.

Do not be concerned about achieving total relaxation. Maintain a passive, matter-of-fact attitude and allow relaxation to occur at its own pace. Try to ignore distracting thoughts or stimuli by not concentrating on them; simply return to repeating "one." Practice relaxation techniques once or twice a day, but not within 2 hours after meals because digestion seems to interfere with the relaxation response.

Progressive relaxation technique Form of relaxation therapy (developed by Jacobson) in which the person alternately tenses and relaxes all voluntary muscle groups progressively from toes to head to elicit a response opposite to that of anxiety.

Visualization (visual imagery, guided imagery) Effective means of deepening relaxation and desensitizing a real-life situation that is generally met with stress and tension (e.g., taking an exam). The individual is instructed to imagine with all the senses a mental picture or image of the feared or troubling situation, based on past memory of the event. The person is then instructed as follows:

1. Relax self in own usual manner.

2. Breathe slowly and deeply several times, concentrating on the feeling of the body as it relaxes.

3. Experience the tension draining from every part of the body, beginning with the feet and working its way upward.

4. Take the time to enjoy the feeling of being totally relaxed (e.g., the warm, tingling sensations).

5. Now, picture self in a favorite place, one that brings peace, joy, or tranquility, and visualize the details. (For example, for an ocean, imagine the waves and foamy whitecaps, smell the sea air, and feel the breeze on your face and the warm sand under your feet.)

Visual imagery combines positive experiences with actual or perceived negative events or situations in an effort to desensitize the trauma of the negative event and/or correct cognitive distortions surrounding the event. It is often combined with relaxation techniques to enhance its effectiveness.

Strategic therapy Part of the *communication theory*, strategic therapy is a unique departure from medical model–based approaches. It is based on the approach of one of its founders, Gregory Bateson, an anthropologist whose position is that behavior makes sense in the context in which it occurs and that behavior is continually being shaped and reinforced by the person's support system (significant others), and vice versa (the *interactive context* of behavior). A strategic therapist always examines the problem behavior in the context of the surrounding behaviors. There are variations of strategic therapy (e.g., solution-focused therapy and brief therapy), and all trace their beginnings to the groundbreaking work of Gregory Bateson, Don Jackson, Paul Watzlawick, John Weakland, and Richard Fisch at the Mental Research Institute in Palo Alto, California, in the 1950s and 1960s. The Palo Alto group attempted to reduce treatment time. They studied the change process and examined problem formulation and maintenance in human systems and how best to promote change in those systems.

Assertiveness training   Component of behavior therapy and a process by which an individual learns to communicate needs, refuse requests, and express both positive and negative feelings in an open, honest, direct, and appropriate manner. Individuals who use assertive responses stand up for their own rights and also respect the rights and dignity of others. A major focus in assertiveness training is the right to choose one's responses in any given situation, which allows the individual to experience control over behavior. Acquisition of power over one's behavior decreases anxiety.

The following is a comparison of assertive, aggressive, and acquiescent behaviors:

Assertive
- Stands up for rights and respects those of others.
- Uses expressive, directive, self-enhancing speech.
- Chooses appropriate words and actions.

Aggressive
- Stands up for rights but abuses those of others.
- Speaks in demeaning or attacking manner.
- Fails to monitor or control words or actions.

Acquiescent
- Does not stand up for own rights.
- Accepts the domination and bullying of others.
- Performs unwanted tasks and feels victimized.

Examples of Assertive Behaviors
1. "I" messages: "I need," "I feel," "I will."
2. Eye contact: looking directly into the eyes of the person while making or refusing a request.
3. Congruent verbal and facial expressions: making certain that the facial expression matches the intent of the spoken message. A serious message accompanied by laughter could negate the credibility of the message.

Example of Assertive Plan for Change
1. Target the behavior that the client wants to change, for example, how to say "no" and mean it.
2. List approximately 10 situations in which it is difficult to say "no," and order them from least to most difficult.
3. Practice saying "no," using the least threatening method first and working up to more challenging situations: imagery, tape recorder, feedback, role playing, and practice in actual situations.
4. Say "no" as the first word in the practice response, since it is a clear message without excuses or apologies.

5. Follow with a clear, concise, declarative statement, such as, "I will not rearrange my schedule. I need my day off."
6. Use eye contact appropriate to the intent of the verbal message.

Assertiveness training is most often done in small group sessions and has been described in detail in a variety of textbooks.

Desensitization   The object of desensitization is to lessen the negative impact of a frightening or troubling object, thought, or event by exposing the individual to the object, thought, or event in a progressive, least to most threatening manner. The following is an example of desensitization in a student with text anxiety:
1. Instruct student to write down all the thoughts surrounding the test-taking event.
2. Request student to isolate the irrational thoughts, for example, "I'm sure to fail"; "All tests are tricky"; "I can never find enough time to study."
3. Inform student that irrational thoughts set up conflicts that result in anxiety.
4. Engage student in a discussion that helps transform irrational thoughts into rational ones.
- "You cannot predict failure; you can choose to study, which will increase your chances for success."
- "All tests are not tricky; why would a teacher put effort into devising trick questions that would result in mass failure?"
- "You have to make time to study. Time is not found, it is structured, and it is time worth spending because it has to do with a career goal."
5. Instruct the student to write down three or four rational thoughts and commit them to memory.
- "I will pass this exam because I will make the time to study for it."
- "I cannot control the content of the exam, but I can control my choice of answers."
- "My career is important to me, and I will make the time to study."
- "Studying will enhance my chances of passing the test."
6. Practice a test-taking scenario with the individual, using the following steps:
   a. Visualize the usual routine on the morning of the exam.
   b. Experience the examination scene in a relaxed state.
   c. Repeat learned rational thoughts to self, in a calm, optimistic manner.
   d. Experience the incidents that generally cause tension (being late, confronting tense classmates), and envision self reacting to them in a calm, accepting manner.
   e. Focus on relaxed feeling state and optimistic thoughts of doing the best to pass the exam.
   f. Continue to envision going in to take the exam.

g. Imagine sitting down and holding onto the pencil, and experience the "feel" of the chair and pencil.

h. Experience relaxation and mental alertness.

i. Practice going through the exam questions, beginning with question number 1, taking time to read the question calmly and respond to it. Look at the distractors, feeling confident that the choice made was the correct one.

j. Concentrate totally on the exam as question number 2 is read. This time, experience the situation of not being able to find the correct answer, even after reviewing the distractors. Mark question number 2 in the margin and calmly proceed to question number 3. After responding to number 3, return to number 2 and answer it. Proceed in this manner, in a relaxed and confident state.

Desensitization is best performed after experiencing the relaxation response (see *Benson's relaxation response*). The scenario may be taped for convenience. Desensitization techniques may be used with clients who are able to tolerate such exercises during times of tension or mild to moderate anxiety. Behavioral therapists use systematic desensitization strategies to help clients with phobic disorders and obsessive-compulsive disorders.

Psychoanalytic therapy Type of therapy (developed by Sigmund Freud and his followers) that focuses on repressed, intrapsychic conflicts that are produced through interactions among three theoretic constructs of the mind: the *id* (storehouse of all unconscious material), the *ego* (problem solver or mediator, which lies mostly in the conscious), and the *superego* (conscience or moral system, which lies in both the conscious and unconscious). Psychoanalysis employs insight-oriented techniques such as free association and dream analysis to explore the meanings behind behaviors. Childhood experiences are discussed in depth because they are believed to be at the root of adult "neuroses." The goal of psychoanalytic therapy is to help the client clarify the psychologic meaning of events, feelings, and behavior and to gain insight into why one behaves or feels a certain way. This type of therapy is a lengthy process that may take as long as 10 years for some individuals.

Gestalt therapy *Gestalt*, which means "the whole," is based on gestalt psychology. The therapist helps the individual become aware of the "total self" and "the world" that surrounds him or her. Gestalt theory (developed by Fritz Perls) explains the "here and now" in that it emphasizes self-expression, self-exploration, and self-awareness in the present. Awareness of feelings is the major focus of therapy, and this awareness renders the individual capable of change, which leads to problem solving and problem resolution. One Gestalt technique is to have the person vent feelings toward an empty chair in which an imagined significant person sits. Gestalt techniques can be applied to individuals and groups and are used with high-functioning persons.

Client-centered therapy Humanistic approach developed by Carl Rogers in which the therapist encourages expression of feelings through reflection and clarification. Some transference and countertransference are allowed in this approach as the therapist demonstrates unconditional acceptance of client and his/her feelings in a nonjudgmental manner. The goals for the individual are (1) acceptance of own feelings, (2) to gain a positive self-regard, and (3) self-acceptance. Inherent in this theory is the belief that growth and change can take place at any time. This type of therapy can be done with individuals or in groups. The group approach is called *Rogerian group therapy*.

Family therapy; family systems therapy Specific mode of intervention for the purpose of establishing open communication and healthy family interactions. Family therapy, based on the *family systems theory*, is built on the premise that the family (whole) is more than the sum of its parts (the individual family members). Family therapy is most often warranted when the member with the presenting symptom (identified client) signals the presence of pain or dysfunction within the whole family. The therapist works to help family members identify and express their thoughts and feelings, define family roles and rules, experiment with more productive styles of relating, and restore strength to the family system.

Group therapy Facilitation of psychotherapy with several clients at the same time in the same session. It may emphasize examination of the interpersonal relationships between group members. Groups may be *homogeneous* (people with similar problems, or of the same sex or age) or *heterogeneous* (people with different problems or of both sexes or various ages). Ten curative factors of group therapy, as described by I.D. Yalom, are (1) imparting of information, (2) instillation of hope, (3) universality, (4) altruism, (5) the corrective recapitulation of the primary family group, (6) development of socializing techniques, (7) imitative behavior, (8) interpersonal learning, (9) group cohesiveness, and (10) catharsis. There are many types of group therapies, and many types of therapies can be accomplished in group situations.

Transactional analysis (TA) Type of therapy (developed by Eric Berne) based on the theory that individuals are capable of responding from three distinct ego states (parent, child, and adult) and that successful interpersonal transactions depend on the use of an appropriate combination of these ego states between the communicators.

- *Parent ego state* incorporates feelings and behaviors that are learned from parents or authority figures and may be nurturing or critical.
- *Child ego state* consists of unrefined, childlike emotions or responses that stem from early developmental

life experiences. It may be adaptive (conforming) or free spirited (nonconforming).

- *Adult ego state* is responsible for objective, mature appraisal of reality and has the problem-solving capacity to process data.

A *complementary transaction* occurs when the transactional stimulus and transactional response originate from identical ego states, that is, parent to parent, child to child, or adult to adult. A *crossed transaction* occurs when the transactional stimulus and transactional response originate from different ego states, such as parent to child, adult to parent, or child to adult. Complementary and crossed transactions may be either successful or unsuccessful, depending on the responses of the individuals and the situation.

A major goal of TA groups is to enable members to communicate from the ego state that is appropriate to the situation and the responses of the individuals, thereby decreasing conflict and promoting mature interpersonal relationships.

Psychodrama Method of group psychotherapy (developed by Jacob Moreno) in which the truth is explored through improvised dramatizations of emotionally charged situations and conflicts. During psychodrama the subject (or client) produces a topic to be explored. The director (or therapist) guides the subject through a series of role-playing scenes related to the topic. The use of *auxiliary egos* (or therapeutic aides) is incorporated in the action and may represent significant people relevant to the subject and the chosen topic. The audience closely relates to the drama that takes place on the stage, and a *catharsis* occurs for the subject and the audience. Psychodrama is not a mainstream therapy and is performed with select, high-functioning groups. Sociodrama and role play are forms of psychodrama.

GRIEF

Grief is a painful experience with lifelong consequences in response to real or perceived loss. It is a personal experience with shared symptoms. Grief is not an illness that needs to be cured. It is a normal response to loss and must be experienced rather than suppressed so that healing can take place.

Grief work is the means by which survivors move through the phases of grief. It is a struggle to avoid despair and a willingness to confront the reality of despair. The grieving person strives to move forward with the business of life while expressing and coping with the deeply painful emotions of grieving. The literature reports a clear link between grief and increased vulnerability to physical and mental dysfunction.

Although grief is most often associated with the death of a loved one or even the loss of a treasured pet, it can also occur as a result of other types of losses.

Grief is not reserved solely for survivors of elderly patients who die from age-related illnesses. Grief can descend on anyone.

Grief also manifests myriad physiologic and psychologic responses.

People Experiencing Grief

- A young mother diagnosed with cancer
- A middle-aged husband who gambled the family savings
- A family whose only child is sent to prison
- A parent whose newborn infant is severely retarded
- An elderly woman caring for her husband who has Alzheimer's disease
- A war veteran struggling to cope with traumatic memories

Physiologic Responses to Grief

- Crying or sobbing
- Sighing respirations
- Shortness of breath, palpitations
- Fatigue, weakness, exhaustion
- Insomnia
- Loss of appetite
- Choking sensation
- Tightness in chest
- Gastrointestinal disturbances

Losses Resulting in Grief

- Loss of a valued job or position
- Loss of a business; financial reverses
- Loss of self-esteem or self-worth
- Loss of family or friends to mental illness
- Loss of a helpful therapist or caregiver
- Loss of a body part or function
- Loss of experience, such as inability to have a child

Psychologic Responses to Grief

- Intense loneliness and sadness
- Anxiety or panic episodes
- Difficulty concentrating and focusing
- Disorientation
- Anger or rage (directed inward or toward others)
- Ambivalence and low self-esteem (may be warning of possible suicidality and need for professional help)

PHASES OF GRIEF

Phase I (1 to 3 Weeks): Shock, Numbness, Denial

Well organized, quiet, polite, immobilized

Flat, isolated affect with intermittent periods of sobbing

Person responds with simple statements.

- "I have to go home soon and feed the dog."
- "I must pick up the clothes from the cleaners."
- "I need to water the plants and prepare dinner."

Lack of connection between the loss and its full meaning

Important Tasks of Mourning: Phase I

Ritual of the funeral ceremony

Planning and preparation for family and friends

Seeking comfort and support from family and friends

Feeding the mourners (an important part of the mourning ritual in many cultures)

Interventions: Phase I

Acknowledge the grief; give permission to vent.

- "This is a bad time for you. It's OK to talk about it, it's OK to cry, and it's OK even to be angry at your loss."

Assure the survivor that she or he won't be alone at this time.

- "I'd like to be with you and stay with you for a while."
- "Kay and Sam want to spend time with you, too."
- "We'll all make sure someone is with you every day."

Be calm, warm, and caring; accept his or her anguish even if it is difficult.

Offer to help with family tasks: kids, meals, phone calls.

Involve person in brief familiar tasks.

Engage chaplain or person's clergy as needed or requested.

There is a higher than normal death rate in survivors during the first year of loss. Survivors won't ask for help; they need stimulation, involvement, and company.

Phase II (3 Weeks to 4 Months): Yearning and Protest, Anger, Confrontation

Intensity of grief heightens.

Person experiences full impact of distress and has no peace.

Headaches and restlessness or agitation may occur.

Person bargains with God or fates: "If only I had another chance" (may also be part of Phase I).

Person expresses feelings of "going crazy" or "losing mind."

Somatic complaints (cannot eat/sleep) are common.

Person is preoccupied with the dead.

Person is unable to concentrate or focus on work or school.

Anger expressed over the loss: "Why did this have to happen?"

Self-pity expressed: "Why did this happen to me?"

Regret expressed: "I should have been a better sister."

Person searches for the deceased and revisits places often visited by deceased.

Interventions: Phase II

Be direct: "How are you sleeping?"

Focus on person's feelings; show acceptance.

Determine person's ability to function, eat, and perform activities of daily living.

Assess person's ambivalence; suicide ideation.

Establish your availability.

Make appointments to visit person on a regular basis.

- "I'll be visiting you every day just to talk or listen or have a meal with you."
- "I'll phone you regularly; so will Jim or Alice."

Phase III (4 to 14 Months): Apathy, Aimlessness, Disorganization, Despair

Difficulty "getting back into the swing of things."

Preoccupation, dreams, or hallucinations may prevail.

Normal

Survivor perceives the deceased person as dead (reinforcing reality and finality of death).

Smells perfume or shaving lotion of deceased.

Discusses deceased as being *both good and bad.*

Talks about *good and bad times* together.

Laughs about the good times shared.

Sleeps and eats better.

Displays more energy and interest in usual activities.

Dysfunctional

Survivor sees or hears the deceased person as still living; unable to "let go."

Experiences scary, vivid, threatening hallucinations.

Idealizes deceased as perfect, not deserving to die.

Has sleep disturbances with nightmares about deceased.

Suggests he or she should have died instead of deceased.

Expresses desire to join deceased because "life is not worth living" (suicidal ideation).

Demonstrates significant weight loss (6 to 10 lb).

States has no energy or interest in usual activities.

Exhibits symptoms of depression (*DSM-IV-TR* criteria).

Nearly two thirds of persons in a major study continue to experience Phase III a year after the death or other loss.

Phase IV (14 Months Throughout Rest of Life): Recovery, Resolution, Acceptance

Survivor is slowly but surely becoming more involved in life.

Reorganization of life evolves out of the chaos of grief

- Camping trip is planned with the kids.
- Previous habits resume, such as little irritations, glimpses of previous sense of humor.

Affect still reverts to sadness with talk of the deceased person, but there are moments of tenderness as well.

Energy is more plentiful and directed toward life.

Scents of deceased are gone; survivor may wish for them back on occasion.

Life seems tolerable, although it may never reach the heights of joy before the loss.

There may still be bouts of immense sadness and even panic, but they will go away.

Dreams are more pleasant and may occasionally include deceased, but there are no more dreams of seeing deceased as dead or threatening.

Memories are warm, with intellectual integration of the loss.

Reestablishment of the survivor's previous life is evident.

Interventions: Phase IV

Contact the survivor, especially at key times.

Share memories of the deceased.

Acknowledge the long, painful process of grieving.

Continue to assess for signs of hidden depression or suicidality.

Assess for ambivalence, low self-esteem, or internalized rage.
- "Life is not worth living."
- "My wife was so good; I'm so bad."

ANTICIPATORY GRIEF: PREMOURNING, PREDEATH

Anticipatory grief is associated with the anticipation of a predicted death or loss. Examples include grieving for persons with a long-term or life-threatening illness and grieving for elderly relatives whose life functions are deteriorating.

Positive aspects of anticipatory grief include the opportunity to resolve relationships, to prepare survivors for the loss, and to work on spiritual reconciliation.

Negative aspects of anticipatory grief include increased stress on caregivers, resentment and anger caused by ambivalent relationship, hopelessness or powerlessness, and depression.

Interventions in Anticipatory Grief

Allow caregivers time to come to terms with the inevitable loss.

Offer empathy and information about the illness when the client is ready.

Identify sources of support, such as grief groups.

Be available to listen and assess signs of depression.

The anguish that caregivers feel during anticipatory grief does not substitute for postdeath grief.

CHRONIC SORROW

Chronic sorrow is a form of grief that is a response to ongoing loss, such as chronic mental or physical illness. It includes characteristics of other types of grief as well.

Interventions in Chronic Sorrow

Acknowledge the demands of the illness on caregivers.

Recognize caregiver behavior patterns as ongoing grief responses.

Assess the phases of grief and intervene accordingly.

Discuss the diagnosis and expected outcomes with the family and caregiver.

Dispel the myth that it is the family's fault (to avoid blame and guilt).

Promote adaptive coping skills among family members.

Enhance communication among the family, caregiver, and client (to prevent burnout, exhaustion, depression).

Help family and caregiver develop realistic expectations (to avoid despair and promote hope).

SUMMARY OF THEORIES OF GRIEF

Lindemann

Grief is manifested by predictable psychologic and somatic symptomatology. *Acute mourning* (feeling or expressing grief or sorrow) is characterized by somatic distress, preoccupation with the deceased person's image, guilt, hostile reactions, and loss of patterns of conduct. *Dysfunctional* or "morbid" grief reactions are distortions of some aspect of "normal grief." The duration of grief and the development of dysfunctional grief depend on the success of grief work.

Kübler-Ross

Elisabeth Kübler-Ross's stages of dying (denial, anger, bargaining, depression, and acceptance) are often applied to grief (Table C-1 on p. 354). The initial response to loss may include denial, anger, and bargaining. *Denial* is characterized by refusal to accept loss. *Anger* may initially be directed at health care staff and later at the person who died. *Bargaining* and denial are often mixed in a futile attempt to reverse reality. *Depression* tends to be the longest phase and, in dysfunctional grief, may become chronic and meet criteria for major depression. Acceptance of the loss is a gradual process that includes aspects of previous stages. Grieving individuals may not reach acceptance.

Bowlby

Grief and loss are characterized first by *numbness*, during which the loss is recognized but not necessarily felt as real. Numbness is followed by *yearning and searching*, in which the individual yearns for the loved one and protests the loss. In the third phase, *disorganization and despair*, the loss is real, and intense emotional pain and cognitive disorganization occur. *Reorganization*, the final phase, is characterized by a gradual adjustment to life without the deceased person.

Engel

The initial response to loss is shock and disbelief. Awareness and meaning of the loss develop during the first year of mourning. Eventually the relationship is resolved and put into perspective (Table C-2 on p. 355).

Shneidman

Conceptualizing less structure and fewer stages than other theorists of grief, Shneidman views the expression of grief as dependent primarily on an individual's personality or

Table C-1	Kübler-Ross's Stages of Grieving	
Stage	**Behavioral Responses**	**Nursing Implications**
Denial	Person refuses to believe that loss is happening. With death or trauma, may actually block the memory of the incident or momentarily believe it has not occurred. Is unprepared to deal with practical problems, such as prosthesis after loss of leg. May assume artificial cheerfulness to prolong denial.	Verbally support client's denial for its protective function. Examine own behavior to ensure not sharing in client's denial.
Anger	Client or family may direct anger at nurse or hospital staff about matters that normally would not bother them. There may be an acute sense of unfairness, fear, anger, and even rage. Questions may arise, such as "Why me?" or "How could you die and leave me alone?"	Help client understand that anger is a normal response to feelings of loss and powerlessness. Avoid withdrawal or retaliation with anger; do not take anger personally. Deal with needs underlying any angry reaction. Provide structure and continuity to promote feelings of security. Allow client as much control as possible over life.
Bargaining	Person seeks to bargain to avoid loss. The bargain may be struck with God, the deceased, or oneself. May express feelings of guilt or fear of punishment for past sins, real or imagined.	Listen attentively, and encourage client to talk to relieve guilt and irrational fears. If appropriate, offer spiritual support.
Depression	Person grieves over what has happened and what cannot be. May talk freely (e.g., reviewing past losses such as money or job) or may withdraw. Acknowledges feelings, allows nurturing by self or others, and moves forward in the process.	Allow client to express sadness. Communicate nonverbally by sitting quietly without expecting conversation. Convey caring by touch. Help support persons understand importance of being with client in silence.
Acceptance	Person comes to terms with loss. Depression has been lifted; loss is acknowledged. May have decreased interest in surroundings and support persons as loss is no longer focal point. May wish to begin making plans (living will, prosthesis, altered living arrangements). Is now free to move forward.	Help family and friends understand client's decreased need to socialize and need for short, quiet visits. Encourage client to participate as much as possible in the treatment program.

style of living. An individual who goes through life feeling depressed and guilty is likely to grieve similarly. A person who avoids emotional investments with others also tends to try to avoid grief.

Theory Synthesis

Grief tends to occur in several phases. The initial response to loss may be shock, numbness, denial, or other attempts to defend against the reality and pain of loss. This initial phase is followed by painful psychologic and physical *disequilibrium*, which in the case of dysfunctional grief, may last indefinitely. The third phase of resolution or *recovery* is a gradual process in which the good days begin to outnumber the bad. Ultimately, although not forgotten, the rela-

tionship with the deceased is resolved and put into perspective.

TIPS FOR HELPING SURVIVORS

1. Listen; say little.
2. Avoid clichés such as, "Everything will be fine," or "I know how you must feel."
3. Be there for the long term, not just for the funeral or memorial service.
4. Include the survivors in the first holiday after the loss.
5. Remember the anniversary of the death in a special way (a call, card, flower).
6. Love the survivors and accept them.

Table C-2	**Engel's Stages of Grieving**
Stage	**Behavioral Responses**
Shock and disbelief	Refusal to accept loss Stunned feelings Intellectual acceptance but emotional denial
Developing awareness	Reality of loss begins to penetrate consciousness Anger may be directed at hospital/nurses Crying and self-blame
Restitution	Rituals of mourning (funeral)
Resolving the loss	Attempts to deal with painful void Still unable to accept new love object to replace lost person May accept more dependent relationship with support person Thinks over and talks about memories of the dead person
Idealization	Produces images of dead person that are almost devoid of undesirable features Represses all negative and hostile feelings toward deceased May feel guilty and remorseful about past inconsiderate or unkind acts to deceased Unconsciously internalizes admired qualities of deceased Reminders of deceased evoke fewer feelings of sadness Reinvests feelings in others
Outcome	Behavior influenced by several factors, such as importance of lost object as source of support, degree of dependence on relationship, degree of ambivalence toward deceased, number and nature of other relationships, and number and nature of previous grief experiences (which tend to be cumulative)

Spirituality as a Dimension of the Person

People are composed of multidimensional facets that include physical, cognitive, affective, relational, and spiritual. To ignore any of these components eliminates a critical part of a person's humanness, with significant consequences to the total life experience.

Although everyone has a spiritual dimension, spirituality is expressed in many ways, both formally and informally. Spirituality is an integral part of the person's identity. It is a critical thread that connects people together, binds cultures, and gives meaning to nature and the universe. Through the spiritual dimension, a person can make sense of powerful life experiences that might otherwise be confusing or devastating, and the person can use them in life-sustaining ways. Spirituality addresses some of the core images and beliefs a person holds regarding humanity, the divine, and the relationship between them.

▌ DESCRIPTIONS OF TERMS

Spirituality

- The search for the sacred and the holy
- The need to experience the divine or higher power
- The desire to find meaning in the universe that transcends a physical or finite existence

Spirituality may be expressed through (but is not limited to) religion and religious rituals. It may also be expressed in music, art, poetry, dance, and storytelling.

Religion

- A formal, organized system that uses a set of rituals, practices, and ceremonies through which a specific community can express spiritual beliefs
- A less formal, less organized system that enables a more diverse community to express individualized spiritual beliefs and practices

Religious expression may also include music, art, literature, and dance, as well as religious rituals, practices, and ceremonies, or regular participation in a congregation with a specific understanding of religious history and future.

Major Types of Formal Religions

- Christianity
- Buddhism
- Taoism
- Judaism
- Islam

New Age religions (or *spirituality*) refer to a collection of individual practices that are largely unconnected to formal communities but still offer meaning and enlightenment to some individuals.

Faith

- The ability to draw on spiritual resources without physical or empiric proof
- An internal certainty that comes from one's own experiences with the divine

Goals of Spirituality

- Provide an image of the divine.
- Provide an image of humanity.
- Provide understanding of the relationship between the divine and humanity.
- Examine thoughts of divine punishment, reward, or neutrality.
- Give belief and meaning to life.
- Give a sense of duty, vocation, calling, or moral obligation.
- Examine one's experience of the divine and sacred.
- Cope with situations that conflict with spiritual understanding.
- Provide spiritual rituals and practices.
- Provide a community of faith.
- Provide authority and guidance for a system of belief, meaning, and ritual.

Faith, although only a part of spirituality, is an essential component. Through faith, a deep, individual spirituality can be mobilized to assist in the challenges and celebrations of life.

SPIRITUALITY IN MENTAL HEALTH

In the treatment of mental disorders, it is imperative to address the spiritual dimension of a person. For many individuals with mental disorders, spirituality offers a powerful sense of hope in the face of devastating, chronic illness.

For those who experience rejection by family and friends because of the impact of the diagnosis on their relationships, spirituality can help maintain a sense of connection and belonging. A healthy spirituality can provide a sense of love and acceptance in the face of loneliness and abandonment. Spirituality can also evoke a sense of peace and calm in individuals whose illnesses create feelings of internal chaos and confusion.

The spiritual images and beliefs that can be healing and sustaining for some individuals may seem punitive and threatening to others because of the nature of their mental disorder. These people may be troubled and tormented by a distorted or negative view of religion and spirituality as a result of severe anxiety, irrational guilt, deep depression, or psychosis.

Some individuals who experience mental illness may become hyperreligious and preoccupied with religious rituals and practice. They may spend inordinate amounts of time praying, chanting, or reading religious doctrine. Others may believe that they are so evil they deserve to be punished by God or the devil and may even require suicide precautions. Left unattended, these individuals may harm themselves or, at the very least, be unable to comply with treatment, which could delay the therapeutic healing process.

ROLE OF THE CHAPLAIN IN MENTAL HEALTH

As a result of the obvious need for spiritual guidance, the chaplain role is becoming more common in the mental health arena. These ministers of spirituality are generally multidenominational, which allows them to address the spiritual needs of many individuals who request or require their services. Chaplains who work in the mental health setting recognize the boundaries between the need for spiritual guidance and the mental disorder, which may provoke a negative view of religion or an unhealthy preoccupation. They collaborate closely with the psychiatric staff as a critical part of the therapeutic team. They may be involved in patient groups, provide individual counseling, facilitate in-services, or offer nondenominational spiritual services for those patients who are interested.

STAGES OF FAITH IN SPIRITUAL PRACTICE AND INTERVENTIONS

Impartial Individual

Religiously impartial persons (30% of the population) generally are not involved or minimally involved in faith communities and have only a casual acquaintance with faith community practices. They tend to do only things that interest them.

Interventions. Appropriate interventions are well-known scripture, hymns, psalms, or readings such as Psalm 23, the poem "Footprints," the Serenity Prayer, the Lord's Prayer, "Amazing Grace," and "Beautiful Savior." Alcoholics Anonymous, Narcotics Anonymous, and other materials may also be helpful.

Institutional Individual

Regular church attendees (40% of the population) who adhere to institutional rules largely adopt a "good person/bad person" concept in their view of spirituality.

Interventions. Include the previous interventions, as well as visits from the minister and members of the local spiritual community. Normal use of prayer, anointing, and laying on of hands is also acceptable. Prayer books and music specific to the denomination, congregation, or faith are also appropriate.

Individual Seeker

Some people (20% of the population) challenge the formal religious community and many of their beliefs and tenets. They seek new or personal answers to questions, problems, or crises. On the surface, they seem to be impartial in regard to faith.

Interventions. Individualized, creative, and varied approaches may encompass historic elements from Eastern and Western spiritual traditions, including meditation, healing touch, devotional readings, communal prayer, and a variety of music. The individual is the best guide in selecting the spiritual resources at this stage.

Integrated Individuals

Faith is internalized for religiously integrated persons, who accept and obey the rules of religion and spirituality (10% of the population). They may not belong to formal faith communities and can often be seen as teachers or mystics.

Interventions. Many of the traditional rituals, rites, and expressions of formal spirituality noted for the institutional individual are appropriate, but with an increased internal meaning. The integrated individual may have the need to leave a spiritual legacy.

SUMMARY OF SPIRITUALITY

Spirituality helps individuals cope with major common issues such as fear, death, and other losses by providing a sense of hope and meaning to experiences that would otherwise be devastating. Having a spiritual understanding that one's connection with the universe is more than physical may help to ease the fear and pain of loss. Feeling connected to the divine eases loneliness, grief, abandonment, and alienation and offers a feeling of unconditional acceptance for one's unique place in life. Spirituality allows people to make sense of the mystery of life and death and of other phenomena that are not within human control. It offers the hope and strength to celebrate life, while consciously acknowledging the reality of illness and tragedy.

Spirituality is a key component of the human experience that can ease the pain of mental and physical illness, enhance treatment, and facilitate the healing process.

Crisis and Crisis Intervention

Crisis has been defined in many ways, but regardless of the definition, it can be viewed as a turning point. From a psychiatric–mental health nursing view, *crisis* can be defined as "a state of psychologic disequilibrium that results from an individual's inability to problem-solve a situation or event (real or perceived) that involves change, loss, or threat (psychologic, biologic, social, cultural, spiritual)." Inherent in a state of crisis is the individual's failure to resolve the problem after using previously learned coping strategies and techniques and/or automatic defense mechanisms (denial, repression, suppression).

As a further result of the crisis state, the person's behavior, affect, and cognitive ability are disrupted. Symptoms include anxiety, powerlessness, helplessness, depression, and varying degrees of mental, emotional, and behavioral disorganization and acting out.

TYPES OF CRISIS

Developmental Crisis

Sometimes referred to as *maturational* or *internal* types of crisis, developmental crises represent events that are built into normal periods of human growth and development, as follows:

- Birth of a normal baby
- Graduation from school
- Marriage
- Timely death of an elderly parent

These events can usually be anticipated. Crisis can occur around the events if a person is unprepared for the amount of change that is required to complete role responsibilities associated with the event or situation or if the person perceives that the event represents a major loss. Symptoms, as described previously, may result.

Situational Crisis

Situational crises are usually unanticipated events in the process of everyday life and have external rather than internal sources. The unexpected events usually require immediate change and response, and often the person is unable to negotiate the event, resulting in crisis and include the following:

- Divorce
- Job change
- Rape, robbery, other victimization
- Death of loved one by accident

INFLUENCING FACTORS

The resolution of a crisis may be affected by the following factors:

- Individual's perception of the event
- Past experience with similar events
- Capacity to accept the need to change
- Motivation to change
- Cognitive abilities
- Control of mood or affect
- Coping style
- Personality traits
- External support system (availability, genuine concern)
- Person's ability to engage support systems

CRISIS INTERVENTION

Crisis intervention is an effective, short-term therapy that focuses only on immediate problems to be resolved. The primary goal of intervention is to return the individual to either the precrisis level of function or, ideally, to a higher level of function because of new skills that were learned in the process of resolving the crisis.

Therapist's Role

The therapist must remember that crisis has a dual nature. It is, according to ancient Chinese teachings, both a time of danger and threat and a time of opportunity. This belief holds today. Because a person in crisis cannot solve the problem by previously known and used methods, at this vulnerable time she or he is open to suggestions and willing to learn new skills that provide an opportunity for growth and change.

A crisis counselor is an active participant rather than a passive listener during the crisis intervention process. Working through a step-by-step methodology, the client is assisted out of the seeming maze. Although crisis will resolve without intervention, the result of an unsuccessful resolution can be diminished levels of function and possible disorder in the form of mental, emotional, physical, spiritual, or social disruption. The client usually benefits from a caring and educated guide.

Active Intervention Process

1. Stay focused in the present. Do not allow digressions or unrelated material to interfere. For example, redirect the client who discusses past problems that are not directly related. (Client may need additional therapy for other problems later.)
2. Discuss the client's positive actions and strengths during the crisis. For example, reinforce all positive attempts the client made to resolve the problem. A strength always to reinforce is that the client sought help.
3. Direct the client when necessary. For example, a disorganized client has taken alcohol to alter mood before the therapy session and is preparing to drive home. The nurse tells the client to call a family member for a ride home to avoid accident or arrest.
4. Allow and encourage client to express feelings for relief.
5. Encourage client to express thoughts. While verbalizing, the client will begin to formalize thoughts. Guide the client in the problem-solving process. (Use nursing process.)
6. Help the client name techniques that were tried and discuss new options and alternative approaches for solving the problem.
   - "What else could you have done instead?"
   - "Did you try . . . ?"
   - "Some people have done . . . in similar situations. Is that something you could do?"
   - "What has worked in the past for some people is . . . ."
7. Assist the client to identify and connect with support people and agencies.

Although crisis intervention is traditionally completed within 6 weeks, clinicians today are sometimes pressured by managed care organizations to complete the process in a much briefer time frame. If necessary, clients who have other psychiatric problems are referred to subsequent therapies after the brief crisis therapy has ended. Before crisis therapy with a client ends, the therapist does the following:

- *Summarize:* Review, with client participation, the components of the client's crisis. Summarize all action taken and action proposed by the client in the near future. Review learned skills.
- *Anticipatory planning:* Evaluate the client's understanding of the process and content of this crisis and his or her readiness and ability to manage future similar events.
- *Praise:* Genuinely praise the client's efforts to engage in resolution of this crisis, and offer hope without giving any false reassurance.

Guidelines for Seclusion and Restraint Based on JCAHO Standards

Rationale: To prevent injury or death to aggressive clients, other clients, and staff and to prevent the destruction of property and the environment. Knowledge of the client's history of violence and awareness of behaviors that indicate risk for violence are critical factors in the prevention of violence.

NURSING ASSESSMENT

Client demonstrates behaviors that are aggressive or potentially destructive to self or others. Behaviors may be subtle or obvious, verbal or nonverbal.
Examples of verbal behaviors:
- Shouting obscenities
- Threats to self or others

Examples of nonverbal behaviors:
Sudden changes in behavior, such as a client who has been reasonably calm suddenly becoming agitated or a client who has been reasonably active suddenly becoming quiet or withdrawn; psychomotor agitation that increases in intensity; clenched fists; hand-to-fist pounding; angry, wild-eyed facial expression; clenched jaw; pacing back and forth in an agitated manner; bumping carelessly into walls, furniture, or people in the environment.

Plan of Action and Rationale

Immediately inform key staff of client's aggressive behavior *to prevent harm or injury to client, other clients, and staff.* (Never leave an aggressive client unattended or attempt to control a potentially dangerous client without qualified help.)

Plan to approach the client on a continuum, using the least restrictive to most restrictive measures as a model for intervention.

Model for Intervention

Verbalize methods to help client maintain control and dignity.
Medicate client as necessary.
Seclude.
Restrain.

Interventions and Rationale

Intervene as soon as the client begins to act in an aggressive manner, and attempt to identify sources leading to aggressive behavior, if possible, *to resolve volatile issues and prevent escalation of behaviors.*

Verbal Interaction

Approach client in a clam, direct, nonchallenging manner *to assure client that staff is in control in increase client's control and trust in staff.*

Offer client the opportunity to control self, indicating that if this is not possible, staff will assist in helping to control client until he or she can regain control, *to ensure security and safety of client and others in the environment.*

Inform clients that his or her concerns will be addressed as soon as the client regains control *to reinforce staff's expectations that client will regain control and to promote trust.*

If client calms down at any time during the verbal interaction, quietly accompany client to an area of decreased stimulation *to decrease anxiety and exert least restrictive measures whenever possible.*

If client's behavior fails to respond to verbal intervention, prescribed medication may be required *to continue to use least restrictive measure.*

INTERVENTIONS AND RATIONALE IN THE USE OF SECLUSION POLICY

On determining the necessity for the use of a seclusion room, obtain the physician's written order or, in an emergency, obtain the written order from the charge nurse and secure the order from the attending physician within a reasonable period of time. (All orders for the use of a seclusion room must comply with individual state laws.)

The charge nurse documents the justification for use of the seclusion room, which includes the following:
- Events leading up to the need for seclusion
- Other interventions used prior to seclusion

- Purpose for the use of seclusion
- Clinical justification for length of seclusion time

Procedure

Explain procedure and purpose of the seclusion to client before placement in the seclusion room *to inform and support the client and reduce anxiety.*

Escort the client into the seclusion room in a calm, direct manner that does not cause discomfort, harm, or pain *to ensure the client's safety and preserve his or her dignity.* (The charge nurse should be present to observe this procedure.)

Check the client every 15 minutes with qualified staff person *to ensure safety and provide support, reassurance, and opportunities for the client to vent feelings.*

Supervise the client's nutrition, hygiene, grooming, and elimination needs *to ensure the client's comfort and safety.* (Bathroom privileges should be offered at least every 2 hours.)

Clear the seclusion room of all articles or utensils that the client might use to harm self or others *to ensure safety of client and others.* (Food should be served in plastic dishes.)

Regulate number of people who enter the seclusion room *to reduce stimulation and provide consistent, therapeutic relationships.* (Only the physician, nurses, and primary therapist should have access to the seclusion room.)

Ensure safe exit of client in case of emergency (fire, disaster) *to ensure client's safety.* (The seclusion room door should open automatically when the alarm is sounded.)

Provide Continual Documentation

Nursing documentation includes the following:

- Factors, events, and client behaviors prior to seclusion
- Other interventions used prior to seclusion
- Time the physician and/or charge nurse was notified and the time client was seen for purpose of seclusion order
- Name of nurse who accompanied client to seclusion room
- Name of staff person who supervised and checked client
- Client's response to seclusion room
- Time that client is removed from seclusion room

Notify physician, medical directory, and all appropriate administrative personnel *to inform key people of the client's status.*

Approach the client and offer him or her the opportunity to talk *to allow ventilation of feelings about seclusion.*

▌ RESTRAINT

Rationale: To provide temporary external controls for clients who cannot provide their own internal controls in the unit or in the seclusion room and whose behavior may result in injury to the client or others. Restraints are applied only after less restrictive measures have failed.

Policy

Obtain a physician's written order or, in an emergency situation, a registered nurse's order after he or she has observed and assessed client *to provide adequate justification for use of (leather) restraints and comply with state laws.*

Documentation (Mandatory for Restraint Order)

Events leading up to restraint
Rationale for the use of restraint
Length of time client is to be restrained
Justification for length of time

Notification of attending physician and others in accordance with state mental health laws *to ensure adequate documentation of restraint order, provide ongoing communication, and comply with laws that protect client's rights.*

Procedure (Supervised by Qualified Charge Nurse)

Provide an adequate number of trained staff members *to prevent injury to clients and staff.*

Use a minimum amount of restraints *to ensure client's safety with the least amount of control.*

Explain to client briefly and simply the reason for use of restraints *to assure client that staff is in control.*

Set up restraints on bed in seclusion room (should be done in advance, although restrains are never left unattended) *to ensure organized application of restraints and promote safety.*

Apply (leather) restraints to all four extremities in a manner that will control client but will not cause undue physical or emotional discomfort *to control client, prevent injury to client or staff, and maintain client's dignity as much as possible.*

Inform client as simply as possible, in a manner-of-fact way, what is happening and why *to facilitate client's understanding without offering own biases and interpretation:*

"You are being restrained so you will have time to control your behavior."

"We're concerned that your behavior will harm you or others."

Refrain from unnecessary authoritative or condescending remarks *to prevent undue anger or shame.*
Examples of nontherapeutic statements:
"We warned you that this would happen."
"This is for your own good."

Check the client every 15 minutes with a qualified staff person *to prevent isolation and assure client of staff concerns.*

Provide relief from restraints at least every 2 hours *to promote comfort and maintain muscle tone.*

Examples:
- Allow client to perform active range-of-motion exercises (if safe to remove restraints).

or

- Provide passive range-of-motion exercises on each extremity every 2 hours (if unsafe to remove restraints).

Offer circulation and skin condition as often as necessary *to maintain circulatory function and prevent skin breakdown.*

Offer fluids and nutrition *to maintain dietary and hydration needs.*

Document the following by registered nurse:
- Events leading up to need for restraint
- Least restrictive measures attempted (including medication) before restraint
- Response of client to least restrictive measures
- Statement that registered nurse was present when client was placed in restraints
- Specific individual who ordered use of restraints
- Whether the client was examined before being placed in restraints

- Exact time restraints were applied
- Exact time client was removed from restraints for relief periods
- Summary of client's response to restraints and relief periods
- Exact time client was removed from restraints and client's behavior at that time.

Postrestraint Procedures

Notify those individuals required by law *to comply with state laws.*

Notify attending physician *to inform physician and plan subsequent care.*

Release client from restraints immediately in case of fire or other disaster *to ensure client's safety.*

Approach client and provide opportunity to talk (registered nurse). *Clients who have just been released from restraints may need to discuss their thoughts and feelings.*

Discuss procedure and feelings about procedure with staff members involved in restraint of the clients *to clarify own and other's perceptions and vent feelings among trusted colleagues.*

Glossary

abuse Maladaptive pattern of substance use leading to problems in psychosocial, biologic, cognitive, perceptual, and spiritual/belief dimensions of life.

acquired immunodeficiency syndrome (AIDS) The syndrome of opportunistic infections that occur as the final stage of infection by the human immunodeficiency virus (HIV).

acting out Reaction of the client's life experiences, relationships with significant others, and resultant unresolved conflicts; may include but not limited to destructive actions.

active listening Communication skill in which the nurse or therapist illustrates active versus passive listening responses toward the client; incorporates such behaviors as appropriate eye contact, general leads ("I hear you," "please go on," "uh-huh"), and occasional nodding of the head; demonstrates respect, interest, and caring toward the client. Techniques should be used with discretion rather than in a continuous, exaggerated manner.

addiction Cluster of cognitive, behavioral, and physiologic symptoms characterized by physical dependence, tolerance, and psychologic dependence on a drug or substance. The addicted person is emotionally dependent on the drug or substance, is able to obtain a desired effect from a specific dosage, and experiences withdrawal symptoms when he or she ceases to take the drug or substance. The person is generally in a state of chronic or recurrent intoxication. *substance dependence.*

affect Emotional range attached to ideas, outwardly manifested.

Appropriate affect Emotional tone in harmony with the accompanying idea, thought, or verbalization.

Blunted affect Disturbance manifested by a severe reduction in the intensity of affect.

Flat affect Absence or near absence of any signs of affective expression.

Inappropriate affect Incongruence between the emotional feeling tone and the idea, thought, or speech accompanying it.

Labile affect Rapid changes in emotional feeling tone, unrelated to external stimuli.

AIDS-dementia complex Severe mental changes (dementia) that may be associated with AIDS.

akathisia One of the classes of nontherapeutic effects caused by neuroleptic drugs; thought to be a result of the blockade effect of these drugs on the neurotransmitter dopamine. Signs include motor restlessness, subjective sense of anxiety, and inability to lie down or sit still; classified as an extrapyramidal symptom.

akinesia Delay or slowness in beginning and carrying through voluntary motor movements and sudden or unexpected stops in motion; extrapyramidal symptom often seen in clients with Parkinson's disease.

akinesthesia Inability to sense movement.

alcoholism Chronic disorder characterized by dependence on alcohol, repeated excessive use of alcoholic beverages, development of withdrawal symptoms on reducing or ceasing alcohol intake, morbidity that may include cirrhosis of the liver, and decreased ability to function socially and vocationally; now believed to be a disease with strong genetic links.

alienation Inability to identify with family, peer group, society, or culture; often associated with schizophrenia.

ambivalence Coexistence of two opposing feelings, impulses, or attitudes directed toward the same person, object, or situation at the same time.

anhedonia Inability to experience pleasure; in major depression, noted as loss of pleasure in activities or experiences that the client deemed as pleasurable or enjoyable before the onset of the depressed episode.

anorexia nervosa Eating disorder primarily affecting adolescent girls and young adult women and characterized by a pathologic fear of becoming fat, a distorted body image, excessive dieting, and emaciation. No loss of appetite occurs until late stages.

anticholinergic effects Nontherapeutic effects in specific areas of the autonomic nervous system caused by the use of neuroleptic medications. Symptoms may include dry mouth, constipation, blurred vision, dry mucous membranes, and urinary retention. Effects may be temporary and relieved by adjustment of prescribed medication.

anxiety Nonspecific, unpleasant feeling of apprehension, discomfort, and, in some cases, dread and impending doom manifested physically by motor tension, autonomic hyperactivity, or hyperattentiveness. Symptoms prompt the person to seek relief. Anxiety can be communicated interpersonally.

apathy Lack of interest and blunting of affect in conditions that would normally stimulate interest or elicit feeling or emotion.

appearance State, condition, manner, or style in which a person or object manifests itself outwardly. In the context of conducting a mental health assessment, the client's appearance involves hygiene, grooming, posture, and general behavior; may include cosmetics.

assaultive behavior Act of being physically aggressive toward another person; a violent attack on another individual that may lead to harm or injury (may be an attempt to do violence with or without battery).

autistic Referring to private, individual thoughts, ideas, and affects derived from internal drives, wishes, and hopes; most often seen in persons diagnosed with schizophrenia who, in the course of their disorder, may experience a private reality rather than the shared reality of the external world.

automatic thoughts In cognitive therapy theory, thoughts that are unwilled, spontaneous, irrational, and self-deprecating. Cognitive therapy techniques help the individual replace automatic thoughts with rational beliefs based on exercises that challenge their validity.

behavior Any observable, recordable, and measurable move, response, or verbal or nonverbal act demonstrated by an individual.

behavior contract Agreement between the client and staff that clearly delineates expected client behaviors and outcomes.

behavior modification Method of treatment, deconditioning, or reeducation based on the principles of Ivan Pavlov and developed further by B. F. Skinner, the goal of which is to change an individual's behavior patterns and responses through techniques that manipulate stimuli.

behavior therapy Treatment that focuses on modifying observable behavior by manipulating the environment or the behavior; focuses on the effects rather than the cause; derived from pavlovian conditioning and useful in the treatment of phobic and obsessive-compulsive disorders; *systematic desensitization* is an example.

bioenergetics Strategies for reducing muscle tension by releasing feelings through physical exercises and verbal techniques.

biofeedback Therapeutic technique used to gain conscious control over unconscious body functions, such as blood pressure and heart rate, to achieve relaxation or relief of stress-related physical symptoms. Self-monitoring equipment is used to measure body functions.

bizarre delusion Fixed belief held by the individual that involves a phenomenon that the individual's culture would regard as totally implausible, such as being controlled by a dead person.

blackouts *Anterograde amnesia*, most often experienced by alcoholics and those with an organic brain syndrome; may result from dehydration of brain tissue. The individual retains consciousness with the memory loss.

blocking or thought deprivation Sudden pause in the train or stream of one's thoughts, most likely caused by unconscious emotional conflicts; noted in persons with schizophrenia.

body image Individual's concept of the size, shape, and physical mass of his or her body and its parts; internalized perception of the physical appearance.

chronic mentally ill Population whose persistent dysfunctional behavior may be attributed to a psychiatric disorder, regardless of specific diagnosis or living situation.

circumstantiality Interruption in the stream of thought caused by excessive associations of an idea reaching the conscious level; characterized by extraneous thinking in which the individual digresses into unnecessary details and inappropriate thoughts before communicating a central idea; may serve to avoid an emotionally charged area.

clanging Speech pattern in which sounds govern the choice of words, as in rhyming or punning. Words often simulate a "clanging" tone; noted most often in persons with schizophrenia, mania, or autism.

clinical specialist in psychiatric nursing Graduate of a master's program that provides specialization in the clinical area of psychiatric–mental health nursing and that qualifies graduates to obtain certification (by examination) by the American Nurses' Association and by some states.

codependence Behaviors that characterize an individual's reliance on the impaired behavior of a spouse or partner as a way to meet own needs for survival, security, and control. A common example is a person's codependence on the partner's alcoholism or drug abuse. Codependence can result in enabling, in which the partner engages in behaviors that perpetuate the affected person's impairment.

cognition Pertaining to the mental processes that include knowing, thinking, learning, judging, and problem solving.

concrete communication Literal interpretation of meanings; inability to think or communicate in an abstract or conceptual manner; may be a sign of departure from reality or preoccupation with a delusion.

confabulation Fabrication of facts or events in response to questions regarding situations that are not recalled by the individual because of memory impairment; most notable in organic mental disorder, in which the person attempts to fill in the memory gaps with unrelated information. Confabulation is *not* lying.

confidentiality Treating information divulged by a client as private, unless it reveals the client's intent to harm self or others. In such a case, only persons qualified to help the client may be notified, with the client's knowledge of the purpose and intent. Confidentiality conveys respect.

confrontation Process by which a client is told something about self by a nurse-therapist that encourages self-examination; also used to clarify an inconsistency or incongruence between what the client says and does.

congruent Accordant states; for example, *mood congruent* means that the person's visible emotional state correlates with his or her mood or feeling state.

constricted Narrowed or restricted range, as in emotion; for example, a "constricted affect."

coping strategy Learned techniques used by individuals to reduce tension, stress, and anxiety; for example, deep-breathing techniques, relaxation exercises, visual imagery, and thought substitution. (See Appendix E.)

crisis Sudden change in a person's life situation or status in which customary methods of coping or problem solving fail or are inadequate; also called a *state of disequilibrium* for which a person may need outside help. The crisis may be a turning point in the person's life.

crisis counseling Brief counseling sessions (5 to 6 weeks) in which specific strategies focus on the issues surrounding the crisis; may be individual, group, or family oriented.

culture Learned values, beliefs, perceptions, and behaviors of specific groups of people. Nurse-therapists value cultural differences and recognize mental disorders within the context of their individual cultures.

decompensate Decline or deterioration of areas of mental or physical functioning; a loss of ability to maintain adequate or appropriate psychologic defenses that may result in anxiety, depression, or psychosis.

deep-breathing technique Stress reduction technique in which the act of deep, slow inhalations moves the diaphragm downward and fills the lungs with air, followed by slow exhalations. Oxygen slows the heart rate, which reduces the individual's physiologic and psychologic symptoms of anxiety. (See Appendix B.)

defense mechanisms (ego defense mechanisms) Psychoanalytic term for coping mechanisms, also called *mental mechanisms*. Operations are initiated at an unconscious level by the ego to protect the organism from anxiety by preventing conscious exposure of a noxious, threatening conflict. Defense mechanisms may be used adaptively or maladaptively and should not be challenged until the person demonstrates that he or she can function without them. Some mechanisms are conscious.

delirium Clouded state of consciousness; decreased sensorium; reduction in clarity of awareness of the environment, accompanied by a reduced capacity to shift, focus, and sustain attention to environmental stimuli; may be reversible, depending on the underlying disease process.

delirium tremens (DTs) Acute psychotic state usually occurring during reduction or cessation of alcohol intake after a prolonged or copious intake of alcohol; characterized by tremors, hallucinations, and seizures; requires immediate treatment; may be life threatening. DTs are severe withdrawal from alcohol.

delusion Fixed belief unrelated to the client's cultural and educational background, improbable in nature, and not influenced or changed by reason or contrary experience; categorized as a thought disorder.
Bizarre delusion Absurd belief, such as being controlled by a dead person.
Mood-congruent delusion Delusion with mood-appropriate content.
Mood-incongruent delusion Delusion with mood-inappropriate content.
Somatic delusion False belief involving a body's parts or functions.

Delusion of grandeur Exaggerated conception of importance.
Delusion of persecution False belief that one is being persecuted.
Delusion of reference False belief that others' behavior refers to oneself; derived from ideas of reference in which one falsely thinks he or she is being discussed.
Delusion of control False feeling that one is being controlled by others.
Paranoid delusion Oversuspiciousness, leading to persecutory delusions.
Delusion of nihilism False feeling that self, others, or the world is nonexistent.
Delusion of poverty False belief that one lacks material possessions.

denial Defense mechanism demonstrated by avoidance of disagreeable realities by the mind's refusal to acknowledge them at a conscious level; may or may not be adaptive, depending on the information being denied.

depersonalization Alteration in the perception or experience of the self in which one's usual sense of reality is temporarily lost or changed. Feeling as if one is detached, in a dreamlike state, or an outside observer of one's mind and body, rather than a participant; may lead to withdrawal.

derailment Gradual or sudden deviation in train of thought without blocking.

derealization Feeling of being disconnected from the environment, that the world is not real; may be manifested by a feeling that the environment has changed and may be associated with depersonalization. Distortion of spatial relationships occurs so that the environment becomes unfamiliar.

dereistic thinking Thought processes that are not based in an external, commonly accepted reality. *Dereism* generally means a disconnection with reality and logic and occurs just before autistic thinking, when the person then engages in private, idiosyncratic thoughts and ideas that are derived from internal drives and desires; seen in clients with schizophrenia. The terms *dereistic thinking* and *autistic thinking* are often used interchangeably.

disorientation Lack of awareness of time, place, or person.

displacement Defense mechanism in which an individual discharges or displaces pent-up feelings and emotions on persons or objects that are less threatening than the source; may or may not be adaptive, depending on the situation.

dissociation Defense mechanism that protects the self from awareness of feelings that threaten to produce overwhelming anxiety by denying the existence of those feelings.

DRGs (diagnosis-related groups) List of medical conditions that are grouped in categories on which prospective hospital costs and payments are calculated; intended to predict use of resources.

drug holidays Carefully planned and managed withdrawal from psychotropic medications; may be executed to reduce nontherapeutic effects; most often done with neuroleptic medications.

dual diagnosis Coexistence of two or more mental disorders where one diagnosis is substance related;

for example, major depression and alcohol dependence.

dysfunctional grief Grief or mourning that is not resolved within an appropriate time and/or demonstration of behaviors that are dysfunctional or inappropriate in accordance with the stages of the grieving process; may result in depression or impaired function.

dysphoria Sense of restlessness, agitation, malaise, or anguish, experienced by persons with depression.

ego-dystonic Feelings or actions that are distressing to the individual or not congruent with the self-image, as in ego-dystonic homosexuality.

ego-syntonic Feelings or actions that are congruent with the individual's self-image even if inconsistent with mainstream society, as in ego-syntonic homosexuality.

electroconvulsive therapy (ECT) Treatment of inducing convulsive seizures via the passage of an electric current through electrodes applied to temporal areas of the head (unilaterally or bilaterally); used most frequently in the treatment of severe depression; also known as *electroshock therapy.*

elopement Departure or flight from a mental health facility by an inpatient, against medical advice (AMA).

empathy Ability to understand the feelings of others, especially clients, as if they were one's own feelings, without losing objectivity, and to accept others' experiences on their terms; differs from sympathy by its lack of condolence, pity, or agreement.

enabler Family member or significant person in an alcoholic or drug addict's life who contributes to the afflicted person's continued use and abuse of the substance; examples include making excuses for the afflicted person and supplying the person with the alcohol or drug.

enmeshment Family pattern characterized by overcontrol, intrusiveness, and interference, usually from parent to child; noted in families of clients with anorexia nervosa.

extrapyramidal side effects (EPSEs) Side effects caused by neuroleptic medications that include three separate classes of effects: parkinsonism, dystonias, and akathisia (see Medications in Chapter 4).

fantasy Sequence of mental images that can be likened to a daydream; may be conscious or unconscious; often cited as a defense mechanism. A person may fantasize to help resolve an emotional conflict or as a means of mental rehearsal. Fantasizing may be adaptive and even beneficial at any age, as long as developmental tasks are being met and the person functions in a manner that reveals the ability to distinguish between fantasy and reality consistent with his or her age-appropriate level.

fear Response that is the same as anxiety but caused by consciously recognized and realistic danger. May also be irrational fear as in phobia.

feedback In communication, method by which one person checks out the verbal or nonverbal communication of another; also a process by which a person offers commentary on another's performance; useful in the therapeutic process.

fetal alcohol syndrome (FAS) Physical or mental defects noted in infants of mothers who used or abused alcohol during their pregnancies.

fight or flight Response to stress of aggression (fight) or withdrawal (flight), provoked in part by the effects of the autonomic nervous system.

flat affect Lack of emotional range or expression; also referred to as *flattened affect.*

flight of ideas Almost continuous flow of rapid speech with abrupt changes from topic to topic; most often observed during manic episodes of bipolar disorder in which the person's thoughts and ideas accelerate to an unintelligible degree. Distinguished from the *looseness of associations* observed in clients with schizophrenia in that flight of ideas is generally more based in reality than the internally stimulated thoughts revealed in the fragmented pattern of loose associations. However, flight of ideas may reach a level of psychosis in the form of grandiose or paranoid delusions; may be perpetuated by stressful stimuli.

general systems theory Conceptual framework that can be applied to living systems or people and that integrates the biologic and social sciences logically with the physical sciences. The theory views individuals as open systems that can influence and be influenced by all other systems.

goal-directed thinking Flow of ideas and associations initiated by a problem or task that leads toward a reality-based conclusion. According to Kaplan and Sadock (1998), thinking is "normal" when a logical sequence of events occurs.

grief (mourning) Sadness appropriate to an actual loss, characterized by specific behaviors that occur in stages of the grieving process in an acceptable time period. In *functional grief* the individual is able to perform activities of daily living in a progression congruent with the stages of the grieving process.

hallucination Perceptual disorder that may involve any of the five senses (auditory, visual, olfactory, gustatory, tactile) and occurs in the absence of external stimuli.

here-and-now interactions Interpersonal communications that deal with current problems and issues that are either "on the spot" or recent enough to affect the individual's present situation.

heterosexuality Preference for sexual activity with a partner of the opposite gender.

holistic Pertaining to totality or the whole; for example, the health profession subscribes to the philosophy of *holism,* viewing the individual as an integrated whole whose parts share an organic and functional relationship.

homelessness Absence of housing that may involve movement from one temporary shelter to another because of financial crisis or emergency or, in the more extreme form, the term refers to street dwellers (the "homeless").

homicidal State characterized by one person's verbal or behavioral threats to harm or kill another person; requires immediate intervention.

homophobia Irrational fear of homosexuals and homosexuality, generally stemming from myths and stereotypes.

homosexual panic Extreme anxiety and agitation as a result of emerging repressed homosexual impulses.

homosexuality Preference for sexual activity with a partner of the same gender.

human immunodeficiency virus (HIV) Virulent virus that causes acquired immunodeficiency syndrome (AIDS); consists of an extremely tiny, double-layered shell, filled with proteins, surrounding a bit of ribonucleic acid (RNA).

hyperactivity (hyperkinesis) Restless, overactive motor movement and behavior; may be aggressive or destructive; seen in children with hyperactive conditions or people experiencing a manic episode.

hypervigilance Increased state of guardedness or watchfulness; may be a sign of escalating anxiety or agitation; may involve scanning behaviors as well.

identification Defense mechanism that involves the desire or wish to emulate another person and to assume the characteristics of that person. Most notable in adolescence, when identification with peers is an important part of growth and development. It actually begins, however, in early childhood (ages 3 to 6), when identification with the parent of the same gender is a critical developmental task.

illogical thinking Thinking that contains erroneous conclusions, irrational ideas, or internal contradictions.

illusions Sensory misperceptions or misinterpretations of actual environmental stimuli. Affects all the senses, but visual and auditory illusions are much more common than tactile, olfactory, and gustatory illusions; may occur as a result of sleep-wake alterations.

inappropriate affect Affect that is incongruent with the content of the client's verbalizations or ideas.

incoherence Running together of thoughts with no logical connections, resulting in disorganized thought processes.

insight Understanding of relationships that sheds light on or helps solve a problem; recognition of sources of emotional difficulty; understanding of the motivational forces behind actions, thoughts, and behaviors; self-knowledge.

intellectualization Defense mechanism that consists of ruminating about philosophic or theoretic data or overusing intellectual or scholarly processes to avoid closeness to one's emotions or expressions; serves to constrain instinctual drives; constitutes an interruption of the stream of thought.

introjection Defense mechanism that begins in infancy and involves the incorporation of traits, qualities, and characteristics of significant persons; more intense than identification, which is more like imitation.

irrational thinking Thinking that is not based on a universally accepted reality; illogical thinking.

judgment Ability or capacity to make a decision based on sound problem solving of a given situation; exercise or demonstration of objective, wise actions.

labile affect Pattern of observable behaviors that express emotion characterized by repeated, rapid, abrupt shifts.

lesbianism Sexual activity between females.

lethality assessment Systematic method of assessing a client's suicide risk or potential.

limit setting Reasonable setting of boundaries and parameters for client behavior to provide control and safety; often used with children and adolescents.

loosening of associations Flow or stream of thought that is characterized by vague, fragmented, unfocused, and illogical speech patterns; notable in persons with schizophrenia; listed in Kaplan and Sadock (1998) as a disturbance in structure of associations of thought; generally based on the client's inner repertoire of thought patterns.

magical thinking Belief that one's thoughts, words, or actions will produce an outcome that defies normal laws of cause and effect; the belief that one's words have the power to make things happen; occurs in schizophrenia. For example, a client may believe his or her thoughts can cause earthquakes.

malingering Simulation of illness with no evidence of organic pathology.

masochism (sexual masochism) Need to experience emotional or physical pain, in reality or in fantasy, to become sexually aroused.

meditation Method of achieving a state of deep rest and increasing α-wave brain activity that allows the individual to focus on one thing at a time for the purpose of attaining inner peace and emotional harmony.

mental disorder "A clinically significant behavioral or psychological syndrome or pattern . . . typically associated with painful symptom . . . or impairment, in one or more important areas of functioning" (DSM-IV-TR, 2001).

mental status examination Record of current findings that includes the description of a client's appearance, behavior, motor activity, speech, alertness, mood, cognition, intelligence, reactions, views, and attitudes.

milieu Therapeutic environment; the client's immediate environment.

milieu therapy Purposeful use of people, resources, and events that take place in the client's therapeutic environment (milieu) for the promotion of optimal functioning in activities of daily living, interpersonal interactions, growth and development, and the ability to manage self-care on discharge.

mood Feeling state or prolonged emotion that influences the whole of one's psychic life. Mood is a subjective state.

mood congruence State in which the mood is congruent or consistent with the person's affect and thought processes. For example, a person demonstrates a saddened affect and expresses feelings of sadness appropriate to the mood.

mood incongruence State in which the mood is incongruent or inconsistent with the person's affect or verbal content. For example, a person expresses feelings of happiness yet outwardly manifests a sad affect and verbalizes content that is pessimistic and negative.

mood-congruent delusion Delusion in which the content is appropriate with the mood of the individual. For example, a person expresses feelings of self-importance and elation and states that he or she is the savior of humanity.

mood-incongruent delusion Delusion in which the content is mood inappropriate. For example, a person expresses elation and exhilaration but speaks of the world ending.

NANDA Acronym for the North American Nursing Diagnosis Association, an organization made up of nurses who were instrumental in the construction of the NANDA Taxonomy and who are responsible for reviewing, studying, and accepting specific nursing diagnoses that cover all clinical practice areas.

neologism Newly coined word that generally indicates a formal thought disorder; often seen in schizophrenia.

neuroleptic Another term for medications known as *antipsychotics.*

neuroleptic malignant syndrome (NMS) Infrequent yet extremely critical condition in clients who are undergoing neuroleptic drug treatment. Symptoms include diaphoresis, muscle rigidity, and hyperpyrexia and are believed to result from dopamine blockade in the hypothalamus; may be fatal.

neurotransmitter Chemical found in the nervous system (e.g., norepinephrine, serotonin, dopamine) that facilitates the transmission of nerve impulses across synapses and between neurons; implicated in affective and schizophrenic disorders.

orientation Conscious awareness of person, place, and time.

orientation phase Initial phase of a one-to-one relationship, which is begun by establishing contact with the client.

paraphrasing Therapeutic communication skill in which the nurse restates what she or he has heard the client communicating; provides an opportunity to test the nurse's understanding of what the client is attempting to communicate and allows the client to hear his own words repeated.

passive-aggressive behavior Behavior characterized by sarcasm, procrastination, or resistance to requests made by others; a covert use of aggression.

passive-aggressive personality disorder Pervasive pattern of resistance to demands for adequate performance in social and occupational settings. Resistance may take the form of "forgetfulness," intentional inefficiency, stubbornness, dawdling, or procrastination.

perception Awareness of objects and relations following peripheral sensory stimulation. A hallucination is an example of a false sensory perception because it is not associated with actual external stimuli.

perseveration Psychopathologic repetition of the same word or idea in response to different questions; considered a disturbance in the structure of thought associations; noted in organic mental disorders and schizophrenia.

personality Unique and distinctive human quality that defines and determines the essence of a person's character; what a person is really like; comprises deeply ingrained patterns of behavior known as *personality traits.*

play therapy Therapy used with children generally between ages 3 and 12 years. The child reveals problems on a fantasy level through the use of dolls, puppets, clay, and other toys and materials. The child is encouraged, with the help of the therapist, to act out feelings such as anger, fear, hostility, and frustration. The therapist may intervene to explain to the child his or her responses and behaviors in language that the child can comprehend.

polypharmacy Mixing of multiple medications; noted in the elderly population, who tend to have a wide variety of medical problems. May have negative effects if over-used.

posture Body stance, position of the limbs, or carriage of the body as a whole. In the mental health assessment the client's posture is an important indicator of general well-being.

poverty of speech Restriction in the amount of speech used by an individual; considered a disturbance in the speed of thought associations.

primary gain Obtaining relief from anxiety by the use of a defense mechanism to keep an internal need or conflict out of conscious awareness.

problem solving Specific form of intellectual activity that involves critical thinking to help an individual deal with a complex situation he or she may not be able to handle with past learned skills. Problem-solving strategies consist of the following sequential steps: observation, definition, preparation, analysis, ideation, incubation, synthesis, evaluation, and development. The nursing process is an example of a systematic set of complex cognitive and behavioral steps in which problem-solving methods are applied.

projection Defense mechanism in which an individual projects onto others unwanted or undesirable characteristics of self.

projective identification Placement of one's aggressive feelings onto another, thereby justifying one's expressions of anger and self-protection.

psychiatric nursing Specialty within the nursing profession in which the focus of the nurse is directed toward the promotion of mental health, the prevention of mental distress, early identification of and intervention in emotional problems that can lead to dysfunctional behaviors and mental disorders, and follow-up care to minimize long-term effects of mental illness.

psychiatry Practice and science of diagnosing and treating mental disorders.

psychology Science of the mind or mental state and processes.

psychomotor Pertaining to a response involving both psychologic and motor components.

psychomotor agitation Agitated motor activity.

psychomotor retardation Generalized slowing of psychologic and physical activity, frequently as a symptom of severe depression.

psychopharmacology Branch of pharmacology that deals with the psychologic effects of drugs.

psychopharmacotherapy Use of psychoactive drugs in the symptomatic treatment and management of psychiatric disorders.

psychosis State in which a person's capacity for recognizing reality and communicating and interacting with others is impaired, thereby greatly diminishing the person's ability to deal with life demands; may be associated with several mental disorders; includes thought disorders (delusion), sensory perceptual alterations (hallucinations, illusions), and extremes of affect.

psychosocial Pertaining to the interaction between psychologic and social factors.

psychotherapy Treatment of psychologic disorders or dysfunctions using a professional technique such as psychoanalysis, group therapy, or behavioral therapy.

psychotropic drugs Chemicals that alter feelings, emotions, and consciousness in a variety of ways; used in the practice of psychiatry to treat a wide range of mental and emotional illnesses.

rationalization Defense mechanism in which a person justifies ideas, actions, or feelings with seemingly acceptable explanations or reasons.

reaction formation Defense mechanism in which an individual expresses opposite feelings, attitudes, or behaviors toward another person or situation than what would normally be expressed under the circumstances, while repressing unacceptable feelings.

recidivism Tendency to relapse into a previous mode of behavior. For the client with a mental or emotional disorder, recidivism focuses on exacerbation of symptoms and relapse of illness.

regression Retreating to past developmental levels of behavior, generally in an attempt to reduce overwhelming anxiety; may be used as a defense mechanism.

repression Defense mechanism in which unacceptable feelings are kept out of conscious awareness; also an operative force in the use of other defense mechanisms; necessary for emotional survival of the organism.

resistance Reluctance or opposition by the individual to examine anxiety-producing aspects of self. The person uses automatic defenses (denial, repression) and learned techniques (arriving late for appointments; worsening symptoms after admission to avoid exploration in group therapy) to avoid personally unacceptable realizations.

restitution Negation of a previous, intolerable conscious act or experience to relieve or reduce feelings of guilt; also called *undoing*.

role playing Reenactment of an experience for the purpose of gaining understanding and alleviating emotional distress. The drama and energy involved in role playing can produce a cathartic effect.

scapegoat Person within a family who is the recipient of the negative emotions experienced by various family members.

self-concept Composite of ideas, perceptions, and attitudes an individual develops about self, based on value systems that develop primarily as a result of responses from significant others.

self-disclosure Sharing personal feelings and experiences with others. The nurse and other professionals need to use judgment as to when and how much to disclose to the client.

self-esteem Feelings of self-worth stemming from the individual's positive or negative beliefs about being valuable and capable.

self-help groups Organized groups that provide support through group interactions between people experiencing the same type of problem, event, or situation; for example, Alcoholics Anonymous (AA).

separation-individuation The process of identifying oneself as different from the primary nurturer while maintaining an emotional attachment to that person. An important task of early growth and development.

sleep disorders Chronic disturbance of sleep patterns; include dyssomnia; amount, quality, or timing of sleep; parasomnia; and events occurring during sleep (e.g., nightmares).

somatization Conversion of mental states or experiences into bodily symptoms; associated with anxiety.

splitting Defense mechanism that prevents a person from integrating the good and the bad aspects of the self or of the person's image of another person. The person thus views self or others as either all good or all bad at any given time and acts accordingly, failing to integrate the positive and negative qualities into a cohesive image. A hallmark symptom in borderline personality disorder.

stereotypy Continuous repetition of speech or physical activity; noted in persons with organic mental disorders and schizophrenia.

stress Broad class of experiences in which a demanding situation taxes a person's physical and emotional resources, resulting in a series of adaptive responses by the organism.

stressor Stimulus perceived by the individual or the organism as challenging, threatening, or damaging.

sublimation Defense mechanism that involves rechanneling consciously intolerable or socially unacceptable impulses or behaviors into activities that are personally or socially acceptable. Urges may be of a sexual or aggressive nature.

suicidal gesture More serious warning than suicidal ideation or threat; involves an action that suggests the act of suicide may be imminent.

suicidal ideation Verbalized thought or idea that indicates a person's desire toward self-harm or self-destruction; requires immediate intervention.

suicidal threat Statement of suicidal intent accompanied by behavior changes that reflect suicidal ideation.

suicide attempt Serious suicide try involving definite risk. The outcome often depends on the circumstances and is not within the person's control.

suppression Willful or conscious act of putting a thought, idea, or feeling out of one's mind for a variety of reasons, with the ability to recall the thought, idea, or feeling at will.

suspiciousness Pronounced attitude of doubt regarding the trustworthiness, intent, or motives of others; may include objects or situations as well.

tardive dyskinesia Most frequent serious untoward effect of antipsychotic drug therapy. Usually an irreversible and late-onset complication, it is characterized by the presence of abnormal, stereotyped, rhythmic movements of the limbs and torso; tongue protrusion; and chewing movements. May affect any muscle in the body, including the diaphragm; can occur after abrupt termination of the drug, after reduction in dosage, or after long-term, high-dose therapy. Incidence may be minimized with judicious dose management, drug holidays, and administration of antiparkinsonian drugs.

therapeutic alliance Conscious relationship between a helping person and a client in which each agrees to work with the other to help the client resolve problems and concerns.

therapeutic community (milieu) Environment in which a hospitalized client works through problems and concerns with the help of therapists in a variety of areas. Traditional hierarchical structure and authority figures are minimized. (Originally attributed to Maxwell Jones.)

therapeutic use of self Ability of a nurse or other health professional to use learned theory, clinical experience, and self-awareness to benefit the client and to explore one's personal impact on others.

thinking Process that consists of a goal-directed flow of ideas, symbols, and associations initiated by a problem and leading in a logical fashion toward a reality-based conclusion.

thought blocking Sudden stopping of a thought or idea in midstream; an interruption in the train of thinking, unconscious in origin. A disturbance in speed of associations.

thought broadcasting Belief that one's thoughts, as they occur, are broadcast from one's head to the external world; disturbance in thought content.

thought disorder Thinking characterized by loosened associations, neologisms, and illogical constructs; includes disturbances in the form, structure, and content of thought.

thought insertion Belief that thoughts that are not one's own are being inserted into one's mind.

thought withdrawal Belief that thoughts have been removed from one's head.

trust Feeling of confidence that another person will behave in ways that are beneficial; a feeling of safety regarding another person's intentions and motives.

undoing See *restitution*.

validation Communication skill that helps the client confirm or deny the content or intent of his or her statement.

verbigeration (polyphasia) Repetition of meaningless words or phrases; disturbed motor behavior as it relates to speech.

violence Behavior instituted by an individual that threatens or inflicts harm or injury to persons or property.

voluntary commitment Legal process by which a client chooses to be admitted to a mental health facility and signs a paper to that effect.

waxy-flexibility Term used to describe a catatonic person who maintains the position in which he or she has been placed. The movement of the limbs has been described by caregivers as feeling "waxlike."

Wernicke-Korsakoff syndrome Disorder of the central nervous system most often associated with alcoholism and characterized by confusion, disorientation, and memory loss with confabulation; related to thiamine deficiency. Named after Karl Wernicke and Sergei Sergeivich Korsakoff.

"word salad" Incoherent mixture of words and phrases consisting of real and imaginary words, lacking comprehension; occurs in severe states of schizophrenia.

writ of habeas corpus Means by which a client can challenge the legality of his or her detention in a mental health facility.

References

TEXTS AND JOURNALS

Current

20 Million Worldwide, Li, Y Metal, Gamma secretase inhibitors & presentation, *Nature* 405:694, 2002.

Ackerman S et al: Generating in midlife and young adults, *Int J Aging Hum Dev* 5(1):17, 2000.

Aguilera D: *Crisis intervention: theory and methodology*, ed 8, St Louis, 1998, Mosby.

Alexopoulos G et al: Vasular depression hypothesis, *Arch Gen Psychiatry* 54:915, 1997.

American Academy of Child and Adolescent Psychiatry: Practice parameters for assessment and treatment of children and adolescents with depressive disorders, *J Am Acad Child Adolesc Psychiatry* 37:63, 1998.

American College of Neuropsychopharmacology: *Race may be a factor in schizophrenia heredity*, 2001, The College.

American Nurse Editorial: Are we ready to respond?: assessing nursing preparedness, *Am Nurse* 33(6):15, 2002.

American Nurses Association: Pharmacology guidelines for psychiatric mental health nurses, In *Psychiatric mental health nursing psychopharmacology project*, Washington, 1994, ANA Publishing.

American Nurses Association: *A statement of psychiatric mental health clinical nursing practice and standards of psychiatric mental health clinical nursing practice*, Washington, 2000, ANA Publishing.

American Nurses Association, International Society of Psychiatric—Mental Health Nurses: *Scope and standards of psychiatric mental health nursing practice*, Washington, 2000, ANA Publishing.

American Psychiatric Association: *Diagnostic and statistical manual of mental disorders*, ed 4, Washington, 2000, The Association.

American Psychiatric Association: *National partnership for workplace mental health*, 2001, The Association.

American Psychiatric Nurses Association: *Seclusion and restraint: position statement and standards of practice*, 2001, The Association.

Andersen K et al: Do non-steroidal anti-inflammatory drugs decrease the risk of Alzheimer's disease? *Neurology* 45:1441, 1995.

Andrews J: Adolescent and family predictors of physical aggression, communication, and satisfaction in young adult couples, *J Consult Clin Psychol* 68(2):195, 2000.

Arnold LE, Jensen PS: Attention-deficit disorders. In Kaplan H, Sadock B, editors: *Comprehensive textbook of psychiatry*, New York, 1995, Williams & Wilkins.

Aronson M et al: Attention deficits and autistic spectrum problems in children exposed to alcohol during gestation, *Dev Med Child Neurol* 39:583, 1997.

Arthur D: Alcohol early intervention: a nursing model for screening and intervention strategies, *A NZ J Ment Hlth Nurs* 6:93, 1997.

Axelson J: *Counseling in a multicultural society*, Belmont, 1999, Wadsworth.

Bachrach L: The state of state mental hospitals, *Psychiatr Serv* 47:1071, 1998.

Baker C et al: Connecting conversations of caring: recalling the narrative to clinical practice, *Nurs Outlook* 42:65, 1994.

Barber S: Helping children and families deal with psychological aspects of disaster, *J Pediatr Hlth Care* 16(1):36, 2002.

Barbey MD, Roose SP: SSRI safety in overdose, *J Clin Psychiatry* 59(suppl 15):42, 1998.

Bartel S et al: Community based long term care for older persons with severe, persistent mental illness, *Psychiatr Serv* 50(9):1189, 1999.

Bateman A, Fonagy P: Effectiveness of partial hospitalization in treatment of borderline personality disorder, *Am J Psychiatry* 156(10):1563, 1999.

Baum A, Posluszny D: Health psychology: mapping behavioral contributions to health and illness, *Annu Rev Psychol* 50:137, 1999.

Beck J, Stanley M: Anxiety disorders in the elderly, *Behav Ther*, 28:83, 1997.

Beeson P et al: Rural mental health at the millennium. In Manderscheid R, Henderson M: *Mental health in the United States*, Washington, 1998, U.S. Government Printing Office.

Beiser M et al: Biological and psychosocial predictors of job performance following a first episode of psychosis, *Am J Psychiatry* 15:857, 1994.

Bickman L et al: Long term effects of a system of care of children and adolescents, *J Behav Health Serv Res* 26:185, 1999.

Boomsa J, Dingemans CAJ, Dassen TWN: The nursing process in crisis-oriented psychiatric home care, *J Psychiatr Ment Hlth Nurs* 4:295, 1997.

Bornstein R: Implicit and self attributed dependency needs in dependent and histrionic personality disorders, *J Pers Assess* 71(1):1, 1998.

Borson S, Raskin M: Clinical features and pharmacologic treatment of behavior symptoms of Alzheimer's disease, *Neurology* 45:17, 1997.

Brady KT, Randall CL: Gender differences in substance use disorders, *Psychiatr Clin North Am* 22:241, 1999.

Brawman-Mintzer O et al: Somatic symptoms in generalized anxiety disorder with and without co-morbid psychiatric disorders, *Am J Psychiatry* 151:930, 1994.

Brunton K: Stigma, *J Adv Nurs* 26:891, 1997.

Busse E, Blazer, D, editors: *The American Psychiatric Press textbook of geriatric psychiatry,* ed 2, Washington, 1996, American Psychiatric Press.

Cadoret R, Widmer R: Development of depressive symptoms in elderly following onset of severe physical illness, *J Fam Pract* 27:71, 1988.

Campbell SB: *Psychiatric disorder in preschool children,* New York, 1990, Guilford.

Cantwell DP: ADHD treatment with nonstimulants. In *Psychiatry psychopharmacology,* Washington, 1994, AACAP Press.

Capson S et al: Alzheimer's like neurodegeneration in aged anti-nerve growth factor in transgenic mice, *Proceeds of Nation Academy of Science* 97:6826, 2000.

Carman M: The psychology of normal aging, *Psychiatr Clin North Am* 20:15, 1997.

Carpenito LJ: *Nursing diagnosis: application to clinical practice,* ed 8, Philadelphia, 2000, JB Lippincott.

Cassady SL et al: Spontaneous dyskinesia in subjects with schizophrenia spectrum personality, *Am J Psychiatry* 155:70, 1998.

Center for Mental Health Services: *Cultural competence standards in managed care mental health services,* Rockville, Md, 1998, The Center.

Centers for Disease Control: Trends in sexual risk behavior among high school students in the United States, *MMWR* 47:749, 1998.

Charney D: Depression anxiety disorders, *NARSAD Res Newslett* 14(1):42, 2002.

Chen N, Davis JM: *Evidence of efficacy of risperidone in schizophrenia,* presented at American Psychiatric Nurses Association meeting, October, 2001, Reno, Nevada.

Chernomas WM: Experiencing depression: women's perspectives in recovery, *J Psychiatr Ment Hlth Nurs* 4:393, 1997.

Coccaro EF: Clinical outcome of psychopharmacologic treatment of borderline and schizotypal personality disordered subjects, *J Clin Psychiatry* 59(suppl 1):30, 1998.

Cohen G: Do health science concepts influence care? The case for new landscape of aging, *Am J Geriatr Psychiatry* 6:273, 1998.

Cole M, Bellavance F: The prognosis of depression in old age, *Am J Geriatr Psychiatry* 5:4, 1997.

Coleman D: *Emotional intelligence,* New York, 1995, Bantam.

Conwell Y: *Suicide and schizophrenia: risk factors and preventive strategies in psychiatry and mental health,* 1998.

Corrigan P, Penn D: Lessons from social psychology on discrediting psychiatric stigma, *Am Psychol* 54:765, 1999.

Crowe M: An analysis of the sociopolitical context of mental health nursing practice, *A NZ J Ment Hlth Nurs* 6:59, 1997.

Davie JK: The nursing process. In Thelan L et al, editors: *Critical care nursing: diagnosis and management,* St Louis, 2000, Mosby.

Davis PC et al: The brain in older persons with and without dementia: finding on MR, PET and SPECT images, *AJR Am J Roentgenol* 162:1267, 1994.

De Oliveira IR et al: Risperidone versus haloperidol in the treatment of schizophrenia: a meta-analysis comparing their efficacy and safety, *J Clin Pharm Ther* 21:349, 1996.

DiClemente R, Hansen W, Ponton L: Adolescents at risk: a generation in jeopardy. In *Handbooks of adolescent health risk behavior,* New York, 1996, Plenum Press.

Dulcan M, Martini D: *Child and adolescent psychiatry,* Washington, 1999, American Psychiatric Press.

Esman AH: Child abuse and multiple personality disorder (letter), *Am J Psychiatry* 151:948, 1994.

Faraone S et al: Bipolar and antisocial disorders among relatives of ADHD children, *Am J Med Genet* 81(1):108, 1998.

Felitti V et al: Relationship of child abuse and household dysfunctions to many of the leading causes of death in adults, *Am J Prev Med* 14:245, 1998.

Fingeld D: Alcohol treatment for women in rural areas, *J Am Psychiatr Nurs Assoc* 8:2, 2002.

Fink M: Catatonia: syndrome or schizophrenia subtype? Recognition and treatment, *J Neural Transm* 108(6):637, 2001.

Fink M, Taylor MA: The many varieties of catatonia, *Eur Arch Psychiatry Clin Neurosci* 251(suppl 1):8, 2001.

Fink M: We should treat neuroleptic malignant syndrome as catatonia, *J Clin Psychopharmacol* 20(2):257, 2000.

Foa EB, Davidson JRT, Frances A, et al: Expert consensus treatment guidelines for posttraumatic stress disorder: a guide for patients and families, reprint, *J Clin Psychiatry* 60(suppl 16), 1999.

Foreman M, Wakefield M, Culp K, et al: Delirium in elderly patients: an overview of the state of the science, *J Gerontol Nurs* 2001.

Fortinash K, Worret PH: *Psychiatric nursing care plans,* ed 3, St Louis, 1999, Mosby.

Fraser M et al: Effectiveness of family preservation services, *Soc Work Res* 21:138, 1997.

Frederick J: Instruments of assessment of auditory hallucinations, *Arch Psychiatr Nurs* 12:255, 1998.

Frese F, Davis W: The consumer survivor movement, recovery, and consumer professionals, *Professional Psychology: Research and Practice* 28:243, 1997.

Friedman R et al: Prevalence of serious emotional disturbances in children and adolescents, *Mental health*, Washington, 1998, U.S. Government Printing Office.

Gallo J: Depression without sadness, *J Am Geriatr Soc* 45:570, 1997.

Gamble C, Brennan G: *Working with serious mental illness: a manual for clinical practice*, Philadelphia, 2000, Bailliere Tindall in association with The Royal College of Nursing, Harcourt Publishers Limited.

Gazzaniga M et al: *Cognitive neuroscience: the biology of the mind*, New York, 1998, WW Norton.

Glazer W: Extrapyramidal side effects, tardive dyskenesia and atypicality, *J Clin Psychol* 61:16, 2000.

Goisman R et al: Psychosocial treatment prescriptions for geralized anxiety disorder, panic disorder, and social phobia, *Am J Psychiatry* 156:1819, 1999.

Goodwin FJ, Ghaemi SN: The impact of mood stabilizers on suicide in bipolar disorder, *CNS Spectrum* 5(2):12, 2000.

Gordis E: Research on alcohol problems, *Phi Kappa Phi J* 79(4):24, 1999.

Gordon M: *Nursing diagnosis: process and applications*, ed 3, St. Louis, 2000, Mosby.

Gorman J: Post traumatic stress disorder, *NARSAD Res Newslett* 14(1):42, 2002.

Gournay K et al: Dual diagnosis: severe mental health problems and substance abuse/dependence: a major priority for mental health nursing, *J Psychiatr Ment Hlth Nurs* 4:89, 1997.

Grilo CM et al: Personality disorders in adolescents with major depression, substance use disorders, and coexisting major depression and substance use disorders, *J Consult Clin Psychol* 65:328, 1997.

Gustafson DH et al: Impact of a patient centered computer based health information support system, *Am J Prev Med* 16:1, 1999.

Haber J: Policy and politics: phoenix rising from the ashes, a mental health opportunity, *J Am Psychiatr Nurs Assoc* 8(1):108, 1998.

Harwood H et al: *The economic cost of alcohol and drug abuse in the United States*, Rockville, Md, 1998, United States Department of Health and Human Services.

Hillis SD et al: Adverse childhood experiences and sexually trasmitted disease in men and women, *Pediatrics* 106, 2000.

Hoffman SB, Platt CA: *Comforting the confused: strategies for managing dementia*, ed 2, New York, 2000, Springer.

Hogstel MD: *Geropsychiatric nursing*, ed 2, St Louis, 1995, Mosby.

Huang TL: *Neuoleptic malignant syndrome associated with long-term clozapine treatment: report of a case and results of a clozapine rechallenge*, Kaoshiung, Taiwan, 2001, Department of Psychiatry, Chang Gung Memorial Hospital.

Institute for Health and Aging: *Chronic care in America: a 21st century challenge*, Princeton, NJ, 1996, Robert Wood Johnson Foundation.

Jeste DV et al: *Risperidone and olanzapine in elderly patients with schizophrenia and schizoaffective disorder*, presented at the American Nurses Association Meeting, October, 2001, Reno, Nevada.

Johnson M, Maas M, Moorhead S: *Iowa outcomes project: nursing outcomes classification (NOC)*, ed 2, St Louis, 2000, Mosby.

Kaplan H: *The comprehensive textbook of psychiatry*, ed 6, Baltimore, 1995, Williams & Wilkins.

Kaplan H, Sadock B: *Synopsis of psychiatry—behavioral science—clinical psychiatry*, ed 8, Baltimore, 1998, Williams & Wilkins.

Keltner NL, Folks DG: *Psychotropic drugs*, ed 3, St. Louis, 2001, Mosby.

Kendler KS, Gardner CO: Boundaries of major depression: an evaluation of DSM-IV criteria, *Am J Psychiatry* 155:172, 1998.

Kent J et al: Clinical utility of selective serotonin reuptake inhibitors in anxiety, *Biol Psychiatry* 44:812, 1998.

Kessler R et al: Lifetime comorbidities between social phobia and mood disorders in the United States national comorbidity survey, *Psychol Med* 29:555, 1999.

Kim J et al: Racial differences in health status and health behaviors of older adults, *Nurs Res* 47(4):243, 1998.

Lambert EW, Wahler RG, Andrade AR, et al: Looking for the disorder in conduct disorder, *J Abnor Psychol* 110(1), 2002.

Lefly II: Perspectives of families regarding confidentiality and mental illness, In Gates J, Arons B (editors): *Privacy and confidentiality in mental health care*, Baltimore, 2000, Brookes Publishing.

Lehman A: Managing schizophrenia: interventions and outcomes, *Disease Management and Health Outcomes* 1:286, 1997.

Lehman A: Patterns of useful care for schizophrenia, *Schizophr Bull* 24:11, 1998.

Leininger M: What is transcultural nursing and culturally competent care? *J Transcul Nurs* 10(1):9, 1999.

Lepola I, Vanhanen L: The patient's daily activities in acute psychiatric care, *J Psychiatr Ment Hlth Nurs* 4:29, 1997.

Levin J: Sexual addiction, *National Forum* 79(4):33, 1999.

Lyon B: Social support as TLC: the great elixir, *Reflections on Nursing Leadership/Sigma Theta Tau International* 4:36, 2001.

Majoribanks D: Ethnicity, birth order and family environment, *Psycholog Rep* 84(3):758, 1999.

McCaffery M, Pasero C: *Pain: a clinical manual*, St Louis, 1999, Mosby.

McCaffrey G: The use of leisure activities in a therapeutic community, *J Psychiatr Ment Hlth Nurs* 5:53, 1998.

McCarthy B: Chronic sexual dysfunction: assessment intervention and realistic expectations, *J Sex Educat Ther* 22(2):51, 1997.

McCay E et al: Sexual abuse comfort scale: a scale to measure nurses' comfort to respond to sexual abuse in psychiatric populations, *J Psychiatr Ment Hlth Nurs* 4:361, 1997.

McCloskey J, Bulechek G, editors: *Iowa intervention project: nursing intervention classification (NIC),* ed 3, St. Louis, 2000, Mosby.

McGuinness T et al: Becoming responsible teens: promoting health of adolescents in foster care, *J Am Nurs Assoc* 8(3):92, 2002.

McNicol T: The impact of drug-exposed children on family foster care, *Child Welfare* 78:184, 1999.

Meeks S, Murell S: Mental illness in late life, *Psychol Aging* 12:296, 1997.

Menzies V, Farrel SP: Schizophrenia tardive dyskensia and the abnormal involuntary movement scale (AIMS), *J Am Psychiatr Nurs Assoc* 8(2):52, 2002.

Meyer JM: *Practical issues in psychiatry: metabolic effects of atypical antipsychotic therapy,* Morrisville, Pa, 2002, MediCom Worldwide, Inc.

Miller J, Striver P: *The healing connection: how women form relationships in therapy and life,* Boston, 1997, Beacon Press.

Mitrushina et al: A comparison of cognitive profiles in schizophrenia and other psychiatric disorders, *J Clin Psychol* 52:177, 1996.

Monohan J et al: Coercion in the provision of mental health services, *Research in Community and Mental Health* 10:13, 1999.

Montgomery SA: Understanding depression and its treatment, *J Clin Psychiatry* 61(6):3, 2001.

Mosby's medical, nursing, and allied health dictionary, ed 6, St. Louis, 2002, Mosby.

Mujica R, Weiden P: Neuroleptic malignant syndrome after addition of haloperidol to atypical antipsychotic, *Am J Psychiatry* 158:650, 2001.

Mulbauer S: Experience of stigma by families with mentally ill members, *J Am Psychiatr Nurs Assoc* 8(3):67, 2002.

Murray S et al: Screening families with young children for child maltreatment potential, *Pediatr Nurs* 26:47, 2000.

Mylant M et al: Adolescent children of alcoholics: vulnerable or resilient? *J Psychiatr Nurs Assoc* 8(2):57, 2002.

Nahas Z et al: SPECT and PET in neuropsychiatry, *Primary Psychiatry* 5(3):52, 1998.

Nasar S: *A beautiful mind: a biography of John Forbes Nash,* New York, 1998, Simon & Schuster.

Neese J: Utilization of mental health services among rural elderly, *Arch Psychiatr Nurs* 13(1):31, 1999.

Neziroglu FA, Yaryura-Tobias JA: A review of congitive-behavioral and pharmacological treatment of body dysmorphic disorder, *Behav Modif* 21:324, 1997.

North American nursing diagnosis: definitions and classification (NANDA Taxonomy), Philadelphia, 2002, North American Nursing Diagnosis Association.

Nottelmann ED, Jensen PS: Comorbidity of disorders in children and adolescents: developmental perspectives. In *Advances in clinical child psychology,* vol 17, New York, 1995, Plenum.

Nutt D: Brain mechanisms of social anxiety disorder, *J Clin Psychiatry* 59:4, 1998.

O'Brien L, Flote J: Providing nursing care for a patient with borderline personality disorder: a phenomenological study, *A NZ J Ment Hlth Nurs* 6:1997.

Pargament K: *The psychology of religion and coping: theory, research, practice,* New York, 1995, Basic Books.

Pasternak R: The post treatment illness course of depression in bereaved elders, *Am J Geriatr Psychiatry* 5:5, 1997.

Patterson T et al: Quality of well being in late life psychosis, *Psychiatry Res* 63:169, 1996.

Paulhus D et al: Birth order effects on personality and achievement within families, *Psychol Sci* 10(6):482, 1999.

Payton J et al: Social and emotional learning: promoting mental health and reducing risk behavior in children and youth, *J Sch Health* 70:179, 2000.

Penn D, Martin J: The stigma of severe mental illness: some potential for solutions for a recalcitrant problem, *Psychiatr Q* 69:235, 1998.

Peplau HE: Interpersonal relations: a theoretical framework for application in nursing practice, *Nurs Sci Q* 5(1):13, 1992.

Phelan J: Psychiatric illness and family stigma, *Schizophr Bull* 24:115, 1998.

Raingruber B: Recognizing, understanding, and responding to familiar responses, *Perspect Psychiatr Care* 35(2):5, 1999.

Reas DL et al: Duration of illness predicts outcome for bulimia nervosa, *Int J Eat Disord* 27:428, 2002.

Regier D, Burke J: Epidemiology. In Sadock B, Sadock V, editors, *Comprehensive textbook of psychiatry,* vol 7, Philadelphia, 2000, Lippincott Williams & Wilkins.

Regier D et al: Prevalence of anxiety disorders and their comorbidity with mood and addictive disorders, *Br J Psychiatry* 34:24, 1998.

Reynolds C, Kupfer D: Depression and aging: a look to the future, *Psychiatr Serv* 50:1167, 1999.

Rizos A: *Adverse drug events (ADE),* San Diego, 2002, Sharp HealthCare Medication Education for Nurses, Physicians, and Pharmacists.

Rocio M et al: Suppression of psychoative effects of cocaine by active immunization, *Nature* 378:727, 1995.

Rogers S: Empirically supported comprehensive treatments for young children with autism, *J Clin Child Psychol* 27:168, 1998.

Rogers S et al: Donepezil improves cognition and global functions in Alzheimer's disease, *Arch Intern Med* 158:1021, 1998.

Rosenbeck R: Principles of priority setting in mental health services and implications for the least well off, *Psychiatr Serv* 50:63, 1999.

Rosse RB et al: Gaze discrimination in pateints with schizophrenia: preliminary report, *Am J Psychiatry* 151:919, 1994.

Roy-Byrne PP: Generalized anxiety and mixed anxiety-depression: association with disability and health care utilization, *J Clin Psychiatry* 57(suppl 7):86, 1996.

Rudorfer M et al: Electroconvulsive therapy. In Kay J, Leiberman J, editors: *Psychiatry*, Philadelphia, 1997, WB Saunders.

Rutter M et al: Genetics and child psychiatry, *J Psychol Psychiatry* 40:3, 1999.

Salzman C: ECT, research and professional ambivalence, *Am J Psychiatry* 155(1):1, 1998.

Sattler J: *Clinical and forensic interview of children and families*, San Diego, 1998, Jerome Sattler, Publisher.

Schenk D et al: Immunization with amyloid beta attenuates Alzheimer's disease-like pathology in PDAPP mouse, *Nature* 400:173, 1999.

Schnelle J: Developing behavioral rehabilitative intervention for long term care, *J Am Geriatr Soc* 46:771, 1998.

Schulz SC et al: Treatment and outcomes in adolescents with schizophrenia, *J Clin Psychiatry* 59(suppl 1):50, 1998.

Schwartz D: *Frail elderly: disease management strategies and programs*, Atlanta, 2001, National Health Information, LLC.

Secker J: Current conceptualization of mental health prioirities, *Health Education Research* 13(1):57, 1998.

Seclusion and restraint: position statement and standards practice, *J Am Psychiatr Nurs Assoc* 8(2):66, 2002.

Shaffer D, Craft L: Methods of adolescent suicide prevention, *J Clin Psychiatry* 60:71, 1999.

Shaffer H: On the nature and meaning of addiction, *National Forum* 79(4):9, 1999.

Sharts-Hopko N: Health and illness concepts for cultural competence with Japanese clients, *J Cultur Divers* 3(3):74, 1996.

Shea CA et al: *Advanced practice nursing in psychiatric and mental health care*, St Louis, 1999, Mosby.

Sheehan D et al: The mini-international psychiatric interview (MINI), *J Clin Psychiatry* 5:22, 1998.

Sheline Y: Hippocampal atrophy in major depression, *Mol Psychiatry* 1:298, 1996.

Simon GE, VonKorff M: Suicide mortality among patients treated for depression in an insured population, *Am J Epidemiol* 147:155, 1998.

Simon R: Psychiatry and the law: taking the "sue" out of suicide: a forensic psychiatrist's perspective, *Psychiatric Ann* 30:6, 2000.

Skeketee G et al: The psychosocial treatment interview of anxiety disorders: a method for assessing psychotherapeutic procedures in anxiety disorders, *J Psychother Pract Res* 6:194, 1997.

Smith H, Thomas SP: Violent and non-violent girls, *Issues in Mental Health Nursing* 21:547, 2000.

Solomon A: *The noonday demon: an atlas of depression*, 2001.

Solomon J, George C: *Attachment disorganization*, New York, 1999, The Guilford Press.

Souder E, O'Sullivan P: Nursing documentation versus cognitive status in hospitalized medical patients, *Appl Nurs Res* 13(1):31, 2000.

Spirito A: Individual therapy techniques with adolescent suicide attempters, *Crisis* 18:62, 1997.

Standards Committee, *Canadian standards of psychiatric and mental health nursing*, ed 2, 1998, Canadian Federation of Mental Health Nurses.

Steadman H et al: Violence by people discharged from acute psychiatric in-patient facilities and by others in the same neighborhood, *Arch Gen Psychiatry* 55:393, 1998.

Suzuki A et al: Association of the taqI: a polymorphism of the dopamine d2 receptor gene with predisposition to neuroleptic malignant syndrome, *Am J Psychiatry* 158:10, 2001.

Tanguay P: Pervasive and developmental disorders: 10 year review, *J Am Acad Child Adolesc Psychiatry* 39:1079, 2000.

Thomas SP: Teaching healthy anger management, *Perspectives in Psychiatric Care* 37:41, 2001.

Torrey E, Fuller BJ: *Surviving schizophrenia*, ed 4, New York, 2001, Harper Trade.

Trygstad, L: Behavioral management of persistent auditory hallucinations in schizophrenia, *J Am Psychiatr Nurs Assoc* 8(3):92, 2002.

Tucker J: From zero tolerance to harm reduction, *National Forum* 79(4):15, 1999.

United States Department of Health and Human Services: *Mental health: a report of the surgeon general*, Rockville, Md, 1999, The Department.

United States Department of Health and Human Services: *Health people 2010*, ed 2, Washington, 2000, U.S. Government Printing Office.

United States Public Health Service: *Report on the surgeon general's conference on children's mental health*, Washington, 2000, Department of Health and Human Services.

Valente S: Social phobia, *J Am Psychiatr Nurs Assoc* 8(3):67, 2002

Van der Kolk et al: *Traumatic stress: the overwhelming experience on the mind, body, and society*, New York, 1996, Guilford Press.

Vastag B: Bioterrorism threat calls: revisiting research protections, *JAMA* 287:21, 2002.

Vogel H et al: Double trouble in recovery: self help for people with dual diagnosis, *Psychiatr Rehabil J* 2:356, 1998.

Wahl O: Mental health consumers experience of stigma, *Schizophr Bull* 25(3):467, 1999.

Walters V: New strategies for old problems: tardive dyskinesia, *Schizophr Res* 28:231, 197.

Wang P: Hazardous benzodiazepine regimens in the elderly: effects of half-life, dosage, and duration on risk of hip fracture, *Am J Psychiatry* 158(6):892, 2001.

Weiden PJ, Miller AL: Which side effects really matter? Screening for common and distresing side effects of antipsychotic medications, *J Psychiatr Pract* 2001.

Wheeler S, Lord L: Denial: a conceptual analysis, *Arch Psychiatr Nurs* 13(6):311, 1999.

Wolf MS et al: Alzheimer's gamma secretase/protease, *Biochemistry* 38:4720, 1999.

Wyatt R: Neurodevelopmental abnoramlties in schizophrenia: a family affair, *Arch Gen Psychiatry* 53:11, 1996.

Wysoke A: Standards of care, *J Am Psychiatr Nurs Assoc* 7:166, 2001.

Yarcheski A et al: Emotions in early adolescence, *Nurs Res* 48:317, 1999.

Young A: Addictive drugs and the brain, *National Forum* 79(4):9, 1999.

Zalewski C et al: A review of neuropsychological differences between paranoid and non-paranoid schizophrenia patients, *Schizophr Bull* 24:127, 1998.

Zarit S: *The hidden victims of Alzheimer's disease: families under stress,* New York, 1985, New York University Press.

Zwanger P, Marcus A, Boerner RJ, et al: Lithium intoxication after administration of (AT.sub.1) blockers, *J Clin Psychiatry* 62:208, 2001.

Classics and Standards

Al-Anon: *The 12 steps and traditions of Al-Anon family groups,* New York, 1973, Al-Anon.

Alberti R, Emmons M: *Your perfect right: a guide to assertive behavior,* ed 2, San Luis Obispo, Ca, 1974, Impact.

Bandura A: *Principles of behavior modification,* New York, 1969, Holt, Rinehart, Winston.

Bandura A: *Social Learning Theory,* Englewood Cliffs, NJ, 1977, Prentice-Hall.

Bateson G, Jackson D, Haley J, et al: Toward a theory of schizophrenia, *Behavior Sci* 1:251, 1956.

Beattie M: *Codependent no more,* New York, 1992, Harper Collins.

Beck A: *Cognitive therapy and emotional disorder,* New York, 1979, New American Library.

Beers C: *A mind that found itself,* New York, 1908, Lonmans, Green and Co.

Benson H: *The relaxation response,* New York, 1975, William Morrow.

Berne E: *Games people play,* New York, 1964, Grove.

Bleuler E, Zinkin J, translator: *Dementia praecox of the group of schizophrenias,* New York, 1950, International Universities Press.

Bolby J: *Attachment,* New York, 1969, Basic Books.

Bolby J: *Attachment and loss: separation, anxiety, and anger,* New York, 1973, Basic Books.

Bolby J: *Loss: sadness and depression,* New York, 1980, Basic Books.

Bowen M: *Family therapy in clinical practice,* New York, 1978, Jason Aronson.

Burnside I: Listen to the aged, *Am J Nurs* 1975.

Ellis A: *Reason and emotion in psychotherapy,* New York, 1962, Lyle Stuart.

Ellis A: *Feeling better, getting better, staying better,* Atascaderoa, Calif, 2001, Impact Publishers.

Ellis A, Harper R: *A new guide to rational living,* Hollywood, 1976, Wilshire.

Engel G: Grief and grieving, *Am J Nurs,* 1964.

Erikson E: *Childhood and society,* New York, 1950, WW Norton.

Erikson EH: *Childhood and society,* revised, New York, 1964, WW Norton.

Erikson EH: *Identity, youth and crisis,* New York, 1968, WW Norton.

Fagan C: Psychotherapeutic nursing. In *Psychiatric-mental health nursing: contemporary readings,* New York, 1978, D Van Nostrand.

Freud S: *New introductory lectures on psychoanalysis,* New York, 1933, WW Norton.

Freud S: *Problem of anxiety,* New York, 1936, Basic Books.

Fromm-Reichmann F: *Principles of intensive psychotherapy,* Chicago, 1960, University of Chicago Press.

Goodwin FJ, Jamison KR: *Manic depressive illness,* New York, 1990, Oxford University Press.

Haley J: *Problem solving theory,* New York, 1976, Harper & Row.

Hays JS, Larson KH: *Interacting with patients,* New York, 1963, Macmillan.

Holmes TH, Rahe RH: The social readjustment rating scale, *J Psychom Res* 1967.

Horney K: *New ways in psychoanalysis,* New York, 1939 WW Norton.

Horney K: *Our inner conflicts,* New York, 1939, WW Norton.

Jacobson E: *Progressive relaxation,* Philadelphia, 1938, JB Lippincott.

Jellinek EM: *The disease concept of alcoholism,* New Haven, 1960, Hills-House Press.

Jones E, editor: *Collected papers of Sigmund Freud,* New York, 1959, Basic Books.

Kanner L: To what extent is early infantile autism determined by constitutional inadequacies? *Proc Assoc Res Nerv Ment Dis* 33:378, 1954.

Klein M: A contribution to the psychogenesis of manic-depressive states. In *Contributions to psychoanalysis,* London, 1934, Hogarth.

Kübler-Ross E: *On death and dying,* New York, 1969, Macmillan.

Kübler-Ross E: What is it like to be dying? *Am J Nurs* 1971.

Lange A, Jakubowski P: *Responsible assertive behavior: cognitive/behavioral procedure for trainers,* Champaign, Ill, 1976, Research Press.

Lindemann E: Symptomatology and management of acute grief 1994 (classical article), *Am J Psychiatry* 151 (suppl 6):155, 1994.

Mace NL, Rabins PV: *The 36 hour day: a family guide to caring for persons with Alzheimer's disease, related dementing illnesses, and memory loss in later life,* Baltimore, 1981, Johns Hopkins University Press.

Maslow AH: *Toward a psychology of being,* New York, 1968, D Van Nostrand.

Maslow AH: *Motivation and personality,* New York, 1970, Harper & Row.

Masters W, Johnson V: *Human sexual response,* Boston, 1966, Little, Brown.

Masterson JF: Psychotherapy of borderline and narcissistic disorders: establishing a therapeutic alliance (a developmental, self, and object relations approach), *Personality Disorders* 4:182, 1990.

May R: *The meaning of anxiety,* New York, 1950, Ronald Press.

Minuchen S: *Families and family therapy,* Cambridge, Mass, 1976, Harvard University Press.

Minuchen S, Fishman HC: *Family therapy techniques,* Cambridge, Mass, 1981, Harvard University Press.

Peplau HE: *Interpersonal relations in nursing,* New York, 1952, GP Putnam.

Peplau HE: Process and concept of learning. In Burd S, Marshall M, editors: *Clinical approaches to psychiatric nursing,* New York, 1963, Macmillan.

Perls F: *In and out of the garbage pail,* Lafayatee, Ca, 1969, Real People Press.

Rogers C: Characteristics of a helping relationship, *Pers Guid J,* 1958.

Rogers C: *On becoming a person,* Boston, 1961, Houghton Mifflin.

Rogers C: *A way of being,* Boston, 1980, Houghton Mifflin.

Selye H: *The stress of life,* New York, 1956, McGraw-Hill.

Selye H: *The stress of life,* revised, New York, 1976, McGraw-Hill.

Selye H: *Stress without distress,* New York, 1974, New American Library.

Sullivan HS: *Conceptions of modern psychiatry,* New York, 1953, WW Norton.

Sullivan HS: *The interpersonal theory of psychiatry,* New York, 1953, WW Norton.

Sullivan HS: *Schizophrenia as a human process,* New York, 1962, WW Norton.

Travelbee J: *Interpersonal aspects of nursing,* ed 2, Philadelphia, 1971, FA Davis.

Torrey EF: *Surviving schizophrenia: a family manual,* New York, 1983, Harper & Row.

Wolpe J: *The practice of behavior therapy,* ed 2, New York, 1973, Pergamon.

Yalom ID. *The theory and practice of group psychotherapy,* ed 3, New York, 1985, Basic Books.

Zung W: A self-rating depression scale, *Arch Gen Psychiatr* 12:63, 1965.

Zung W: Prevelance of clinical significant anxiety in a family practice setting, *Am J Psychol* 143:1471, 1986.

INTERNET WEBSITES

Agency for Health Care Policy and Research: www.AHCPR.com

Alzheimer's Disease Education and Referral Center: www.alzheimer's.org/pubs/progoo.htm

Alzheimer's Disease Research Center at the University of California, San Diego: www.adrc.ucsd.edu

American Medical Association's Code for Medical Ethics: www.ama-assn.org/ethics

American Nurses Association: www.nursingworld.org

American Psychiatric Nurses Association: http://apna.org

BC Family: www.bcfamily.com

Bipolar Child Newsletter: www.bipolarchild.com

Centers for Disease Control and Prevention: www.cdc.gov

Gale Encyclopedia of Medicine: www.findarticles.com

Governement and Law: The Library of Congress: www.lcweb.loc.gov

Group Dynamics and Skills for Leading Groups: www.princeton.edu

Guide for resources and education: http://mentalhelp.net

Health Care Finance Administration Regulations for Seclusion and Restraint: www.hcva.gov

Library of Congress, Legislative Updates: http://thomas.loc.gov

Mental Health information: www.psychiatrymedscape.com

Micromedex Healthcare Series, The Care Notes System: http://sharpnet/mdxcgi/cn

National Alliance for Research of Schizophrenia and Depression: www.narsad.org

National Association for the Mentally Ill: www.nami.org

National Institutes for Health: www.NIH.gov

National Institutes for Mental Health: www.NIMH.gov

National Library of Medicine (NLM): www.ncbi.nlm.nih.gov

National Rural Health Association: www.nrharural.org

Nursing Center: www.nursingcenter.com

Nursing Center Library, Journal Articles: www.nursingcenter.com/library/journal

Nursing Diagnosis and Assessment: www.cybernurse.com/books/nursingassessment.html

Nursing Theory: www.healthsci.clayton.edu/eichelberger/nursing.hotmail

Teen Health: www.teenwirc.com

Women's Health Research: www.women'shealth.org/NIHM/htm

VIDEOS

Antianxiety agents, Cypress, Ca, 2000, Medcom, Inc.

Antidepressant agents, Cypress, Ca, 2000, Medcom, Inc.

Antipsychotic agents, Cypress, Ca, 2000, Medcom, Inc.

Fidaleo RA: *Suicide: strategies for assessing and decreasing lethality,* 2001, Sharp HealthCare Office of Continuing Medical Education (CME).

Mood stabilizing agents, Cypress, Ca, 2000, Medcom Inc.

Suicide in in-patient settings: intervention strategies, Irvine, CA, 1997, Concept Media.

Suicide in in-patient settings: overview and assessment, Irvine, CA, 1997, Concept Media.

Index

Page numbers followed by f indicate figures; t, tables; b, boxes.

Index